The Wiley Blacl
Handbook of tne
Psychology of
Occupational Safety
and Workplace Health

The Wiley Blackwell Handbook of the Psychology of Occupational Safety and Workplace Health

Edited by Sharon Clarke, Tahira M. Probst, Frank Guldenmund, and Jonathan Passmore

WILEY Blackwell

This paperback edition first published 2020

© 2016 John Wiley & Sons, Ltd

Registered Office
John Wiley & Sons Ltd, The Atrium, Southern Gate, Chichester, West Sussex, PO19 8SQ, UK

Editorial Offices
350 Main Street, Malden, MA 02148-5020, USA
9600 Garsington Road, Oxford, OX4 2DQ, UK
The Atrium, Southern Gate, Chichester, West Sussex, PO19 8SQ, UK

For details of our global editorial offices, for customer services, and for information about how to apply for permission to reuse the copyright material in this book please see our website at www.wiley.com/wiley-blackwell.

The right of Sharon Clarke, Tahira M. Probst, Frank Guldenmund, and Jonathan Passmore to be identified as the author(s) of the editorial material in this work has been asserted in accordance with the UK Copyright, Designs and Patents Act 1988.

Library of Congress Cataloging-in-Publication data is available:

Paperback (9781119140795)

Cover Design: Wiley
Cover Image: © busypix/Getty Images

Set in 9.5/11pt Galliard by Aptara Inc., New Delhi, India

10 9 8 7 6 5 4 3 2 1

Contents

About the Editors

Jonathan Passmore (Series Editor) is the Professor of Coaching and Behavioural Change at Henley Business School, University of Reading and a professor of psychology at the University of Evora, Portugal. He is a chartered psychologist, holds five degrees, and has an international reputation for his work in coaching and leadership, including being listed by Thinkers50 as one of the top 10 coaches in the world. He has published widely books on the themes of leadership, personal development and change, and served as editor for the *Association for Coaching* book series. He speaks widely at conferences across the world and has published over 100 journal papers and book chapters.

Sharon Clarke is Professor of Organizational Psychology,Head of Division and Deputy Head of School at Alliance Manchester Business School, University of Manchester, UK. Her research interests are in occupational safety, health and wellbeing, particularly safety leadership, climate and culture. She is currently Editor-in-Chief of the *Journal of Occupational and Organizational Psychology* and Associate Editor at the *Journal of Occupational Health Psychology*. She is also on the Editorial Board of the International Journal of Stress Management.

Tahira M. Probst is a Professor of Psychology at Washington State University Vancouver, USA. Her research focuses on occupational health and safety, with a particular interest in the psychosocial antecedents of accident underreporting. She is currently Editor-in-Chief of *Stress & Health* and an Editorial Board member of the *Journal of Occupational Health Psychology, Occupational Health Science, Military Psychology* and the *Journal of Business and Psychology*.

Frank Guldenmund is Ass. Professor in the Safety Science and Security Group at Delft University of Technology, the Netherlands. He works primarily in the field of occupational, process and nuclear safety, where he focusses on human behaviour in a technological environment. Within this context he developed an interest in the topic of safety culture, into which he has conducted research for two decades. He has been Associate Editor of *Safety Science* for many years.

About the Contributors

Tom Bellairs is a doctoral student at the University of Alabama. He examines how employees approach their work in the context of how they view their future at work. He earned a BS from the United States Air Force Academy and an MBA from the University of Southern California.

Andrea Bishop, PhD is a Postdoctoral Fellow at the School of Nursing, Dalhousie University with the Strengthening Transitions in Paediatric Care Team. Dr Bishop's research interests focus on patient engagement in patient safety and transitions in care, organizational patient safety culture, and knowledge translation.

Michael J. Burke is the Lawrence Martin Chair in Business at Tulane University. He received his PhD in Psychology from Illinois Institute of Technology. His current research focuses on the efficacy of workplace safety interventions, the development of procedures for assessing inter-rater agreement, and psychological and organizational climate.

Francesco Cangiano is a PhD candidate in Organisational Behaviour at the UWA Business School. Francesco received a Masters in Social and Organisational Psychology from the University of Exeter and has a BSc in Organisational Psychology. His main research areas include proactive work behavior, employee well-being, and work motivation.

Nik Chmiel is Professor of Psychology, Head of the Department of Psychology and Counselling, and Director of the People and Well-Being in the Everyday Research (POWER) Centre at the University of Chichester, UK. He is a past president of the European Association of Work and Organizational Psychology (EAWOP).

Stacey M. Conchie is a Lecturer in Psychology at Lancaster University, UK. Her research focuses on the role of interpersonal trust in shaping interactions within high-risk contexts; namely industry and security.

Arla Day is Canada Research Chair and Full Professor of Industrial/Organizational Psychology at Saint Mary's University, Halifax, Canada. Her research and consulting address issues of healthy workplaces, occupational stress, employee well-being, and work–life balance. Arla chairs the Nova Scotia Psychological Healthy Workplace Program, and she is Associate Editor of the *Journal of Occupational Health Psychology.*

Maureen F. Dollard, PhD is Professor of Work and Organisational Psychology and Director of the Asia Pacific Centre for Work Health and Safety at the University of South Australia. She is President of the Asia Pacific Academy for Psychosocial Factors at Work, Co-chair of the International Commission on Occupational Health (ICOH-WOPS) Scientific Committee, and Chair of the ICOH-WOPS 2014 congress.

Ståle Einarsen is Professor of Work and Organizational Psychology from the University of Bergen and Head of the Bergen Workplace Bullying Research Group (BBRG). He is a pioneer in workplace bullying research where he has published extensively over the last 20 years. Ståle is also the co-editor of two international volumes on workplace bullying.

Mark Fleming, PhD is the CN Professor of Safety Culture at Saint Mary's University, in Halifax, Nova Scotia, Canada. He has over 20 years of experience in health and safety research. Currently, Mark's research includes investigating methods for measuring and improving safety culture, safety motivation, safety leadership, and rail safety.

Rhona Flin, PhD, FBPsS, FRSE, FRAeS holds the Chair of Applied Psychology, University of Aberdeen (www.abdn.ac.uk/iprc) and is a member of the Safety Advisory Committee, Military Aviation Authority. She studies human performance in high-risk industries, current projects on safety culture, safety leadership, non-technical skills, and surgeons' intra-operative decision-making.

Jeff Foster is Vice President of Science at Hogan Assessment Systems. His team completes over 100 criterion-related, generalization of validity, and customized validity studies annually. Dr Foster previously worked in selection and assessment for Anheuser-Busch while earning his PhD in Industrial and Organizational Psychology at the University of Missouri-St. Louis.

Carla Santos Fugas has a PhD in Psychology, specializing in Work and Organizational Psychology. As a Researcher at ISCTE-IUL Business School, she has published in the domain of health psychology, social norms, and safety behaviors. She combines academic research with practice in Safety and Health at Work Management.

E. Scott Geller, PhD Alumni Distinguished Professor at Virginia Tech, Blacksburg, Virginia, is Director of the Center for Applied Behavior Systems in the Department of Psychology. He is also Senior Partner of Safety Performance Solutions, a leading-edge training and consulting firm for occupational health, safety, leadership, sustainability, and culture improvement.

A. Ian Glendon is Associate Professor, School of Applied Psychology, and a member of the Behavioral Basis of Health Program, and the Work and Organizational Wellbeing Research Centre, Griffith University, Queensland, Australia; he has published more than 100 scientific papers, book chapters, and books on aspects of risk and safety, including the third edition of *Human Safety and Risk Management* (2015, with Sharon Clarke).

Mark A. Griffin is Professor of Organizational Psychology and Director of the Centre for Safety at the University of Western Australia. He received his PhD in Industrial/

Organizational Psychology from the Pennsylvania State University. His research includes areas such as leadership, safety, work performance, organizational climate, and work stress.

Gudela Grote is Professor of Work and Organizational Psychology at the ETH Zurich. She received her PhD at the Georgia Institute of Technology in Atlanta, USA. Her research addresses the individual and organizational management of uncertainty, for example in medical and software development teams, and human resource management practices related to well-being, safety, and performance.

Sara Guediri, PhD is a Lecturer in Organizational Psychology at Manchester Business School, University of Manchester. Her research focuses on leadership, workplace safety, and employee well-being. She is a member of the Society for Industrial and Organizational Psychology (SIOP) and the European Association of Work and Organizational Psychology (EAWOP).

Jonathon R. B. Halbesleben is the HealthSouth Chair of Health Care Management in the Department of Management in the Culverhouse College of Commerce at the University of Alabama. He received his PhD in Industrial/Organizational Psychology from the University of Oklahoma. His research explores employee well-being and work–family issues.

Isabelle Hansez is Full Professor of Work and Organizational Psychology at the University of Liège (Belgium) where she leads the Human Resources Development Unit. She has an extended experience in psychosocial risks and well-being assessment in organizations, including safety outcomes in high-risk sectors. This practical experience is in line with the adaptation of the Job Demands-Resources framework to safety issues in collaborative research with Professor Nik Chmiel.

Thomas Helson is a student at Saint Mary's University, Halifax, Canada. His research interests are in occupational health psychology, with much of his work involving workplace health promotion, assessing healthy workplaces, employee well-being, and leadership development.

Helge Hoel is Professor of Organisational Behaviour at Manchester Business School, University of Manchester. He has contributed to a number of books, articles, and reports on workplace bullying, harassment, and violence, including commissioned works for the European Foundation for the Improvement of Living and Working Conditions and the International Labour Organization (ILO).

Patti Jordan is a Professor of Professional Practice at Texas Christian University. She earned her PhD in Business Administration from Oklahoma State University. Patti spent 30 years working in various roles in the manufacturing arena including working in the steel and airline industries. During her career in industry she was instrumental in implementing safety programs to improve the safety of the work area and behavior of the employees.

E. Kevin Kelloway is the Canada Research Chair in Occupational Health Psychology and a Professor of Psychology at Saint Mary's University. As a prolific researcher, he is a Fellow of the Association for Psychological Science, the Canadian Psychology Association, the International Association for Applied Psychology, and the Society for Industrial and Organizational Psychology.

Gil Luria is a Senior Lecturer and Department Chair in the Department of Human Services, the Faculty of Social Welfare and Health Sciences at the University of Haifa. He conducts research on occupational safety with the focus on organizational climate, leadership, stress, and organizational interventions. He received his PhD from the Faculty of Management at the Technion–Israel Institute of Technology.

Daniel W. Makhan holds a MSc in Ergonomics from Loughborough University in the UK and a MBA from Saint Mary's University in Halifax, Canada. As a Certified Human Factors Professional, Daniel brings systems thinking to business through human-centred design and management disciplines to make the workplace better, safer, and more profitable.

Stephen B. Nichols is Manager of International Research at Hogan Assessment Systems. He focuses on providing research expertise to Hogan's multinational partners and international distributors. His experiences have led to collaborations with researchers from over 50 countries. Stephen earned his MS in Industrial and Organizational Psychology at Missouri State University.

Morten Birkeland Nielsen is Senior Researcher at the Norwegian National Institute of Occupational Health and Professor in Work and Organizational Psychology at the University of Bergen, Norway. His research interests include occupational health and safety, workplace bullying and harassment, leadership, personality, and research methodology. Morten is Associate Editor of *Work & Stress* and an editorial board member of *Scandinavian Psychologist*.

Michael P. O'Driscoll is Professor of Psychology at the University of Waikato in New Zealand, where he convenes the postgraduate program in Organisational Psychology. His primary research interests focus on job-related stress (including the effects of bullying at work), coping and psychological well-being, work–life balance, and well-being of older workers. He is Associate Editor of *Stress & Health* and the *New Zealand Journal of Psychology*, and serves on the editorial boards of several international academic journals.

Sharon K. Parker is a Winthrop Professor at the UWA Business School, University of Western Australia. She is an Australian Research Council Future Fellow and a leading international scholar on the topics of proactivity and work design. Professor Parker has published over 60 refereed journal articles, 40 book chapters, two books, and numerous technical and practitioner publications.

Zechariah J. Robinson, senior undergraduate honors student is Coordinator of Research for the Center for Applied Behavior Systems, and Undergraduate Supervisor for the Behavioral Neuroscience Lab, at Virginia Tech. He has authored/coauthored 13 professional conference presentations and three publications, and was awarded Senior of the Year for the College of Science.

Maree Roche is a Senior Lecturer in Psychology (Organisational) at the University of Waikato in New Zealand. Her primary research interests focus on employee psychological well-being and leadership. She is the author of several journal articles and book chapters. She is Co-editor of the *New Zealand Journal of Human Resource Management*, and provides consulting services to organizations on employee well-being and leadership.

Wilmar B. Schaufeli is Full Professor of Work and Organizational Psychology at Utrecht University, The Netherlands, and Distinguished Research Professor at Leuven University, Belgium. He is a Fellow of the European Academy of Occupational Health Psychology and was awarded "Highly Cited Researcher" by Thomson Reuters, ranking among the top 1 percent of most cited researchers in psychology (www.wilmarschaufeli.nl).

Sílvia Agostinho Silva is Associate Professor in the Department of Human Resources and Organizational Behavior at Instituto Universitário Lisboa (ISCTE- IUL). Her research on work psychology applied to safety and health focuses on work culture, climate, and norms. She has coordinated research projects and collaborated with several companies on workplace health promotion.

Mickey B. Smith is a Visiting Assistant Professor of Management at the University of Southern Mississippi. He earned his PhD in Management from Oklahoma State University. His research focuses on the interactions among individual, group, and organizational factors that influence employee performance.

Caitlin E. Smith Sockbeson is a PhD student in Organizational Behavior at Tulane University. After graduating from Spring Hill College, she worked in the publishing industry for six years before pursuing her PhD. Her research interests include diversity in the workplace, influence and political behavior, and performance management.

Toon W. Taris is Full Professor of Work and Organizational Psychology at Utrecht University, The Netherlands, and heads the Department of Psychology of that university. Since 2013 he has served as Editor-in-Chief of *Work & Stress*, one of the leading journals in occupational health psychology.

Paul J. Taylor is Professor of Psychology at Lancaster University, UK, and Professor of Human Interaction at Twente University, the Netherlands. Supported by over £4m of funding, Paul's research combines experimental, archival, and field methods to understand the workings of human interaction and the strategies that promote cooperation. Read more at: www.pauljtaylor.com.

J. Craig Wallace is the William S. Spears Chair in Business Administration at Oklahoma State University. He earned his PhD in Industrial/Organizational Psychology from the Georgia Institute of Technology. His research focuses on the intersection of individual-level theories of motivation, emotion, and cognition with higher-level constructs, such as leadership and climate, to better explain and predict important outcomes.

Helena E. Woodcock gained her PhD from the University of Liverpool, UK, in 2013. Her research interests are in the repair of employees' trust in management; specifically, identifying both the verbal and non-verbal behavioral strategies that are effective at maintaining a workable relationship.

Jennifer H. K. Wong is currently pursuing her PhD in Industrial-Organizational Psychology at Saint Mary's University. She completed her MSc in Applied Psychology from the same university in 2012. Jennifer takes on a multidisciplinary approach to occupational health and safety by incorporating methods and theories from related areas of research.

Amy Zadow holds a Masters in Work and Organisational Psychology. She is a Research Assistant and PhD candidate at the Asia Pacific Centre for Work Health and Safety at the University of South Australia. She has presented at the International Forum for Quality and Safety in Healthcare, the European Academy of Occupational Health Psychology, the International Congress of Applied Psychology, and the International Commission on Occupational Health.

Dieter Zapf is Professor of Work and Organizational Psychology and Scientific Director, Center for Leadership and Behavior in Organizations (CLBO) at the Johann Wolfgang Goethe-University Frankfurt, Germany, and Visiting Professor at Manchester Business School, Manchester, UK. His research interests include stress at work, workplace bullying, older workers, job analysis, human errors, job satisfaction, emotional labor, service interactions, and customer satisfaction.

Foreword

The editors of this volume, Sharon Clarke, Tahira M. Probst, Frank Guldenmund, and Jonathan Passmore, each have distinct areas of expertise within occupational health and safety. They have brought together an exceptional team of international experts on occupational health and safety to provide a comprehensive set of essays that mirror the state of knowledge and practice in occupational health psychology.

The focus of occupational health psychology is to develop and maintain a safe and healthy work environment for all workers – not only to protect the workers themselves from accident and injury but to prevent negative effects in the work environment from affecting their families and communities. Occupational health psychology was initially conceptualized as a multidisciplinary field bringing together expertise in work and organization psychology, social psychology, clinical psychology, safety, engineering, occupational nursing and medicine, human factors and ergonomics, and organizational science to name a few of the relevant areas of expertise.

In the early years of occupational health psychology, much of the underlying framework drew on occupational stress as a psychological mechanism for understanding the effects of work on employee health and well-being. As is readily apparent from this volume, the field has grown to draw on most areas of psychology in contributing to our knowledge of detrimental effects of work on employees' safety, health, and well-being, as well as their families. Additionally, it is becoming increasingly clear that work can have positive effects on people by giving their lives a sense of meaning, purpose, and accomplishment. The contributions of the team of international experts included in this volume reflect the theoretical progress in occupational health psychology. This international representation among the contributors is important given the globalization of work organizations.

As the field of occupational health psychology grows and matures, it is imperative to integrate the findings from the theoretical investigations of factors influencing workers' safety, health, and well-being into interventions appropriate for the workplace. Such interventions are becoming increasingly designed and evaluated according to sound scientific principles and this volume dedicates a major section to presenting the theoretical basis and empirical evidence for safety and health interventions. This bridges the "supposed gap" between science and practice providing practical implications for the development and maintenance of a safe and healthy work environment for all workers and their families.

This volume provides an integration of multiple perspectives on occupational health and safety, primarily from an occupational health psychology view, attending to issues at the individual, job, group/team, organizational, and societal level. Further, the contributions to the volume provide a science and practice perspective.

Lois E. Tetrick, PhD
Professor of Psychology
George Mason University
Fellow – European Academy of Occupational Health Psychology
Fellow – Society for Industrial and Organizational Psychology
Fellow – American Psychological Association
Fellow – Association for Psychological Science
Founding Member – Society for Occupational Health Psychology

Series Editor Preface

Welcome to this fourth book in the Wiley Blackwell Industrial and Organizational Psychology series. This title in the series focuses on health and safety and builds on the previous three titles in the series on leadership and change, coaching and mentoring, and training and development.

In recent years we have seen a growing development in our understanding of accidents and how organizations can draw on our understanding of human psychology to improve on safety outcomes. The same is true of occupational health, which is now a significant feature in many organizational human resources policies.

We believe this series differs in four ways from other titles in the field. Firstly, the focus for the title is aimed at the academic researcher and student, as opposed to the practitioner, although scholar practitioners may also find this an interesting read. The aim of this book is to offer a comprehensive coverage of the main topics of inquiry within the domain and in each of these to offer a comprehensive critical literature review of the main topic areas. Each chapter is thus an attempt to gather together the key papers, book chapters and ideas and to present these for the serious researcher, student, and academic as a starting point for research in the key topics of I/O psychology in a focused (10,000 word) chapter. The book thus aims to operate as a starting point for any in depth inquiry into the field.

Secondly, while many books take a UK/European or a US/North American approach with contributors drawn predominantly from one continent or the other, in this series we have made strenuous efforts to create an international feel. For each title in the series we have drawn contributors from across the globe, and encouraged them to take an international, as opposed to national or regional focus. Such an approach creates challenges: challenges in terms of language and spelling, but also in the way ideas and concepts are applied in each country or region. We have encouraged our contributors to highlight such differences. We encourage you as the reader to reflect on these to better understand how and why these differences have emerged and what implications these have for your research and our deeper understanding of the psychological constructs which underpin these ideas.

Thirdly, the chapters avoid offering a single perspective, based on the ideas of the contributor. Instead we have invited leading writers in the field to critically review the literature in their areas of expertise. The chapters thus offer a unique insight into the literature in each of these areas, with leading scholars sharing their interpretation of the literature in their area.

Finally, as series editor I have invited contributors and editors to donate their royalties to a charity. Given the international feel for the title we selected an international charity – Railway Children – a charity that supports runaway and abandoned children across the world. This means approximately 10 percent of the cover price has been donated to charity and with this small contribution we collectively hope to make the world a slightly better place.

With any publication of this kind there are errors; as editors we apologies in advance for these.

Jonathan Passmore
Series Editor, I/O Psychology

Railway Children

Railway Children supports children alone and at risk on the streets of India, East Africa, and here in the UK. Children migrate to the streets for many reasons, but once there they experience physical and sexual abuse, exploitation, drugs, and even death. We focus on early intervention, getting to the street kids before the street gets to them, and where possible we reunite them with their families and communities.

In addressing the issue we work through our three step change agenda to:

- Meet the immediate needs of children on the streets – we work with local organizations to provide shelter, education, or vocational training, counseling and, if possible, reintegration to family life.
- Shift perception in the local context – we work with local stakeholders to ensure that street children are not viewed as commodities to be abused and exploited, but as children in need of care and protection.
- Hold governments to account – if we are to see a long-term, sustainable change for the children with whom we work, we must influence key decision-makers, ensuring that provisions for safeguarding children are made within their policies and budgets.

Last year we reached over 27,000 children; 14,690 of these were in India where we reunited 2,820 with their families. In the UK we launched our research, "Off the Radar," which revealed the experiences of over 100 of the most detached children in the UK. Many of these children received no intervention either before leaving home or once they were on the streets. We have made recommendations that include emergency refuge for under 16s and a wrap-round of other services, such as Misper schemes, local helplines, outreach and family liaison to allow children and young people to access interventions in a variety of ways.

To find out more about our work, or to help us support more vulnerable children, please go to www.railwaychildren.org.uk or call 00 44 1270 757596.

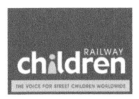

1

The Psychology of Occupational Safety and Workplace health

Sharon Clarke, Tahira M. Probst, Frank Guldenmund, and Jonathan Passmore

Occupational health and safety remains a critical issue for academics and practitioners alike, given the impact that occupational accidents and work-related ill-health has on individuals, families, organizations, and societies worldwide. Despite the significant advances that have been made in disciplines such as occupational health psychology, safety science, and industrial ergonomics, workplace fatalities and deaths resulting from work-related diseases remain a global issue. The International Labour Organization (ILO, 2014) estimates that over 2.3 million fatalities are caused by occupational accidents and work-related diseases per annum; in addition, occupational injuries (requiring absence of three days or more from work) result from over 313 million non-fatal occupational accidents each year. Given the significant proportion of our lives that we spend working, research and practice into occupational safety and workplace health and well-being can also provide insight into ways in which the world of work can have positive benefits, in terms of satisfaction, challenge, and achievement.

This edited volume takes an integrative approach to health and safety in organizations, bringing together a collection of chapters from renowned contributors. Their fields of expertise range from personality and individual differences to risk management at a societal level. We examine key topics in the health and safety literature, both from the specific perspective of occupational safety (e.g., personality, social norms, and leadership) and workplace health and well-being (e.g., job demands, long work hours, and workplace aggression), and also from a consideration of the intersection of these two areas (e.g., safety workarounds and organizational climate). The first two parts of this volume consider those factors that influence occupational health and safety and the subsequent challenges; in the third part, we examine the practical implications for individuals and organizations, with a particular focus on the design and implementation of interventions

The Wiley Blackwell Handbook of the Psychology of Occupational Safety and Workplace Health, First Edition. Edited by Sharon Clarke, Tahira M. Probst, Frank Guldenmund, and Jonathan Passmore. © 2016 John Wiley & Sons Ltd. Published 2020 by John Wiley & Sons Ltd.

in organizations, and the broader context within which such interventions take place. Interventions are examined from a variety of perspectives, from the micro level (e.g., behavioral safety and training) through to a macro-level approach (e.g., psychosocial safety climate and organizational culture). In this part, we explore the challenges of managing health and safety in safety-critical environments (e.g., patient safety culture) and the wider context of the risk society.

The first part focuses on occupational safety. Traditionally, research and practice in occupational safety has been dominated by technical, engineering, and human factors approaches. In this volume, we examine the influences on occupational safety from a psychological perspective, considering factors at an individual, team, job, and organizational level that impact upon the work environment and employees' behavior. Recent research in this area has highlighted the importance of the psychological perspective and emphasized the range of factors that influence workplace safety (e.g., Clarke, 2010; Nahrgang, Morgeson, & Hofmann, 2011). This section comprises six chapters, which explore the following topics: personality and individual differences; behavior as a mediator of personality on safety outcomes; role of social norms at group level; safety leadership; role of coworker and leader trust; job design and safety behavior.

In Chapter 2, Smith, Jordan, and Wallace discuss how personality and other individual differences (e.g., cognition, age, and experience) influence an employee's ability to respond to organizational hazards. They provide a historical overview, from the early conceptualization of "accident proneness" (Greenwood & Woods, 1919), to the Big Five personality characteristics (Costa & McCrae, 1992) and their ability to predict safety behavior and safety outcomes, including accidents and injuries. Although a useful typology, Smith et al. discuss personality traits that fall outside of the Big Five, such as those comprising core self-evaluations (self-esteem, generalized self-efficacy, locus of control, and emotional stability; Judge, Locke, & Durham, 1997). They extend the discussion to consider the role of self-regulation, focusing on regulatory focus as a dual-path motivational phenomenon (Higgins, 1997) in which individuals tend to approach or avoid outcomes by applying promotion or prevention strategies; those who have a greater tendency toward prevention strategies also tend to have higher scores on safety performance. Their review is suggestive of motivational mechanisms underlying safety performance (a theme which is picked up repeatedly in the following chapters). A number of individual differences not only affect the safety-related behavior that people engage in, but also their ability to cope with stressors (e.g., hardiness). The chapter highlights how age and experience influence accident liability (e.g., a lack of "know-how" makes younger workers particularly vulnerable) and type of job (e.g., level of cognitive or physical demands) interacts with individual differences (e.g., physiological and psychological factors) to influence safety behavior and accident liability. Smith et al. emphasize the role of "mindfulness" as important but understudied in relation to safety (another theme which will reappear in later chapters of this volume).

In Chapter 3, Foster and Nichols consider the mediating effects of behavior on the relationship between personality and workplace safety. The chapter focuses on the complexities of this relationship, and considers how multiple personality traits and combinations of traits (including sub-facets of the Big Five) best predict safety-related behavior. They explore how different patterns of traits are associated with different behaviors, including a detailed examination of the six safety-related behaviors identified by Hogan and Foster (2013) as critical to a high level of safety performance and how personality relates to these behaviors. While some facets are important predictors of safety behaviors, others are essentially irrelevant. There are a number of underlying psychological mechanisms by which personality can influence safety, including its influence on individuals' response to stress (as discussed in Part II of this volume). Based on their review, Foster and Nichols discuss how individual differences in personality should be taken into account in relation to the design and delivery of safety training (as discussed further in Part III of this volume). Although the authors have focused on safety in this chapter, they also highlight implications for the design of tailored interventions aimed at improving health and well-being: in terms of individual participation in health programs, such as health screening (see also Chapter 17 on Workplace Health Promotion in Part III).

Although individual-level factors have an important influence on employee behavior, this behavior takes place within a social and organizational context. Social psychological theories emphasize the importance of understanding this context as one cannot fully understand behavior, without consideration of the social context (Johns, 2006). In most organizational settings, this comprises coworkers, supervisors, and managers, each of whom has an influence on individuals' behavior. The following chapters consider the effects of the social context on safety behavior, in terms of social norms, leadership, and the role of interpersonal trust.

In Chapter 4, Silva and Fugas consider the influence of peer norms on safety and health at work. Whereas the previous two chapters in this part take the individual as the primary unit of analysis, in this chapter we shift to consider the group. Silva and Fugas draw on social and organizational psychology to discuss social influence, in terms of the subjective norms or pressure that people perceive from important others to exhibit, or not exhibit, a specific behavior. They distinguish between two types of norm – those that are descriptive (reflecting what is commonly done) and injunctive (reflecting what is approved/disapproved). There are affective and cognitive motivations for perceiving that one has to conform to group behavior. The reference groups are those that are psychologically significant to the individual's attitudes and behaviors. Silva and Fugas also discuss the difference between local norms and global norms, where the former are more proximal. It is important to understand the role of coworker norms not only in relation to occupational safety, but also workplace health and well-being. This chapter discusses the influence of social norms on a range of risk behaviors that affect health and safety, such as healthy eating, smoking, and risky driving behaviors. The authors review the empirical research, which has shown that coworkers' descriptive safety norms are a major differentiating variable in proactive safety behaviors. Coworkers' norms play a critical role in risk perception and management, determining which behaviors are safe or unsafe, and reinforcing those behaviors.

In Chapter 5, Wong, Kelloway, and Makhan focus on the role of supervisors and managers on employee safety behavior. They review the research evidence, which shows that leaders have a significant influence on workplace safety, and examine the effects of different leadership styles on safety outcomes, especially transformational leadership style (Bass, 1985). In addition, Wong et al. discuss the role of active transactional leadership as a positive influence in relation to safety (due to the increased emphasis on monitoring compliance and correcting errors before they lead to safety incidents); other complementary models of leadership, such as "empowering leadership" (a style of leadership associated with psychological empowerment; Martínez-Córcoles et al., 2011) which focuses on the role of leaders developing self-management skills in their subordinates; and the role of leader–member exchange (LMX) where a high LMX relationship between leader and subordinate facilitates the influence of leaders on employee safety behaviors. Wong et al. discuss mediating and moderating influences on how leadership impacts on occupational safety behavior, including safety climate, perceived organizational support, role stressors, and individual-level factors of trust and motivation. In terms of practical implications, the authors introduce the SAFER model of safety leadership, which provides explicit guidance in terms of leader behaviors.

In Chapter 6, Conchie, Woodcock, and Taylor discuss the importance of interpersonal trust in the creation of a safe work environment. They highlight that trust is important in increasing employee engagement in safety, willingness to comply with management requests, and propensity to take the initiative. Trust may also be misplaced and actually detract from the critical vigilance required for high levels of safety performance. In their review of the research evidence, Conchie et al. discuss trust as a mechanism for facilitating the effects of a transformational leader on employee behaviors, leading to employees engaging in safety-related behavior. They extend their discussion by considering not only trust in the leader, but also the employee being trusted by the leader. Trust is related to aspects of safety culture, such as open communication and organizational learning; a lack of trust can create a climate of blame and fear, which leads employees to be concerned about "covering their backs" and stifles organizational learning. They highlight the "fragility" of trust and the difficulties associated with rebuilding trust. Furthermore, Conchie et al. discuss strategies for rebuilding trust and their relative effectiveness in different circumstances.

In the final chapter of this part, we examine the influence of job-related and organizational factors on safety behavior. In Chapter 7, Chmiel and Hansez examine these broader contextual factors with particular reference to their influence on violations and errors. Reason's (1990) classification of human error, captures both unintentional actions (slips, lapses, and mistakes) and intentional deviations from safety procedures (violations); both types of unsafe act are associated with accident involvement and occupational injuries. The authors use the General Accident Case Scenario (Wagenaar, Hudson, & Reason, 1990) to illustrate how errors and violations relate to accident involvement and extend their discussion to consider the underlying psychological processes involved. In terms of antecedents, Chmiel and Hansez discuss General Failure Types (GFTs) as precursors of accidents and which fall into three categories: Physical environment; Human behavior; and Management. The effects of organizational and job related factors are mediated by psychological processes, including energy depletion (such as burnout), motivational processes (such as work engagement), instrumental processes, and social exchange. They argue that different types of behavior have different antecedents and psychological processes linking them.

The second part focuses on workplace health and well-being. Within the field of occupational health psychology, theories of occupational stress and the impact of stress on employees' health and well-being, constitutes a major area of research. The first chapter in this part (Taris & Schaufeli) focuses on one of most influential frameworks, the Job Demands-Resources (JDR) model (Demerouti et al., 2001), which conceptualizes job demands and job resources within the work environment, and how these factors affect health and well-being over time. Other stress theories are drawn upon to discuss the effects on health and well-being in this part; the chapter by Nielsen et al. draws on the transactional model of stress (Lazarus & Folkman, 1984) to examine the effects of workplace aggression, and chapters by Cangiano and Parker, and Halbesleben and Bellairs, both draw on conservation of resources (COR) theory (Hobfoll, 1989) to examine the effects of proactivity and safety workarounds respectively. In this part we address some of the contemporary challenges in the workplace that have an impact on health and well-being, including long work hours (O'Driscoll & Roche) and workplace aggression (Nielsen et al.). Although certain demands within the workplace can act to erode physical and psychological well-being, individual differences in how employees manage their jobs will also impact their health; for example, those who are more proactive tend to "craft" their jobs, with proactivity having the potential to both improve and damage health (as discussed by Cangiano & Parker).

In Chapter 8, Taris and Schaufeli provide a review of the research conducted in relation to the JDR framework, which links job demands and job resources to health, well-being, and other outcomes. The initial focus of the model was on burnout, but it has been extended to consider further outcome variables; there is empirical evidence to support the relationships predicted by the model in relation to burnout, such that high job demands are associated with high levels of fatigue and exhaustion, and lack of resources associated with withdrawal. The model was later revised to extend outcomes from the specific concept of burnout to strain more generally. Later development of the model also recognized that in relation to interactions between job demands and job resources, these may be mediated by a variety of different pathways, in contrast to the two specific pathways (strain and motivation) which mediated the main effects of job demands and job resources, respectively. In their review, Taris and Schaufeli note that although most empirical evidence is drawn from self-report cross-sectional data, more recently longitudinal studies have also provided support for the assumptions of the revised JDR model; however, they also highlight that over longer time periods where there is long-term stability in some variables, such as work engagement and job resources, the expected results have not been consistently demonstrated. The chapter discusses other extensions of the model, such as the inclusion of personal resources, as well as job resources; that is, extending the model to include individual-level factors, as well as environmental factors. Personal resources relate to resilience and the ability to impact upon the environment. Taris and Schaufeli discuss the different ways of incorporating personal resources into the JDR model including as a potential confound (as personal resources are related to both work characteristics and work outcomes). Finally, the chapter provides some practical discussion of how the JDR model can be used as the theoretical basis for interventions in organizations, and also the development of individual-level strategies to improve the content of one's job to make it more interesting and enjoyable (such as job crafting, Wrzesniewski & Dutton, 2001).

In Chapter 9, O'Driscoll and Roche discuss the relationship between work hours and well-being. They consider not only how many hours are spent working, but also how work is done. In their review of the research evidence, they highlight that there is no simple relationship between work hours and well-being, but a complex relationship, which can be mitigated by a number of factors. They note that there is an overall global trend toward working longer hours. Physical health may be affected as longer work hours mean greater exposure to job demands, reduced time available for recovery, as well as activities that contribute to a healthy lifestyle, such as fitness and exercise. Indeed, O'Driscoll and Roche highlight that research evidence suggests a significant association between long work hours and a variety of health symptoms and increased risk of developing serious health problems; although buffering effects come from control over work hours and social support. O'Driscoll and Roche also consider how changes in technology have affected our working lives, and so our health and well-being. For example, mobile technology may allow increases in autonomy and flexibility, but also allows more work to be undertaken in non-work hours, leading to the blurring of work and non-work boundaries. In addition, working in virtual teams across time zones can lead to negative health effects. The chapter discusses ways of coping with the effects of long work hours, including job crafting and mindfulness.

In Chapter 10, the impact of exposure to workplace aggression on health and well-being is discussed by Nielsen, Hoel, Zapf, and Einarsen. The chapter focuses on work-place aggression, defined in terms of experienced or enacted negative behaviors, rather than the intention to cause harm, which is often difficult to identify. This applies to psychological aggression, which includes abusive supervision, incivility, bullying, and social undermining. Nielsen et al. review a robust body of research evidence which suggests that exposure to workplace aggression leads to short-term experience of stress emotions, and in the longer term, to negative effects on health and well-being, including anxiety, depression, burnout, and physical symptoms. As mental health issues can also act as an antecedent of exposure to aggression, this can lead to a negative cycle of ongoing health problems. Nielsen et al. extend their discussion by considering mediating and moderating effects on the relationship between workplace aggression and health, including state negative affect and perceived victimization at an individual level, and perceived justice at an organizational context. Moderating variables examined include: individual characteristics and personality (such as core self-evaluations), coping strategies, and job resources (such as social support and leadership).

In Chapter 11, Cangiano and Parker consider proactivity, where employees undertake self-initiated and future oriented actions to change and improve themselves or their work environment. The chapter focuses specifically on the relationship between proactivity and health. Cangiano and Parker describe proactive behavior as anticipating and taking control of the situation; thus, it is a way of behaving rather than a set of behaviors. The underpinnings of proactivity are motivational: linking to both self-determination theory (Ryan & Deci, 2000) and the motivation to develop autonomy, competence, and relatedness; and also broaden-and-build theory (Fredrickson, 2001) and the motivation of positive energized feelings, vigor, and work engagement. Cangiano and Parker develop and discuss a model that considers both the potential benefits and costs of proactivity in terms of individual health and well-being, via two pathways, one motivational and the other resource-depletion. They argue that the first pathway can lead to a positive gain spiral, which enhances resilience and ability to cope with stressors, leading to better health and well-being; however, the second pathway may lead to depletion of resources, resistance from supervisors and coworkers, and destructive criticism which erodes self-efficacy. Cangiano and Parker extend their model through the consideration of the moderating role of feedback and extrinsic motivation. From an organizational perspective, proactive employees need to be supported in order to avoid potential negative impacts on health and well-being.

Most research on the JDR model has focused on outcomes related to employee health and well-being, but the model has also been considered as a framework for understanding occupational safety (Nahrgang et al., 2011). Although the relationship between occupational safety and employee well-being is rarely examined, the chapter by Halbesleben and Bellairs considers one psychological mechanism (safety workarounds) underlying the relationship between burnout and safety outcomes. At an organizational level, both health and safety outcomes share common antecedents, in terms of organizational structure and climate. The chapter by Guediri and Griffin considers organizational climate in relation to occupational health, safety and well-being, including a discussion of facet-specific climates and how these climates relate to each other.

Previous chapters in this part have considered some of the major job and individual-level factors that act as antecedents to workplace health and well-being, and the psychological mechanisms involved in this relationship. In Chapter 12, Halbesleben and Bellairs consider the behavioral impact of employee well-being on occupational safety. The chapter reviews the research that has linked exposure to work stressors directly to accidents and injuries, and also indirectly via negative health and well-being. Halbesleben and Bellairs develop a model that highlights two pathways for linking well-being to safety behavior – one motivational pathway and one health-impairment pathway. The chapter focuses on safety workarounds as the behavioral mediator between employee well-being and safety outcomes. Workarounds, which involve working in a way that was not originally designed or intended, can have both positive and negative consequences. Organizational anteced-ents relate to HRM issues, such as staffing and individual-level factors also play a role, particularly self-efficacy. Halbesleben and Bellairs suggest that a loss spiral may develop over time, as the experience of work injuries leads to a decline in health and well-being, which in turn increases vulnerability to injuries.

Chapter 13 by Guediri and Griffin broadens the discussion by considering the role of organizational factors and their influence on health and safety in the workplace. Organiza-tional climate is defined as a summary profile of formal and informal policies, practices and procedures; it reflects the "atmosphere" within an organization. Guediri and Griffin discuss the need to integrate micro and macro approaches to health and well-being. Organizational climate is related to employee well-being, with the research evidence suggesting that leader-ship and job-related aspects of climate are most strongly associated. The chapter highlights a number of specific climates that have been linked to health and well-being, and the role of strategic climates, and whether these can come into conflict. Guediri and Griffin also consider the role of organizational climate in relation to safety, and differentiate between safety culture and safety climate. With a focus on the latter, they discuss the development of this concept, including the research work on measurement, and stability across samples and over time. They review the research evidence that safety climate acts as a leading indicator; with longitudinal studies demonstrating the effects of safety climate on safety outcomes, particularly at a group level. The chapter also reviews research that integrates occupational health and safety variables.

The third and final part picks up on the challenges discussed in the preceding two sec-tions, which consider some of the most significant factors that influence health and safety in organizations. In Part III we consider the different approaches that are adopted for the design and implementation of interventions. These may be implemented at an in-dividual level, by targeting workplace behavior. The first chapter (Geller & Robinson) in this part discusses behavioral safety, which is a specific approach based on reinforcement theory; the second chapter (Burke & Smith Sockbeson) examines safety training, which aims to improve knowledge and motivation, and so behavior. Both of these approaches tackle the direct antecedent of accidents and injuries at work – the behavior of employ-ees "at the sharp end." Behavioral safety and safety training remain the most popular interventions undertaken by companies to improve organizational safety performance. Another point of leverage is at group level; given the discussion on social context and importance of relationship with supervisor, Luria looks at group-level safety climate and supervisor interventions. A large number of interventions have been developed to improve workplace health and well-being – these range from those targeted at changing specific behaviors (e.g., physical exercise, stress management) to those that aim to re-move stressors from the workplace (e.g., job redesign). The chapter on workplace health promotion (Day & Helson) considers interventions that target individual behavior, as well as contextual factors. A broad approach that addresses the role of managerial and organizational factors is discussed in relation to concept of "psychosocial safety climate" (Zadow & Dollard).

In Chapter 14, Geller and Robinson discuss behavioral safety as a means for improving occupational safety in organizations. This approach is based on the principles of applied behavioral science, which relate to the work of the behavioral psychologist, B.F. Skinner. The chapter provides an overview of research and practice in the area of behavior-based safety (BBS). The authors discuss the BBS approach to improving safety, where the focus is on changing specific behaviors, so that unsafe behaviors are replaced with safe ones. Internal states, such as attitudes and beliefs, are not the target of the intervention, but often change in line with behaviors. Although the focus is on changing behavior, the methodology of behavioral analysis can be used to identify factors influencing behavior in the work environment, including managerial and organizational factors. The chapter discusses examples of the effective use of BBS as a safety intervention and the challenges of maintaining behavioral change in the long-term.

Chapter 15 (Burke & Smith Sockbeson) reviews safety training interventions, most of which are designed to change safety knowledge and/or safety motivation, in order to change subsequent behavior (often defined in terms of compliance and participation). The chapter discusses the effectiveness of training across different outcomes (knowledge, motivation, performance) and types of delivery (more and less engaging). Although there is a smaller evidence base, Burke and Smith Sockbeson also consider the effectiveness of training in terms of health and safety outcomes. In an extension of their discussion, they examine moderators of the relationship between safety training and safety-related outcomes, including unit level safety climate, and broader aspects of culture. The implications for the design of training interventions are discussed, such as the relative costs associated with more engaging training versus benefits in terms of safety outcomes. Further issues include the length of time over which training affects behavior, and the spacing of refresher training.

In Chapter 16, Luria focuses on group-level safety climate, and discusses group processes from a multilevel perspective. Organizational safety climate captures the top-down pro-safety influences in the organization and measures employee perceptions regarding safety policies, procedures, and practices in the work environment. Employees are able to perceive safety climate at both organizational and group levels; climate is reflected in employees' shared perceptions at these different levels. The chapter discusses a multilevel model of safety climate, in which group-level climate mediates the effects of organizational climate on employees' behavior. Luria discusses the psychological processes by which shared perceptions develop and highlights the important role played by coworkers, in relation to sense-making processes, and leaders, in relation to sense-giving processes. The discussion is extended through consideration of mediators and moderators of the relationship between safety climate and safety outcomes; the existence of different facet-specific climates and how these co-exist; and the implications for safety. The chapter also covers context-specific safety climates, such as road safety. There is a focus on interventions targeted at supervisors' behavior, which in turn influences group-level climate and employees' safety behavior. A review of the research on such interventions has shown that this is a promising approach.

Previous chapters have looked at interventions designed specifically to improve safety in the workplace. Most of these have been focused at changing employee behavior by directly targeting behavior (through BBS programs) or the immediate antecedents of safety knowledge and motivation (through training). More recently, there has been interest in group-level interventions which target leader behavior and subsequently group-level climate. Similar approaches have been adopted in relation to workplace health promotion (WHP), and these programs are discussed within Chapter 17 by Day and Helson. These include smoking cessation, alcohol consumption, stress reduction, and promoting healthy behaviors and lifestyles (such as healthy eating, physical fitness, and exercise). The effectiveness of these programs in the improvement of health and well-being is reviewed. Although targeted at individual level, such programs have more wide-ranging effects, including work outcomes, potentially decreasing job stress and improving work culture. Programs are not just targeted at changing at-risk behavior, but also at health promotion and prevention, e.g., companies offering health screening. As discussed previously (in Chapter 13), it is important to recognize the broader context and consider organizational factors in relation to health. Day and Helson note that organizational-level changes are less well documented in the literature, but generally multi-component programs are most effective. The chapter reviews the business case for WHP and examines factors that influence the success of WHP in organizations, in terms of individual, program, and organizational characteristics.

As discussed in previous chapters, an organizational approach can be effective in managing workplace health and safety. In Chapter 18, Zadow and Dollard define psychosocial safety climate (PSC) as the organizational context preceding the development of risky work conditions that lead to poor psychological health; PSC extends existing work stress theories and provides guidance for the design of interventions. Zadow and Dollard argue that PSC defines the organizational context and management practices that precede the individual job demands and job resources (as articulated in the JDR model), meaning that it is possible to intervene at the organizational level to impact employees' psychological well-being and health. PSC has a direct effect on adverse work conditions, and also moderates the effects of work environment on health and well-being. Zadow and Dollard advocate the need for interventions to address the cause of the adverse work conditions using a primary prevention approach to target the organizational context, and discuss how to design interventions based on these principles and provide some examples of these interventions in practice. These focus on a participatory approach; for example, the use of workgroups to develop action plans as part of an overall socially coordinated workplace stress reduction system, endorsed by upper management.

Finally, we focus on health and safety in high-risk environments and safety-critical organizations, where there are particular challenges to managing health and safety. Firstly, Guldenmund discusses the concept of organizational safety culture, which is critical to high reliability organizations (HROs; Weick & Sutcliffe, 2007). Safety culture has been largely considered in relation to occupational safety, but there are also different forms of safety, such as patient safety (in healthcare organizations) and process safety (in some industrial organizations, such as oil and gas) to be taken into account in such discussions. Safety culture is discussed in relation to healthcare and patient safety (Bishop, Fleming, & Flin). Operating in high-risk environments is characterized by uncertainty; as discussed by Grote, managing uncertainty is essential for safety-critical organizations. Taking a broader perspective on risk management, the final chapter (Glendon) considers a range of contemporary risk issues.

In Chapter 19, Guldenmund discusses the nature of safety culture (which was introduced earlier in Chapter 13, where the concept of organizational safety culture was differentiated from the similar, but distinct concept of organizational safety climate). Safety culture is an especially important concept for understanding how to develop and maintain organizational safety in high-risk environments, where high safety standards are critical (such as nuclear power plants, oil and gas platforms, aviation, etc.). Guldenmund discusses different safety culture models and the use of safety culture assessments. He distinguishes between different perspectives on culture – that it is something that an organization "is," reflecting its fundamental values and beliefs, and something it "has," which can be measured, and can be changed. Safety culture is understood as that part of organizational culture that is concerned with organization members' specific meanings, symbols and behaviors around safety. The chapter highlights different methodologies for safety culture assessment, for example approaches include qualitative methodologies, such as case studies and grounded theory, which produce "rich" descriptions. Such assessments provide insight into the nature of a company's underlying safety culture, which may be compared with its own mission statements, or to industry norms. Questionnaires can be used to identify dimensions and so pinpoint the company in the cultural space. Some approaches advocate structural and behavioral changes to move the company's culture toward a more generative or mature safety culture. The chapter considers ways of influencing safety culture.

Healthcare organizations are responsible not only for the occupational health and safety of their employees, but also the well-being and safety of their patients. Chapter 20 by Bishop, Fleming, and Flin, discusses the concept of "patient safety culture," which is defined as an integrated pattern of individual and organizational behavior, based upon shared beliefs and values, that continuously seeks to minimize patient harm that may result from the processes of care. Bishop et al. discuss the dimensions of patient safety culture, and ways in which these may be developed in healthcare organizations, for example, effective communications and teamwork. They also discuss common barriers to improving safety culture, such as a "blame and shame" culture and the importance of a systems approach to the improvement of safety culture, such as ensuring continuity of care. The chapter presents safety culture measurement tools that are used in practice and reviews research conducted using these instruments.

In high-risk environments, the concept of uncertainty is an important one, and critical for understanding how individuals, teams, and organizations function effectively and safely. In Chapter 21, Grote defines uncertainty as "the absence of information and more specifically, the difference between the amount of information required to perform a task and the amount of information already possessed by the organization." She argues that the focus has been on risk, but this has shifted to uncertainty, with the recognition that organizations, especially those in safety-critical environments, need to have both stability and flexibility. Safety culture depends on systems of meanings, so can provide stability, in situations characterized by uncertainty. However, effective safety management means that an organization needs to have the flexibility to respond to situations, not only by reducing or maintaining uncertainty, but in some circumstances, increasing uncertainty (e.g., speaking up in a critical situation). The chapter considers work on uncertainty at individual, team, and organizational levels.

The final chapter takes a broader perspective, locating our discussions around health and safety within the context of risk management, and drawing on the concepts of uncertainty and safety culture, as discussed in the previous three chapters. In Chapter 22, Glendon discusses how a risk management approach has impinged upon the wider societal and governmental context within which organizations operate, and highlights the importance of risk management in an increasingly risk-averse society. The chapter discusses ways in which organizations can better manage decision-making around risk (e.g., through the use of storytelling) and strategies for effective risk communication and managing risk behaviors. Glendon notes that transportation is a key area in relation to risk management, and risk-related problems (e.g., fatigue, shift work, regulation) can be common across different forms of transportation. The chapter addresses current and future challenges for risk management.

References

Bass, B. M. (1985). *Leadership and performance beyond expectations.* New York, NY: Free Press.

Clarke, S. (2010). An integrative model of safety climate: Linking psychological climate and work attitudes to individual safety outcomes using meta-analysis. *Journal of Occupational and Organizational Psychology, 83*(3), 553–578.

Costa, P. T., Jr., & McCrae, R. R. (1992). Four ways five factors are basic. *Personality and Individual Differences, 13*(6), 653–665.

Demerouti, E., Bakker, A. B., Nachreiner, F., & Schaufeli, W. B. (2001). The job demands-resources model of burnout. *Journal of Applied Psychology, 86*(3), 499–512.

Fredrickson, B. L. (2001). The role of positive emotions in positive psychology: The broaden-and-build theory of positive emotions. *American Psychologist, 56*(3), 218.

Greenwood, M., & Woods, H. M. (1919). The incidence of industrial accidents upon individuals with special reference to multiple accidents. Report no. 4. Industrial Fatigue Research Board, London.

Higgins, E. T. (1997). Beyond pleasure and pain. *American Psychologist, 52*, 1280–1300.

Hobfoll, S. E. (1989). Conservation of resources: A new attempt at conceptualizing stress. *American Psychologist, 44*(3), 513.

Hogan, J., & Foster, J. (2013). Multifaceted personality predictors of workplace safety performance: More than conscientiousness. *Human Performance, 26*(1), 20–43.

International Labour Organization (2014). *Safety and health at work: A vision for sustainable prevention.* http://www.ilo.org/safework/info/publications/WCMS_301214/lang–ja/index.htm (accessed May 10, 2015).

Johns, G. (2006). The essential impact of context on organizational behavior. *Academy of Management Review, 31*(2), 386–408.

Judge, T. A., Locke, E. A., & Durham, C. C. (1997). The dispositional causes of job satisfaction: A core evaluations approach. *Research in Organizational Behavior, 19*, 151–188.

Lazarus, R. S., & Folkman, S. (1984). *Stress, appraisal and coping.* New York, NY: Springer.

Martínez-Córcoles, M., Gracia, F., Tomás, I., & Peiró, J. M. (2011). Leadership and employees' perceived safety behaviors in a nuclear power plant: A structural equation model. *Safety Science, 49*(8–9), 1118–1129.

Nahrgang, J. D., Morgeson, F. P., & Hofmann, D. A. (2011). Safety at work: A meta-analytic investigation of the link between job demands, job resources, burnout, engagement, and safety outcomes. *Journal of Applied Psychology, 96*(1), 71–94.

Reason, J. T. (1990). *Human error.* Cambridge: Cambridge University Press.

Ryan, R. M., & Deci, E. L. (2000). Self-determination theory and the facilitation of intrinsic motivation, social development, and well-being. *American Psychologist, 55*(1), 68.

Wagenaar, W. A., Hudson, P. T. W., & Reason, J. T. (1990). Cognitive failures and accidents. *Applied Cognitive Psychology, 4*(4), 273–294.

Weick, K. E., & Sutcliffe, K. M. (2007). *Managing the unexpected: Assuring high performance in an age of complexity.* San Francisco, CA: Jossey-Bass.

Wrzesniewski, A., & Dutton, J. E. (2001). Crafting a job: Revisioning employees as active crafters of their work. *Academy of Management Review, 26*(2), 179–201.

Part I
Occupational Safety

2
Personality and Individual Differences

Mickey B. Smith, Patti Jordan, and J. Craig Wallace

Throughout the world, every 15 seconds over 160 workers have a work-related accident and one worker dies from work-related accidents or disease. According to the International Labour Organization (ILO, 2014), the workplace claims over 2.3 million employees' lives each year in which 350,000 are fatal accidents. ILO estimates that poor safety and health practices account for 4 percent of global Gross Domestic Product each year. According to the Bureau of Labor Statistics (2012), nearly 3 million employees in the private sector in the United States incurred non-fatal injuries and illnesses from job-related accidents in 2012 costing companies over $51.8 billion. More than 2.8 million of the nearly 3 million were due to workplace injuries and over half of these cases were of a serious nature that involved days away from work, job transfer, or restrictions. In the United Kingdom, the Health and Safety Executive (2014) reported a fatality rate of 0.44 deaths per 100,000 workers, which was 19 percent lower than the average amount of deaths in the past five years. A similar trend was observed in the occurrence of non-fatal injuries in which there was around a 4 percent decrease from the previous year.

In the twenty-first century, employee health and safety continues to be in the forefront of organizational initiatives, so much so that performance management systems commonly incorporate safety performance as a metric of overall job performance. In addition, companies are experiencing a heightened request by customers to audit their health and safety programs, which makes safety performance a competitive advantage. Due to the pressure of keeping their employees healthy and safe, companies are continually seeking new means to improve their safety programs and performance. In order to evaluate safety-related competencies, employers also assess applicant predispositions toward safety. The implication here is that individual characteristics can be used to predict unsafe behaviors and accidents. This chapter focuses on the individual characteristics that mold workers' safety behavior.

The Wiley Blackwell Handbook of the Psychology of Occupational Safety and Workplace Health, First Edition. Edited by Sharon Clarke, Tahira M. Probst, Frank Guldenmund, and Jonathan Passmore. © 2016 John Wiley & Sons Ltd. Published 2020 by John Wiley & Sons Ltd.

We have structured this chapter across several topics in the personality and individual differences literatures. We begin with a timeline-based review of key personality traits appearing in the occupational health and safety literature. We then move beyond personality by discussing how individual differences in cognition, age, and experience influence an employee's ability to respond to organizational hazards. We then discuss physiological predictors of safety outcomes, and provide several examples of behavior related to individual differences that lead to accidents and injuries. In the next section, we evaluate current gaps in the research. We discuss underrepresented areas of research and describe the recent shift from a singular lens of safety outcomes to multilevel interactional safety psychology, which includes the workplace environment and employee experiences at work. Each of the preceding sections offers opportunities for future research, thus we describe two potential areas of research that are not included elsewhere in the chapter: subfacet-based personality traits and rethinking safety outcomes. Finally, we offer some closing commentary on the direction of personality and individual differences research in the area of occupational health and safety.

Personality Traits and Individual Differences: An Overview

Great strides have been made in the study of individual differences and safety outcomes. The earliest study of safety predictors included concepts of proneness. Accident proneness was the earliest of these traits and has been studied in industry for almost a century. Accident proneness refers to an enduring or stable personality characteristic that predisposes an individual toward accidents (Haddon, Suchman, & Kline, 1964). Others defined accident proneness as a predisposed response to occupational hazards and stress (Arbous & Kerrich, 1951; Engel, 1991; Greenwood & Woods, 1919; Mintz & Blum, 1949). Additional proneness constructs have been studied in relation to occupational accidents and safety behaviors (e.g., boredom proneness: Game, 2007; cognitive failure: Wallace & Vodanovich, 2003; see also Foster & Nichols, Chapter 3, this volume). Recently however, the majority of research has shifted to the Big Five (Hogan & Foster, 2013).

Personality is one of the most studied topics in the fields of organizational psychology and management. However, in comparison with perceptions of and attitudes toward safety, dispositional variables (e.g., personality) have received far less attention in the occupational health and safety literature (Clarke, 2006). Nonetheless, enough research exists to warrant recent meta-analyses summarizing the general relationships among personality traits and safety outcomes (Christian, Bradley, Wallace, & Burke, 2009; Clarke, 2006). In terms of personality, researchers commonly focus their work on the Big Five (i.e., conscientiousness, neuroticism, extraversion, agreeableness, openness to experience). However, other traits and individual difference variables impact safety outcomes (Cellar, Nelson, Yorke, & Bauer, 2001). Risk-taking (Harrell, 1995), locus of control (Janicak, 1996), self-efficacy (Cellar, Yorke, Nelson, & Carroll, 2004), impulsiveness (Hansen, 1988), hardiness (Hystad & Bye, 2013), trait mindfulness (Zhang, Ding, Li, & Wu, 2013), and cognitive ability (Ford & Wiggins, 2012) have been studied as predictors of employee and organizational safety outcomes.

Recently, the research lens has shifted again. Fewer researchers are focusing solely on personality traits and individual differences in the prediction of safety behaviors and workplace accidents. The recent trend is to employ an interactionist perspective by acknowledging the combined effects of person factors and components of the environment (Christian et al., 2009). Thus, it is common to find studies incorporating factors such as safety climate (Neal, Griffin, & Hart, 2000; Zohar, 1980, 2000; see also Guediri & Griffin,

Chapter 13, and Luria, Chapter 16, this volume). In this chapter, we provide an overview and timeline of the personality-safety literature and discuss where this research will benefit in the future.

Early Safety-Related Personality Factors

Prior to the 1880s, workplace safety was not recognized as an important component to the organizational bottom-line. When workers were injured, employers would blame the actions of the employees and argue that workers assumed risk of injury as a component of employment. With little regard to employee safety, efficiency was the primary goal. Beginning in the late nineteenth century, industrial organizations faced added pressure to minimize accidents and injuries caused by exorbitantly dangerous working conditions. When companies began to realize the high cost related to workplace accidents, they began to focus specifically on occupational safety. The early focus was to make the work environment safer. It would take nearly two decades for the first psychological predictor of workplace accidents and injury to emerge. Accident proneness was the one of the first personality traits to be studied in occupational safety (Greenwood & Woods, 1919).

Accident proneness was a personality trait thought to explain the disproportionate distribution of accidents in the workplace (Farmer & Chambers, 1929; Visser, Pijl, Stolk, Neeleman, & Rosmalen, 2007). Greenwood and Woods (1919) recorded accident rates within a British factory. The authors observed that the majority of workplace accidents could be attributed to a small proportion of the workforce. They suggested the notion of unequal initial liability, which Farmer and Chambers (1929) described as accident proneness. In the following decades, accident proneness was both championed and criticized by occupational safety researchers. Using percentage-based distributions and Poisson regression analysis, early researchers found a skewed distribution in the occurrence of accidents (Farmer & Chambers, 1929). Essentially, these researchers found that most accidents involved the same small group of workers leading them to theorize the existence of two personality traits: accident free and accident prone. This early work indicated that those who were involved in an accident were more likely to be involved in subsequent accidents. Greenwood and Woods (1919) found a strong positive correlation between certain individuals and their frequency of accidents.

In 1926, Newbold found the same relationship among a large sample of workers in 13 factories. She concluded that this finding was indicative of a stable personality characteristic and personal tendency. Newbold's work offered initial support for a psychological disposition to cause or incur workplace accidents (Haddon et al., 1964). Farmer and Chambers continued to investigate accident proneness by developing a set of personality tests, which measured factors such as perceptual motor, intelligence, mechanical aptitude, and preservation. Their psychomotor test showed indications that accident proneness existed. However, their assertion that this test could be used for screening applicants was found to be unwarranted. The misinterpretation of their findings provided managers with a reason to blame employees for accidents, downplaying the organization's ability and responsibility to create a safe work environment.

In the 1940s, the study of accident proneness continued to grow. However, scholars began to criticize accident proneness as being tautological and capitalizing on non-normal distributions and other methodological biases (Arbous & Kerrich, 1951). By the late 1980s, over twenty separate research studies had been performed revealing little on how accident-involved workers differed from those with no accidents (Hansen, 1988). For instance, Wagenaar and Groeneweg (1987) questioned the validity of accident proneness tests. However, despite the conclusions of these studies, the belief that accident prone-ness can be tested continues to cycle in and out of favor within the occupational safety literature (Visser et al., 2007).

In their meta-analysis, Visser and colleagues (2007) took a slightly different approach to study accident proneness. The authors concluded that certain clusters of people did in fact experience multiple accidents and injuries. The authors determined that accident proneness did exist, but they could only observe it at the group level. Thus, accident proneness could be attributed to group characteristics. The authors offered several reasons for the lack of findings at the individual level. Of chief concern, prior literature lacked a clear definition of accident proneness, and without a clear construct definition, it is impos-sible to establish construct validity. Nonetheless, the cyclical trends in prior work indicate that accident proneness will remain a controversial predictor of accident involvement and workplace stress (Day, Brasher, & Bridger, 2012).

The Big Five in Occupational Safety Research

Beyond accident proneness, safety scholars began to include high-order constructs of personality – namely the Big Five, which originated with the research of D. W. Fiske (1949) and was later expanded by other researchers (Barrick & Mount, 1991; Goldberg, 1990; McCrae & Costa, 1987; Norman, 1963). The Big Five is comprised of extraver-sion, agreeableness, conscientiousness, emotional stability or neuroticism, and openness to experience or intellect (Costa & McCrae, 1992; John, 1990).

When applied to the workplace, extraverted employees are more likely to engage in so-cial interaction than their introverted counterparts. These employees require stimulation and have a higher capacity for positive emotion. Agreeableness describes an employee's orientation toward accepting the opinions of others. Employees high in agreeableness avoid conflict and tend to go along with the crowd. Conscientious employees are observant of their surroundings, cognizant of goals, and dependable. These employees are more likely to set and commit to goals. Emotional stability and neuroticism speak to an individual's ability to cope with psychological stress and control excessive urges. Neurotic employees are more likely to react negatively and impulsively to stressful situ-ations. Openness to experience or intellect captures an individual's tendency to seek out new opportunities and experiences. Some research suggests that these five factors can be utilized to predict both individual and organizational performance and impact em-ployee satisfaction, work motivation, and other job performance measurements (Barrick & Mount, 1991).

Many studies have used the Big Five as predictors of work-related outcomes (Cellar et al., 2001, 2004; Clarke & Robertson, 2005; Conte & Jacobs, 2003; Hansen, 1988; Salgado, 2002; Thoresen, Bradley, Bliese, & Thoresen, 2004). Research performed by Hogan and Foster (2013) concluded that out of the Big Five, conscientiousness consist-ently predicted safety-related outcomes reinforcing the research of others in this area (Cellar et al., 2001; Christian et al., 2009; Wallace & Vodanovich, 2003). Conscientious-ness is believed to be a good predictor of safety-related criteria, because individuals who are less attentive and ignore policies and procedures are more likely to have accidents and injuries (Hogan & Foster, 2013). The evidence is less clear for the other Big Five factors but studies have shown employees low in emotional stability, low in agreeableness, high in extraversion, and high in openness are more likely to engage in unsafe behavior (Cellar et al., 2004; Cellar, Nelson, & Yorke, 2000; Clarke, 2006; Clarke & Robertson, 2005, 2008; Hansen, 1988; Smillie, Yeo, Furnham, & Jackson, 2006).

Two meta-analyses found mixed or negligible results. Clarke and Robertson (2008) found weak evidence for relationships between each of the Big Five factors and accident involvement, except for extraversion. Both neuroticism ($M_\rho = .30$) and low agreeableness ($M_\rho = .05$) were positively correlated with accident involvement. However, the authors cautioned readers to take into consideration the high variability among their findings. Also, several of the effects were likely situation specific suggesting the need to incorporate moderators (e.g., climate, leadership). In a subsequent meta-analysis, Christian et al. (2009) tested a mediation model where personality factors were distal predictors of safety performance, which led to safety outcomes. It should be noted that Christian and colleagues separated safety performance from safety outcomes (i.e., accidents, injuries). The authors found a significant mean correlation between safety performance and conscientiousness ($M_\rho = .18$). They also found a significant mean correlation between safety outcomes and conscientiousness ($M_\rho = -.26$). All other relationships were not significantly different from zero. In their meta-analysis, Christian and colleagues also tested for effects between the propensity to take risks and locus of control. We will discuss these findings along with other personality traits beyond the Big Five. Overall, conscientiousness is the only Big Five trait to consistently hold as a predictor of safety performance. This is in line with research in other areas that finds conscientiousness to positively relate to job performance (Barrick & Mount, 1991).

A promising area of research has taken the Big Five and combined the traits to create personality-based safety traits (Hogan & Foster, 2013). The authors created six safety-related performance dimensions that they claimed would better capture effects on safety performance than the general five-factor model (see Foster & Nichols, Chapter 3, this volume). The six dimensions comprise compliance, confidence, emotional stability, vigilance, cautiousness, and trainability. The authors hypothesized positive relationships between each of the factors (as well as the composite battery) and safety performance, and their predictions were supported. Additionally, the highest relationship existed between the composite battery and safety performance. This is an exciting development in the use of personality to predict safety performance and outcomes. Other opportunities exist in the personality-safety research area. Particularly, there are additional personality traits beyond the Big Five that may have an important impact on safety performance and safety outcomes.

Additional Personality Traits that Influence Safety Outcomes

Although the largest area of the literature has been dedicated to the Big Five, other personality traits appear in the occupational safety literature (Clarke, 2011). For instance, Christian and colleagues (2009) also tested the relationships between locus of control and risk-taking and safety performance and safety outcomes. Harrell (1995) studied the role of risk-taking in accident involvement finding that risk-taking was positively related to accident involvement (see also Foster & Nichols, Chapter 3, this volume). Janicak (1996) found that locus of control was a predictor of accident involvement when jobs were hazardous. Both risk-taking and locus of control are captured in the higher-order personality construct of core self-evaluations (CSE: Judge, Locke, & Durham, 1997). Additionally, traits related to self-regulation (e.g., regulatory focus) offer more nuanced views of how individual traits lead to safety behaviors.

Core self-evaluations

Core self-evaluation (CSE) is a multidimensional construct consisting of self-esteem, generalized self-efficacy, locus of control, and emotional stability (Judge et al., 1997). Self-esteem and generalized self-efficacy have been shown to be highly correlated, thus those with a positive self-image tend to also have a general belief that they can accomplish tasks (Judge, Locke, Durham, & Kluger, 1998). Locus of control is one of the more potent predictors of individual behavior as it relates to perceptions of an individual's influence over the environment (Judge & Bono, 2001; Rotter, 1966). Emotional stability, which is also a factor of the Big Five (i.e., neuroticism), is defined as an individual's ability to control emotional reactions in stressful situations. We discussed the role of emotional stability earlier in the chapter, so we focus here on the other three factors of CSE.

Locus of control is the degree to which an individual feels in control of a given situation as opposed to having no control and being at the whim of the environment (Rotter, 1966). Individuals with an internal locus of control (internals) feel that they have more control over life situations than what is determined by the environment. Externals are those individuals who feel that they are at the whim of the environment. Therefore, Christian and colleagues (2009) expected locus of control (i.e., a higher score describes an internal) to positively relate to safety performance and negatively relate to safety outcomes (accidents and injuries). In line with their hypotheses, locus of control was positively related to safety performance (M_ρ = .35) and negatively related to safety outcomes (M_ρ = −.26). These findings suggest that internals are more likely to take responsibility for safety outcomes. Internals typically take a more proactive stance when setting safety goals (Clarke, 2011). Externals, however, are less likely to focus on preventing safety outcomes because they believe that accidents are caused by factors in the environment, of which they have little control.

As Clarke (2011) observed, we know less about the roles self-esteem and generalized self-efficacy play in preventing accidents and injuries and promoting safety behaviors. Based upon CSE theory, individuals with a high CSE are those with a positive self-image. Therefore, high CSE corresponds with high self-esteem and high generalized self-efficacy. High CSE employees feel that they have the ability to successfully control and cope with tasks across various job-related situations. Based upon work that has demonstrated a moderate to strong positive relationship between CSE and general job performance (Judge, Erez, Bono, & Thoresen, 2003), high CSE employees are intrinsically motivated by achieving self-determined goals. We expect individuals with high self-regard and strong perceptions of ability to be motivated to set personal goals that align with safety standards and strive to achieve those goals.

Similar to a neurotic individual, risk takers are impulsive, thrill seeking, and likely to engage in unsafe behaviors. In their meta-analysis, Christian and colleagues (2009) expected propensity to take risks to be negatively related to safety performance and positively related to safety outcomes. Risk-taking was negatively related to safety performance (M_ρ = −.28). The authors did not find a significant relationship between risk-taking and safety outcomes.

Self-regulation: regulatory focus, self-control, self-efficacy

Self-regulation describes a field of motivation research that seeks to demonstrate the internal processes that drive goal attainment. Because of space limitations, we cannot provide a comprehensive review of the constructs in the literature as they relate to occupational health and safety, thus we focus our discussion on trait regulatory focus (i.e., regulatory orientation: Higgins, 1997, 1998), self-control (Baumeister, Vohs, & Tice, 2007), and self-efficacy (Bandura, 1997). Each of these factors influences attainment of work-related goals.

Higgins (1997) defined regulatory focus as a dual-path motivational phenomenon. His theory was that individuals were motivated to either approach or avoid outcomes by applying promotion or prevention strategies. Promotion-focused individuals seek out opportunities for success. They have an inherent need for growth and nurturance. Therefore, promotion-focused individuals employ strategies that increase the likelihood of achieving goals and avoiding errors of omission. Prevention-focused individuals are concerned with duty, security, and responsibility (Crowe & Higgins, 1997). These individuals engage strategies that are focused on preventing mistakes or making errors of commission. There is some debate as to how regulatory focus should be conceptualized, whether it is a trait or dependent upon the situation (Brockner & Higgins, 2001; Wallace, Johnson, & Frazier, 2009). Scholer and Higgins (2008) suggest that both operationalizations are correct and exist within the hierarchy of regulatory focus theory. We focus our discussion on trait regulatory focus, which Higgins (1997, 1998) referred to as regulatory orientation.

Regulatory orientation is the general tendency to view situations as either opportunities to succeed (promotion orientation) or a chance to fail (prevention orientation). There is a substantial amount of literature on how regulatory focus strategies influence task performance, extra-role performance, and safety outcomes. Across these outcomes, the findings are pretty consistent in that promotion strategies lead to increased task performance and extra-role performance (Brockner & Higgins, 2001; Scholer & Higgins, 2008). However, those who engage prevention strategies typically have higher safety performance scores, including fewer accidents and injuries (Wallace et al., 2009). Wallace and colleagues created the *Regulatory Focus at Work Scale*, which is a combination of trait and state regulatory focus. The RFWS measures specific behaviors and attitudes toward following regulations and accomplishing as much as possible. The authors' use of the RFWS reified observations of prior studies by finding that promotion-focused employees had lower safety performance ratings, and prevention-focused employees were rated higher.

Safety performance is an amalgamated construct measured by supervisor ratings, reported accidents and injuries, and self-report. When employees engage prevention strategies, their supervisor-rated performance increases because they are perceived to be careful and are less likely to make mistakes that could lead to injury. These employees are involved in fewer accidents and suffer fewer injuries, and they are less likely to self-report accidents and injuries because they see this as a potential risk for reprimand. Promotion strategies create an interesting scenario for safety performance. Wallace and colleagues (2009) found a negative relationship between trait promotion focus and safety performance. Promotion strategies involve seeking opportunities and acting on those opportunities without regard for potential loss. Safety performance is highly loss-driven, in that when an error is committed the potential loss could be as harmless as an alarm sounding, but as serious as potential death. Promotion-focused employees are commonly perceived to be more likely to take risks, particularly when they are nearing goal attainment (Förster, Higgins, & Idson, 1998). Consequently, promotion strategies can be equated to risk-taking in that promotion strategies create greater opportunities for failure, which promotion-focused employees disregard.

Self-control is a self-regulatory phenomenon that is dependent upon psychological resources (Baumeister et al., 2007; Hagger, Wood, Stiff, & Chatzisarantis, 2010; Muraven & Baumeister, 2000). We include it in this chapter as people vary in terms of the availability of resources, that is, some people have more self-control than others. Self-control is relevant in a discussion of safety for two reasons. First, differences among individuals' self-control create separate scenarios for safety performance. Second, self-control is dependent upon a limited pool of resources, which is depleted by daily job-related tasks. Employees high in self-control are more likely to take their time in performing dangerous tasks. However, regardless of how much self-control an employee possesses, stressors requiring self-control that occur throughout the work day will deplete resources to the point of self-control failure (Muraven & Baumeister, 2000). Surprisingly, we found little research investigating self-control or self-control failure and safety performance. However, research in other areas may suggest probable findings for safety performance.

Muraven and Slessareva (2003) found an interesting trend in performance related to self-control failure. In their study, the authors found that resource depletion and motivation jointly influence subsequent performance. This interaction suggests that resource depletion, which should lead to self-control failure, does not always lead to poorer performance. Instead, when employees are sufficiently motivated, declines in performance due to self-control failure can be mitigated. These effects were further supported by evidence found in a meta-analysis that supported a partial-depletion model (Hagger et al., 2010). This model suggests that people can actually manage ego depletion by conserving resources when they know of subsequent tasks requiring self-control.

Employees must show self-control in the workplace, regardless of the safety context. When the job involves hazardous or dangerous tasks, self-control becomes even more important. Safety protocols, procedures, and trained behaviors create a system that should minimize accidents and injuries. Employees lacking in self-control, or who are likely to experience self-control failure, are more likely to exert reduced effort and take shortcuts. Also, these employees may not attend to smaller but important details of their work. In either case, a lack of self-control poses serious implications for employee safety performance.

We finish the section of self-regulation's impact on safety performance with self-efficacy. Self-efficacy is one of the most studied motivational constructs in the organizational sciences, and its implications for employee performance are well documented (Gist, 1987; Stajkovic and Luthans, 1998). Self-efficacy is an individual's belief that he/she can perform a specific task, which can differ between individuals facing the same task (Bandura, 1997). Bandura's self-efficacy differs from the general self-efficacy component of CSE in that it is a belief targeted at specific tasks (Bandura, 2012).

Stajkovic and Luthans (1998) found overall positive effects between self-efficacy and job performance ($r = .38$). They concluded that self-efficacy focused on job performance was indicative of employees setting specific goals, which were both challenging and attainable. In line with goal-setting theory, employees high in self-efficacy, who self-manage the creation of goals, are intrinsically motivated to attain those goals (Locke & Latham, 2002). Sitzmann and Yeo (2013) found similar results in their study of the directionality of the self-efficacy–performance relationship ($r = .40$). However, the authors found this result when controlling for directionality (i.e., past performance predicts self-efficacy). In both cases, self-efficacy was moderately and positively related to performance.

Efficacious beliefs concerning safety lead employees to set goals that are conducive to reducing accidents and injuries. These employees believe that they can appropriately follow safety standards (DeJoy, 1996). These employees also appear to view job demands as challenges that can be overcome, thus reducing job-related strain (Schaubroeck & Merritt, 1997; see also Taris & Schaufeli, Chapter 8, this volume). Similar to the observed effects of locus of control and conscientiousness, employees high in safety-related self-efficacy will take responsibility for achieving safety performance standards, be intrinsically motivated to achieve those goals, and experience less stress related to job demands. To date, there has been a lack of research investigating the self-efficacy–safety relationship. This is an opportunity for future researchers.

Hardiness

Kobasa (1979) defined hardiness as a tendency to find meaning in stressful situations. Similar to several of the Big Five factors, hardiness is a multidimensional construct consisting of control, challenge, and commitment (Bartone, 1995; Hystad & Bye, 2013; Maddi & Kobasa, 1984). Control, which is similar to locus of control (Rotter, 1966), reflects an individual's general belief that he/she has the ability to control outcomes and respond appropriately to stressful situations. Challenge can be thought of as a tendency to interpret stressful situations as an opportunity to succeed. Commitment describes the tendency to be devoted and invested in goals. Employees high in hardiness attend to safety goals and are committed to achieving those goals, particularly in hazardous or stressful situations (Hystad & Bye, 2013).

Researchers have studied hardiness in several employee populations (e.g., seafarers on cargo ships: Hystad & Bye, 2013; soldiers: Britt, Adler, & Bartone, 2001), but only a few studies have investigated hardiness in relation to occupational safety. Hystad and Bye (2013) found that hardiness positively related to safety behaviors onboard cargo ships ($r = .28$). The authors also looked at the interaction of personal values with hardiness finding that safety behaviors were consistently high when employees were high in hardiness, regardless of whether they valued openness or conservation. In fact, when hardiness was low, the rate of safety behaviors increased in the conservation condition, but fewer safety behaviors were still reported in this condition.

We were unable to find additional studies that included hardiness as a predictor of safety outcomes. However, hardiness has a rich history in both the personality literatures and health care (e.g., nursing, patient safety) literatures (Abdollahi, Talib, Yaacob, & Ismail, 2014; Kobasa, 1979). Although we do not include a review of this research here, those interested in pursuing hardiness research in the occupational safety realm would benefit from a detailed review of each of those fields of study.

Beyond Personality: Individual Differences and Safety Outcomes

People differ in more than psychological traits. Characteristics ranging from intelligence, skill sets, experience, lifestyle, past experience, and other physiological characteristics influence safety performance and safety outcomes (Chau et al., 2011). In this section, we focus on three areas of study in the occupational safety literature. First, we discuss the impact that cognition has on occupational safety. We also examine the existing literature on demographic factors such as age, experience, and gender. Finally, we address additional physiological characteristics that make employees more susceptible to injuries or accidents.

Cognition: cognitive ability, cognitive failure, safety knowledge

Knowledge and the ability to think critically about one's job are imperative for performance. Both of these factors are commonly used in the selection of employees. Indeed, organizations continue to utilize intelligence tests for various occupations. Ford and Wiggins (2012) deemed those occupations as requiring high cognitive abilities. In occupations with physical hazards that also require high cognitive ability, injury rates were exceedingly high. Thus, jobs that are dangerous and require critical thinking, deep understanding, and the ability to move quickly from one task to the other provide increased opportunity for accidents and injuries. Employees who work in these occupations must possess the requisite knowledge and cognitive ability.

Providing knowledge through training, onboarding, and display materials (e.g., safety poster) is one of the larger functions of human resource management. Knowledge-based selection tests are beneficial in determining existing knowledge, but modern safety standards change frequently in the event of an accident, disaster, or legal development. Additionally, providing knowledge about their job and how it fits within the overall production process is a core component in involvement-based HR initiatives (Lawler, 1986; Vandenberg, Richardson, & Eastman, 1999). In this instance, safety knowledge is a job resource employees possess to meet the demands of a dangerous job (Nahrgang, Morgeson, & Hofmann, 2011). Furthermore, employees who possess a working understanding of safety protocols and standards have the basis for compliance.

Simply possessing a working understanding of safety standards will not prevent accidents and injuries. Employees must be able to take that knowledge and apply it. Cognitive ability and cognitive failure are two aspects of applied cognition in the workplace. Cognitive ability is typically defined in terms of intelligence or critical thinking. Research on the effects of cognitive ability and workplace performance has provided mixed results, particularly concerning accident involvement. At the occupational level, when cognitive ability demands are high, injuries are more likely to occur in hazardous jobs (Ford & Wiggins, 2012). This suggests that complex and hazardous jobs that require employees to possess high cognitive ability are also jobs with higher incident rates. However, Kotzé and Steyn (2013) found negligible effects between cognitive ability and workplace accident involvement at the employee level. This suggests that the complexity of a job, and the resulting demands on cognitive ability, may be washing away the inverse effect between cognitive ability and accident involvement.

Wallace and Vodanovich (2003) defined cognitive failure as "a breakdown in cognitive functioning that results in a cognitively based mistake or error in task execution" (p. 316). In their study, cognitive failure negatively related to workplace safety behavior and positively related to accident involvement. Cognitive failure also moderated the effect of conscientiousness, strengthening the negative effect of conscientiousness on accident involvement and strengthening the positive effect of conscientiousness on safety behaviors.

Experience/age

So far we have discussed behavior and psychological individual differences that contribute to workplace safety. However, other individual characteristics, such as, age, education level, job knowledge, and time on job have been shown to play a role in safety outcomes. In a study by Chau and colleagues (2011) of approximately 20,000 workers, the lack of know-how and lack of job knowledge was related to age and accident rate. Injuries due to lack of know-how were more represented in younger employees (<30 years of age) with an odds ratio of 1.45 (p < .05) and lack of knowledge with an odds ratio of 2.06 (p < .01). This study showed 25 percent of injuries were due to the lack of know-how or knowledge in which almost half were among younger workers. In other studies, inexperience has also been linked to the increase risk of injury among teenagers and temporary workers (Driscoll, Ansari, Harrison, Frommer, & Ruck, 1994; Jacobsson & Schelp 1987; Nola et al., 2000). The higher risk in young employees has been studied by numerous scholars (including, Bazroy, Sahai & Soudarssanane, 2003; Bhattacherjee et al., 2003; Brett 2004; Chau et al., 2002; Cloutier 1994; McCaig, Burt, & Stussman, 1998) who measured know-how and job knowledge.

As a worker continues to do the same job day after day, the risk of boredom increases. Boredom is: "an unpleasant, transient affective state in which the individual feels a pervasive lack of interest in and difficulty concentrating on the current activity" (Fisher, 1993, p. 396). Studies have shown that boredom may be moderated by differences in age, gender, intelligence, and tenure (Drory, 1982; Hill, 1975; Stagner, 1975). Young intelligent males high in tenure and extroverts both show a low threshold for boredom (O'Hanlon, 1981). Task-related boredom research indicates that boredom often arises from perceived or actual constraints on behavior – constraints that may be imposed by organizational policies and procedures, the lack of clear expectations, and by an individual's sense of duty (regulatory focus) (Fenichel, 1951; Fisher, 1993; Iso-Ahola & Weissinger, 1990). Bored workers have reported increasing fatigue and an increased number of lapses or moments of transient inattention, which have clear implications for both individual and organizational safety and have been associated with increased injuries and accidents in industrial settings (Branton, 1970; Cox, 1980; Drory, 1982; Game, 2007). Boredom can also affect a worker's capacity to respond quickly to important events and information, which increases the risk of accidents or injuries in highly safety-critical industries such as aviation, nuclear energy, chemical processing, and steel manufacturing (Hopkin, 1990).

Another area of interesting research with regard to age and experience is the study of bias. Self–other bias is the tendency to think that other people are responsible for their accidents and at the same time perceive that factors in the environment cause one's own accidents (Lingard, 2002). Similar to locus of control, self–other bias likely influences the effectiveness of safety protocols, because individuals attribute accidents and injuries to others or the environment instead of taking accountability. Another form of bias is optimism bias, which is the tendency to believe negative events are more likely to affect one's peers than oneself also referred to as "it won't happen to me" (Weinstein, 1984). Studies have shown that lack of experience can lead to an increase in optimism bias (Dejoy, 1989). Optimism bias is important in the context of occupational safety because how workers perceive and respond to danger and risk is critical to improving the management of safety in the workplace. For instance, if people think that the injuries or accidents are less likely to happen to them versus others, efforts to promote and improve safety may be ignored. Dispositional optimism, the belief and expectation of good things happening in the future has been shown to influence the level to which workers care for the safety of others (Roberts & Geller, 1996), yet no linkage has been found between poor safety behavior and dispositional optimism. A study by Caponecchia (2010) found evidence that optimism bias continues to exist in the occupational safety and health domain. The study showed workers continue to believe events such as suffering a life-threatening injury, causing an injury to someone else, or being harmed after not using protective equipment are less likely to happen to oneself than to others. This has serious implications on the education, awareness, and climate implemented by organizations. Understanding how a behavior-based safety program will improve safety behavior can mean the difference between the program being effective or just a waste of time and resources (see Geller & Robinson, Chapter 14, this volume). Consideration of how optimism bias can be reduced and how workers can see the personal relevance of safety information and policies should be emphasized.

Physiological Characteristics

Individual differences can also include physiological characteristics such as health status, obesity, presence of diseases, and lifestyle factors such as smoking, alcohol abuse, drug use, and lack of physical activity, which are all known to increase the risk of injury and accidents (Chau, Gauchard, Siegfried, Benamghar, Dangelzer, Français, & Mur, 2004; Chau et al., 2011; Gauchard, Chau, Mur, & Perrin, 2001; Gauchard et al., 2003; Härmä, Tenkanen, Sjöblom, Alikoski, & Heinsalmi, 1998). This is especially evident when physical job demand is high (Chau et al., 2008). Numerous studies over the past several decades in this area have been performed. Table 2.1 is a summary of the results.

Table 2.1 Studies examining physiological characteristics associated with heightened risk of accidents.

Physiological characteristics	Finding	Researcher(s)
Aging/balance control	The lack of balance control has been linked to increased risk of falls. Since balance control requires central processing of information from visual, vestibular, and somatosensory systems that create the motor responses, such as gaze control and posture stabilization, damage to any one of these postural systems increase the risk of falls.	Gauchard et al. (2003) Vouriot et al. (2004)
Aging/inactivity	Lower physical strength means older workers are at greater risk of injury when work is physically demanding and requires more strength than skill.	Chau, Bhattacherjee, & Kunar (2009) Khlat, Jusot, & Ville (2009) Mathiowetz, et al. (1985)
Aging/job demand	Studies show a positive correlation between cumulative job demand and injury rate among workers over the age of 45 when controlling for other factors.	Chau et al. (2009)
Alcohol	Alcohol abuse was found to be associated with a higher injury risk.	Chau et al. (2009)
Alcohol	In a 2003 study of railway workers, the daily use of alcohol was strongly linked to stepping down from a railcar among railway workers (adjusted odds ratio 6.2).	Gauchard et al. (2003)
Drug Abuse	Many working people smoke and used medication or other licit psychoactive substances and alcohol in order to cope with work-related stressors, which is more common among manual or blue collar workers.	Peretti-Watel et al. (2009)
Drug abuse	Blue collar or manual workers who have poorer working conditions may lead to physical and mental disturbances resulting in the use of psychotropic drugs. These workers are also more likely to use tobacco.	Peretti-Watel et al. (2009)
Drug abuse	Cumulative job stress is common and is associated with increased risk of psychotropic drug use. Physical job demands lead to fatigue and the development of work-related stress reactions, psychological overload, and health problems.	Peretti-Watel et al. (2009)
Drug abuse	Workers with short-term employment and occupational demands are subject to a higher risk for alcohol abuse and smoking with high gender and age disparities.	Legleye, Peretti-Watal, Baumann, Beck, & Chau (2009)
Drug, alcohol/balance control	Smoking, alcohol, and drug use also alter balance control and therefore increase the risk of falls.	Chau et al. (2008) Gauchard et al. (2003)

Hearing & cognitive disability	Hearing disability may be a risk factor for injuries by preventing the affected individual from hearing various sounds or warning messages in the workplace. Cognitive disability may impair thinking, concentration, attention, orientation, problem solving, or memory. Both hearing and cognitive disabilities have been reported as risk factors for falls.	Vouriot et al. (2004)
Hearing & cognitive disability	Hearing disorders have been shown to affect injury rate when moving objects are involved (adjusted odds ratio of 2.0) because of the reduced noise perception, particularly warning messages.	Vouriot et al. (2004)
Inactivity	The risk was higher among train drivers. The lack of physical activity such as playing sports and gardening was also linked to high risk of injury for railway workers.	Gauchard et al. (2003)
Obesity	Obesity was more common among older workers than among younger workers with a 2.7-fold increased injury risk for workers older than age 45.	Chau et al. (2009)
Obesity	Obese workers are at greater risk of falls requiring prolonged sick leave and of injury in environments with high ergonomic demands.	Gauchard et al. (2003) Froom, Melamed, Kristal-Boneh, Gofer, & Ribak (1996)
Obesity	Musculoskeletal disorders were risk factors for injury in all age groups but more pronounced in workers aged ≥45	Chau et al. (2009)
Obesity	Studies have shown overweight workers (BMI >25) have a higher risk of falls in construction jobs.	Chau et al. (2004)
Obesity	Obesity (BMI >30) has been linked to fall injuries and required time off of 8 days or more among railway workers but did not affect the overall number of falls.	Gauchard et al. (2003)
Sleeping disorders	Sleeping disorders have been linked to increase risk of accidents under certain conditions. For workers with less than 6 hours per day of sleep and no use of sleeping pills, the risk factor was moderate (odds ratio of 1.7) and when sleeping pills were used the risk factor increased (odds ratio of 2.8). However, when sleeping pills were used and the worker received less than 6 hours per day of sleep the risk of injury significantly increased with an odds ratio of 10.	Chau et al. (2002)
Smoking	Increased risk of non-fatal occupational injuries among both active and passive smokers working in small-to-medium size manufacturing companies in Japan.	Nakata et al. (2006)
Smoking	In workers aged <30, smoking was the factor that influenced injury rate the most. Being male, smoking, and abusing alcohol were associated with a higher risk of injury for all age groups.	Chau et al. (2009)

By no means is Table 2.1 a complete list of all studies performed regarding individual physiological characteristics and work safety outcomes, but rather an overview to how each worker has numerous factors that contribute to their safety-related behavior at work. When evaluating worker safety, it is important to consider both psychological and physiological factors to determine the level of risk and the types of prevention programs that might be most effective. For physiological factors, especially those related to workers' health and well-being, job demand can impact the injury rate for workers with certain conditions as seen in this chapter.

Gaps in Knowledge

Occupational health and safety research is extensive, but there remain several avenues for research, particularly in regard to personality and individual differences. Studies have shown that one of the main causes of accidents is inattention or lack of mindfulness about one's circumstances and surroundings (Gomez, 2013). Many believe workplace safety is a state of mind. In recent years, mindfulness has become a targeted area of research in studying workplace safety. Mindfulness has been defined as a present-focused awareness and attention with an open attitude regarding ongoing events and experiences (Bishop et al., 2004). Mindfulness has been studied in the areas of well-being (Brown, Ryan, & Creswell, 2007), cognitive flexibility (Moore & Malinowski, 2009), control of risk behavior (Lakey, Campbell, Brown, & Goodie, 2007), and interpersonal relationships (Dekeyser, Raes, Leijsssen, Leysen, & Dewulf, 2008). However, little is known regarding mindfulness and organizational and individual performance and safety outcomes. Research has demonstrated that mindfulness can stimulate sustained attention, cognitive flexibility, situational awareness, and better metacognitive skills (Bishop et al., 2004; Moore & Malinowski, 2009; Schmertz, Anderson, & Robins, 2009). These skills are necessary to promote positive safety behavior.

Researchers believe mindfulness can improve safety behavior for several reasons. First, mindful workers are more likely to avoid cognitive failure, the involuntary lapse which can cause accidents because one loses awareness of external surroundings and internal processes (Herndon, 2008; Reason, Manstead, Stradling, Baxter, & Campbell, 1990). Second, mindful individuals are concerned with their perceived behaviors and are better at controlling their risky behavior (Lakey et al., 2007). Thus, mindful people are less likely to violate rules and procedures purposefully, such as taking shortcuts (Zohar & Erev, 2007). Mindful workers also have a tendency to be more aware of their coworkers' behavior and the potential risks in the environment because mindfulness can impede automatic or categorical thinking, biased judgment and habitual reactions (Bishop et al., 2004; Brown et al., 2007). Finally mindfulness has been linked to empathy, improved social skills, and improved interpersonal relationships; therefore, a mindful person is more likely to exhibit safety participation behavior showing more capabilities and willingness to ensure safety participation (Brown et al., 2007; Zhang et al., 2013).

Zhang and Wu (2014) investigated the influence of dispositional mindfulness on operators' safety behavior. These participants worked in nuclear power plant control rooms. The authors established a positive relationship between dispositional mindfulness (β = .32, p < .001) and safety performance. Mindfulness predicted safety performance beyond that attributed to conscientiousness. Finally, the authors investigated the moderating roles of experience and intelligence. They measured these variables by comparing operators who were more experienced or intelligent (one standard deviation above the mean) and found that the effect of mindfulness in predicting safety performance was greater when experience was above average and intelligence was above average. While this study has limitations, it does expand our knowledge of the influence dispositional mindfulness has on safety behavior and provides merit for further studies in this area.

We lack an understanding of how negative individual characteristics, such as dark triad personality traits (Machiavellianism, narcissism, psychopathy), will affect safety behavior. The study of counterproductive work behavior (CWB), which are volitional acts intended to harm individuals or the organization (Spector & Fox, 2005), includes a dimension that evaluates unsafe behavior (Gruys & Sackett, 2003). Research by Wu and Lebreton (2011) demonstrated a link between CWB and the dark triad. Team and group research has also shown the negative influence of aberrant personality traits on variables such as team potency, performance, satisfaction, and cohesion, but few have focused on group and organizational outcomes.

The real-world implications of understanding the relationship between safety performance and dark personality traits are numerable. In recent years, workplace safety was seen a whole new dimension with the increase of workplace violence and deaths. Employers are not just responsible for work safety as it pertains to their jobs, but must also ensure the employee is not exposed to workplace violence. Thus, understanding how dark personality traits may manifest themselves into situations in which safety is jeopardized will allow organizations to prevent such acts from occurring.

Personality and individual differences can be powerful predictors of subsequent behaviors. However, factors from the environment create contexts and situations that influence the personality–behavior relationships. Work-related experiences (e.g., engagement) and workplace climate are two situational factors that influence employee safety behavior. Employee engagement has become a vital topic as employers seek to retain good employees and increase employee satisfaction and well-being. Creating a trusting relationship with employees can have implications beyond organizational effectiveness but also create a safe work environment. Nahrgang and colleagues (2011) found that engagement motivated employees to comply with procedures and was negatively related to accidents and injuries; adverse events and unsafe behavior was positively related to working safely. They believe by creating a supportive environment, organizations will not just achieve a safer workplace but will also increase the motivation and health of their employees. This meta-analysis provided insight into how engagement and organizational support can effect safety behavior, while also calling for additional research.

Hoffman and Morgeson (1999) found evidence which suggested that individuals are more likely to commit to safety and engage in open communication about safety when perceived organization support is high and there is a high quality relationship with their leader. For the past 30 years research on safety climate has found a strong relationship between safety climate and safety outcomes, however, research to develop a better theoretical understanding of the antecedents, mediators, and moderators of this relationship is needed (Zohar, 2010). Research has shown that quality leadership enhances the engagement, motivation, commitment, and involvement of workers to improve work and performance outcomes (Avolio, Gardner, Walumbwa, Luthans, & May, 2004; Avolio & Luthans, 2006; Gardner, Avolio, Luthans, May & Walumbwa, 2005). However, little is known regarding how managers demonstrate their commitment to safety and how their commitment motivates their followers (Eid, Mearns, Larsson, Laberg, & Johnsen, 2012). One specific area of interest is how advances in leadership theory and Psychological Capital (PsyCap) can improve our understanding of the role of organizational support as a mechanism that affects safety outcomes. PsyCap is a form of positive organizational behavior defined as "an individual's positive psychological state of development involving four criteria of self-efficacy, optimism, hope and resilience" (Luthans, Avolio, Avey, &

Norman, 2007). A 2012 review by Eid and colleagues hypothesized that authentic leadership will positively relate to Psychological Capital and the PsyCap variables will mediate the relationship between safety climate and safety outcomes. They suggest future research to better understand the impact of indirect and direct leadership processes on individual safety behavior and organizational safety outcomes.

Future Research

Facet-based personality and individual differences

To date, sparse and inconclusive findings exist regarding individual differences, beyond personality, associated with safety performance. In 2009, Christian and colleagues were the first to support a fully mediated model showing multiple individual constructs contribute to the prediction of safety performance. Their model included safety-related predictors such as, safety climate, personality, safety knowledge, and motivation. However, data was limited on the number of personality variables focusing on a single dimension of conscientiousness. To expand our knowledge in this area, Hogan and Foster are developing a multi-faceted safety predictor scale which includes several dimensions: (a) following rules, (b) being steady under pressure, (c) controlling temper, (d) being vigilant, (e) avoiding risk, and (f) being responsive to training and feedback (Hogan & Foster, 2013). Their research provides grounds for reevaluating the role of personality characteristics in a safety-related context.

Managers understand the importance of individual characteristics as antecedents of unsafe safety behavior, however identifying the actual relationship between personality and performance has been difficult to identify. Taking one dimension at a time limits our ability to develop a broad factor scale. Hogan and Foster suggest a multi-facet approach enhances our understanding of how to predict safety behavior by creating meaningful facets to assess a range of safety-related performance dimensions.

Rethinking safety outcomes

A meta-analysis performed by Christian and colleagues in 2009 suggested that both the person and the situation are important factors related to workplace safety. The authors suggested one research avenue might be to examine how person and situation factors interact to influence safety. They suggested one way to approach the issue of person–situation interactions is with Schneider's (1987) attraction–selection–attrition model, which suggests that individuals are differentially attracted to, selected for, and retained within different work environments on the basis of their values, personality, and other individual differences. For example, thrill-seeking people may be more likely to seek out high-risk jobs. To the extent that risk-seeking individuals congregate in riskier environments, the organizational climate may become socially constructed to lead to riskier decisions and actions.

Christian and colleagues (2009) also suggest the need for further research in identifying safety outcome criteria. Today, most studies assess accidents in terms of the number of recordable accidents as defined by regulators, meaning the injury requires more than first aid or time off work. While it is apparent when these types of injuries occur, an accident has taken place, the lack of a recordable injury does not mean an accident did not take place. With the push for organizations to reduce their number of recordable accidents, first aid is usually the first line of defense to avoid having to report the accident as recordable. This form of accident is referred to as non-recordable accidents or near misses.

Clearly, when an injury has occurred, an accident has also taken place. Christian and associates suggest by recognizing that injuries are less common than accidents, future research could investigate how situational factors might moderate individual difference (predictor) relationships with accidents and injury criteria. For example, workers low in conscientiousness might be more likely to cause an accident but because of required protective equipment and clothing may not be injured by the accident. Therefore, they encourage future research that examines microaccidents, or accidents requiring only basic first aid treatment (Zohar, 2000, 2002; Christian et al., 2009).

Conclusion

This chapter focused on the implications of various personality and individual difference factors on safety behavior, performance, and outcomes. Occupational safety research continues to evolve providing organizational leadership with more tools and concepts to improve safety performance. In this chapter, we hoped to provide a general summary of the expansive research on individual differences and occupational health and safety. Due to space limitations, we admit that this is only a small window into a growing area of research. As research continues to build our understanding of the psychological causes of unsafe behavior by employees, the need for research in personality and individual differences continues to grow. While studies show promise, research demonstrates that testing employees for unsafe traits is still a work in progress. Most safety managers agree that employee behavior causes accidents (Smith, 2007). But several questions remain, such as what influences behavior, how much of it is situational and how much of it is the individual underlying traits, and to what extent can organizational leadership, climate, or culture influence how employees view safety, participate in safety programs, and act in a safe manner.

The human dynamics of an organization include behaviors, attitudes, cognitions, and the context; therefore, an organization's safety program must address each of these factors. Throughout this chapter we touch on many of the areas that influence safety from an individual level. We discussed predictors of safety-related outcomes, such as the Big Five personality dimensions, regulatory focus, and several other individual constructs. We explored research on "safety traits" such as accident proneness, the strength and direction of various dispositional predictors of accidents, and how personality, along with other variables, explain safe and unsafe behavior. We discussed the impact of regulatory focus (promotion vs. prevention) has on individual motivation and attitudes toward safety in the workplace and concluded that prevention focused individuals are more likely to possess good safety behavior. Taken together, the research contends that personality and individual differences influence safety outcomes. We hope that scholars and practitioners will build from our summary of prior research and focus specifically on the different opportunities we present for future research. Although we described two larger areas of future research, we also proposed opportunities within each section. These are incremental steps, but valuable nonetheless.

References

Abdollahi, A., Talib, M. A., Yaacob, S. N., & Ismail, Z. (2014). Hardiness as a mediator between perceived stress and happiness in nurses. *Journal of Psychiatric and Mental Health Nursing, 9,* 789–796.

Arbous, A. G., & Kerrich, J. E. (1951). Accident statistics and the concept of accident-proneness. *Biometrics, 7,* 340–432.

Avolio, B. J., Gardner, W. L., Walumbwa, F. O., Luthans, F., & May, D. R. (2004). Unlocking the mask: A look at the process by which authentic leaders impact follower attitudes and behaviors. *The Leadership Quarterly, 15*, 801–823.

Avolio, B. J., & Luthans, F., (2006). *High impact leader: Moments matter in authentic leadership development*. New York, NY: McGraw-Hill.

Bandura, A. (1997). *Self-efficacy: The exercise of control*. New York, NY: Freeman.

Bandura, A. (2012). On the functional properties of perceived self-efficacy revisited. *Journal of Management, 38*, 9–44.

Barrick, M. R., & Mount, M. K. (1991). The big five personality dimensions and job performance: A meta-analysis. *Personnel Psychology, 44*, 1–26.

Bartone, P. T. (1995, June). *Development and validation of a short hardiness measure*. Paper presented at the annual meeting of the American Psychological Society, Washington, DC.

Baumeister, R. F., Vohs, K. D., & Tice, D. M. (2007). The strength model of self-control. *Current Directions in Psychological Science, 16*, 351–355.

Bazroy, J., Roy, G., Sahai, A., & Soudarssanane, M. B. (2003). Magnitude and risk factors of injuries in a glass bottle manufacturing plant. *Journal of Occupational Health, 45*, 53–59.

Bhattacherjee, A., Chau, N., Sierra, C. O., Legras, B., Benamghar, L., Michaely, J. P., & Mur, J. M. (2003). Relationships of job and some individual characteristics to occupational injuries in employed people: A community-based study. *Journal of Occupational Health, 45*, 382–391.

Bishop, S., Lau, M., Shapiro, S., Carlson, L., Anderson, N., Carmody, J., et al. (2004). Mindfulness: A proposed operational definition. *Clinical Psychology: Science and Practice, 11*, 230–241.

Branton, P. (1970). A field study of repetitive manual work in relation to accidents at the work place. *International Journal of Production Research, 8*, 93–107.

Brett, Y. B. (2004). Accidents du travail et maladies professionnelles. *Face au Risque, 399*, 13–19.

Britt, T. W., Adler, A. B., & Bartone, P. T. (2001). Deriving benefits from stressful events: The role of engagement in meaningful work and hardiness. *Journal of Occupational Health Psychology, 6*, 53–63.

Brockner, J., & Higgins, E. T. (2001). Regulatory focus theory: Implications for the study of emotions at work. *Organizational Behavior and Human Decision Processes, 86*, 35–66.

Brown, K., Ryan, R., & Creswell, J. (2007). Mindfulness: Theoretical foundations and evidence for its salutary effects. *Psychological Inquiry, 18*, 211–237.

Bureau of Labor Statistics. (2012). Workplace injury and illness summary. http://www.bls.gov/news.release/osh.nr0.htm (accessed June 14, 2015).

Caponecchia, C. (2010). It won't happen to me: An investigation of optimism bias in occupational health and safety. *Journal of Applied Social Psychology, 40*, 601–617.

Cellar, D. F., Nelson, Z. C., & Yorke, C. M. (2000). The five-factor model and driving behavior: Personality and involvement in vehicular accidents. *Psychological Reports, 86*, 454–456.

Cellar, D. F., Nelson, Z. C., Yorke, C. M., & Bauer, C. (2001). The five-factor model and safety in the workplace: Investigating the relationships between personality and accident involvement. *Journal of Prevention & Intervention in the Community, 22*, 43–52.

Cellar, D. F., Yorke, C. M., Nelson, Z. C., & Carroll, K. A. (2004). Relationships between five factor personality variables, workplace accidents, and self-efficacy. *Psychological Reports, 94*, 1437–1441.

Chau, N., Bhattacherjee, A., & Kunar, B. M. (2009). Relationship between job, lifestyle, age and occupational injuries. *Occupational Medicine, 59*, 114–119.

Chau, N., Bourgkard, E., Bhattacherjee, A., Ravaud, J. F., Choquet, M., & Mur, J. M. (2008). Associations of job, living conditions and lifestyle with occupational injury in working population: a population-based study. *International Archives of Occupational and Environmental Health, 81*, 379–389.

Chau, N., Gauchard, G. C., Siegfried, C., Benamghar, L., Dangelzer, J. L., Français, M., & Mur, J. M. (2004). Relationships of job, age, and life conditions with the causes and severity of occupational injuries in construction workers. *International Archives of Occupational and Environmental Health, 77*, 60–66.

Chau, N., Lemogne, C., Legleye, S., Choquet, M., Falissard, B., & Fossati, P. (2011). Are occupational factors and mental difficulty associated with occupational injury? *Journal of Occupational and Environmental Medicine, 53*, 1452–1459.

Chau, N., Mur, J. M., Benamghar, L., Siegfried, C., Dangelzer, J. L., Français, M., & Sourdot, A. (2002). Relationships between some individual characteristics and occupational accidents in the construction industry: A case–control study on 880 victims of accidents occurred during a two-year period. *Journal of Occupational Health, 44*, 131–139.

Christian, M. S., Bradley, J. C., Wallace, J. C., & Burke, M. J. (2009). Workplace safety: A meta-analysis of the roles of person and situation factors. *Journal of Applied Psychology, 94*, 1103–1127.

Clarke, S. (2006). The relationship between safety climate and safety performance: A meta-analytic review. *Journal of Occupational Health Psychology, 11*, 315–327.

Clarke, S. (2011). Accident proneness: Back in vogue? In S. Clarke, R. J.Burke, & C. L. Cooper (Eds.), *Occupational health and safety: Psychological and behavioral challenges* (pp. 95–117). Farnham, UK: Gower.

Clarke, S., & Robertson, I. T. (2005). A meta-analytic review of the Big Five personality factors and accident involvement in occupational and non-occupational settings. *Journal of Occupational and Organizational Psychology, 78*, 355–376.

Clarke, S., & Robertson, I. T. (2008). An examination of the role of personality in work accidents using meta-analysis. *Applied Psychology, 57*, 94–108.

Cloutier, E. (1994). The effect of age on safety and work practices among domestic trash collectors in Quebec. *Safety Science, 17*, 291–308.

Conte, J. M., & Jacobs, R. R. (2003). Validity evidence linking polychronicity and Big Five personality dimensions to absence, lateness, and supervisory performance ratings. *Human Performance, 16*, 107–129.

Costa, P. T., Jr, & McCrae, R. R. (1992). Four ways five factors are basic. *Personality and Individual Differences, 13*, 653–665.

Cox, T. (1980). Repetitive work. In C. L. Cooper & R. Payne (Eds.), *Current concerns in occupational stress* (pp. 23–41). Chichester, UK: John Wiley & Sons, Ltd.

Crowe, E., & Higgins, E. T. (1997). Regulatory focus and strategic inclinations: Promotion and prevention in decision-making. *Organizational Behavior and Human Decision Processes, 69*, 117–132.

Day, A. J., Brasher, K., & Bridger, R. S. (2012). Accident proneness revisited: The role of psychological stress and cognitive failure. *Accident Analysis & Prevention, 49*, 532–535.

DeJoy, D. M. (1989). The optimism bias and traffic accident risk perception. *Accident Analysis & Prevention, 21*, 333–340.

DeJoy, D. M. (1996). Theoretical models of health behavior and workplace self-protective behavior. *Journal of Safety Research, 27*, 61–72.

Dekeyser, M., Raes, F., Leijssen, M., Leysen, S., & Dewulf, D. (2008). Mindfulness skills and interpersonal behaviour. *Personality and Individual Differences, 44*, 1235–1245.

Driscoll, T. R., Ansari, G., Harrison, J. E., Frommer, M. S., & Ruck, E. A. (1994). Traumatic work related fatalities in commercial fishermen in Australia. *Occupational and Environmental Medicine, 51*, 612–616.

Drory, A. (1982). Individual differences in boredom proneness and task effectiveness at work. *Personnel Psychology, 35*, 141–151.

Eid, J., Mearns, K., Larsson, G., Laberg, J. C., & Johnsen, B. H. (2012). Leadership, psychological capital and safety research: Conceptual issues and future research questions. *Safety Science, 50*, 55–61.

Engel, H. O. (1991). Accident proneness and illness proneness: A review. *Journal of the Royal Society of Medicine, 84*, 163–164.

Farmer, E., & Chambers, E. G. (1929). A study of personal qualities in accident proneness and proficiency. Industrial Health Research Board Report 55, Medical Research Council.

Fenichel, O. (1951). On the psychology of boredom. In R. Rapaport (Ed.), *Organization and pathology of thought* (pp. 349–361). New York, NY: Columbia University Press.

Fisher, C. D. (1993). Boredom at work: a neglected concept. *Human Relations, 46*, 395–417.

Fiske, D. W. (1949). Consistency of the factorial structures of personality ratings from different sources. *Journal of Abnormal and Social Psychology, 44,* 329–344.

Ford, M. T., & Wiggins, B. K. (2012). Occupational-level interactions between physical hazards and cognitive ability and skill requirements in predicting injury incidence rates. *Journal of Occupational Health Psychology, 17*(3), 268.

Förster, J., Higgins, E. T., & Idson, L. C. (1998). Approach and avoidance strength during goal attainment: Regulatory focus and the "goal looms larger" effect. *Journal of Personality and Social Psychology, 75,* 1115–1131.

Froom, P., Melamed, S., Kristal-Boneh, E., Gofer, D., & Ribak, J. (1996). Industrial accidents are related to relative body weight: the Israeli CORDIS study. *Occupational and Environmental Medicine, 53,* 832–835.

Game, A. M. (2007). Workplace boredom coping: Health, safety, and HR implications. *Personnel Review, 36,* 701–721.

Gardner, W. L., Avolio, B. J., Luthans, F., May, D. R., & Walumba, F., 2005. Can you see the real me? A self-based model of authentic leader and follower development. *Leadership Quarterly, 16,* 343–372.

Gauchard, G., Chau, N., Mur, J. M., & Perrin, P. (2001). Falls and working individuals: Role of extrinsic and intrinsic factors. *Ergonomics, 44,* 1330–1339.

Gauchard, G. C., Chau, N., Touron, C., Benamghar, L., Dehaene, D., Perrin, P., & Mur, J. M. (2003). Individual characteristics in occupational accidents due to imbalance: A case–control study of the employees of a railway company. *Occupational and Environmental Medicine, 60,* 330–335.

Gist, M. E. (1987). Self-efficacy: Implications for organizational behavior and human resource management. *Academy of Management Review, 12,* 472–485.

Goldberg, L. R. (1990). An alternative "description of personality": The Big-Five factor structure. *Journal of Personality and Social Psychology, 59,* 1216–1229.

Gomez, R. (2013). ADHD and Hyperkinetic Disorder Symptoms in Australian adults: Descriptive scores, incidence rates, factor structure, and gender invariance. *Journal of Attention Disorders.* Advanced online publication. http://jad.sagepub.com/content/early/2013/04/29/1087054713485206.abstract (accessed June 14, 2015).

Greenwood, M., & Woods, H. M. (1919). *The incidence of industrial accidents upon individuals with special reference to multiple accidents.* Report no. 4. Industrial Fatigue Research Board, London.

Gruys, M. L., & Sackett, P. R. (2003). Investigating the dimensionality of counterproductive work behavior. *International Journal of Selection and Assessment, 11,* 30–42.

Haddon, W., Suchman, E. A., & Klein, D. (1964). *Accident research: Methods and approaches.* New York, NY: Harper & Row.

Hagger, M. S., Wood, C., Stiff, C., & Chatzisarantis, N. L. D. (2010). Ego depletion and the strength model of self-control: A meta-analysis. *Psychological Bulletin, 136,* 495–525.

Hansen, C. P. (1988). Personality characteristics of the accident involved employee. *Journal of Business and Psychology, 2,* 346–365.

Härmä, M., Tenkanen, L., Sjöblom, T., Alikoski, T., & Heinsalmi, P. (1998). Combined effects of shift work and life-style on the prevalence of insomnia, sleep deprivation and daytime sleepiness. *Scandinavian Journal of Work, Environment & Health,* 300–307.

Harrell, W. A. (1995). Factors influencing involvement in farm accidents. *Perceptual and Motor Skills, 81,* 592–594.

Health and Safety Executive (2014). Workplace injury: All industries. http://www.hse.gov.uk/statistics/causinj/index.htm (accessed June 14, 2015).

Herndon, F. (2008). Testing mindfulness with perceptual and cognitive factors: External vs. internal encoding, and the cognitive failures questionnaire. *Personality and Individual Differences, 44,* 32–41.

Higgins, E. T. (1997). Beyond pleasure and pain. *American Psychologist, 52,* 1280–1300.

Higgins, E. T. (1998). Promotion and prevention: Regulatory focus as a motivational principle. *Advances in Experimental Social Psychology, 30,* 1–46.

Hill, A. B. (1975). Work variety and individual differences in occupational boredom. *Journal of Applied Psychology, 60*, 128–131.

Hofmann, D. A., & Morgeson, F. P. (1999). Safety-related behavior as a social exchange: the role of perceived organizational support and leader–member exchange. *Journal of Applied Psychology, 84*, 286–296.

Hogan, J., & Foster, J. (2013). Multifaceted personality predictors of workplace safety performance: More than conscientiousness. *Human Performance, 26*, 20–43.

Hopkin, V. D. (1990). The human factor aspects of single manning. *Journal of Navigation, 43*, 346.

Hystad, S. W., & Bye, H. H. (2013). Safety behaviours at sea: The role of personal values and personality hardiness. *Safety Science, 57*, 19–26.

International Labour Organization. (2014). Safety and health at work. http://ilo.org/global/topics/safety-and-health-at-work/lang–en/index.htm (accessed June 14, 2015).

Iso-Ahola, S. E., & Weissinger, E. (1990). Perceptions of boredom in leisure: Conceptualization, reliability and validity of the Leisure Boredom Scale. *Journal of Leisure Research, 22*, 1–177.

Jacobsson, B., & Schelp, L. (1987). One-year incidence of occupational injuries among teenagers in a Swedish rural municipality. *Scandinavian Journal of Social Medicine, 16*, 21–25.

Janicak, C. A. (1996). Predicting accidents at work with measures of locus of control and job hazards. *Psychological Reports, 78*, 115–121.

John, O. P. (1990). The "Big Five" factor taxonomy: Dimensions of personality in the natural language and in questionnaires. In L. A. Pervin (Ed.), *Handbook of personality: Theory and research* (pp. 66–100). New York, NY: Guilford Press.

Judge, T. A., & Bono, J. E. (2001). Relationship of core self-evaluations traits – self-esteem, generalized self-efficacy, locus of control, and emotional stability – with job satisfaction and job performance: A meta-analysis. *Journal of Applied Psychology, 86*, 80–92.

Judge, T. A., Erez, A., Bono, J. E., & Thoresen, C. J. (2003). The core self-evaluations scale: Development of a measure. *Personnel Psychology, 56*, 303–331.

Judge, T. A., Locke, E. A., & Durham, C. C. (1997). The dispositional causes of job satisfaction: A core evaluations approach. *Research in Organizational Behavior, 19*, 151–188.

Judge, T. A., Locke, E. A., Durham, C. C., & Kluger, A. N. (1998). Dispositional effects on job and life satisfaction: The role of core evaluations. *Journal of Applied Psychology, 83*, 17–34.

Khlat, M., Jusot, F., & Ville, I. (2009). Social origins, early hardship and obesity: a strong association in women, but not in men? *Social Science & Medicine, 68*, 1692–1699.

Kobasa, S. C. (1979). Stressful life events, personality, and health: An inquiry into hardiness. *Journal of Personality and Social Psychology, 37*, 1–11.

Kotzé, M., & Steyn, L. (2013). The role of psychological factors in workplace safety. *Ergonomics, 56*, 1928–1939.

Lakey, C., Campbell, W., Brown, K., & Goodie, A. (2007). Dispositional mindfulness as a predictor of the severity of gambling outcomes. *Personality and Individual Differences, 43*, 1698–1710.

Lawler, E. E. (1986). *High-involvement management: Participative strategies for improving organizational performance.* San Francisco, CA: Jossey-Bass.

Legleye, S., Peretti-Watal, P., Baumann, M., Beck, F., and Chau, N. (2009, June). Associations between demanding occupational conditions and tobacco, alcohol and cannabis use among French men and women. 39th World Congress of the International Institute of Sociology, Yerevan.

Lingard, H. (2002). The effect of first aid training on Australian construction workers' occupational health and safety motivation and risk control behaviour. *Journal of Safety Research, 33*, 209–230.

Locke, E. A., & Latham, G. P. (2002). Building a practically useful theory of goal setting and task motivation: A 35-year odyssey. *American Psychologist, 57*, 705–717.

Luthans, F., Avolio, B., Avey, J. B., & Norman, S. M., (2007). Psychological capital: measurement and relationship with performance and job satisfaction. *Personnel Psychology, 60*, 541–572.

Maddi, S. R., & Kobasa, S. C. (1984). *The hardy executive.* Homewood, IL: Jones-Irwin.

Mathiowetz, V., Kashman, N., Volland, G., Weber, K., Dowe, M., & Rogers, S. (1985). Grip and pinch strength: normative data for adults. *Archives Physiological Medicine Rehabilitation, 66*, 69–74.

McCaig, L. F., Burt, C. W., & Stussman, B. J. (1998). A comparison of work-related injury visits and other injury visits to emergency departments in the United States, 1995–1996. *Journal of Occupational and Environmental Medicine, 40*, 870–875.

McCrae, R. R., & Costa, P. T. (1987). Validation of the five-factor model of personality across instruments and observers. *Journal of Personality and Social Psychology, 52*, 81.

Mintz, A., & Blum, M. L. (1949). A re-examination of the accident proneness concept. *Journal of Applied Psychology, 33*, 195.

Moore, A., & Malinowski, P. (2009). Meditation, mindfulness and cognitive flexibility. *Consciousness and Cognition, 18*, 176–186.

Muraven, M., & Baumeister, R. F. (2000). Self-regulation and depletion of limited resources: Does self-control resemble a muscle? *Psychological Bulletin, 126*, 247–259.

Muraven, M., & Slessareva, E. (2003). Mechanisms of self-control failure: Motivation and limited resources. *Personality and Social Psychology Bulletin, 29*, 894–906.

Nahrgang, J. D., Morgeson, F. P., & Hofmann, D. A. (2011). Safety at work: A meta-analytic investigation of the link between job demands, job resources, burnout, engagement, and safety outcomes. *Journal of Applied Psychology, 96*, 71.

Nakata, A., Ikeda, T., Takahashi, M., Haratani, T., Hojou, M., Fujioka, Y., & Araki, S. (2006). Non-fatal occupational injury among active and passive smokers in small-and medium-scale manufacturing enterprises in Japan. *Social Science & Medicine, 63*, 2452–2463.

Neal, A., Griffin, M. A., & Hart, P. M. (2000). The impact of organizational climate on safety climate and individual behavior. *Safety Science, 34*, 99–109.

Newbold, E. M. (1926). *A contribution to the study of the human factor in the causation of accidents.* Industrial Fatigue Research Board. Report 34. London, UK: HMSO.

Nola, A., Cattaneo, G., Maiocchi, A., Gariboldi, C., Rocchi, R., Cavallaro, S., & Bassino, P. (2000). Occupational accidents in temporary work. *La Medicina del Lavoro, 92*, 281–285.

Norman, W. T. (1963). Toward an adequate taxonomy of personality attributes: Replicated factor structure in peer nomination personality ratings. *Journal of Abnormal and Social Psychology, 66*, 574–583.

O'Hanlon, J. F. (1981). Boredom: Practical consequences and a theory. *Acta Psychologica, 49*, 53–82.

Peretti-Watel, P., Legleye, S., Baumann, M., Choquest, M., Falissard, B., Chau, N., & Lorhandicap Group (2009). Fatigue, insomnia and nervousness: Gender disparities and roles of individual characteristics and lifestyle factors among economically active people. *Social Psychiatry and Psychiatric Epidemiology, 44*, 703–709.

Reason, J., Manstead, A., Stradling, S., Baxter, J., & Campbell, K. (1990). Errors and violations on the roads: A real distinction? *Ergonomics, 33*, 1315–1332.

Roberts, D. S., & Geller, E. S. (1996). An "actively caring" model for occupational safety: A field test. *Applied and Preventive Psychology, 4*, 53–59.

Rotter, J. B. (1966). Generalized expectancies for internal versus external control of reinforcement. *Psychological Monographs, 80*, 1–28.

Salgado, J. F. (2002). The Big Five personality dimensions and counterproductive behaviors. *International Journal of Selection and Assessment, 10*, 117–125.

Schaubroeck, J., & Merritt, D. E. (1997). Divergent effects of job control on coping with work stressors: The key role of self-efficacy. *Academy of Management, 40*, 738–754.

Schmertz, S., Anderson, P., & Robins, D. (2009). The relation between self-report mindfulness and performance on tasks of sustained attention. *Journal of Psychopathology and Behavioral Assessment, 31*, 60–66.

Schneider, B. (1987). The people make the place. *Personnel Psychology, 40*, 437–453

Scholer, A. A., & Higgins, E. T. (2008). Distinguishing levels of approach and avoidance: An analysis using regulatory focus theory. In A. J. Elliot (Ed.), *Handbook of approach and avoidance motivation* (pp. 489–203). New York, NY: Psychology Press.

Sitzmann, T., & Yeo, G. (2013). A meta-analytic investigation of the within-person self-efficacy domain: Is self-efficacy a product of past performance or a driver of future performance? *Personnel Psychology, 66*, 531–568.

Smillie, L. D., Yeo, G. B., Furnham, A. F., Jackson, C. J. (2006). Benefits of all work and no play: The relationship between neuroticism and performance as a function of resource allocation. *Journal of Applied Psychology, 91,* 139–155.

Smith, S. (2007). Behavior-based safety: Myth or magic? *EHS Today,* October 1. http://ehstoday.com/safety/ehs_imp_75429 (accessed June 14, 2015).

Spector, P. E., & Fox, S. (2005). The stressor-emotion model of counterproductive work behavior. In F. Suzy & P. E. Spector (Eds.), *Counterproductive work behavior: Investigations of actors and targets* (pp. 151–174). Washington, DC: American Psychological Association.

Stagner, R. (1975). Boredom on the assembly line: Age and personality variables. *Industrial Gerontology, 2,* 23–24.

Stajkovic, A. D., & Luthans, F. (1998). Self-efficacy and work-related performance: A meta-analysis. *Psychological Bulletin, 124,* 240–261.

Thoresen, C. J., Bradley, J. C., Bliese, P. D., & Thoresen, J. D. (2004). The Big Five personality traits and individual job performance growth trajectories in maintenance and transitional job stages. *Journal of Applied Psychology, 89,* 835–853.

Vandenberg, R. J., Richardson, H. A., & Eastman, L. J. (1999). The impact of high involvement work processes on organizational effectiveness: A second-order latent variable approach. *Group & Organization Management, 24,* 300–339.

Visser, E., Pijl, Y. J., Stolk, R. P., Neeleman, J., & Rosmalen, J. G. (2007). Accident proneness, does it exist? A review and meta-analysis. *Accident Analysis & Prevention, 39,* 556–564.

Vouriot, A., Gauchard, G., Chau, N., Benamghar, L., Lepori, M. L., Mur, J. M., & Perrin, P. (2004). Sensorial organisation favouring higher visual contribution is a risk factor of falls in an occupational setting. *Neuroscience Research, 48,* 239–247.

Wagenaar, W. A., & Groeneweg, J. (1987). Accidents at sea: Multiple causes and impossible consequences. *International Journal of Man-Machine Studies, 27,* 587–598.

Wallace, J. C., Johnson, P. D., & Frazier, M. L. (2009). An examination of the factorial, construct, and predictive validity and utility of the regulatory focus at work scale. *Journal of Organizational Behavior, 30,* 805–831.

Wallace, J. C., & Vodanovich, S. J. (2003). Workplace safety performance: Conscientiousness, cognitive failure, and their interaction. *Journal of Occupational Health Psychology, 8,* 316.

Weinstein, N. D. (1984). Why it won't happen to me: Perceptions of risk factors and susceptibility. *Health Psychology, 3,* 431.

Wu, J., & Lebreton, J. M. (2011). Reconsidering the dispositional basis of counterproductive work behavior: The role of aberrant personality. *Personnel Psychology, 64,* 593–626.

Zhang, J., Ding, W., Li, Y., & Wu, C. (2013). Task complexity matters: The influence of trait mindfulness on task and safety performance of nuclear power plant operators. *Personality and Individual Differences, 55,* 433–439.

Zhang, J., & Wu, C. (2014). The influence of dispositional mindfulness on safety behaviors: A dual process perspective. *Accident Analysis & Prevention, 70,* 24–32.

Zohar, D. (1980). Safety climate in industrial organizations: Theoretical and applied implications. *Journal of Applied Psychology, 65,* 96–102.

Zohar, D. (2000). A group-level model of safety climate: Testing the effect of group climate on microaccidents in manufacturing jobs. *Journal of Applied Psychology, 85,* 587–596.

Zohar, D. (2002). The effects of leadership dimensions, safety climate, and assigned work priorities on minor injuries in work groups. *Journal of Organizational Behavior, 23,* 75–92.

Zohar, D. (2010). Thirty years of safety climate research: Reflections and future directions. *Accident Analysis and Prevention, 42,* 1517–1522.

Zohar, D., & Erev, I. (2007). On the difficulty of promoting workers' safety behaviour: Overcoming the underweighting of routine risks. *International Journal of Risk Assessment and Management, 7,* 122–136.

3

The Mediating Effects of Behavior

Jeff Foster and Stephen B. Nichols

Introduction

Due to improvements in technology and working conditions, some have concluded that human error is responsible for most work accidents and injuries in developed countries (Reason, 1990). Despite related arguments that certain individuals may be more accident prone than others (Perrow, 1984), research has failed to uncover specific individual characteristics responsible for large portions of variance in safety outcomes. In this chapter, we explain the role personality plays in organizational safety and why research examining direct links between individual personality variables and safety-related criteria often produces inconsistent results.

First, we discuss previous research examining personality and its relationship to safety-related outcomes, behaviors, and performance ratings. Next, we explain how combinations of personality scales, or the use of personality subscales or facets, can be stronger predictors of safety-related criteria. Finally, we discuss and illustrate how specific behaviors mediate relationships between personality and safety-related criteria. This final point is critical in explaining relationships between personality and safety criteria and helps explain why existing research has often found inconclusive, or even contradictory, results. To demonstrate the importance of focusing on subscales and possible mediation, we define a model of six behaviors critical to organizational safety across settings and outline how specific personality facets predict each of these behaviors. We conclude with suggestions for using this information to improve safety training and by outlining recommendations for future research.

The relationship between personality and organizational safety is complex. Although a number of researchers have examined potential linear relationships between individual personality variables and a variety of safety-related outcomes, most stop at reporting correlations. While informative, such relationships often fail to account for the complete influence of personality on organizational safety. Instead, combinations of personality scales and facets (i.e., subscales) are more predictive of safety-related criteria (Hogan & Foster, 2013).

The Wiley Blackwell Handbook of the Psychology of Occupational Safety and Workplace Health, First Edition. Edited by Sharon Clarke, Tahira M. Probst, Frank Guldenmund, and Jonathan Passmore. © 2016 John Wiley & Sons Ltd. Published 2020 by John Wiley & Sons Ltd.

Table 3.1 FFM scales and definitions.

Scale	Definition
Extraversion	The degree to which a person is outgoing and talkative.
Agreeableness	The degree to which a person is rewarding to deal with and pleasant.
Conscientiousness	The degree to which a person complies with rules, norms, and standards.
Emotional Stability	The degree to which a person appears calm and self-accepting.
Openness	The degree to which a person seems creative and open-minded.

And as with other predictors such as climate and motivation, the relationship between personality and objective safety outcomes (e.g., accidents and injuries) is often mediated by on-the-job behaviors (Christian, Bradley, Wallace, & Burke, 2009).

For example, a number of researchers have found significant correlations between measures of Conscientiousness and safety-related criteria (Cellar, Yorke, Nelson, & Carroll, 2004; Clarke, 2006; Clarke & Robertson, 2005, 2008; Demerouti, 2006; Dudley, Orvis, Lebiecki, & Cortina, 2006; Liao, Arvey, Butler, & Nutting, 2001; Wallace & Chen, 2006; Wallace & Vodanovich, 2003). Conscientiousness is one factor in the Five Factor Model (FFM) of personality (Digman, 1990; Goldberg, 1992; John, 1990). This model is based on decades of factor analytic work examining relationships between the adjectives we use to describe others. Table 3.1 presents FFM scales and definitions.

Conscientiousness relates to a person's reputation for working hard, following rules, and attending to details. Despite being the most widely studied FFM scale in the area of safety, research has also found relationships between each of the other FFM measures and safety-related criteria. For example, individuals who are prone to stress and anxiety (low Emotional Stability), are direct or unfriendly (low Agreeableness), easily tire of mundane tasks (high Openness), or seek attention from others (high Extraversion) have all been found to engage more often in unsafe behaviors (Cellar, Nelson, & Yorke, 2000; Cellar et al., 2004; Clarke, 2006; Clarke & Robertson, 2005, 2008; Hansen, 1988; Liao et al., 2001; Smillie, Yeo, Furnham, & Jackson, 2006). A range of personality characteristics, therefore, can influence organizational safety.

Using data for nearly 900 employees from 12 organizations, Hogan and Foster (2013) conducted a meta-analysis examining relationships between personality and supervisory safety performance ratings. They found that Conscientiousness ($\rho = .21$) and Emotional Stability ($\rho = .20$) were the strongest FFM predictors of safety behaviors. However, the strongest overall predictor was a composite of multiple personality facets ($\rho = .31$) selected to predict a range of safety-related behaviors (e.g., complying with rules, remaining vigilant while performing mundane tasks). Furthermore, safety-related behaviors fully mediated relationships between personality measures and objective safety outcomes (e.g., accidents and injuries). Such complexity in the relationship between personality and organizational safety has four implications.

First, comprehensive personality inventories, such as those representing the FFM, predict organizational safety better than single, narrow measures. Multiple FFM scales predict a variety of work-related criteria, including teamwork (Driskell, Goodwin, Salas, & O'Shea, 2006; O'Neill & Allen, 2011), leadership (Hogan & Judge, 2013; Judge, Bono, Ilies, & Gerhardt, 2002), negotiation (Sharma, Bottom, & Elfenbein, 2013), sales-related criteria (Sitser, van der Linden, & Born, 2013), training assessments (Dean, Conte, & Blankenhorn, 2006), and overall job performance (Barrick & Mount, 1991; Barrick, Mount, & Judge, 2001; Hogan, Hogan, & Roberts, 1996; Hogan & Holland, 2003; Tett, Jackson, & Rothstein, 1991).

For example, consider teamwork. Although being nice and respectful of others (high Agreeableness) predicts teamwork ratings, other characteristics are also important, such as remaining calm during pressure or crisis (high Emotional Stability) and following rules and procedures (high Conscientiousness). Therefore, a measure of interpersonal interactions might capture some variance in teamwork ratings, but will fail to capture variance associated with other characteristics. The same is true for safety. Although Conscientiousness might have the most stable relationship with organizational safety, individual studies should include comprehensive personality measures to identify additional characteristics that also predict safety.

Second, combinations of personality facets are more predictive of organizational safety than broad personality scales (Hogan & Foster, 2013). In other words, while the use of multiple FFM scales may increase prediction, the same or better results can be achieved by using only their most predictive facets. This not only maximizes prediction with fewer items, but provides more precise information concerning which components of personality predict behaviors.

To compare the prediction of FFM scales to their facets, Woo, Chernyshenko, Stark, and Conz (2014) coded Openness scales and subscales from over a dozen personality instruments into six general facets. They found that individual facets were generally more predictive of performance ratings than factor-level Openness. Furthermore, different facets often predicted different behaviors. For example, curiosity was the strongest predictor of training performance but virtually unrelated to leadership ratings. In contrast, ingenuity was the strongest predictor of leadership but had little association with training. Although curiosity and ingenuity are clearly related, curiosity suggests an openness to learning and exploring new ideas, which is more beneficial to learning new skills, while ingenuity suggests applying new ideas to work, which is more representative of leadership. Although both are facets of Openness, curiosity and ingenuity predict different outcomes.

We often view safety in terms of a single outcome: the number of reported incidents over a period of time. However, not only are accidents and injuries as diverse as the behaviors that cause them, different components of personality predict different behaviors. For example, whereas some facets are most predictive of rule following, others are most predictive of crisis management. To understand relationships between personality and organizational safety, we must identify which facets predict which behaviors.

Third, research that fails to account for safety-related behaviors cannot illustrate how personality impacts overall organizational safety or provide adequate guidance for improving safety. Although a number of behaviors impact safety, it is unlikely these behaviors are equally impactful across all jobs and settings. Given that different personality facets predict different behaviors, it is also unlikely that the same personality characteristics will be equally important across all jobs and settings.

Consider the following safety-related behaviors: responding to crises and remaining vigilant. Research shows that crisis management is more closely linked to facets related to self-confidence (Schwebel, Severson, Ball, & Rizzo, 2006) while vigilance is more closely linked to facets related to boredom proneness and a need for stimulation (Dahlen, Martin, Ragan, & Kuhlman, 2005; König & Waller, 2010). Although some jobs might require both, it is reasonable to assume that (a) crisis management is more important for jobs where one must react to changing or unforeseen circumstances, and (b) vigilance is more important for jobs that involve working alone and focusing on a specific mundane task over long periods of time. Therefore, self-confidence may be more important for first responders who must quickly and effectively react to different situations while vigilance is more important for factory workers who operate machinery performing high-speed tasks. Studies examining relationships between personality and safety outcomes are likely to find different results in these two settings. Consequently, researchers can only expect to develop sufficient a priori hypotheses concerning relationships between personality characteristic and safety if they first identify the behaviors critical to safety in a specific setting. Furthermore, such information is necessary to explain why personality influences safety in such settings and how to use this information to influence behaviors that improve organizational safety.

Finally, researchers are only beginning to realize the importance of mediating variables in the relationship between personality and safety. Researchers have identified mediators that influence relationships between personality and other work-related criteria, such as communication and team outcomes (Macht, Nembhard, Kim, & Rothrock, 2014), adaptability and service performance (Prentice & King, 2013), alertness and entrepreneurial outcomes (Sambasivan, Abdul, & Yusop, 2009), strategic flexibility and firm performance (Nadkarni & Herrmann, 2010), and goal orientation and both sales performance (McFarland & Kidwell, 2006) and leadership effectiveness (Hendricks & Payne, 2007).

The focus on behaviors as mediators of personality/safety relationships is relatively new (e.g., Christian et al., 2009; Hogan & Foster, 2013). Although we can learn from studies reporting correlations between personality scales and a range of safety-related criteria, we need more research that also includes facet-level personality and behavioral measures. Existing research has identified six behaviors that are critical for organizational safety across a variety of jobs and settings (Hogan & Foster, 2013). These include: (1) complying with rules, (2) avoiding unnecessary risks, (3) remaining vigilant, (4) responding appropriately to safety threats, (5) managing stress, and (6) adhering to training. The combinations of personality characteristics that predict these behaviors are as unique as their potential consequences.

Following Rules

Following rules is one of the most obvious behaviors that influence safety. Griffin and Neal (2000) defined rule compliance as "core safety activities that need to be carried out by individuals to maintain workplace safety" (p. 349). Similarly, others have identified links between safety and both rule compliance (e.g., Gyekye & Salminen, 2005) and its counterpart, deviance (e.g., Frone, 1998).

Some safety-related rules target accident prevention, such as required rest periods for employees, limits for operating equipment within proper thresholds, and instructions to only use tools for approved purposes. Others focus on tracking accidents or minimizing their impact. For example, across two field studies, Probst, Graso, Estrada, and Greer (2013) found that considerations of future safety consequences, which focused on reporting injuries, near misses, conducting pre-job inspections, and using protective equipment, predicted a variety of safety-related outcomes such as motivation, attitudes, behaviors, and injuries. Rules associated with reporting and minimizing accidents may be just as important as those aimed at avoiding them.

A number of personality scales predict rule following. Although some research efforts have focused only on Conscientiousness (e.g., Postlethwaite, Robbins, Rickerson, & McKinniss, 2009), others have taken a more comprehensive approach and found that additional FFM scales, such as Agreeableness and Extraversion (negative), also predict rule compliance in different settings (Collins & Schmidt, 1993; Mulder, 1971; Shiner, 2000; Shiner, Masten,

& Roberts, 2003). Based on results from 13 studies examining relationships between FFM scales and counterproductive work behaviors, Salgado (2002) found that Conscientiousness, Agreeableness, and Openness predicted a lack of deviant behaviors. While Conscientiousness was the strongest predictor, Agreeableness was also related to rule compliance across all settings while Openness was negatively related in at least some settings.

Similarly, Johnson and Foster (2010) report meta-analytic results that align both scale and factor scores from the Hogan Personality Inventory (HPI; Hogan & Hogan, 2007) with supervisory ratings of 62 work-related behaviors. Their results provide an opportunity to compare factor-level predictors to facets in the prediction of rule compliance. Mirroring previous research, they report that Conscientiousness is the single best predictor of supervisory ratings of rule compliance. At the facet level, the components of Conscientiousness most highly related to rule compliance are avoiding trouble and lacking impulsivity; facets relating to integrity, such as acting morally and virtuously, are less predictive. Finally, facets associated with achievement orientation, a common component of many Conscientiousness scales in FFM-based inventories, such as the NEO-PI-R (Costa & McCrae, 1992) and the BFI (John & Srivastava, 1999), are generally the least predictive. These results indicate that in the eyes of supervisors, rule compliance is primarily the result of acting carefully and avoiding trouble. In contrast, while one may extol rule compliance as a virtue, it might not be as strongly predicted by virtuous intentions if such intentions lead to breaking rules perceived as wrong or unethical. Finally, striving to reach goals and achieve power, a component shared by many Conscientiousness scales, has little to do with rule following. Such distinctions are important because they show that, in terms of predicting supervisory ratings of rule compliance, not all Conscientiousness facets are equally important.

Further, Johnson and Foster (2010) found that Emotional Stability and Agreeableness are positively related to rule compliance, while Extraversion is negatively related. An examination of facet-level results shows these correlations are driven primarily by empathy and maintaining an even temper for Emotional Stability, being considerate and tolerant for Agreeableness, and a lack of showing off for Extraversion. Again, these results point to specific characteristics that drive rule compliance. For example, although being witty and engaging is also a component of Extraversion, it has almost no relationship with rule compliance.

Facet-level results help illustrate how practitioners can use personality to facilitate safety training (see Burke & Smith Sockbeson, Chapter 15, this volume). Rather than simply encouraging individuals to follow organizational rules, it is helpful to know which individual characteristics are most likely to lead individuals astray. Someone who tends to act without thinking might benefit most from training focused on gathering information prior to making decisions. In contrast, an individual who is more careful before acting, but shows little aversion to being reprimanded, might benefit most from training focused on the justifications for and consequences of potential offences. The key to using personality to facilitate training is first identifying an individual's potential risk factors and then tailoring training content to focus on those factors. Individuals with more risk factors relating to rule compliance are generally more likely to discard organizational policies and procedures. However, if an individual lacks such factors relating to rule compliance, he or she may still be more likely to exhibit other behaviors that could undermine organizational safety.

Avoiding Unnecessary Risks

In some fields, such as sales and finance, risk taking may be viewed as a standard job component that can lead to a variety of outcomes, some of which are positive and encouraged (e.g., Basak & Makarov, 2012; Gaba & Kalra, 1999; Piercy, 2010). But with safety, risk is most commonly viewed as an antecedent to avoidable accidents and injuries. A number of researchers have found relationships between risk taking and safety outcomes (Lind, 2008; Paul & Maiti, 2007). In a study including data on over 10,500 accidents from employees representing 25 organizations, Pierce (2005) found that risk takers were about twice as likely to experience accidents and injuries compared with their risk avoidant counterparts. Similar results show risk taking also increases accidents and injuries in other domains such as driving (Bell, Amoroso, Yore, Smith, & Jones, 2000; Rajalin, 1994), cycling (Bacchieri, Barros, dos Santos, & Gigante, 2010), and health care as evidenced by emergency room visits (McLeod et al., 2003).

In examining results from 312 urban dwellers, Fyhri and Backer-Grøndahl (2012) found that personality might not only impact risk taking, but how individuals perceive risk. Emotional Stability and Agreeableness were both negatively correlated with perceptions of risk associated with public transportation. Similarly, Soane, Dewberry, and Narendran (2010) showed that perceived costs and benefits mediated relationships between personality and risk-related choices. Research also reveals links between personality and non-work-related safety behavior. Fischer and Frewer (2008) found that optimism and internal locus of control predicted behaviors related to food preparation safety such as checking the temperature of meat and keeping food cool when transporting it home. Similarly, Kornelis, De Jonge, Frewer, and Dagevos (2007) showed locus of control also predicts what type of information consumers attend to when they have questions about food safety.

Nicholson, Soane, Fenton-O'Creevy, and Willman (2005) describe risk taking as an amalgam of FFM scales combining high Extraversion, Openness, and Emotional Stability with low Agreeableness and Conscientiousness. Weller and Tikir (2011) found similar results for Conscientiousness and Extraversion and a number of risk-related outcomes such as risk taking, risk perception, and the perceived benefits of risk. They uncovered similar relationships between risk-related outcomes and an additional personality factor represented in the HEXACO personality model (see Lee & Ashton, 2005), Honesty/Humility, indicating that risk taking is associated with a desire for personal gain or sense of self-importance.

Johnson and Foster (2010) found that Extraversion, as measured by the HPI Ambition scale, is the best single predictor of supervisory ratings of managing risk. It should be noted, however, that scores on the HPI Ambition scale are highly correlated with a number of achievement orientation facets commonly considered part of Conscientiousness in other FFM inventories (Goldberg, 2008). An examination of facet-level results reveals that the relationship between Ambition and risk management is primarily driven by a desire to reach individual goals, outperform others, and displaying confidence when interacting with others. The least predictive facet concerns satisfaction with one's place in life. These results indicate that supervisors view goal oriented and driven employees as most effective at successfully managing risk. Openness also predicted risk management, driven primarily by facets relating to sensation seeking and idea generation. Unlike Ambition, where all facets showed at least some positive relationship with risk taking, a number of Openness facets – being analytical, enjoying games, and showing an interest in culture – had no relationship with supervisory ratings of risk management.

Results from Johnson and Foster (2010) indicate that supervisors generally associate effective risk management with drive, ambition, and intellectual curiosity. These results stand in contrast, however, to research finding that accidents and injuries are more closely associated with Emotional Stability and Agreeableness, and appear to directly contradict results relating to Honesty/Humility (Weller & Tikir, 2011), which indicate that personal drive and ambition lead to more accidents and injuries. One likely reason for these contradictions is that the Johnson and Foster (2010) samples are overly representative of managerial and professional positions and may not, therefore, generalize well to a range of entry-level jobs. It is possible that being driven and intellectually curious might have negative safety-related consequences for entry-level or blue collar positions where safety more directly impacts an employee's health and well-being, but are seen as drivers of appropriate risk taking to seek rewards for professional and managerial jobs. Perhaps more than any other safety-related behavior, risk taking, and its consequences, likely varies across jobs and organizations.

This diversity of findings emphasizes the need to evaluate risk as it relates to specific safety-related behaviors for specific jobs. Again, within specific contexts, practitioners can use personality to identify individual risk factors and tailor safety training to individuals based on their individual characteristics as they relate to these factors. While behaviors associated with a variety of facets under Ambition might drive risk management across higher-level jobs, such behaviors might not be beneficial in settings where the only way to safely manage risk is to avoid it entirely (Cekada, Janicak, & Ferguson, 2009).

Although it is useful to identify relationships between FFM scales and risk taking, such relationships do not tell as complete a story as facet-level results. Results from Johnson and Foster (2010) not only mirror previous research finding relationships between sensation seeking and risk taking (Curran, Fuertes, Alfonso, & Hennessy, 2010; Nicholson et al., 2005; Schwebel et al., 2006; Scott-Parker, Watson, King, & Hyde, 2012), but also show that this single characteristic likely accounts for the majority of the variance shared between Openness and risk taking, while other components of Openness are relatively unimportant. Trainers, therefore, would likely benefit more from focusing on sensation seeking than other facets of Openness. In contrast, several facets related to Ambition might drive risk taking, but the consequences of such behaviors may vary across jobs. To exploit personality as it pertains to risk taking, trainers must first identify the individual characteristics associated with risky behaviors for specific jobs and then assess individuals on these characteristics.

Remaining Vigilant

Maintaining focus is especially important for jobs that require operating, observing, or working near potentially dangerous machinery or materials. A number of researchers have reported relationships between boredom proneness and safety-related behaviors (e.g., Dahlen et al., 2005; Frone, 1998). Although vigilance is important for jobs with varied tasks, it might be particularly important for jobs that require focusing on one action over long periods of time (König & Waller, 2010).

Rose, Murphy, Byard, and Nikzad (2002) examined relationships between a number of FFM scales and vigilance in college students. They found that individuals who were high on Conscientiousness and low on Extraversion produced fewer incorrect responses during a 12-minute vigilance task. Individuals high on Conscientiousness were also more receptive to changes in stimuli while those low in Emotional Stability reported more frustration with the task. However, on a similar task with another college student sample, Burton et al. (2010) found that vigilance for college students was predicted by low Emotional Stability, low Extraversion, and low Agreeableness. Furthermore, for men, they found that Conscientiousness had a negative relationship with vigilance. These contradictory results suggest that the relationship between personality and vigilance might vary across settings.

Others have examined more complex relationships between personality and vigilance. For example, Barbato et al. (2013) found that, during long periods without sleep, introverts reported a greater impact of sleep deprivation on vigilance than did extraverts.

When examining boredom proneness (McGiboney & Carter, 1988; Vodanovich & Kass, 1990; Vodanovich, Wallace, & Kass, 2005), researchers have uncovered relationships with a number of outcomes such as non-class related student activities (Mann & Robinson, 2009), personally destructive or harmful behaviors (Boden, 2009), job mistakes and intent to leave (Mann, 2012), and perceived organizational support and job performance (Watt & Hargis, 2010).

Similar to Rose et al. (2002), Johnson and Foster (2010) found that high Conscientiousness and low Extraversion predicted supervisory ratings of vigilance. Relationships between Conscientiousness and vigilance were driven almost entirely by a need to be planful and organized. Relationships between Extraversion and vigilance were driven primarily by negative relationships with liking crowds and entertaining others. These results indicate that vigilance might be higher for individuals who prefer organization and to avoid potentially distracting stimuli. As one might expect, individuals who prefer to focus on specific activities are generally better at doing so.

The potential training implications are twofold. First, because individuals who do not like to focus on one task are generally poorer at doing so, organizations would benefit from measuring vigilance as part of selection systems or focusing training programs on methods for sustaining attention. Second, the contradictory nature of research findings suggests that contextual factors relating to task and setting likely moderate the relationship between personality and vigilance. For example, boredom proneness may be more predictive for long-term tasks than those requiring focused attention for only short periods of time; or a need for planning may be more predictive for tasks where one must attend to changing details than for tasks that involve monitoring repetitive processes.

Responding Appropriately to Threats

Unlike behaviors focused on accident prevention, responding appropriately to threats involves quick reactions to thwart or reduce the impact of accidents once they occur. Such reactions are precipitated by confidence in one's ability to deflect threats or minimize damage. Bandura (1997) defined self-efficacy as an individual's belief in his or her ability to manage a situation. In work settings, self-efficacy has been viewed as both an antecedent and outcome of other work-related variables. The same is true for safety. Safety researchers have found that self-efficacy predicts a range of outcomes, such as safety attitudes, safety-related motivation, and safety behaviors (Hsu, Lee, Wu, & Takano, 2008; Newman, Griffin, & Mason, 2008). In contrast, Mullen and Kelloway (2009) suggest that safety-related self-efficacy could be an effective outcome measure for assessing training effectiveness.

A number of studies have identified links between confidence and responsiveness to safety-related situations. For example, Roberts et al. (2014) found that nurses and physicians reported a lack of confidence – in both recognizing the need for and effectively acting – as the number one barrier to implementing rapid response systems when facing respiratory or cardiac crises. In a review of how emergency service planning can account for ad-hoc volunteers, Scanlon, Helsloot, and Groenendaal (2014) outline examples of bystanders saving lives by responding to disasters before emergency personnel arrive. Similarly, Beck, Ohmer, and Warner (2012) argue for the importance of collective efficacy amongst neighbors to prevent and respond to neighborhood violence.

Researchers have also examined relationships between FFM scales and various forms of self-efficacy. Thoms, Moore, and Scott (1996) found that all but Openness from the FFM predicted an individual's confidence in participating in self-managed work groups.

Similarly, Spurk and Abele (2011) revealed positive relationships between all FFM scales except for Agreeableness and occupational self-efficacy, which reflects one's confidence in his or her ability to perform well within a given occupation. In relation to emotions, which have implications for a variety of organizational and individual outcomes (Barsade & Gibson, 2007; Brief & Weiss, 2002; Elfenbein, 2007; Weiss & Cropanzano, 1996), Pool and Qualter (2012) found that emotional self-efficacy was related to all five FFM scales. These results suggest that a variety of personality characteristics influence confidence across tasks and settings. However, findings that all five FFM scales influence self-efficacy are too general to be of much use. Instead, it is important to examine results at the facet level.

Results from Johnson and Foster (2010) mirror previous findings in that HPI scales representing each FFM factor are significantly related to supervisory ratings of self-efficacy. However, Ambition accounts for more than three times the variance in supervisory ratings (over 17 percent) than any other HPI scale, indicating that confidence is most closely aligned with the desire to set and achieve difficult and meaningful personal goals. Furthermore, all six subscales under Ambition (i.e., competitiveness, self-assurance, accomplishment, leadership, identity, and no social anxiety) contributed to supervisory ratings of an employee's confidence. Facet-level results from other HPI scales were more diverse (Johnson & Foster, 2010). For example, the most predictive component of Emotional Stability was an absence of regret over one's previous actions and decisions. Other important facets were components of Extraversion relating to needing variety and showing off, components of Agreeableness relating to enjoyment from being around others, and components of Openness relating to seeking stimulus, displaying creativity, and being able to easily recall information. Coupled with relationships with Ambition, these results suggest that four general components of an individual's behavior contribute to others' perceptions of his or her self-efficacy. Supervisors generally view employees as confident if they (a) set and strive toward personal goals, (b) appear comfortable when interacting with others, (c) actively seek variety and new stimulus, and (d) are comfortable recalling information and voicing new ideas.

Such insight offers two implications. First, some individuals are naturally more adept at responding to a crisis than others. When selecting individuals for positions that require crisis management, organizations would benefit from using reliable personality instruments that measure characteristics related to self-efficacy. Second, training programs might benefit from not only focusing on procedures related to crisis response but also developing trainee confidence. This could facilitate methods for training individuals who are not otherwise predisposed to respond in the time required to prevent or react effectively to a crisis.

Managing Stress

While crisis response involves reacting to threats, controlling one's emotions concerns avoiding behaviors that can create new threats. While anger and hostility are related to careless behavior (Schwebel et al., 2006), individuals who are more likely to respond effectively to stress are also more likely to engage in safe behaviors (Clarke & Robertson, 2005; Liao et al., 2001; Smillie et al., 2006).

A number of researchers have linked emotional intelligence and maturity to safety-related outcomes such as psychological safety, conflict management, and safety attitudes. For example, Harper and White (2013) linked group psychological safety to team members' levels of emotional perception, emotional management, emotional facilitation, and emotional understanding. These results indicate that teams comprised of members higher in certain emotional intelligence components are more willing to discuss potentially emotion-laden issues, such as errors or poor practices by a member. Desivilya and Yagil (2005) showed that group members' emotions toward one another, if negative, could lead to dominating or avoiding styles of conflict management, as opposed to cooperative styles such as integrating or compromising when emotions were more positive. Jeffries (2011) posited a theoretical model where emotional intelligence and moral maturity influence one's attitude toward an act, which in turn influences behavioral intentions and subsequent behavior Finally, at their most extreme, emotional outbursts can lead to violent and dangerous behaviors (Geddes and Callister, 2007; Geddes & Stickney, 2011). In contrast, displaying appropriate emotions can help facilitate safety compliance (Li, Jiang, Yao, & Li, 2013) and create and maintain a safer work environment (Codier, 2014; Sunindijo & Zou, 2013).

Research illustrates how personality can influence organizational safety through individual responses to stress. Emotional Stability, which is often called Neuroticism when negatively oriented, is negatively correlated with work stress (Balducci, Fraccaroli, & Schaufeli, 2011; De Fruyt, 2002). Furthermore, Lucas, Weidner, and Janisse (2012) found that rather than simply reporting more stress, individuals low on Emotional Stability may be more susceptible to the influence of work stress. Not only did more neurotic participants report greater stress levels in response to stressors, they reported lower levels of stress than their more emotionally stable counterparts in the absence of stressors. Similarly, Bakker, Van Der Zee, Lewig, and Dollard (2006), found the Emotional Stability was the only consistent predictor of three components of burnout for volunteer counselors, and that this relationship increased as the number of negative experiences increased. These results suggest a complex relationship between Emotional Stability and work-related stress.

Bakker et al. (2006) found that, for those reporting a high number of negative experiences, Agreeableness also predicted two components of burnout: Depersonalization and Personal Accomplishment. Furthermore, Extraversion predicted Personal Accomplishment for all participants. Likewise, Mitchelson (2009) found that, although Emotional Stability was the strongest predictor of self-reported work–family strain for a diverse sample of working adults, Agreeableness and Conscientiousness also had significant negative relationships with self-reported strain. And in a sample of over 3,500 Finns, Törnroos et al. (2013) found that all five FFM scales were related to self-reported work strain.

Similarly, Johnson and Foster (2010) found that while Emotional Stability from the HPI was the strongest predictor of supervisory ratings of managing stress, components of other FFM scales also played a role. The strongest facet-level predictors from Emotional Stability related to concern for others, an absence of worry, remaining calm, and being even tempered. Other predictive facets included characteristics such as being easy going and tolerant of others from Agreeableness, and striving for perfection and acting with a sense of personal effectiveness from Conscientiousness. These results indicate that supervisors associate a number of distinct individual characteristics with stress tolerance, such as maintaining a cool and collected demeanor, being accepting of faults and differences in others, and acting with a sense of purpose. Trainers, therefore, may not only benefit from activities aimed at helping individuals remain calm and composed when stressed, but also on activities aimed at relying on others' diverse talents and skills and maintaining focus on specific outcomes or objectives.

Responding to Training

Being able to learn from and then adhere to safety training can relate to any of the previous five behaviors, but is unique in how it relates to structured, organized safety training. For example, following rules is important, but only as important as an individual's ability and motivation to first learn those rules. A number of researchers have found that safety training can reduce accidents and injuries (Burke et al., 2006; Burke et al., 2011; Geller, 1996; Sinclair et al., 2003; Vrendenburgh, 2002; see also Burke & Smith Sockbeson, Chapter 15, this volume). Research has also found that forcing individuals to participate in training programs can have negative consequences (DePasquale & Geller, 1999), which emphasizes the need for active engagement and participation in training programs.

In their widely cited meta-analysis, Barrick and Mount (1991) reported that Extraversion, Conscientiousness, and Openness are the strongest predictors of training proficiency. Ziegler et al. (2014) expanded on these findings by examining relationships between FFM scales and training performance for over 5,000 individuals within four job families. Although they found that facets from the same three FFM scales were related to training proficiency for at least one job family, they also found that (a) relationships varied across job families and (b) that facets were often more predictive of training proficiency than their corresponding factor-level scales. Johnson and Foster (2010) found that supervisory ratings of self-development were most strongly associated with facets relating to achievement orientation such as competitiveness, self confidence, and displaying leadership tendencies. One component of Emotional Stability, which related to an absence of regret over past mistakes, also predicted self-development. Additional predictive facets from Openness involved an enjoyment of intellectual games, displaying a good memory, and an interest in education.

Facet-level results from Ziegler et al. (2014) and Johnson and Foster (2010) offer suggestions for tailoring training programs based on individual differences. First, although naturally curious individuals are likely going to be more open to and engaged in training, it might be beneficial for others if trainers clearly outline how training will impact and improve their ability to obtain desired goals. In other words, trainers should be clear about how the training will benefit each participant. Second, trainers may need to encourage some trainees to discard previous mistakes and focus on future goals and objectives. Finally, for less ambitious individuals, trainers may first need to help them set clear goals tied to the training and to recognize the importance of those goals. In general, trainers would benefit from understanding that some individuals will naturally create or easily migrate toward training goals while others will benefit from information outlining how training benefits them.

Safety Training Implications

Focusing on behaviors that mediate the relationship between personality and organizational safety not only offers important insight into the nature of these relationships, but provides guidance for developing interventions to improve safety. The key to such interventions is to identify and focus on individual risk factors. Zierold, Welsh, and McGeeney (2012) offer insight into the potential benefits of such customization by examining safety attitudes among teenage employees. Although young workers accounted for a disproportionately large percentage of workplace injuries, they were also among the least receptive to safety training, often referring to it as boring and claiming it reflected little more than common sense practices. This response was likely exaggerated because, as the researchers report, "in most cases all workers received the same type of training" (p. 1289). Zierold et al. (2012) concluded by recommending practitioners construct tailored training programs for teen audiences.

Such programs are likely to be even more effective if tailored to the personality of individuals in the audience. For example, although research demonstrates consistent personality differences across age groups and/or generations, these differences often account for only a small percentage of variance in scores across adult samples (Wong, Gardiner, Lang, & Coulon, 2008). Similarly, Yang (2014) mirrored findings by Foster and Meyer (2012) concerning individual values, showing that generational membership typically accounted for less than one percent of the variance across individuals in a variety of personality measures. She concludes that these findings "challenge the practical implication of generational stereotypes and suggest that talent managers attend to individual differences beyond generational membership in management practice" (p. 5). In other words, although small generational differences in personality and values exist, trainers cannot tell much about specific individuals simply from their age.

In contrast, research linking personality characteristics to safety-related behaviors offers information trainers could use to pinpoint individual characteristics associated with safety risk and tailor programs to individuals based on these characteristics. Although, some individuals will be more receptive to training than others, trainers could use personality assessment to identify and work with individuals who require more guidance to recognize how training will benefit them. Also, simply emphasizing behaviors, such as following rules or remaining vigilant, may not be as effective as first identifying characteristics that lead to these behaviors and then implementing tailored strategies for addressing these characteristics. For example, extraverts might benefit more from training centered on how to maintain focus over long periods while introverts may benefit more from training centered on the need to respond quickly and appropriately to stressful situations.

The relationships between personality, behavior, and safety also have implications for non-work-related safety. Research has found links between personality measures and a variety of non-organizational safety-related criteria, such as driving-related criteria (e.g., Adrian, Postal, Moessinger, Rascle, & Charles, 2011; Chen, 2009; Curran et al., 2010; Guo & Fang, 2013; Machin & Sankey, 2008) and drug and alcohol use (e.g., Cyders, Flory, Rainer, & Smith, 2009). For example, Paaver et al. (2013) found that a program targeting risky driving behaviors benefits individuals with specific genetic markers linked to impulsivity but not individuals who lacked such markers.

Similarly, research in other fields related to health and wellness could benefit from the organizational safety literature. A number of researchers have argued that targeted health care interventions tailored to individuals are more effective than generic interventions (e.g., D'Amore, 2013; Jordan, 2013; Noar, Benac, & Harris, 2007; Siest & Schallmeiner, 2013). Furthermore, a growing body of research has found relationships between personality and health-related behaviors, indicating that personality may provide one means of tailoring individual health care programs. For example, Armon and Toker (2013) found that Conscientiousness, Extraversion, Openness, and Emotional Stability predicted the likelihood that employees would participate in multiple, employer-paid, health screenings. They conclude that "personality traits should be taken into consideration in the planning and implementation of health-promoting interventions" (p. 452). They do not, however, have the evidence needed to suggest how to take personality into account when planning such interventions. As with most research examining relationships between personality and outcomes of interest, an important next step is collecting additional data concerning relationships between personality and specific behaviors that proceed the outcome (e.g., scheduling appointments in advance, marking them on a calendar, discussing health screening with others). In this case, we might hypothesize that individuals high on Extraversion would benefit most from discussing health screening with others while those low on Conscientiousness would benefit most from scheduling appointments in advance and marking them on their calendar. Additional research is needed to determine the likelihood that such hypotheses are correct.

Similarly, Dutta-Bergman (2003) examined reactions to communications concerning AIDS prevention among college students. They found that high self-monitors react more strongly to functional communications, which focus on the practical implications of protective methods, while low self-monitors react more strongly to social appeals, which focus on favorable views of using protective methods. These results suggest the best way to appeal to someone at the individual level is to tailor that appeal according to the individual's personality, or more specifically in this case, the degree to which they self-monitor. However, the impact of tailored communications on AIDS prevention can only be deduced through additional research including prevention-related behaviors and their outcomes. In other words, Dutta-Bergman's (2003) results offer a promising first step in linking personality to AIDS prevention, but additional data are required to determine how practitioners can use this information to encourage preventive behaviors.

Much like organizational safety research, the impact of personality on interesting outcomes in other fields requires an examination of multiple variables that include personality, behaviors, and outcomes. Only by understanding the impact of individual characteristics on critical behaviors can we begin to use these relationships to create tailored training programs. Furthermore, although initial research examining higher-order factors, such as those represented by the FFM, is a promising way to uncover potential relationships with outcomes of interest, further research at the facet level is often more informative and useful when determining how to explain these relationships and shape individual behaviors.

Future Research

Research examining relationships between personality, behaviors, and safety outcomes offers a number of promising directions for future efforts aimed at better understanding how personality influences safety-related behaviors and how practitioners can use this information to improve organizational safety. We encourage the continual examination of these relationships and offer the following suggestions for improving our knowledge of personality and organizational safety.

First, our review of safety-related behaviors is not comprehensive. Research should continue to examine additional safety-related behaviors and the personality characteristics that drive them. Examples may include knowledge sharing (Nesheim & Gressgard, 2014), active participation in safety practices (Neal & Griffin, 2006; Neal, Griffin, & Hart, 2000), and setting and adhering to safety goals (Grouzet et al., 2005; Shafer, 2008). Furthermore, Hogan and Foster (2013) demonstrated that the best predictors of safety outcomes across a range of jobs are comprised of personality facets selected to predict multiple safety behaviors. For example, they found that individuals scoring in critically low ranges on two or more safety predictor scales were about twice as likely to have accidents or injuries compared with those with critical scores on zero or one safety scale. In other words, the chances of having an accident or injury increase for individuals who are at risk on multiple behaviors. The examination of additional safety-related behaviors, therefore, could aid development of scales that better predict safety across a range of industries, organizations, and jobs.

Second, research should focus on identifying which safety-related behaviors are most critical in different settings. We expect additional work in this area would indicate that a number of organizational, environmental, and job-related factors moderate relationships between personality and organizational safety. A consideration of what safety-related behaviors are most critical for different jobs indicates that such moderators likely exist. For example, following rules (e.g., traffic laws, required rest periods) and vigilance (i.e., remaining attentive over long periods of time) might be the most critical safety-related behaviors for long haul truck drivers. The same might be true for other transportation-related jobs such as locomotive engineers and airline pilots. In contrast, responding to training and reacting appropriately to crisis might be the most important behaviors for many service-related positions such as first responders. Although any safety-related behavior likely plays some role in predicting safety outcomes for any job, it is probable that the strength of these relationships varies across jobs based on context and task requirements. As a result, the relative importance of different personality antecedents predictive of safety-related behaviors will also vary.

Third, additional evidence concerning personality and safety-related behaviors across jobs would help inform better methods safety-related job analysis. Most current research focuses on relationships between personality and safety outcomes for job incumbents, meaning we only know what characteristics lead to accidents and injuries after they occur. Further examination of the organizational and job characteristics that moderate relationships between personality and safety would help practitioners identify critical individual characteristics related to safety, and then either select for or focus training around those characteristics, to better prevent accidents and injuries before they occur.

Questions also remain about the relationship between a leader's personality and organizational safety. Thoms and Venkataraman (2002) found that leaders who were higher on Conscientiousness and Extraversion experienced fewer accidents within their groups. Although these findings parallel results for individuals where Conscientiousness is negatively related to accidents and injuries, they are the reverse of individual-level results for Extraversion. In other words, components of Extraversion such as showing off and seeking attention are negatively related to safety for individual employees. In contrast, Thoms and Venkataraman (2002) found that Extraversion for leaders was positively related to safety, perhaps because extraverted leaders are more likely to communicate with and attend to employees. Again, this emphasizes the need for focusing on specific facets of personality as they relate to safety-related behaviors in different contexts. Future research should determine if other components and behaviors relating to role or task requirements moderate relationships between leader personality and safety.

Other variables may also moderate relationships between personality and organizational safety. For example, a number of researchers have found that personality and safety climate both contribute when predicting a variety of outcomes such as relational conflicts (Chi & Huang, 2010), individual performance (Baba, Tourigny, Wang, & Liu, 2009), and both productivity and safety performance (Wallace & Chen, 2006). These results not only provide additional evidence of the complexity between personality and organizational safety, but show that by focusing more on mediating behaviors, we might help clarify why a variety of contextual variables moderate these relationships. In other words, we might better identify which characteristics moderate relationships between personality and organizational safety if we first identify which behaviors are most critical in different situations.

Finally, research demonstrating the value of behaviors as mediators and contextual factors as moderators of relationships between personality and organizational safety can help inform other areas. The value of such an approach also extends beyond traditional personality measures to other individual differences such as cognitive ability and personal history (demographics, biodata, etc.). Most organizational interventions aim at either selecting individuals who exhibit important job-related behaviors or at shaping the behaviors of current employees to help align their activities with organizational goals. Unfortunately, when examining the impact of these interventions, we too often look only at relationships between the predictor measures and outcomes while ignoring the behaviors that shape these relationships.

Conclusions

The most significant advances to organizational safety have focused on working conditions, equipment, and implementing safety-related processes and procedures for high-risk jobs. However, despite these advances, accidents and injuries continue to occur even in the most regulated and strict environments. This has led to an increase in research examining individual characteristics that may cause accidents and injuries. Such a view inevitably leads to an examination of personality that, by definition, is the study of the individual differences that drive behaviors and shape the impressions we make on others (Hogan & Kaiser, 2010).

Although primarily stagnant throughout earlier decades dominated by behavioral approaches to psychological research, the study of personality and individual differences in the workplace built momentum throughout the 1980s and witnessed a dramatic increase in both acceptance and published research following the emergence of the FFM (Digman, 1990; Goldberg, 1992; John, 1990), along with a number of subsequent meta-analyses linking personality to performance ratings across jobs and organizations (Barrick & Mount, 1991; Barrick et al., 2001; Hogan et al., 1996; Hogan & Holland, 2003; Tett et al., 1991). Only recently, however, have multiple researchers extended the examination of personality and job behaviors into the realm of organizational safety.

There are a number of advantages to examining relationships between broad personality scales, such as those representing the FFM model, and other constructs. One advantage is that any study examining individual differences would likely benefit from the inclusion of personality as a potential mechanism for strengthening or better explaining results among other variables. A second advantage is that many self-report FFM inventories are short and easy to administer. Examples include the Big Five Mini Markers (Saucier, 1994) and the NEO-FFI (McCrae & Costa, 2004), both of which are only 40 and 60 items respectively, designed to take about 5–10 minutes to complete, and provide reliable results for all FFM scales. The potential downside of including such measures is minimal. The potential upside, however, is that personality data can help supplement nearly any research activity relying on data from individuals or, more importantly, a comparison of individual differences to other variables of interest.

Personality factors, which are often referred to as traits, predict a range of outcomes such as mortality, health, job performance, training, organizational performance, leadership, creativity, teamwork, and counterproductive performance and behaviors (Hough & Oswald, 2008). But while short FFM scales might be useful for discovering general relationships between personality and other variables of interest, research consistently shows facets are more predictive than broad factors for a variety of outcomes (e.g., Christiansen & Robie, 2011; Paunonen & Ashton, 2001). Although broad factors are useful for examining potential relationships between personality and other constructs, they often fall short of fully capturing or explaining these relationships. As McAdams (1995) stated when considering the value of factors for describing individuals, "A person cannot be known without knowing traits. But knowing traits is not enough" (p. 371).

Nowhere are relationships between personality and behaviors more important than with organizational safety. Unlike many other work-related areas, poor safety can have disastrous consequences extending well beyond the individuals involved. Not only is safety critically important to the health and well-being of individual workers, the costs associated with one accident can displace countless employees. And while accidents continue to exist in even the most well structured and regulated environments, the primary remaining threat to organizational safety is human actions and errors. To help eliminate threats, we must know what drives unsafe behaviors so we can improve selection and safety training.

There are three keys to using personality to improve organizational safety: (a) identifying behaviors that are most critical to safety for individual jobs, (b) identifying specific and narrow personality characteristics that drive these behaviors, (c) using this information to create tailored practices for selecting out individuals with these characteristics or create training aimed at mitigating their influence. Given the low base rates of accidents and injuries in most organizations, it is difficult to predict the often unusual combination of rare and unforeseen events that lead to a single tragic outcome. Furthermore, the circumstances and actions leading to such events are often as diverse as the individual characteristics that drive them. This not only makes accidents and injuries harder to predict, but emphasizes the need to minimize human error by understanding the role of personality in organizational safety.

References

Adrian, J., Postal, V., Moessinger, M., Rascle, N., & Charles, A. (2011). Personality traits and executive functions related to on-road driving performance among older drivers. *Accident Analysis and Prevention, 43*, 1652–1659.

Armon, G., & Toker, S. (2013). The role of personality in predicting repeat participation in periodic health screening. *Journal of Personality, 81*, 452–464.

Baba, V. V., Tourigny, L., Wang, X., & Liu, W. (2009). Proactive personality and work performance in China: The moderating effects of emotional exhaustion and perceived safety climate. *Canadian Journal of Administrative Sciences/Revue Canadienne Des Sciences De L'Administration, 26*, 23–37.

Bacchieri, G., Barros, A. J., dos Santos, J. V., & Gigante, D. P. (2010). Cycling to work in Brazil: Users profile, risk behaviors, and traffic accident occurrence. *Accident Analysis and Prevention, 42*, 1025–1030.

Bakker, A. B., Van Der Zee, K. I., Lewig, K. A., & Dollard, M. F. (2006). The relationship between the Big Five personality factors and burnout: A study among volunteer counselors. *Journal of Social Psychology, 146*, 31–50.

Balducci, C., Fraccaroli, F., & Schaufeli, W. B. (2011). Workplace bullying and its relation with work characteristics, personality, and post-traumatic stress symptoms: An integrated model. *Anxiety, Stress and Coping, 24*, 499–513.

Bandura, A. (1997). Editorial. *American Journal of Health Promotion, 12*, 8–10.

Barbato, G., Costanzo, A., Monica, C. D., D'Onofrio, P., Cerrato, F., & De Padova, V. (2013). Effects of prolonged wakefulness: The role of period3 genotypes and personality traits. *Psychological Reports, 113*, 540–551.

Barrick, M. R., & Mount, M. K. (1991). The Big Five personality dimensions and job performance: A meta-analysis. *Personnel Psychology, 44*, 1–26.

Barrick, M. R., Mount, M. K., & Judge, T. A. (2001). Personality and performance at the beginning of the new millennium: What do we know and where do we go next? *International Journal of Selection and Assessment, 9*, 9–30.

Barsade, S. G., & Gibson, D. E. (2007). Why does affect matter in organizations? *Academy of Management Perspectives, 21*, 36–57.

Basak, S., & Makarov, D. (2012). Difference in interim performance and risk taking with short-sale constraints. *Journal of Financial Economics, 103*, 377–392.

Beck, E., Ohmer, M., & Warner, B. (2012). Strategies for preventing neighborhood violence: Toward bringing collective efficacy into social work practice. *Journal of Community Practice, 20*, 225–240.

Bell, N. S., Amoroso, P. J., Yore, M. M., Smith, G. S., & Jones, B. H. (2000). Self-reported risk-taking behaviors and hospitalization for motor vehicle injury among active duty Army personnel. *American Journal of Preventive Medicine, 18*, 85–95.

Boden, J. (2009). The devil inside: Boredom proneness and impulsive behavior. *Critical Studies, 33*, 203–226.

Brief, A. P., & Weiss, H. M. (2002). Organizational behavior: Affect in the workplace. *Annual Review of Psychology, 53*, 279–307.

Burke, M. J., Salvador, R. O., Smith-Crowe, K., Chan-Serafin, S., Smith, A., & Sonesh, S. (2011). The dread factor: How hazards and safety training influence learning and performance. *Journal of Applied Psychology, 96*, 46–70.

Burke, M. J., Sarpy, S. A., Smith-Crowe, K., Chan-Serafin, S., Salvador, R. O., & Islam, G. (2006). Relative effectiveness of worker safety and health training methods. *American Journal of Public Health, 96*, 315–324.

Burton, L., Pfaff, D., Bolt, N., Hadjikyriacou, D., Silton, N., Kilgallen, C., Cofer, J., & Allimant, J. (2010). Effects of gender and personality on the Conners Continuous Performance test. *Journal of Clinical and Experimental Neuropsychology, 32*, 66–70.

Cekada, T., Janicak, C., & Ferguson, L. (2009). Preventing occupational fatalities: A review of findings from a recent industry forum. *Professional Safety, 54*, 29–32.

Cellar, D. F., Nelson, Z. C., & Yorke, C. M. (2000). The Five-Factor model and driving behavior: Personality and involvement in vehicular accidents. *Psychological Reports, 86*, 454–456.

Cellar, D. F., Yorke, C. M., Nelson, Z. C., & Carroll, K. A. (2004). Relationships between Five Factor personality variables, workplace accidents, and self-efficacy. *Psychological Reports, 94*, 1437–1441.

Chen, C. (2009). Personality, safety attitudes and risky driving behavior: Evidence from young Taiwanese motorcyclists. *Accident Analysis and Prevention, 41*, 963–968.

Chi, S. S., & Huang, C. (2010). Safety climate and relational conflict in the eyes of team members: Examining the role of need for closure. *Social Behavior and Personality: An International Journal, 38*, 103–114.

Christian, M. S., Bradley, J. C., Wallace, J. C., & Burke, M. J. (2009). Workplace safety: A meta-analysis of the roles of person and situation factors. *Journal of Applied Psychology, 94*, 1103–1127.

Christiansen, N. D., & Robie, C. (2011). Further consideration of the use of narrow trait scales. *Canadian Journal of Behavioural Science/Revue Canadienne Des Sciences Du Comportement, 43*, 183–194.

Clarke, S. (2006). The relationship between safety climate and safety performance: A meta-analytic review. *Journal of Occupational and Health Psychology, 11*, 315–327.

Clarke, S., & Robertson, I. T. (2005). A meta-analytic review of the Big Five personality factors and accident involvement in occupational and non-occupation settings. *Journal of Occupational and Organizational Psychology, 78*, 355–376.

Clarke, S., & Robertson, I. T. (2008). An examination of the role of personality in work accidents using meta-analysis. *Applied Psychology: An International Review, 57*, 94–108.

Codier, E. (2014). Making the case for emotionally intelligent leaders. *Nursing Management, 45*, 44–48.

Collins, J. M., & Schmidt, F. L. (1993). Personality, integrity, and white collar crime: A construct validity study. *Personnel Psychology, 46*, 295–311.

Costa, P. T., Jr., & McCrae, R. R. (1992). *Revised NEO Personality Inventory (NEO-PI-R) and NEO Five-Factor Inventory (NEO-FFI): Professional manual.* Odessa, FL: Psychological Assessment Resources.

Curran, M. F., Fuertes, J. N., Alfonso, V. C., & Hennessy, J. J. (2010). The association of sensation seeking and impulsivity to driving while under the influence of alcohol. *Journal of Addictions and Offender Counseling, 30*, 84–98.

Cyders, M. A., Flory, K., Rainer, S., & Smith, G. T. (2009). The role of personality dispositions to risky behavior in predicting first-year college drinking. *Addiction, 104*, 193–202.

D'Amore, F. (2013). The doctor and the patient: Doing too much or too little. *Italian Journal of Medicine, 7*, 135–137.

Dahlen, E. R., Martin, R. C., Ragan, K., & Kuhlman, M. M. (2005). Driving anger, sensation seeking, impulsiveness, and boredom proneness in the prediction of unsafe driving. *Accident Analysis and Prevention, 37*, 341–348.

Dean, M. A., Conte, J. M., & Blankenhorn, T. R. (2006). Examination of the predictive validity of Big Five personality dimensions across training performance criteria. *Personality and Individual Differences, 41*, 1229–1239.

De Fruyt, F. (2002). A person-centered approach to P-E Fit questions using a multiple-trait model. *Journal of Vocational Behavior, 60*, 73–90.

Demerouti, E. (2006). Job characteristics, flow, and performance: The moderating role of conscientiousness. *Journal of Occupational Health Psychology, 11*, 266–280.

DePasquale, J. P., & Geller, E. (1999). Critical success factors for behavior-based safety. *Journal of Safety Research, 30*, 237–249.

Desivilya, H. S., & Yagil, D. (2005). The role of emotions in conflict management: The case of work teams. *International Journal of Conflict Management, 16*, 55–69.

Digman, J. M. (1990). Personality structure: Emergence of the Five-Factor model. *Annual Review of Psychology, 41*, 417–440.

Driskell, J. E., Goodwin, G. F., Salas, E., & O'Shea, P. G. (2006). What makes a good team player? Personality and team effectiveness. *Group Dynamics: Theory, Research, and Practice, 10*, 249–271.

Dudley, N. M., Orvis, K. A., Lebiecki, J. E., & Cortina, J. M. (2006). A meta-analytic investigation of conscientiousness in the prediction of job performance: Examining the intercorrelations and the incremental validity of narrow traits. *Journal of Applied Psychology, 91*, 40–57.

Dutta-Bergman, M. J. (2003). The linear interaction model of personality effects in health communication. *Health Communication, 15*, 101–116.

Elfenbein, H. A. (2007). Emotion in organizations: A review and theoretical integration. In A. Brief & J. Walsh (Eds.), *Academy of Management Annals* (Vol. 1, pp. 371–457). Amsterdam, The Netherlands: Elsevier.

Fischer, A. R., & Frewer, L. J. (2008). Food-safety practices in the domestic kitchen: Demographic, personality, and experiential determinants. *Journal of Applied Social Psychology, 38*, 2859–2884.

Foster J., & Meyer, K., (2012). *Generational and cultural effects on values using the MVPI*. Paper presented at the 27th Annual Conference of the Society for Industrial and Organizational Psychology, San Diego, CA.

Frone, M. R. (1998). Predictors of work injuries among employed adolescents. *Journal of Applied Psychology, 83*, 565–576.

Fyhri, A., & Backer-Grøndahl, A. (2012). Personality and risk perception in transport. *Accident Analysis and Prevention, 49*, 470–475.

Gaba, A., & Kalra, A. (1999). Risk behavior in response to quotas and contests. *Marketing Science, 18*, 417–434.

Geddes, D., & Callister, R. R. (2007). Crossing the line(s): A dual threshold model of anger in organizations. *Academy of Management Review, 32*, 721–746.

Geddes, D., & Stickney, L. T. (2011). The trouble with sanctions: Organizational responses to deviant anger displays at work. *Human Relations, 64*, 201–230.

Geller, E. S. (1996). *The psychology of safety: How to improve behaviors and attitudes on the job.* Radnor, PA: Chilton Book Company.

Goldberg, L. R. (1992). The development of markers for the Big-Five factor structure. *Psychological Assessment, 4*, 26–42.

Goldberg, L. R. (2008). The Eugene-Springfield community sample: Information available from the research participants. *Oregon Research Institute Technical Report* (Vol. 48). Eugene, OR: Oregon Research Institute.

Griffin, M. A., & Neal, A. (2000). Perceptions of safety at work: A framework for linking safety climate to safety performance, knowledge, and motivation. *Journal of Occupational Health Psychology, 5*, 347–358.

Grouzet, F. M., Kasser, T., Ahuvia, A., Dols, J. M., Kim, Y., Lau, S., ..., & Sheldon, K. M. (2005). The structure of goal contents across 15 cultures. *Journal of Personality and Social Psychology, 89*, 800–816.

Guo, F., & Fang, Y. (2013). Individual driver risk assessment using naturalistic driving data. *Accident Analysis and Prevention, 61*, 3–9.

Gyekye, S. A., & Salminen, S. (2005). Are "good soldiers" safety conscious? An examination of the relationship between organizational citizenship behaviors and perceptions of workplace safety. *Social Behavior and Personality, 33*, 805–820.

Hansen, C. P. (1988). Personality characteristics of the accident involved employee. *Journal of Business and Psychology, 2*, 346–365.

Harper, S., & White, C. (2013). The impact of member emotional intelligence on psychological safety in work teams. *Journal of Behavioral and Applied Management, 15*, 2–10.

Hendricks, J. W., & Payne, S. C. (2007). Beyond the big five: Leader goal orientation as a predictor of leadership effectiveness. *Human Performance, 20*, 317–343.

Hogan, J., & Foster, J. (2013). Multifaceted personality predictors of workplace safety performance: More than conscientiousness. *Human Performance, 26*, 20–43.

Hogan, R., & Hogan, J. (2007). *Hogan personality inventory manual* (3rd edn.). Tulsa, OK: Hogan Assessment Systems.

Hogan, R., Hogan, J., & Roberts, B. W. (1996). Personality measurement and employment decisions: Questions and answers. *American Psychologist, 51*, 469–477.

Hogan, J., & Holland, B. (2003). Using theory to evaluate personality and job-performance relations: A socioanalytic perspective. *Journal of Applied Psychology, 88*, 100–112.

Hogan, R., & Judge, T. (2013). Personality and leadership. In M. G. Rumsey (Ed.), *The Oxford handbook of leadership* (pp. 37–46). New York, NY: Oxford University Press.

Hogan, R., & Kaiser, R. (2010). Personality. In J. C. Scott & D. H. Reynolds (Eds.), *Handbook of workplace assessment: Evidence-based practices for selecting and developing organizational talent* (pp. 81–108). San Francisco, CA: Josey-Bass.

Hough, L. M., & Oswald, F. L. (2008). Personality testing and industrial-organizational psychology: Reflections, progress, and prospects. *Industrial and Organizational Psychology, 1*, 272–290.

Hsu, S. H., Lee, C., Wu, M., & Takano, K. (2008). A cross-cultural study of organizational factors on safety: Japanese vs. Taiwanese oil refinery plants. *Accident Analysis and Prevention, 40*, 24–34.

Jeffries, F. L. (2011). Predicting safety related attitudes in the workplace: The influence of moral maturity and emotional intelligence. *Journal of Behavioral and Applied Management, 12*, 200–216.

John, O. P. (1990). The "Big Five" factor taxonomy: Dimensions of personality in the natural language and in questionnaires. In L. A. Pervin (Ed.), *Handbook of personality: Theory and research* (pp. 66–100). New York, NY: Guilford Press.

John, O. P., & Srivastava, S. (1999). The Big Five trait taxonomy: History, measurement, and theoretical perspectives. In L. A. Pervin & O. P. John (Eds.), *Handbook of personality: Theory and research* (Vol. 2., pp. 102–138). New York, NY: Guilford Press.

Johnson, A., & Foster, J. (2010). *Hogan competency, domain, and job family synthetic validation results from the Hogan Personality Inventory and the Hogan Development Survey.* Tulsa, OK: Hogan Assessment Systems.

Jordan, B. (2013). The role of clinical laboratories in personalized healthcare [Editorial]. *Journal of the International Federation of Clinical Chemistry and Laboratory Medicine, 24*, 1–2.

Judge, T. A., Bono, J. E., Ilies, R., & Gerhardt, M. W. (2002). Personality and leadership: A qualitative and quantitative review. *Journal of Applied Psychology, 87*, 765–780.

König, C. J., & Waller, M. J. (2010). Time for reflection: A critical examination of polychronicity. *Human Performance, 23*, 173–190.

Kornelis, M., De Jonge, J., Frewer, L., & Dagevos, H. (2007). Consumer selection of food-safety information sources. *Risk Analysis, 27*, 327–335.

Lee, K., & Ashton, M. C. (2005). Psychopathy, Machiavellianism, and narcissism in the Five-Factor Model and the HEXACO model of personality structure. *Personality and Individual Differences, 38*, 1571–1582.

Li, F., Jiang, L., Yao, X., & Li, Y. (2013). Job demands, job resources and safety outcomes: The roles of emotional exhaustion and safety compliance. *Accident Analysis and Prevention, 51*, 243–251.

Liao, H., Arvey, R. D., Butler, R. J., & Nutting, S. M. (2001). Correlates of work injury frequency and duration among firefighters. *Journal of Occupational Health Psychology, 6*, 229–242.

Lind, S. (2008). Types and sources of fatal and severe non-fatal accidents in industrial maintenance. *International Journal of Industrial Ergonomics, 11–12*, 927–933.

Lucas, T., Weidner, N., & Janisse, J. (2012). Where does work stress come from? A generalizability analysis of stress in police officers. *Psychology and Health, 27*, 1426–1447.

Machin, M. A., & Sankey, K. S. (2008). Relationships between young drivers' personality characteristics, risk perceptions, and driving behaviour. *Accident Analysis and Prevention, 40*, 541–547.

Macht, G. A., Nembhard, D. A., Kim, J. H., & Rothrock, L. (2014). Structural models of extraversion, communication, and team performance. *International Journal of Industrial Ergonomics, 44*, 82–91.

Mann, S. (2012). Boredom at the checkout: Causes, coping strategies and outcomes of workplace boredom in a supermarket setting. *Journal of Business and Retail Management Research, 6*, 1–14.

Mann, S., & Robinson, A. (2009). Boredom in the lecture theatre: An investigation into the contributors, moderators and outcomes of boredom amongst university students. *British Educational Research Journal, 35*, 243–258.

McAdams, D. P. (1995). What do we know when we know a person? *Journal of Personality, 63*, 365–396.

McCrae, R. R., & Costa, P. T. (2004). A contemplated revision of the NEO Five-Factor inventory. *Personality and Individual Differences, 36*, 587–596.

McFarland, R., & Kidwell, B. (2006). An examination of instrumental and expressive traits on performance: The mediating role of learning, prove, and avoid goal orientations. *Journal of Personal Selling and Sales Management, 26*, 143–159.

McGiboney, G. W., & Carter, C. (1988). Boredom proneness and adolescents' personalities. *Psychological Reports, 63*, 741–742.

McLeod, R., Stockwell, T., Rooney, R., Stevens, M., Phillips, M., & Jelinek, G. (2003). The influence of extrinsic and intrinsic risk factors on the probability of sustaining an injury. *Accident Analysis and Prevention, 35*, 71–80.

Mitchelson, J. K. (2009). Seeking the perfect balance: Perfectionism and work–family conflict. *Journal of Occupational and Organizational Psychology, 82*, 349–367.

Mulder, F. (1971). Characteristics of violators of formal company rules. *Journal of Applied Psychology, 55*, 500–502.

Mullen, J. E., & Kelloway, E. K. (2009). Safety leadership: A longitudinal study of the effects of transformational leadership on safety outcomes. *Journal of Occupational and Organizational Psychology, 82*, 253–272.

Nadkarni, S., & Herrmann, P. (2010). CEO personality, strategic flexibility, and firm performance: The case of the Indian business process outsourcing industry. *Academy of Management Journal, 53*, 1050–1073.

Neal, A., & Griffin, M. A. (2006). A study of the lagged relationships among safety climate, safety motivation, safety behavior, and accidents at the individual and group levels. *Journal of Applied Psychology, 91*, 946–953.

Neal, A., Griffin, M., & Hart, P. (2000). The impact of organizational climate on safety climate and individual behavior. *Safety Science, 34*, 99–109.

Nesheim, T., & Gressgård, L. J. (2014). Knowledge sharing in a complex organization: Antecedents and safety effects. *Safety Science, 62*, 28–36.

Newnam, S., Griffin, M. A., & Mason, C. (2008). Safety in work vehicles: A multilevel study linking safety values and individual predictors to work-related driving crashes. *Journal of Applied Psychology, 93*, 632–644.

Nicholson, N., Soane, E., Fenton-O'Creevy, M., & Willman, P. (2005). Personality and domain-specific risk taking. *Journal of Risk Research, 8*, 157–176.

Noar, S. M., Benac, C. N., & Harris, M. S. (2007). Does tailoring matter? Meta-analytic review of tailored print health behavior change interventions. *Psychological Bulletin, 133*, 673–693.

O'Neill, T. A., & Allen, N. J. (2011). Personality and the prediction of team performance. *European Journal of Personality, 25*, 31–42.

Paaver, M., Eensoo, D., Kaasik, K., Vaht, M., Mäestu, J., & Harro, J. (2013). Preventing risky driving: A novel and efficient brief intervention focusing on acknowledgement of personal risk factors. *Accident Analysis and Prevention, 50*, 430–437.

Paul, P., & Maiti, J. (2007). The role of behavioral factors on safety management in underground mines. *Safety Science, 45,* 449–471.

Paunonen, S. V., & Ashton, M. C. (2001). Big Five factors and facets and the prediction of behavior. *Journal of Personality and Social Psychology, 81,* 524–539.

Perrow, C. (1984). *Normal accidents: Living with high-risk technologies.* New York, NY: Basic Books.

Pierce, F. D. (2005). Personality types and injuries. *Professional Safety, 50,* 42–50.

Piercy, N. F. (2010). Evolution of strategic sales organizations in business-to-business marketing. *Journal of Business and Industrial Marketing, 25,* 349–359.

Pool, L. D., & Qualter, P. (2012). Improving emotional intelligence and emotional self-efficacy through a teaching intervention for university students. *Learning and Individual Differences, 22,* 306–312.

Postlethwaite, B., Robbins, S., Rickerson, J., & McKinniss, T. (2009). The moderation of conscientiousness by cognitive ability when predicting workplace safety behavior. *Personality and Individual Differences, 47,* 711–716.

Prentice, C., & King, B. E. M. (2013). Impacts of personality, emotional intelligence and adaptiveness on service performance of casino hosts: A hierarchical approach. *Journal of Business Research, 66,* 1637–1643.

Probst, T. M., Graso, M., Estrada, A. X., & Greer, S. (2013). Consideration of future safety consequences: A new predictor of employee safety. *Accident Analysis and Prevention, 55,* 124–134.

Rajalin, S. (1994). The connection between risky driving and involvement in fatal accidents. *Accident Analysis and Prevention, 26,* 555–562.

Reason, J. (1990). *Human error.* Cambridge, UK: Cambridge University Press.

Roberts, K. E., Bonafide, C. P., Paine, C. W., Paciotti, B., Tibbetts, K. M., Keren, R., Barg, F., & Holmes, J. H. (2014). Barriers to calling for urgent assistance despite a comprehensive pediatric rapid response system. *American Journal of Critical Care, 23,* 223–229.

Rose, L. C., Murphy, L. B., Byard, L., & Nikzad K. (2002). The role of the Big Five personality factors in vigilance performance and workload. *European Journal of Personality, 16,* 185–200.

Salgado, J. F. (2002). The Big Five personality dimensions and counterproductive behaviors. *International Journal of Selection and Assessment, 10,* 117–125.

Sambasivan, M., Abdul, M., & Yusop, Y. (2009). Impact of personal qualities and management skills of entrepreneurs on venture performance in Malaysia: Opportunity recognition skills as a mediating factor. *Technovation, 29,* 798–805.

Saucier, G. (1994). Mini-markers: A brief version of Goldberg's unipolar Big-Five markers. *Journal of Personality Assessment, 63,* 506–516.

Scanlon, J., Helsloot, I., & Groenendaal, J. (2014). Putting it all together: Integrating ordinary people into emergency response. *International Journal of Mass Emergencies and Disasters, 32,* 43–63.

Schwebel, D. C., Severson, J., Ball, K. K., & Rizzo, M. (2006). Individual difference factors in risky driving: The roles of anger/hostility, conscientiousness, and sensation-seeking. *Accident Analysis and Prevention, 38,* 801–810.

Scott-Parker, B., Watson, B., King, M. J., & Hyde, M. K. (2012). The influence of sensitivity to reward and punishment, propensity for sensation seeking, depression, and anxiety on the risky behaviour of novice drivers: A path model. *British Journal of Psychology, 103,* 248–267.

Shafer, C. (2008). Preconstruction safety: Plan for safety excellence. *Professional Safety, 53,* 26–31

Sharma, S., Bottom, W. P., & Elfenbein, H. A. (2013). On the role of personality, cognitive ability, and emotional intelligence in predicting negotiation outcomes: A meta-analysis. *Organizational Psychology Review, 4,* 293–336.

Shiner, R. L. (2000). Linking childhood personality with adaptation: Evidence for continuity and change across time into late adolescence. *Journal of Personality and Social Psychology, 78,* 310–325.

Shiner, R. L., Masten, A. S., & Roberts, J. M. (2003). Childhood personality foreshadows adult personality and life outcomes two decades later. *Journal of Personality, 71,* 1145–1170.

Siest, G., & Schallmeiner, E. (2013). Pharmacogenomics and theranostics in practice: A summary of the Euromedlab-ESPT satellite symposium. *Journal of the International Federation of Clinical Chemistry and Laboratory Medicine, 24,* 1–5.

Sinclair, R. C., Smith, R., Colligan, M., Prince, M., Nguyen, T., & Stayner, L. (2003). Evaluation of a safety training program in three food service companies. *Journal of Safety Research, 34,* 547–558.

Sitser, T., van der Linden, D., & Born, M. P. (2013). Predicting sales performance criteria with personality measures: The use of the general factor of personality, the Big Five and narrow traits. *Human Performance, 26,* 126–149.

Smillie, L. D., Yeo, G. B., Furnham, A. F., & Jackson, C. J. (2006). Benefits of all work and no play: The relationship between neuroticism and performance as a function of resource allocation. *Journal of Applied Psychology, 91,* 139–155.

Soane, E., Dewberry, C., & Narendran, S. (2010). The role of perceived costs and perceived benefits in the relationship between personality and risk-related choices. *Journal of Risk Research, 13,* 303–318.

Spurk, D., & Abele, A. E. (2011). Who earns more and why? A multiple mediation model from personality to salary. *Journal of Business and Psychology, 26,* 87–103.

Sunindijo, R. Y., & Zou, P. W. (2013). The roles of emotional intelligence, interpersonal skill, and transformational leadership in improving construction safety. *Australasian Journal of Construction Economics and Building, 13,* 97–113.

Tett, R. P., Jackson, D. N., & Rothstein, M. (1991). Personality measures as predictors of job performance: A meta-analytic review. *Personnel Psychology, 44,* 703–742.

Thoms, P., Moore, K., & Scott, K. (1996). The relationship between self-efficacy for participating in self-managed work groups and the Big Five personality dimensions. *Journal of Organizational Behavior, 17,* 349–362.

Thoms, P., & Venkataraman, R. R. (2002). Relation of managers' personality to accident and injury rates. *Psychological Reports, 91,* 1107–1115.

Törnroos, M., Hintsanen, M., Hintsa, T., Jokela, M., Pulkki-Råback, L., Hutri-Kähönen, N., & Keltikangas-Järvinen, L. (2013). Associations between Five-Factor Model traits and perceived job strain: A population-based study. *Journal of Occupational Health Psychology, 18,* 492–500.

Vodanovich, S., & Kass, S. (1990). A factor analytic study of the boredom proneness scale. *Journal of Personality Assessment, 55,* 115–123.

Vodanovich, S. J., Wallace, J. C., & Kass, S. J. (2005). A confirmatory approach to the factor structure of the boredom proneness scale: Evidence for a two-factor short form. *Journal of Personality Assessment, 85,* 295–303.

Vredenburgh, A. G. (2002). Organizational safety: Which management practices are most effective in reducing employee injury rates? *Journal of Safety Research, 33,* 259–276.

Wallace, C., & Chen, G. (2006). A multilevel integration of personality, climate, self-regulation, and performance. *Personnel Psychology, 59,* 529–557.

Wallace, J. C., & Vodanovich, S. J. (2003). Workplace safety performance: Conscientiousness, cognitive failure, and their interaction. *Journal of Occupational Health Psychology, 8,* 316–327.

Watt, J. D., & Hargis, M. B. (2010). Boredom proneness: Its relationship with subjective underemployment, perceived organizational support, and job performance. *Journal of Business and Psychology, 25,* 163–174.

Weiss, H. M., & Cropanzano, R. (1996). Affective events theory: A theoretical discussion of the structure, causes and consequences of affective experiences at work. In B. M. Staw & L. L. Cummings (Eds.), *Research in organizational behavior: An annual series of analytical essays and critical reviews* (pp. 1–74). Greenwich, CT: JAI Press.

Weller, J. A., & Tikir, A. (2011). Predicting domain-specific risk taking with the HEXACO personality structure. *Journal of Behavioral Decision Making, 24,* 180–201.

Wong, M., Gardiner, E., Lang, W., & Coulon, L. (2008). Generational differences in personality and motivation: Do they exist and what are the implications for the workplace? *Journal of Managerial Psychology, 23,* 878–890.

Woo, S. E., Chernyshenko, O. S., Stark, S. E., & Conz, G. (2014). Validity of six openness facets in predicting work behaviors: A meta-analysis. *Journal of Personality Assessment, 96,* 76–86.

Yang, R., (2014). *Generational and cultural effects on personality using the Hogan Personality Inventory and Hogan Development Survey.* Tulsa, OK: Hogan Assessment Systems.

Ziegler, M., Bensch, D., Maaß, U., Schult, V., Vogel, M., & Bühner, M. (2014). Big Five facets as predictor of job training performance: The role of specific job demands. *Learning and Individual Differences, 29*, 1–7.

Zierold, K. M., Welsh, E. C., & McGeeney, T. J. (2012). Attitudes of teenagers towards workplace safety training. *Journal of Community Health, 37*, 1289–1295.

4

The Influence of Peer Norms

Sílvia Agostinho Silva and Carla Santos Fugas

Humans, as social beings, interact and react to the surrounding social context that shapes the construction of meaning and provides a framework for socially acceptable beliefs, attitudes, needs, individual reasoning, and actions. The social context is, therefore, very important in setting work routines but in new or ambiguous work circumstances its impact will be even greater. Additionally, it is also recognized that the more similar someone is to us, the bigger the impact this person will have on determining our understanding of our environment.

The potential effects of organizational groups on the beliefs, attitudes, and behaviors of their members have been recognized since Hawthorne and Tavistock's classical studies (Hackman, 1992). Groups are used by individuals as sources of data about external reality, especially when other relevant data are not available, and also about themselves.[1] Festinger (1954) suggested that when what constitutes appropriate behavior is uncertain, people come to rely increasingly more on social reality. In an ambiguous situation, the actions of others provide guidelines for behavior. This has become more important recently in modern workplaces, characterized by uncertainty and changes in work design (Tesluk & Quigley, 2003). However, only in the last decade, has a fundamental shift begun as groups, instead of individuals, emerge as a critical unit of analysis in relation to health and safety. Organization and management have also brought new challenges with regard to workers' health and safety.

Although regulatory efforts can make a difference to compliance with formal health and safety rules, this difference is often dwarfed by the influence of social factors. First, in the next sections, an overview of the literature focused on social influence and norms in an attempt to understand more about the normative influences on health and safety, is provided. Second, the role of coworkers as important informational reference groups in influencing health and safety behaviors is discussed.

The Wiley Blackwell Handbook of the Psychology of Occupational Safety and Workplace Health, First Edition. Edited by Sharon Clarke, Tahira M. Probst, Frank Guldenmund, and Jonathan Passmore. © 2016 John Wiley & Sons Ltd. Published 2020 by John Wiley & Sons Ltd.

Social Influence and Norms in the Literature on Organizational and Social Psychology

Social influence is an interpersonal process that changes group members' thoughts, feelings, and behaviors. Influence research began as an attempt to explain group psychology. Social norms are a central theoretical construct that have a long tradition in the field of social psychology, referring to so many of the phenomena and processes included in this discipline. Several theories have developed the assumptions that support this normative approach (e.g., Festinger, 1954; Fishbein & Ajzen, 1975; Latané & L'Herrou, 1996). An overall summary is presented in Table 4.1.

Table 4.1 Theoretical models with critical contributions to the Social Norms Theory.

Theory designation	*Main assumptions*	*Authors*
Social Comparison Theory	Social influence processes stem directly from the drive for self-evaluation and the need for such evaluation being based on comparison with other people.	Festinger, 1954
Theory of Reasoned Action Theory of Planned Behavior	Subjective norms are significant predictors of behavioral intentions. Perceiving that one's social referents expect one to engage in a behavior, should result in a greater likelihood of engaging in that behavior.	Fishbein & Ajzen, 1975; Ajzen, 1991
Integrative Theory of Intergroup Conflict	Real conflicts of group interests not only create antagonistic intergroup relations but also heighten identification with, and positive attachment to, the in-group. The individuals who are members of the opposing groups will behave toward each other as a function of their respective group memberships, rather than in terms of their individual characteristics or inter-individual relationships.	Tajfel, & Turner, 1979
Social Impact Theory	The impact of any source of influence depends on the strength, immediacy, and number of influences involved.	Latané, 1981
Problem Behavior Theory	All behavior emerges out of the structure and interaction of three systems: the behavior (problem and conventional behavior), personality (motivational-instigation, personal belief, and personal control structures), and the perceived environment (distal and proximal structures).	Donovan, Jessor, & Jessor, 1983
Social Identification Theory; Self-categorization Theory	When people define and evaluate themselves in terms of a self-inclusive social category, the joint processes of categorization and self-enhancement come into play. Categorization perceptually accentuates differences between the in-group and out-group and similarities among in-group members (including self) on stereotypical dimensions. Social identity theory was extended to focus more specifically on the role of the categorization process.	Turner, 1982, 1985

Social Learning Theory	People can learn new information and behaviors by watching other people (observational learning, vicarious reinforcement, or modeling).	Bandura, 1986
Focus Theory of Normative Conduct	The impact of social norms on human action can only be properly recognized when researchers separate two types of norms: injunctive norms (what most others approve or disapprove of) and descriptive norms (what most others do); and norms should motivate behavior primarily when they are activated.	Cialdini, Reno, & Kallgren, 1990
Choice Process Theory	People become more emotionally attached to groups which strengthen their generalized sense of control.	Lawler, 1992
Dynamic Social Impact Theory	Extension of the social impact theory. Culture is created and shaped by local social influence as defined by four phenomena: clustering, or regional differences in cultural elements; correlation, or emergent associations between elements; consolidation, or a reduction in variance and continuing diversity.	Latané & L'Herrou, 1996
Subjective Group Dynamics	Subjective group dynamics arise when people respond to deviant individuals within groups in a context involving comparisons between their in-group and an out-group.	Marques, Páez, & Abrams, 1998
Social Norms Theory	People are highly influenced by what they think their peers are doing or thinking and then conform to what they believe is the norm, or social expectation. This perception can cause people to overestimate problem behaviors and underestimate healthy behaviors. These misperceptions tend to increase problem behaviors and decrease healthy behaviors because people act in agreement with what they think is the norm.	Berkowitz, 2003; Perkins, 2003
Theory of Normative Social Behavior	Perceiving that many others engage in a behavior (strong descriptive norms) is likely to motivate individuals to engage in the same behavior if they also believe that social pressures exist to conform (strong injunctive norms).	Rimal, Lapinski, Cook, & Real, 2005

Classic researchers (e.g., Allport, 1924; Asch, 1952; Newcomb, 1953, 1954; and Sheriff, 1936, 1956) confirmed the principle that groups influence their members when they discovered that people's attitudes and outlooks changed when the group's attitudes and outlooks also changed. However, social influence also flows from the individual to the group.

As originally conceived, social norms not only drive behavior but also guide it in direct and meaningful ways. Norms are constructed by evaluating information from three sources: observable behavior, direct (what words mean), and indirect (what words imply) communications and knowledge of the self (Borsari & Carey, 2008). Larimer and

Neighbors' (2003) research indicates that misperceptions of social norms (such as, the *false consensus effect*, Marks & Miller, 1987; the *false uniqueness effect*, Miller & McFarland, 1991; and the *pluralist ignorance*, Prentice & Miller, 1993) may be just as important as accurate norms in influencing individuals' behavior in social groups. These misperceptions occur in relation to problem or risk behaviors, and in relation to healthy or protective behaviors. Workers tend to underestimate their own problem or risk behaviors and to overestimate their healthy or protective behaviors. Thus, correcting misperceptions is likely to result in decreased problem behavior or an increased prevalence of pro-normative behaviors (Rimal, Lapinski, Cook, & Real, 2005).

Several theoretical approaches sustain the normative approach and play a critical role in the understanding of normative conceptualizations, processes, and impacts (see Table 4.1). However, there is, as yet, no definitive scientific theory of social norms and little is known about how and under what conditions social norms affect behaviors (Rimal, 2008).

Conceptualization of social norms

Despite being highly endorsed social influence still continues to raise important concerns. There is a great deal of conceptual ambiguity surrounding the meaning of norms. Researchers have used a myriad of terms to describe the term *norms*.[2] The theory of planned behavior (TPB; Ajzen, 1991), an extension of the theory of reasoned action (TRA; Ajzen & Fishbein, 1980) and one of the most influential theories for the prediction of social and health behaviors conceptualizes social influence in terms of *subjective norm* or pressure that people perceive from important others to exhibit, or not exhibit, a behavior. Subjective norms determined by beliefs about the extent to which important others want them to exhibit a behavior or normative beliefs (e.g., "My coworkers think I should use individual protective equipment") are multiplied by one's motivation to comply with those people's views (e.g., "I generally want to do what my coworkers think I should do"). Subjective norms are proposed to influence behavior through their impact upon intentions (e.g., "I intend to use individual protective equipment"). However, social pressure is rarely so direct or explicit, leading a number of researchers to suggest alternative conceptualizations.

There is an important distinction between two types of social norms. On the one hand, the perception of what is commonly done in a given situation, or *informational influence* and, on the other hand, the perception of what is commonly approved or disapproved of within the culture, or *normative influence* (Deutsch & Gerard, 1955). According to the focus theory of normative conduct (Cialdini, Kallgren, & Reno, 1991; Cialdini, Reno, & Kallgren, 1990; Cialdini & Trost, 1998; Reno, Cialdini, & Kallgren, 1993) the former, corresponds to *descriptive norms* (the norm of the "*is*"), and the latter, to *injunctive norms* (the norm of the "*ought*"). The subjective norm component of the TPB is an injunctive norm because it is related to perceived social pressure. Thus, norms are descriptive, reflecting similarities and also prescriptive, reflecting shared beliefs about appropriate behavior. Two premises are worth noting: first, norms guide action directly only when they are focal (Kallgren, Reno, & Cialdini, 2000), and, second, activating one or the other of the two types of norms produces significantly different behavioral responses (Reno et al., 1993).

Descriptive norms have been extensively emphasized by several prominent social theories of behavior or behavior change, such as: the social learning theory (Bandura, 1986), the problem behavior theory (Donovan, Jessor, & Jessor, 1983) and the social comparison theory (Festinger, 1954). Nevertheless, these theories do not consider descriptive and injunctive norms acting in concert, even though each is likely to be conceptually and motivationally separate and presumably affect behaviors differently (Cialdini et al., 1990;

Rivis & Sheeran, 2003). Ajzen and Fishbein (2005) recommended including both types of normative measures in constructing planned behavior surveys.

The lack of distinction in the literature between these two types of social influence has led to inconsistencies in evaluating normative influences on behavior. Thus, attempting to clarify its conceptualization appears to have some preliminary usefulness for formulating and investigating problems in the health and safety domain.

Social norms influence processes

Social influence results from discovering new information about a situation by observing others' responses and normative influence causes us to feel, think, and act in ways that are consistent with the group's norm (Deutsch & Gerard, 1955). Group norms are informal rules that groups adopt to regulate group members' behavior (Feldman, 1984). These norms may or may not be formal, written, or unwritten (Cialdini, Bator, & Guadagno, 1999). Some groups enforce norms about work behavior that are consistent with the organization's policies, but others do not.

The idea of a norm conveys a feeling of *"oughtness"* about certain behaviors. In this case, the underlying social influence process is probably *public compliance* based on a need for social approval and acceptance (Miniard & Cohen, 1981). The *principle of social proof* (Cialdini, 2001) posits that it is usually in the individual's interest to follow group norms because doing so is beneficial for the individual's survival. Reinforcement of group norms is often achieved by derogating in-group members who deviate from their group's norms (the "black sheep" effect). Members who consistently violate their group's norms are often disliked, assigned lower job status, and in some cases dismissed from the group (Schachter, 1951). Abrams and colleagues (Abrams, Marques, Bown, & Henson, 2000) found that in-group anti-norm deviants were evaluated less favorably than other in-group members and out-group anti-norm deviants who expressed the same attitude. However, individuals obey norms not only because they fear the negative interpersonal consequences resulting from non-conformity, but also to fulfill their own expectations about proper behavior (Turner, 1991). Norms are not simply external constraints but internalized standards. Further, according to Christensen, Rothgerber, Wood, and Matz (2004), compliance with descriptive norms emanating from one's social referents can result in positive emotions. Thus, there are both affective and cognitive motivations for perceiving that one has to conform to group behavior.

Furthermore, individuals construct meaningful and coherent definitions of social situations and validate their conclusions differently, by comparing themselves to others. Traditionally, this type of social influence occurs when individuals internalize and privately accept information from others because the information provides a basis for correct perceptions, attitudes, and beliefs (Asch, 1952; Deutsch & Gerard, 1955; Kelley, 1952). However, people frequently ignore or severely underestimate the extent to which their actions in a situation are determined by the similar actions of others (Cialdini, 2005, 2007). Informational influence also capitalizes on people's willingness to make use of *heuristics* when they make decisions (such as, *"to get along, go along"*). Dual-process models of social cognition suggest that when cognitive resources are limited or when individuals are not motivated to do the cognitive work necessary to weigh up the information available to them, they rely on heuristics, simplifying inferential principles or rules of thumb that generate decisions efficiently (Forsyth, 2013).

The second issue highlighted by the literature on norms is that a social norm does not exist for each and every particular behavior, situation, or group of interacting people. We must think in terms of degrees of *norm-ness* or the process of normative regulation, rather than in terms of a norm as a "thing". The process of perceiving norms is a relational process between two structures, the cognitive structure of the perceiver and the structure of the object perceived. In certain areas a transgression is punished severely, in others it seems to be of little concern. The strength of that influence depends on the nature of the group situation. The characteristics of the situation in which the process of perceiving norms occurs should also be taken into consideration. It should be remembered that we are dealing only with an analogy between a person perceiving an object, in the context of a situation, and an Actor "cognizing" a norm-system constituted by others' role expectations, in the situation generated by a social system. The Return Potential Model (RPM) highlighted that "norms differ greatly with respect to the intensity of approval or disapproval evoked by appropriate or inappropriate behavior" (Jackson, 1965, p. 305). In certain areas of behavior, a transgression is punished severely, in others there seems to be little concern from members of a group concerning how individuals behave. The concept of crystallization measures the degree to which a norm "exists" in a group. When intensity is very low, presumably, there is no norm for that type of behavior. Another condition that might signify the absence of a norm is when there is little agreement among the members of a group in regard to a given area of behavior. Crystallization is a measure of the degree of agreement or consensus that a group has about the amount of approval or disapproval associated to a given area of behavior. High crystallization signifies a great deal of consensus, and low crystallization indicates an absence of consensus. However, the members of a social system may agree in their indifference. A combination of high intensity and high crystallization indicates that the members of the system would feel strongly about the behavior in question and would be in agreement about their feelings (Jackson, 1965). When intensity and crystallization are high, univocal forces or influences are likely to be generated to "push" individuals' behavior in the group-valued direction.

Influence referents

The reference groups are very important in the acquisition of social norms and changing an individual's attitudes and behaviors. The reference groups are groups that are psychologically significant to the individual's attitudes and behaviors. The more credible the reference group is as a source of information about reality, the greater the group's influence on the individual will be. The reference group can have a *comparative* basis, in which the individual compares with others to assess his situation and attributes and a *normative* function in which the individual appropriates the values and norms of the group.

The use of a wide variety of possible informational reference groups and the need to understand their respective influence on personal behaviors has plagued research on social norms for decades. Referent informational influence links norms to specific groups, and these norms have their effect because the group is relevant to the behavioral context. According to Terry, Hogg, and White (1999), norms should focus the referent group on those that are most relevant in the context that is being considered.

Terry and colleagues (e.g., Terry & Hogg, 1996; Terry, Hogg & White, 1999), drawing on self-categorization (e.g., Turner, 1985; Turner, Hogg, Oakes, Reicher, & Wetherell, 1987) and social identity theories (e.g., Hogg & Abraams, 1988; Tajfel & Turner, 1979; Turner, 1982) have shown that identification with a behaviorally relevant group moderates the effects of group norms on the consistency of attitude-behavior. When a social identity is salient, people construct a context-specific group norm from the shared social comparative information that is available. Subjectively, this norm is represented as a group prototype that describes and prescribes beliefs, attitudes, feelings, and behaviors that optimally minimize in-group differences and maximize inter-group differences (*principle of meta-contrast*) (Terry, Hogg, & Duck, 1999). The cognitive process of self-categorization means that there is an assimilation of self to the prototype. In this sense, norms are properties of groups that influence people through self-categorization, rather than simply for social approval in a public context, as implied by the conceptualization of norms from a normative influence approach. The subjective group dynamics (SGD) framework proposes that group members use intragroup differentiation not just to judge the group prototypes, but also to reinforce prescriptive in-group norms (Abrams, Moura, Marques, & Hutchison, 2008).

An individual's behavior is most influenced by individuals that are highly similar to the self, share an important category membership with the self, are referent others, and place the self in a positive light (Miller and Prentice, 1996). Norms from more proximal groups ("*local norms*") are presumably more relevant than from more distal groups ("*global norms*"). A key corollary to the premise that groups influence their members is that the impact of group members on one another depends on their strength or status in the group. According to Sullivan's concept of *parataxic distortion,* the perceiver's past history of relationships with significant figures, as represented in personality, interacts with the relationship between Actor and Other in an immediate situation to produce the resultant perception (Sullivan, 1947). Also, more immediate experience should facilitate an individual's ability to perceive the others' role expectations more accurately. An individual's position in the social structure also affects the volume and type of information available. The greater the amount of information the workers have previously obtained regarding others, the type of activity involved, and in general the social system in which a role is located, the greater their accuracy of perceiving it will be.

Latané's *social impact theory* (Latané, 1981) proposes that when individuals identify the people who have the most impact on them, and as the concept of *immediacy* suggests, these people will be the most influential. In a word, the higher the immediacy, the more influential that person or people will be. Additionally, the dynamic social impact theory (Latané & L' Herrou, 1996), an extension of the social impact theory, explains that people are more influenced by their closest neighbors, and so clusters of group members with similar opinions emerge in groups. *Clustering* is more likely when group members communicate more frequently with members who are close by and less frequently with more distant group members.

Examples of research on norms in the organizational context

A number of studies have been done in the work context revealing the relevance of peer norms for various individual cognitive, affective behavior, and performance outcomes, over the last 30 years. For instance revealing that group norms and coworker norms are important to explaining job satisfaction (O'Reilly & Caldwell, 1985), performance (e.g., Lichtman & Lane, 1983), absenteeism (e.g., Bamberger & Biron, 2007; Biron & Bamberger, 2012), substance abuse (e.g., Bacharach et al., 2007; Frone, 2009; Biron, Bamberger, & Noyman, 2011), intentions and behaviors (e.g., Bang, 2012; Ehrhart & Naumann, 2004; Potocnik, Tordera, & Peiró, 2009; Obschonka et al., 2012; Roberts & Barrett, 2011; Schmidtke, 2007; Whitby et al., 2007), social relations (Thommes, Akkerman, Torenvlied, & Born, 2014), and fit perceptions (e.g., Cooper-Thomas & Wright, 2013). Some of these studies are illustrated below.

There are three contributions highlighting the influence of norms on performance. Lichtman and Lane (1983) conducted the first study that revealed that workgroup norms influenced individual productivity, thus combining the goal setting theory with the social influence theory. A confederate coworker had a critical role in the goal setting and goal feedback in this research. Other studies also made an important contribution to understanding group norms on group effectiveness and efficacy. For instance, by suggesting group task norms as moderators between group cohesiveness and group effectiveness (Langfred & Shanley, 1997; Shanley & Langfred, 1998), namely that high cohesiveness and strong task norms lead to higher group effectiveness (quality and accuracy of the work and the efficiency of unit operations) in military work groups. In another study, the social categorization theory was applied in order to understand the impact of cooperative norms, suggesting that cooperative norms function as a mediator in the relationship between group composition and work outcomes. This was tested both at the individual level and group level (Chatman & Flynn, 2001). It was observed that groups with higher heterogeneity (demographic) led to group norms of lower cooperation, which had a mediation impact on satisfaction and team efficiency and effectiveness. However, this effect changed (becoming lower) over time, due to contacts between members.

In the health domain, the main concern was about the role of norms on substance abuse. For instance, in the USA, Frone (2009) studied the multiple dimensions of the climate of workplace substance abuse that covered substance availability, workplace descriptive norms, and workplace injunctive norms. These climate characteristics were considered as predictors of perceived workplace safety, work strain, and employee morale among employees who do not use alcohol or drugs at work. The results showed that all three dimensions of workplace substance abuse were negatively related to workplace safety, positively related to work strain, and negatively related to employee morale. These results emphasize the relevance of permissive norms about substance abuse at work. In another study about substance abuse, in Israel, Biron et al. (2011) studied the existence of higher substance abuse among those perceiving (a) more permissive drinking norms, (b) lower supervisor ability to handle substance abuse problems, (c) greater exposure to job hazards, and (d) lower levels of coworker interactions. The findings also revealed that permissive drinking norms moderated the associations between the other risk factors and substance abuse, for instance, greater encouragement to use alcohol as a means of tension reduction may occur if employees perceive tolerant norms for drinking.

Research on absenteeism has also highlighted the role of group norms. Bamberger and Biron's (2007) results supported the idea that referent group norms about absenteeism significantly explain excessive absence behavior. Their study also revealed that permissive referent group norms are likely to have a greater impact on the probability of the individual displaying excessive absence when the individual has a more conformist nature. Furthermore, more negative perceptions of the consequences of absenteeism were associated with a lower impact of permissive group norms on excessive absence behavior. Later these authors tested the moderator role of peer absence group norms (Biron et al., 2012). In this study, perceived job hazards and exposure to critical incidents were positively related to subsequent absenteeism, but only under the conditions of more permissive peer absence norms. Moreover, this positive impact of peer norms on absenteeism was amplified among those employees perceiving their supervisor to be less supportive but was attenuated among those viewing their supervisor as more supportive.

In some studies the TPB model was applied to the explanation of intentions. For instance, one study in the Netherlands showed that the attitude toward training participation, subjective norms on training participation, and perceived behavioral control over participating in training had a role in stimulating lower educated workers' training intentions (Sanders, Oomens, Blonk, & Hazelzet, 2011). In another study Obschonka,

Goethner, Silbereisen, and Cantner (2012) combined the TPB with group identification in the understanding of entrepreneurial intentions. Namely, they observed that those were predicted by attitude, social norms, and perceived control and that group identification was negatively associated with perceived control. Additionally, their findings also show that group identification moderated the TPB-intention link. Participants with low group identification based their entrepreneurial intentions not so much on social norms and attitudes but on their own self-initiative and control beliefs. However, entrepreneurial intentions were mainly a function of social norms among participants with high group identification.

Overall, these studies cover very different contexts and focused on specific norms. Most focus at the individual level of analysis and only in some exceptions were they focused at the group level and only occasionally were the coworkers explicitly focused on.

Impact of Coworkers' Norms on Safety and Health at Work

Research in the past 30 years has revealed strong evidence of the impact of peers' norms on health, risk, and safety behaviors in social and health psychology literature, for instance, in promoting environmental preservation behaviors like not littering (e.g., Cialdini et al., 1990), health behaviors like eating well and doing exercise (e.g. Yun & Silk, 2011), inhibiting risk behaviors like smoking (e.g., Vitória, Salgueiro, Silva, & De Vries, 2009, 2011) and driving-related risk behaviors (e.g. Cestac, Paran, & Delhomme, 2011; Cestac, Delhomme, & Paran, 2014; Lajunen & Räsänen, 2004) across generations. Most of these studies used the planned behavior theory (Ajzen, 1991; Ajzen & Fishbein, 2000; 2005) to frame the normative approach.

In this domain, a well-established body of research argues for the consideration of coworkers as a psychologically significant reference group in the behavioral domain of health and safety. Through social interactions between workers who are related to each other psychologically, informational referent groups give rise to shared pro-normative health and safety behaviors and, in that sense, social norms can improve the health and safety of groups and their members. The influence exercised by people at the same level/ status is becoming increasingly important in contemporary worksite settings.

Coworkers are not only a vital element, but they define the work environment (Schneider, 1987). At the group level, coworkers have often been referred to as having a great influence in promoting an environment supportive of health and safety. For instance, coworkers can serve as vehicles for learning, creating, and transmitting knowledge and, by being decentralized structures, coworker groups are more open to sharing and asking for help, and experimenting (Tesluk & Quigley, 2003). Nevertheless, the role of group, and especially coworkers' norms, has been significantly understudied (Fugas, Meliá, & Silva, 2011, 2013; Fugas, Silva, & Meliá, 2012) creating a need for researchers and practitioners to pay more attention to this aspect of safety.

Workers typically feel more committed to their coworkers, than to their organizations, supervisors, or senior managers (Becker, 1992; Lawler, 1992). In fact, the literature on substitutes for leadership (Kerr & Jermier, 1978) has indicated that certain characteristics of subordinates (e.g., experience, skills, and training), the task (e.g., unambiguous, routine), and the organization (e.g., formalization, inflexibility, spatial distance between superiors and subordinates) might reduce the importance of leaders. When people know what to do, how to do it, when they do it, and are rewarded for doing so, the importance of leadership may be reduced (Hofmann & Morgeson, 2002; see also Wong, Kelloway & Makhan, Chapter 5, this volume). It is likely that workers interact more frequently with their coworkers than with supervisors, either because they are more often present during the regular performance of tasks, or because they have the same status, a condition that increases the likelihood of social interaction. Despite their influence, coworkers' norms have received less systematic attention than the influence of managers and so their influence on the workers' behavior has been little explored. The literature on the influence of coworkers is fragmented and numerous questions about the influence of coworkers remain unanswered (Chiaburu & Harrison, 2008).

The discussion that follows focuses on the role of coworkers as a source of important informational referent group norms that affect health and safety in organizations.

Social influences on safety and health

Theories, and their related empirical approach to social norms, have been increasingly used to help formulate a safer and healthier organizational culture, resulting in fewer illnesses, accidents, and injuries. Safety influence literature has essentially been dominated by models that emphasize safety climate, safety leadership, and supervisor and coworker social support (see Guediri & Griffin, Chapter 13; Luria, Chapter 16; Wong, Kelloway & Makhan, Chapter 5, this volume) but, in the last 10 years, a good number of studies covering peer normative influence have been conducted.

Workers know they "*ought*" to comply with safety rules, orders, and standardized procedures, engage in safety initiatives and safety-related citizenship behaviors. They feel compelled to act, in order to maintain health and safety, to prevent accidents and injuries because of sanctions resulting from nonconformity with the peer group. Some groups have a higher degree of normative regulation than others (e.g., nuclear power plant and chemical plant control room teams, surgical teams, and flight crews), reflecting the priority and value of safety to the organization. A significant determinant of the workers' perception of norms is the degree and type of organization being perceived. Coworkers exert control and influence the work environment and act as key players in defining the safety culture of the organization (Grant & Ashford, 2008; see also Guediri & Griffin, Chapter 13; Guldenmund, Chapter 19, this volume). Coworkers also play an important role in initiating and reinforcing both positive and negative safety behaviors. Coworkers' descriptive norms provide a standard from which workers do not want to deviate and act as a magnet for the workers' behavior both above and below the norm. Thus, when coworkers demonstrate a positive orientation toward health and safety, coworkers' perceived descriptive norms can reduce an undesirable behavior (e.g., safety procedure violations) among workers who exhibit that behavior, at a rate above the norm and increase the undesirable behavior among individuals who exhibit that behavior at a rate below the norm.

According to Turner, Chmiel, Hershcovis, and Walls (2010), when coworkers espouse the importance of safe work practices they are reinforcing safe practices and teaching workers that such practices are valued and expected, that is, they are providing opportunities for vicarious learning. If workers receive social cues from coworkers that safety is important, they are more likely to act in accordance with this social information. Therefore, it is recognized that although the organizational context and supervisors are very important for promoting safety and health behaviors at work, there is also a compelling and critical need to include the focus on peers/coworkers. Additionally, it is assumed that a coworker may play an even more critical role if the specific characteristics of the work context, degree of interdependence, interaction frequency, and worker identification, are taken into consideration.

Influence of peer norms on risk and preventive behavior

In the last 16 years studies have been undertaken to understand normative influence on many types of risk and preventive behavior, for instance: risk taking, safety violations, specific safety behaviors (e.g., safe lifting, hoist usage, hand hygiene), intentions, general safety compliance behaviors or safety proactive/participative behaviors (e.g., Colémont & Van den Broucke, 2008; Cullen & Hammer, 2007; Fogarty & Shaw, 2010; Fugas, Meliá, & Silva, 2011; Hinsz, Nickell, & Park, 2007; Jiang, Yu, Li, & Li, 2010; Lawton, 1998; Quick et al., 2008; Singer, Lin, Falwell, Gaba, & Baker, 2009; Sorensen et al., 2011) .

Lawton (1998) presented the first paper that focused on the role of group norms on safety issues, with the intention of distinguishing errors from violations and that was also an attempt to propose a model for understanding violating behavior. In this paper, the author specifically identifies: erroneous violations, situational and exceptional violations, and also routine violations. The theoretical model proposed represents a hierarchy of factors promoting violations which have three main causes, namely: attitudes/motivation, situation/control and rules/knowledge which are explained by organizational culture, organizational and situational factors, and group norms (rules derived from individuals belonging to work groups).

In 2003, Sheeran and Silverman evaluated psychological interventions that were intended to increase attendance at workplace health and safety training courses. The research design considered three intervention types: a motivational intervention based on the theory of planned behavior (thus including norms), a volitional approach for supporting implementation intentions, and a combined intervention (motivational and volitional). The motivational intervention contemplated attitudes, subjective norms, and perceived behavioral control regarding training for increasing intentions to attend. The volitional intervention was aimed at increasing the likelihood of attendance by specifying when and where the training courses would take place. The subjective norm was operationalized in a traditional way with the statement, "Most people who are important to me think that I should attend a university fire training course in the next three months." The experiment was conducted with employees from a large UK university and who had the opportunity to attend a training course related to health and safety (e.g., fire training course). Results showed that the volitional and combined interventions doubled the rate of attendance compared with the motivational and control conditions.

In a study done in a manufacturing company in the USA, Johnson and Hall (2005) conducted the first research applying the theory of planned behavior and including subjective norms to explain a specific safety behavior, safe-lifting behavior. Three items were used to measure subjective norms in this study. For example, "Most people who are important to me would strongly encourage/discourage me to lift materials within my strike zone." Findings revealed that all the variables were important to explain the safe-lifting behavior, both in terms of direct and indirect effects. Perceived behavioral control and intention were the strongest predictors of safe-lifting behavior and subjective norms were also important (although with a lower impact) to explaining intention and behavior (self-reported). Attitudes were not direct predictors but affected behavior and intent via mediating factors (subjective norms and perceived behavioral control). The theory of planned behavior was supported as an effective model explaining safe-lifting behavior. The operationalization of subjective norms did not focus on a specific referent but covered a wider group, "people that are important to me," in this study.

Mullen (2005) proposed a model linking employee willingness to raise safety issues and the contextual variables, Namely, suggesting that the perceived probability of success when raising safety issues and the perception of risk to one's image due to having that initiative would influence employee willingness to raise a safety issue. In turn, perceived organizational support, top management openness, and norms favoring issue identification would affect the employees' perceived probability of success and their perceived image risk. This model was tested in the manufacturing and service industries in Canada. *Perceived norms* were assessed using three items developed by Ashford et al. (1998) that assess norms regarding the communication of issues. The items were slightly modified to ensure that they were appropriate for assessing safety. The items included, "In this organization, safety issues are kept under the table," and "People seldom raise safety issues in this organization."

Top management openness and the norms favoring raising issues were significant predictors of an individual's perceived probability of success and an individual's perceived probability of successfully raising an issue, will be related to his/her willingness to raise an issue. This was indicated by statements such as: "I am confident that I could get management to pay attention to the safety issue," and "I am confident that I could successfully identify the safety issue in my organization." Perceived probability of success, in turn, predicted an individual's willingness to raise a safety issue.

The first empirical study specifically focusing on coworkers' safety norms was carried out by Watson, Scott, Bishop, and Turnbeaugh (2005). This study was conducted in an American company in the steel industry, the predictors of risk behavior and perceived work environment safety considered: trust in the supervisor, coworker safety norms, and management safety values. Coworkers' influence was assessed with four items that measure descriptive norms. The results revealed that employee norms predicted both perceptions of work environment safety and at-risk behavior and trust in supervisor predicted perceptions of a safe work environment, while belief in the management's safety values predicted at-risk behaviors.

In the same year, Westaby and Lowe (2005) published another very innovative paper about young workers' risk-taking orientation and injury by distinguishing different sources of influence and using a longitudinal approach. In this study the authors examined how three sources of social influence (i.e., supervisory, coworker, and parental) had an impact on youths' risk-taking orientation and injury across a wide variety of jobs for youths. Coworker risk taking was assessed using two items that covered perceptions of risk taking among coworkers: "Other people take risks at work" and "My coworkers take risks". The sample included young workers working in various sectors of activity in the USA. Results confirmed the relevance of the social influence variables and also revealed that coworker risk taking was a stronger predictor of risk-taking orientation than supervisory influence.

Rickett, Orbell, and Sheeran's (2006) study is about social-cognitive determinants of hoist usage in two hospitals in the UK. The hypothesis considered person and organization characteristics and motivational variables. In this study the authors considered injunctive norms with a focus on staff coworkers and injunctive norms held by patients as part of the motivational variables. The coworkers injunctive norms were assessed by one item: "How do you think other people who work with you on the wards would react to your using a hoist every time you transfer a dependent patent from sitting to standing in the next 6 weeks?" using two bipolar scales, *discouraging–encouraging* (a) and *unsupportive–supportive* (b). The findings showed that the biographical, occupational context, and motivational variables explained the intention to use a hoist, and intention, in turn, explained the hoist use reported six weeks later. Results revealed that safety practices in the workplace, and particularly hoist use, appear to be normatively driven in that they require negotiation and the support of coworkers and patients and are carried out in a social setting.

More recently, Fogarty and Shaw's (2010) study applied TPB and included group norms for predicting the intention to violate and actual violations. The study was conducted with the Australian Defense Force (Army, Air Force, and Navy) or civilian contractors working for the Australian Defense Force. Seven items were used to measure the participants' perceptions of group safety norms in their study. These items focused on the respondents' beliefs about usual group practices in relation to violations; for example, "Other people in my workplace violate procedures." Findings highlighted the importance of management attitudes and group norms as direct and indirect predictors of violation behavior. This suggests that TPB is a useful tool for understanding the psychological background to the procedural violations often associated with incidents and accidents. In this study, group norms had a strong influence on individual attitudes, violation intentions, and actual violation.

In Portugal, Fugas and colleagues (Fugas, Meliá, & Silva, 2011, 2013; Fugas, Silva, & Melia, 2012) developed a research project that considered socio-cognitive predictors of safety behaviors. This research was also innovative since the authors distinguished the coworkers' descriptive norms from the injunctive norms and also the referents of the group norms (supervisors and coworkers). In 2011 the longitudinal study demonstrated the differences between the supervisors' and coworkers' descriptive and injunctive norms as sources of social influence on compliance and proactive safety behavior. Later, in 2012, these authors showed that the relationship between the organizational safety climate and proactive safety behaviors was mediated by coworkers' descriptive norms and attitudes toward safety. More recently, Fugas, Meliá, and Silva (2013) have revealed in a multivariate profile analysis that the perceived behavioral control was shown to be the variable that best differentiated the groups with safer behaviors from the others. However, results also indicated that coworkers' descriptive safety norms were a major differentiating variable in proactive safety behaviors.

Overall, this body of research has revealed a significant number of studies supporting the significance of normative influence and clearly supporting the significant role of peers for safety and health. This research has been conducted worldwide but is still dominated by American studies that correspond to around 40 percent of the total. The samples cover very different contexts, primary, secondary, and tertiary activity sectors, namely, the service sector (e.g., education, insurance, healthcare), the manufacturing industry (e.g., manufacturing, construction), and the extracting sector (e.g., agriculture). Almost all the studies are intended to understand and predict behaviors, but one study tested intervention approaches. This literature is dominated by an emphasis on subjective norms and the planned behavior theory (approximately 65 percent of the studies).

Furthermore, some diversity in the operationalization of the normative influence is also clear when considering the referent focus (e.g., workers in general, peers, coworkers, workgroups, teams); the type of norms assessed with "simpler" approaches (subjective norms only) or more complete approaches (descriptive and injunctive norms); and normative strength (consensus, crystallization).

Future Research

Considering the state of the art, it is clear that some challenges still exist in terms of making our understanding of the complexity of normative influence more complete. For instance, some issues that clearly require more attention are: the temporal dynamics of this type of influence, the differential and cumulative effects of different referents, levels of analysis, incongruence effects, moderators that condition the influence (e.g., the effects of personal norms), the mediation processes that best explain why these influence occur, the motivations and reasons for breaking norms, the selectivity in rule violations, what happens when norms are dysfunctional and how to change norms. These are only some examples of the opportunities for further research.

The work environment is comprised of variables related to the individual (e.g., personality characteristics, age, gender, and past work experience), workgroup (e.g., size, structure, cohesiveness, goals, and the complexity, ambiguity and importance of their tasks) and the organizational level (e.g., size, and sector/activity). Since social norms are a property of the context in which the individual works, research on social norms should use multilevel models. People who share the same work environment may or not perceive and react to it in the same way. Individual differences may be determined by their shared experiences. Because norms are unit/group properties, the focus of measurement should be at the unit level. When measuring characteristics, common to all unit workers and that have emerged over time from individual member's beliefs, values, and experiences, although these can be measured at the individual level, the study should focus on what happens at the unit level (Klein, Danserau, & Hall, 1994; Kozlowski & Klein, 2000). As has been stated before, only a few studies have taken the group level into account.

There can be all shades of blending of descriptive and injunctive norms. Both types of norms are seen to be located and embedded in the organizational culture, which can vary greatly in the degree to which it impinges upon the system of action, or social system. The incongruences between "What is done" and "What should be done" should be carefully considered by organizations. The perceived incongruences between descriptive and injunctive norms and personal norms (e.g., moral norm), and the incongruences between both and organizational norms are also of enormous empirical interest in the light of the social norms approach, but have not yet been studied. Furthermore, consideration of the organizational context suggests cross-level effects must cover different lateral and hierarchical levels of referents including coworkers (in-group and out-group coworkers), line supervisors (or shop floor supervisors), managers, and top managers, using multilevel and cascade levels (see also Luria, Chapter 16, this volume).

The use of a wide variety of possible specific reference groups, and the need to understand their respective influence on behavior, has plagued research on social norms for years (Miller & Prentice, 1996). The literature on health and safety at work is not an exception, as it uses reference groups that vary in their proximity to the individual. Research has indicated that workers' perceptions become more distorted for groups that they know less well (e.g., top management). The workers' informal peer-reference group typically consists of those individuals in whom the workers place the greatest trust, have the closest work-based bounds, and from whom workers ask for advice and support. This should also be considered in future research.

Since self-perceptions and approval of health and safety behaviors are usually higher than the judgments compared of others, the perceived discrepancies between personal behaviors and the perceived descriptive and injunctive norms of others is also an empirical challenge. Recent research suggests that self–other discrepancies in injunctive norms are larger than those for descriptive norms (Fugas, Meliá, & Silva, 2013). Further, although some evidence suggests that coworkers' descriptive safety norms foster greater proactivity concerning safety when injunctive safety norms are highly crystallized (e.g., Fugas, Meliá, & Silva, 2011), various theoretical issues remain to be formally studied. For instance, future research needs to explore whether crystallization is expected to be higher when workers actually change their minds and come to agree with the group's position (conversion or private acceptance); and inversely, whether crystallization is lower when workers privately disagree with the group, but publicly express an opinion that matches the opinions expressed by the majority of the group (compliance). In addition, research needs to consider if the consistency between descriptive and injunctive safety norms fosters the crystallization of norms.

Moreover, the moderation mechanisms linked with the interaction of social norms with the personal norms or self-identity perceptions, the role of self-categorizations and group identification considering multiple categories, should also be explored. These have already been revealed as being very important in other fields (e.g. Fekadu & Kraft, 2002; Hamilton & White, 2008; Rise, Sheernan, & Hukkelberg, 2010). Other individual variables may determine group normative influence. For instance, it has been suggested that individuals with a prevention focus motivate others to copy social norms more than individuals with a promotion focus (Zhang, Higgins, & Chen, 2011) but this has not been studied very profoundly, nor applied to the field of health and safety. Additionally, these influences should be approached while taking the workers' experience/seniority/expertise into consideration, since some studies have already shown that this variable can maximize (in less experienced workers), or minimize (in the more experienced), normative impacts (e.g., Roberto, Mearns & Silva, 2011). Another critical issue so far unexplored is what happens in the presence of social/organizational anomy. Anomic organizations are those that fail to meet a minimum set of common workplace norms (Hodson, 1999). Norms may be absent or may be more or less "moral," the "dark side" of normative influence (e.g., Robinson, Kiewitz, & Wang, 2014; Schultz, Nolan, Cialdini, Goldstein, & Griskevicius, 2007). Until now it is not clear how these situations are surpassed or not and how they may have a bigger, or smaller, impact on health and safety at work. These kinds of normative organizational contexts are critical for health and safety but still considerably understudied.

Finally, research that aims to understand how to change safety/health/risk norms should be prioritized. Approaches grounded in social and organizational psychology could be used for this purpose, as has been highlighted by recent examples focusing on the minority influence (e.g., Grant & Patil, 2012) and leadership (e.g., Abrams, Moura, Marques, & Hutchison, 2008). Finally, health and safety communication and intervention literature should also be used in order to study campaign design.

Conclusion

This chapter focused on a social influence approach, highlighting social norms and the coworkers' role, to explain workers' health and safety behavior. The basic assumption is that "People as adaptive organisms adjust their behavior and beliefs to the social context" (Salancik & Pfeffer, 1978, p. 226). The social context shapes the construction of meaning, provides a framework for socially acceptable beliefs, attitudes, needs, individual reasoning, and actions. Additionally, it is also recognized that the more similar someone is to us, the bigger the impact this person will have on determining our understanding of our environment. Most of the social interactions at work are between peers and people rely more on their coworkers than on managers to obtain information about behavior norms and standards, for opinions about the workplace, the organization, and their specific job. Coworkers play a key role in helping their peers learn *how and what to do* through ongoing modeling, practice and example. Moreover, coworkers' norms play a critical role in risk perception and management, determining which behaviors are safe or unsafe, and reinforcing those behaviors. Therefore, peer norms may influence employee safety and health in several ways, modeling beliefs, attitudes and behaviors.

The literature on the impact of situational factors on health and safety at work has been dominated by the safety climate theory with the coworkers assuming only residual importance. Although there is strong evidence of the impact of peers' norms on health, risk, and safe behaviors in social and health psychology literature, the literature on safety has not sufficiently explored coworkers as a source of normative and informative influence.

In summary, the social norms theory provides a model for understanding human behavior that has important implications for the promotion of health and safety and the prevention of accidents. Indeed, reviews of this literature document extensive evidence of the pervasiveness of the influence of coworkers. Norms about health and safety represent one potentially important, yet understudied, contextual influence on employee health and safety. Coworker effects may actually result from perceptions of the coworkers' descriptive and injunctive social norms, rather than from their actual behavior. Although significant knowledge has already been gained that emphasizes the relevance of peers' influence on safety and health at work, there are still various avenues open for innovative research, some of which have been exemplified here.

Notes

1. Cooley's (1922) use of the term *looking glass self* highlights the importance of self-knowledge gained from the actions and reactions of others.
2. Norms are also referred in the literature simply as *norms* (Gibbs, 1968; Bendor & Swistak, 2001), *social norms* (Berkowitz, 2003), *social influence* (Rice, 1993) and *normative influences* (Cialdini et al., 1990; Deutsch & Gerard, 1955).

References

Abrams, D., Marques, J. M., Bown, N. J., & Henson, M. (2000). Pro-norms and anti-norm deviance within and between groups. *Journal of Personality and Social Psychology, 78*(5), 906–912.

Abrams, D., Moura, G. R., Marques, J. M., & Hutchison, P. (2008). Innovation credit: When can leaders oppose their group's norms? *Journal of Personality and Social Psychology, 95*(3), 662–678.

Ajzen, I. (1991). The theory of planned behavior. *Organizational Behavior and Human Decision Processes, 50*, 179–211.

Ajzen, I., & Fishbein, M. (1980). *Understanding attitudes and predicting social behavior.* Englewood Cliffs, NJ: Prentice-Hall.

Ajzen, I., & Fishbein, M. (2000). Attitudes and the attitude-behavior relation: Reasoned and automatic processes. In W. Stroebe & M. Hewstone (Eds.), *European review of social psychology* (pp. 1–33). New York, NY: John Wiley & Sons, Inc.

Ajzen, I., & Fishbein, M. (2005). The influence of attitudes on behaviour. In D. Albarracín, B. T. Jonhson, & M. P. Zanna (Eds.) *The handbook of attitudes and attitude change: Basic principles* (pp. 173–221). Mahwah, NJ: Lawrence Erlbaum Associates.

Allport, G. W. (1924). The study of the undivided personality. *Journal of Abnormal and Social Psychology, 19*(2), 132–141.

Asch, S. E. (1952). *Social psychology.* Englewood Cliffs, NJ: Prentice-Hall.

Ashford, S. J., Rothbard, N. P., Piderit, S. K., & Dutton, J. E. (1998). Out on a limb: The role of context and impression management in selling gender-equity issues. *Administrative Science Quarterly, 43*(1), 23–57.

Bacharach, S. B., Bamberger, P. A., & Valerie M. M. (2007). Harassing under the influence: The prevalence of male heavy drinking, the embeddedness of permissive workplace drinking norms, and the gender harassment of female coworkers. *Journal of Occupational Health Psychology, 12*(3), 232–250.

Bamberger, P., & Biron, M. (2007). Group norms and excessive absenteeism: The role of peer referent others. *Organizational Behavior and Human Decision Processes, 103*(2), 179–196.

Bandura, A. (1986). *Social foundations for thought and action: A social cognitive theory.* Englewood Cliffs, NJ: Prentice Hall.

Bang, H. (2012). What prevents senior executives from commenting upon miscommunication in top management team meetings? *Qualitative Research in Organizations and Management: An International Journal, 7*(2), 189–208.

Becker, T. E. (1992). Foci and bases of commitment: Are they distinctions worth making? *Academy of Management Journal, 35*(1), 232–244.

Bendor, J., & Swistak, P. (2001). The evolution of norms. *American Journal of Sociology, 106*(6), 1493–1545.

Berkowitz, A. D. (2003). *The social norms resource book.* Little Falls, NJ: Paper Clip Communications.

Biron, M., & Bamberger, P. (2012). Aversive workplace conditions and absenteeism: Taking referent group norms and supervisor support into account. *Journal of Applied Psychology, 97*(4), 901–912.

Biron, M, Bamberger, P., & Noyman, T. (2011). Work-related risk factors and employee substance use: Insights from a sample of Israeli blue-collar workers. *Journal of Occupational Health Psychology, 16*(2), 247–263.

Borsari, B., & Carey, K. B. (2008). Descriptive and injunctive norms in college drinking: A meta-analytic integration. *Journal of Studies on Alcohol, 64*(3), 331–341.

Cestac, J., Delhomme, P., & Paran, F. (2014). Drive as I say, not as I do: Influence of injunctive and descriptive norms combination on speeding intention among young drivers. *Transportation Research, Part F, 23,* 44–56.

Cestac, J., Paran, F., & Delhomme, P. (2011). Young drivers' sensation seeking, subjective norms, and perceived behavioral control and their roles in predicting speeding intention: How risk-taking motivations evolve with gender and driving experience. *Safety Science, 49*(3), 424–432.

Chatman, J. A., & Flynn, F. J. (2001). The influence of demographic composition on the emergence and consequences of cooperative norms in work teams. *Academy of Management Journal, 44*(5), 956–974.

Chiaburu, D. S., & Harrison, D. A. (2008). Do peers make the place? Conceptual synthesis and meta-analysis of coworker effects on perceptions, attitudes, OCBs, and performance. *Journal of Applied Psychology, 93*(5), 1082–1103.

Christensen, P. N., Rothgerber, H., Wood, W., & Matz, D. C. (2004). Social norms and identity relevance: A motivational approach to normative behaviour. *Personality and Social Psychology Bulletin, 30,* 1295–1309.

Cialdini, R. B. (2001). *Influence: Science and practice* (4th edn.). New York, NY: Harper Collins College.

Cialdini, R. B. (2005). Basic social influence is underestimated. *Psychological Inquiry, 16*(4), 158–161.

Cialdini, R. B. (2007). Descriptive social norms as underappreciated sources of social control. *Psychometrika, 72*(2), 263–268.

Cialdini, R. B., Bator, R. J., & Guadagno, R. E. (1999). Normative influences in organizations. In L. L. Thompson, J. M. Levine, & D. M. Messick (Eds.), *Shared cognition in organizations: The management of knowledge* (pp. 195–211). Mahwah, NJ: Erlbaum.

Cialdini, R. B., Kallgren, C. A., & Reno, R. (1991). A focus theory of normative conduct. *Advances in Experimental Social Psychology, 24,* 201–234.

Cialdini, R. B., Reno, R., & Kallgren, C. A. (1990). A focus theory of normative conduct: Recycling the concept of norms to reduce littering in public places. *Journal of Personality and Social Psychology, 58*(6), 1015–1026.

Cialdini, R. B., & Trost, M. R. (1998). Social influence: Social norms, conformity and compliance. In D. T. Gilbert, S. T. Fiske, & G. Lindzey (Eds.) *The handbook of social psychology* (4th edn., vol. 2, pp. 151–192). New York, NY: McGraw-Hill.

Colémont A., & Van den Broucke, S. (2008). Measuring determinants of occupational health related behavior in Flemish farmers: An application of the Theory of Planned Behavior. *Journal of Safety Research, 39*(1), 55–64.

Cooley, C. H. (1922). *Human nature and the social order.* New York, NY: Scribner's.

Cooper-Thomas, H. D., & Wright, S. (2013). Person–environment misfit: Then neglected role of social context. *Journal of Managerial Psychology, 28*(1), 21–37.

Cullen, J. C., & Hammer, L. B. (2007). Developing and testing a theoretical model linking work–family conflict to employee safety. *Journal of Occupational Health Psychology, 12*(3), 266–278.

Deutsch, M., & Gerard, H. B. (1955). A study of normative and informational social influences upon individual judgment. *Journal of Abnormal and Social Psychology, 51*(3), 629–636.

Donovan, J. E., Jessor, R., & Jessor, L. (1983). Problem drinking in adolescence and young adulthood: A follow-up study. *Journal of Studies on Alcohol, 44*(1), 109–137.

Ehrhart, M., & Naumann, S. E. (2004). Organizational citizenship behavior in work groups: A group norms approach. *Journal of Applied Psychology, 89*(6), 960–974.

Fekadu, Z., & Kraft, P. (2002). Expanding the Theory of Planned Behavior: The role of social norms and group identification. *Journal of Health Psychology, 7*(1), 33–43.

Feldman, D. C. (1984). The development and enforcement of group norms. *Academy of Management Review, 9*(1), 47–53.

Festinger, L. (1954). A theory of social comparison processes. *Human Relations, 7*, 117–140.

Fishbein, M., & Ajzen, I. (1975). *Belief, attitude, intention and behavior: An introduction to theory and research*. Reading, MA: Addison-Wesley.

Fogarty , G. J. & Shaw, A. (2010). Safety climate and the theory of planned behavior: Towards the prediction of unsafe behavior. *Accident Analysis and Prevention, 42*(5), 1455–1459.

Forsyth, D. R. (2013). Social influence and group behavior. In I. B. Weiner (Ed. in-chief) *Handbook of psychology* (Vol. 5, H. Tennen & J. Suls, Eds., pp. 305–328). Hoboken, NJ: John Wiley & Sons, Inc.

Frone, M. R. (2009). Does a permissive workplace substance use climate affect employees who do not use alcohol and drugs at work? A U.S. National study. *Psychology of Addictive Behaviors, 23*(2), 386–390.

Fugas, C. S., Meliá, J. L., & Silva, S. A. (2011). The "is" and the "ought": How perceived social norms influence safety behaviors at work? *Journal of Occupational Health Psychology, 16*(1), 67–79.

Fugas, C. S., Meliá, J. L., & Silva, S. A. (2013). Profiling safety behaviors: Exploration of the socio-cognitive variables that best discriminate between different behavioral patterns. *Risk Analysis, 33*(5), 838–850.

Fugas, C. S., Silva, S. A., & Meliá, J. L. (2012). Another look at safety climate and safety behavior: Deepening the cognitive and social mediator mechanisms. *Accident Analysis and Prevention, 45*, 468–477.

Gibbs, J. (1968). The study of norms. In David Sills (Ed.): *International encyclopedia of the social sciences*, Vol. 11. New York, NY: Macmillan.

Grant, A. M., & Ashford, S. J. (2008). The dynamics of proactivity at work. *Research in Organizational Behavior, 28*, 3–34.

Grant, A. M., & Patil, S. V. (2012). Challenging the norm of self-interest: Minority influence and transitions to helping norms in work units. *Academy of Management Review, 37*(4), 547–568.

Hackman, J. R. (1992). Group influences on individuals in organizations. In M. Dunnett & L. Hough (Eds.), *Handbook for industrial and organizational psychology* (2nd edn., vol. 3, pp. 199–267). Palo Alto, CA: Consulting Psychologists Press.

Hamilton, K., & White, K. M. (2008). Extending the theory of planned behavior: The role of self and social influences in predicting adolescent regular moderate-to-vigorous physical activity. *Journal of Sport & Exercise Psychology, 30*(1), 56–74.

Hinsz, V. B., Nickell, G. S., & Park, E. S. (2007). The role of work habits in the motivation of food safety behaviors. *Journal of Experimental Psychology: Applied, 13*(2), 105–114.

Hodson, R. (1999). Organisational anomie and worker consent. *Work and Occupations, 26*, 292–323.

Hofmann, D. A., & Morgeson, F. P. (2002). The role of leadership in safety. In J. Barling & M. Frone (Eds.), *The psychology of workplace safety* (pp. 159–180). Washington, DC: American Psychological Association.

Hogg, M. A., & Abraams, D. (1988). *Social identifications: A social psychology of intergroup relations and group processes.* London, UK: Routledge.

Jackson, J. (1965). Structural characteristics of norms. In I. D. Steiner & M. Fishbein (Eds.), *Current studies in social psychology* (pp. 301–309). New York, NY: Holt, Rinehart and Winston.

Jiang, L., Yu, G., Li, Y., & Li, F. (2010). Perceived colleagues' safety knowledge/behavior and safety performance: Safety climate as a moderator in a multilevel study. *Accident Analysis and Prevention, 42*(5), 1468–1476.

Johnson, S., & Hall, A. (2005). The prediction of safe lifting behavior: An application of theory of planned behavior. *Journal of Safety Research, 36*(1), 63–73.

Kallgren, C. A., Reno, R. R., & Cialdini, R. B. (2000). A focus theory of normative conduct: When norms do and do not affect behavior. *Personality and Social Psychology, 26*(8), 1002–1012.

Kelley, H. H. (1952). Two functions of reference groups. In G. E. Swanson, T. M. Newcomb, & E. L. Hartley (Eds.), *Readings in social psychology* (2nd edn., pp. 410–414). New York, NY: Holt Rinehart, and Winston.

Kerr, S., & Jermier, J. M. (1978). Substitutes for leadership: Their meaning and measurement. *Organizational Behavior and Human Performance, 22*, 375–403.

Klein, K. J., Dansereau, E., & Hall, R. J. (1994). Levels issues in theory development, data collection, and analysis. *Academy of Management Review, 19*(2), 195–229.

Kozlowski, S. W. J., & Klein, K. J. (2000). A multilevel approach to theory and research in organizations: Contextual, temporal, and emergent processes. In K. J. Klein & S. W. J. Kozlowski (Eds.), *Multilevel theory, research and methods in organizations: Foundations, extensions, and new directions* (pp. 3–90). San Francisco, CA: Jossey-Bass.

Langfred, C. W., & Shanley, M. T. (1997). The importance of organizational context, I: A conceptual model of cohesiveness and effectiveness in work groups. *Public Administration Quarterly, 21*(3), 349–369.

Lajunen, T., & Räsänen, M. (2004). Can social psychological models be used to promote bicycle helmet use among teenagers? A comparison of the Health Belief Model, Theory of Planned Behavior and the Locus of Control. *Journal of Safety Research, 35*(1), 115–123.

Larimer, M. E., & Neighbors, C. (2003). Normative misperception and the impact of descriptive and injunctive norms on college student gambling. *Psychology of Addictive Behaviors, 17*(3), 235–243.

Latané, B. (1981). The psychology of social impact. *American Psychologist, 36*(4), 343–356.

Latané, B., & L' Herrou, T. (1996). Spatial clustering in the conformity game: Dynamic social impact in electronic games. *Journal of Personality and Social Psychology, 70*(6), 1218–1230.

Lawler, E. J. (1992). Affective attachments to nested groups: A choice process theory. *American Sociological Review, 57*(3), 327–339.

Lawton R. (1998). Not working to rule: Understanding procedural violations. *Safety Science, 28*(2), 77–95

Lichtman, R. J., & Lane, I. M. (1983). Effects of group norms and goal setting on productivity. *Group & Organization Studies, 8*(4), 406–420.

Marks, G., & Miller, N. (1987). Ten years of research on the false-consensus effect: An empirical and theoretical review. *Psychological Bulletin, 102*(1), 72–90.

Marques, J. M., Paéz, D., & Abrams, D. (1998). Social identity and intragroup differentiation as subjective social control. In S. Worchel, J. F. Morales, D. Páez, & J.-C. Deschamps (Eds.), *Social identity: International perspectives* (pp. 124–141). New York, NY: Sage.

Miller, D. T., & McFarland, C. (1991). When social comparison goes away: The case of pluralistic ignorance. In J. Suls & T. A. Wills (Eds.), *Social comparison: Contemporary theory and research* (pp. 287–313). Hillsdale, NJ: Erlbaum.

Miller, D. T., & Prentice, D. A. (1996). The construction of social norms and standards. In F. T. Higgins & A. W. Kruglanski (Eds.), *Social psychology: Handbook of basic principles* (pp. 799–829). New York, NY: Guilford.

Miniard, P. W., & Cohen, J. B. (1981). An examination of the Fishbein-Ajzen behavioral intentions model's concepts and measures. *Journal of Experimental Social Psychology, 17*(3), 309–339.

Mullen, J. (2005). Testing a model of employee willingness to raise safety issues. *Canadian Journal of Behavioural Science/Revue canadienne des sciences du comportement, 37*(4), 273–282.

Newcomb, T. M. (1953). An approach to the study of communicative acts. *Psychological Review, 60*(6), 393–404.

Newcomb, T. M. (1954). *Social psychology.* New York, NY: Dryden.

Obschonka, M., Goethner, M., Silbereisen, R. K., & Cantner, U. (2012). Social identity and the transition to entrepreneurship: The role of group identification with workplace peers. *Journal of Vocational Behavior, 80*(1), 147–187.

O' Reilly, C. A., & Caldwell, D. F. (1985). The impact of normative social influence and cohesiveness on task perceptions and attitudes: A social information processing approach. *Journal of Occupational Psychology, 58*(3), 193–206.

Potocnik, K., Tordera, N., & Peiró, J. M. (2009). The role of human resource practices and group norms in the retirement process. *European Psychologist, 14*(3), 193–206.

Prentice, D. A., & Miller, D. T. (1993). Pluralistic ignorance and alcohol use on campus: Some consequences of misperceiving the social norm. *Journal of Personality and Social Psychology, 64*(2), 243–256.

Quick, B. L., Stephenson, M. T., Witte, K., Vaught, C., Booth-Butterfield, S., & Patel, D. (2008). An examination of antecents to coal miners' hearing protection behaviors: A test of the theory of planned behavior. *Journal of Safety Research, 39*(3), 329–338.

Reno, R. R., Cialdini, R. B., & Kallgren (1993). The transsituational influence of social norms. *Journal of Personality and Social Psychology, 64*(1), 104–122.

Rice, R. E. (1993). Using network concepts to clarify sources and mechanisms of social influence. In W. D. Richards, Jr. & G. A. Barnett (Eds.), *Progress in communication sciences* (Vol. 12, pp. 43–62). Norwood, NJ: Ablex.

Rickett , B. Orbell , S. & Sheeran, P. (2006). Social-cognitive determinants of hoist usage among health care workers. *Journal of Occupational Health Psychology, 11*(2), 182–196.

Rimal, R. N. (2008). Modeling the relationship between descriptive norms and behavior: A test and extension of the theory of normative social behavior (TNSB). *Health Communication, 23*(2), 103–116.

Rimal, R. N., Lapinski, M. K., Cook, R. J., & Real, K. (2005). Moving toward a theory of normative influences: How perceived benefits and similarity moderate the impact of descriptive norms on behaviors. *Journal of Health Communication, 10*(5), 433–450.

Rivis, A., & Sheeran, P. (2003). Descriptive norms as an additional predictor in the Theory of Planned Behaviour: A meta-analysis. *Current Psychology: Developmental, Learning, Personality, Social, 22*(3), 218–233.

Rise, J., Sheernan, P., & Hukkelberg, S. (2010). The role of self-identity in the theory of planned behavior: A meta-analysis. *Journal of Applied Social Psychology, 40*(5), 1085–1105.

Roberto, M., Mearns, K., & Silva, S. A. (2011). Work experience and physician's intention to comply with hand hygiene: An extended application of the theory of planned behavior. In A. Caetano, S. A. Silva, & M. J. Chambel (Eds.), *New challenges for a healthy workplace in human services* (Organizational Psychology and Health Care, Vol. 6, edited by W. Schaufeli & J. M. Peiro, pp. 157–170). Munich, Germany: Rainer Hampp Verlag.

Roberts, K. R., & Barrett, B. B. (2011). Restaurant managers' beliefs about food safety training: An application of the theory of planned behavior. *Journal of Foodservice Business Research, 14*(3), 206–225.

Robinson, S. L., Kiewitz, C., & Wang, W. (2014). Coworkers behaving badly. *Annual Review of Organizational Psychology and Organizational Behavior, 1*, 123–143.

Salancik, G. R., & Pfeffer, J. (1978). A social information processing approach to job attitudes and task design. *Administrative Science Quarterly, 23*(2), 224–253.

Sanders, J., Oomens, S., Blonk, R. W. B., & Hazelzet, A. (2011). Explaining lower educated workers' training intentions. *Journal of Workplace Learning, 23*(6), 402–416.

Schachter, S. (1951). Deviation, rejection, and communication. *Journal of Abnormal and Social Psychology, 46*(2), 190–208.

Schultz, P. W., Nolan, J. M., Cialdini, R. B., Goldstein, N. J., & Griskevicius, V. (2007). The constructive, destructive, and reconstructive power of social norms. *Psychological Science*, *18*, 429–434.

Schmidtke, J. M. (2007). The relationship between social norm consensus, perceived similarity, and observer reactions to coworker theft. *Human Resource Management*, *46*(4), 561–582.

Shanley, M. T., & Langfred, C. W. (1998). The importance of organizational context, II: An empirical test of work group cohesiveness and effectiveness in two government bureaucracies. *Public Administration Quarterly*, *21*(4), 465–485.

Sheeran, P., & Silverman, M. (2003) Evaluation of three interventions to promote workplace health and safety: Evidence for the utility of implementation intentions. *Social Science and Medicine*, *56*(10), 2153–2163

Sherif, M. (1936). *The psychology of social norms*. New York, NY: Harper and Brothers (Harper Torchbook edition, 1966).

Sherif, M. (1956). Experiments in group conflict. *Scientific American*, *195*, 54–58.

Schneider, B. (1987). The people make the place. *Personnel Psychology*, *40*(3), 437–454.

Singer, S., Lin, S., Falwell, A., Gaba, D., & Baker, L. (2009). Relationship of safety climate and safety performance in hospitals. *Health Services Research*, *44*(2), 399–421.

Sorensen, J. A., Jenkins, P. L., Emmelin, M., Stenlund, H., Weinehall, L., Earle-Richardson, G. B., & May, J. J. (2011). The social marketing of safety behaviors: A quasi-randomized controlled trial of tractor retrofitting incentives. *American Journal of Public Health*, *101*(4), 678–684.

Sullivan, H. S. (1947). *Conceptions of modern psychiatry*. Washington DC: William A. White Psychiatric Foundation.

Tajfel, H., & Turner, J. C. (1979). An integrative theory of intergroup conflict. In W. G. Austin & S. Worchel (Eds.), *The social psychology of intergroup relations* (pp. 33–47). Monterey, CA: Books-Cole.

Terry, D. J., & Hogg, M. A. (1996). Group norms and the attitude–behavior relationship. A role for group identification. *Personality and Social Psychology Bulletin*, *22*(8), 776–793.

Terry, D. J., Hogg, M. A., & Duck, J. M. (1999). Group membership, social identity, and attitudes. In D. Abrams & M. A. Hogg (Eds.), *Social identity and social cognition*. Oxford, UK: Blackwell.

Terry, D. J., Hogg, M. A., & White, K. M. (1999). The theory of planned behaviour: Self-identity, social identity and group norms. *British Journal of Social Psychology*, *38*(3), 225–244.

Tesluk, P., & Quigley, N. R. (2003). Group and normative influences on health and safety, perspectives from taking a broad view on team effectiveness. In David A. Hofmann & Lois E. Tetrick (Eds.), *Health and safety in organization: A multilevel perspective* (pp. 131–172), Hoboken, NJ: John Wiley & Sons, Inc.

Thommes, K., Akkerman, A., Torenvlied, R., & Born, M. (2014). The dark side of solidarity: Social norms and social relations in the aftermath of strikes. *Industrial Relations Journal*, *45*(4), 348–367.

Turner, J. C. (1982). Towards a cognitive redefinition of the social group. In H. Tajfel (Ed.), *Social identity and intergroup relations* (pp. 15–40). Cambridge, UK: Cambridge University Press.

Turner, J. C. (1985). Social categorization and the self-concept: A social cognitive theory of group behavior. In E. J. Lawler (Ed.), *Advances in group processes: Theory and research*, (Vol. 2, pp. 77–122). Greenwich, CT: JAI Press.

Turner, J. C. (1991). *Social influence*. Buckingham, UK: Open University Press.

Turner, J. C., Hogg, M. A., Oakes, P. J., Reicher, S. D., & Wetherell, M. S. (1987). *Rediscovering the social group: A self-categorization theory*. Oxford, UK: Blackwell.

Turner, N., Chimiel, N., Hershcovis, M. S., & Walls, M. (2010). Life on the line: Job demands, perceived coworker support for safety, and hazardous work events. *Journal of Occupational Health Psychology*, *15*(4), 482–493.

Vitória, P. D., Salgueiro, M. F., Silva, S. A., & De Vries, H. (2009). The impact of social influence on adolescent intention to smoke: Combining types and referents of influence. *British Journal of Health Psychology*, *14*(4), 661–669.

Vitoria, P., Salgueiro, M. F., Silva, S. A., & De Vries, H. (2011). The longitudinal impact of parents and peers influence on adolescents smoking intention and behavior. *British Journal of Health Psychology*, *16*(4), 779–798.

Watson, G., Scott, D., Bishop, J., & Turnbeaugh, T. (2005). Dimensions of interpersonal relationships and safety in the steel industry. *Journal of Business & Psychology*, *19*(3), 303–318.

Westaby, J. D., & Lowe, J. K. (2005). Risk-taking orientation and injury among youth workers: Examining the social influence of supervisors, coworkers, and parents. *Journal of Applied Psychology*, *90*(5), 1027–1035.

Whitby, M., Pessoa-Silva, C. L., McLaws, M.-L., Allegranzi, B., Sax, H., Seto, W. H., Donaldson, L., & Pittet, D. (2007). Behavioural considerations for hand hygiene practices: The basic building blocks. *Journal of Hospital Infection*, *65*(1), 1–8.

Yun, D., & Silk, K. J. (2011). Social norms, self-identity, and attention to social comparison information in the context of exercise and healthy diet behavior. *Health Communication*, *26*(3), 275–285.

Zhang, S., Higgins, E. T., & Chen, G. (2011). Managing others like you were managed: How prevention focus motivates copying interpersonal norms. *Journal of Personality and Social Psychology*, *100*(4), 647–663.

5

Safety Leadership

Jennifer H. K. Wong, E. Kevin Kelloway, and Daniel W. Makhan

Introduction

The notion that organizational leaders play an important role in initiating and maintaining the safety attitudes and behaviors of their subordinates at work is empirically supported by research (for a review see Mullen, Kelloway, & Teed, 2011). This conclusion is derived from a wide range of study designs including intervention studies (e.g., Mullen & Kelloway, 2009) that demonstrate the positive effect of changing supervisors' leadership style on safety outcomes, meta-analyses (e.g., Clarke, 2013) that reveal the reliability of this positive effect across studies, and prevention programs (e.g., Morag & Luria, 2013) that show that the research can be successfully implemented in practice as leader-focused safety initiatives. Given the substantial influence that workplace supervisors have over their employees' safety performance, a focus on "what" leaders can do to foster a safer workplace is warranted. This is the primary goal of this chapter. We review the literature by critically examining the leadership models studied in the context of safety, and follow with a discussion of the organizational and individual mediators and moderators involved. We then discuss current measurement issues and limitations, as well as introduce a new practical safety leadership model that can be used as a framework for future research and application.

Leadership Models and Safety

Historically, early attempts to understand organizational leadership focused on the identification of characteristics or traits of great leaders (Barling, Christie, & Hoption, 2010). Although consistent relationships had emerged from this research such as the relationship between the "Big Five" personality traits and leadership style (Judge & Bono, 2000),

The Wiley Blackwell Handbook of the Psychology of Occupational Safety and Workplace Health, First Edition.
Edited by Sharon Clarke, Tahira M. Probst, Frank Guldenmund, and Jonathan Passmore. © 2016 John Wiley & Sons Ltd. Published 2020 by John Wiley & Sons Ltd.

this approach was fraught with difficulties; extensive research resulted in a seemingly endless list of traits that were hard to interpret as a whole, situational factors were largely ignored, and the usefulness of the knowledge for leadership development was debatable (Northouse, 2012). As a result of these concerns, leadership researchers began to focus on assessing the behaviors of leaders associated with a certain style of leadership (Barling et al., 2010). The earliest statements of leadership as behaviors related to initiating structure (i.e., concern for task) and consideration (i.e., concern for people) continue to have considerable validity (Judge, Piccolo, & Illies, 2004), although more elaborate models of effective leadership have subsequently been developed. Of these latter leadership models, the most extensively researched and well-developed one is the Full Range Leadership Model (Bass, 1985), and in particular, the transformational leadership style.

Transformational leadership

Transformational leadership falls under the Full Range Leadership Model, which was first theorized by Bass (1985) to encompass both transformational and transactional leadership behaviors. The underlying premise of the model is that leadership styles range from high quality (transformational) to poorer quality (transactional), and a leader can use varying degrees of each style of leadership (Bass & Avolio, 1994).

Transactional leadership focuses on the leaders' response to subordinates' actions. It encompasses negative transactions such as a lack of response (i.e., laissez-faire leadership) or punishing behaviors in reaction to rule infractions or substandard performance (i.e., management-by-exception). Furthermore, management-by-exception can be broken down into active or passive. The former is active monitoring and correcting subordinates' mistakes before they occur, and the latter is correcting mistakes after they have already happened. However, Bass (1985) also recognized the role of positive transactions such as providing rewards and recognition based on performance (i.e., contingent reward). In fact, meta-analytical findings demonstrated that contingent reward was considered as an effective form of leadership while laissez-faire leadership was considered as ineffective (Judge & Piccolo, 2004). Judge and Piccolo (2004) did not reach a verdict on management-by-exception leadership style due to inconsistent findings, but they suggested that active management-by-exception had a positive influence on workplace outcomes and passive management-by-exception had a negative influence.

Beyond transactional leadership, the Full Range Leadership Model includes transformational leadership, which is conceptualized as a set of behaviors that motivate subordinates to perform beyond expectations. Transformational leadership has four distinct qualities: being a role model (i.e., idealized influence), inspiring and providing meaningful and challenging work (i.e., inspirational motivation), stimulating subordinates to be creative and innovative in problem solving (i.e., intellectual stimulation), and being aware of subordinates' individual needs for higher achievement and growth (i.e., individualized consideration; Bass, 1985). A great deal of research supports the value of transformational leadership. In Judge and Piccolo's (2004) meta-analysis, transformational leadership was positively related to leadership effectiveness even after controlling for the effects of transactional leadership.

Transformational leadership is linked to a variety of subordinate attitudes such as satisfaction with leadership (Hater & Bass, 1988; Judge & Bono, 2000), trust (Burke, Sims, Lazzara, & Salas, 2007), and psychological safety (Detert & Burris, 2007). It is also associated with various measurements of work performance such as subordinate work motivation (Judge & Bono, 2000), sales performance (Barling, Weber, & Kelloway, 1996), and unit performance (Howell & Avolio, 1993). The effectiveness of transformational leadership is reliable across different research methodologies. For instance, in Barling et al.'s (1996) intervention study, transformational leadership training was found to improve subordinate-rated organizational commitment and actual number of sales. In a laboratory experiment, transformational leadership qualities predicted better performance on a brainstorming task, and this relationship was partially mediated by trust in leader and value congruence (Jung & Avolio, 2000).

The four dimensions of transformational leadership can be rationalized to relate to workplace safety as well. Barling, Loughlin, and Kelloway (2002) proposed that leaders with high levels of idealized influence are more likely to focus on the long-term benefits of safety goals over a short-term focus on productivity pressures. Leaders who challenge their subordinates to work toward a collective goal of safety are considered to have the quality of inspirational motivation. A transformational leader also intellectually stimulates their subordinates to think of novel and innovative ways to adhere to safety. Lastly, showing active interest in subordinates' physical well-being (i.e., individualized consideration) is a characteristic of a good safety leader. Barling et al. (2002) tested their theoretical contemplations using a safety-specific transformational leadership measure that was adapted from the Multifactor Leadership Questionnaire (Bass & Avolio, 1990) to reflect safety-related transformational leadership behaviors. In their first sample of restaurant workers, they found a positive relationship between safety-specific transformational leadership behaviors and safety climate. Furthermore, safety climate fully mediated the relationship between leadership and safety violations, and fewer reported safety violations were linked to a lower rate of injuries (see also Chmiel & Hansez, Chapter 7, this volume). Barling et al. (2002) replicated this predictive model with a sample of young mixed-industry workers, but the best fit of the data was acquired when an additional direct link was placed between safety climate and occupational injuries. Their study showed that safety-specific leadership impacted distal safety outcomes (e.g., injuries) by influencing proximal ones (e.g., safety climate). Distal safety outcomes are important because not only do they signify better well-being of the subordinates but also improvements for the organization's bottom line; fewer reported injuries means fewer human and financial costs for the company (Haccoun & Saks, 1998).

The scale developed by Barling et al. (2002) became the foundation for a study that used it to create a safety-specific transformational leadership training program for managers in long-term care facilities (Mullen & Kelloway, 2009). In the intervention, the leaders received safety-specific transformational leadership training, general transformational leadership training, or no training if they were assigned to the control group. Leaders in the safety-specific training rated themselves higher on safety attitudes and self-efficacy at post-training measures compared with the general training and control groups. As well, subordinates rated these leaders significantly higher on safety-specific transformational leadership. Safety-specific transformational leadership training also impacted subordinates' reports of safety climate, safety participation, safety events, and injuries. However, after controlling for correlations among dependent variables, only the effect of safety-specific transformational training on safety climate remained. Safety climate ratings were significantly higher for both safety-specific transformational leadership and general leadership groups compared with the control group, suggesting that general transformational leadership also had a positive impact on safety outcomes. Mullen and Kelloway (2009) not only verified a causal link between safety-specific transformational leadership and subordinates' perception of safety climate, but also showed that a valid training program can be developed from a measurement of safety-specific transformational leadership.

One particularly interesting study design examined the influence of transformational leadership on moonlighting employees – workers who hold two jobs (Inness, Turner,

Barling, & Stride, 2010). Ratings of transformational leadership predicted safety participation within the job rather than spilling over to predict safety outcomes in the secondary job. Furthermore, this relationship was found after controlling for individual differences of the subordinate (i.e., negative affectivity, conscientiousness), length of work shift, and tenure of position under the supervisor. In sum, transformational leadership does not necessarily have to be safety-specific to influence subordinates' safety performance (e.g., Mullen & Kelloway, 2009), but it does have to be job-specific (Inness et al., 2010).

Transactional and laissez-faire leadership

Despite its popularity, studies with a singular focus on transformational leadership neglect the other half of the Full Range Leadership Model (Bass, 1985), the transactional component. Analyses revealed that safety-specific transformational and passive leadership were empirically distinct from each other and were not simply opposite ends of a single continuum (Kelloway, Mullen, & Francis, 2006). This implies that a leader with safety-related transformational qualities does not necessarily lack transactional qualities. Therefore, a deeper understanding of leadership dynamics can be obtained if transformational leadership is investigated alongside transactional leadership. In fact, when examined concurrently, safety-specific passive leadership explained incremental variance beyond safety-specific transformational leadership for predicting reports of safety violations and injuries (Kelloway et al., 2006). Structural equation modeling further revealed that the two leadership styles have differential effects on safety consciousness and safety climate. Safety-specific transformational leadership was positively associated with these safety outcomes while safety-specific passive leadership was negatively associated with them. The overall model revealed that leadership predicted safety consciousness, which predicted safety climate, safety violations, and finally injuries at work. Even though transformational qualities are critical in leaders, the lack of an active approach to safety appears to be detrimental for both proximal and distal safety outcomes.

Since a leader is considered to have a profile of varying degrees of transformational and transactional leadership styles (Bass & Avolio, 1994), it is presumed that both transformational and transactional qualities can be displayed at the same time. Mullen et al. (2011) described this as "inconsistent" leadership. Inconsistent safety leadership is operationalized as the interaction of high safety-specific transformational and high safety-specific passive leadership. Inconsistency is undesirable because the presence of passive leadership behaviors may attenuate the positive influence of transformational leadership since a mixed message is being conveyed to the subordinates regarding the leader's stance on safety. Mullen et al. (2011) carried out their hypotheses in a sample of employed university students and a sample of healthcare workers. Inconsistent leadership predicted safety compliance in both samples, yet only safety participation in the healthcare workers sample. Safety performance outcomes were rated lower in subordinates who perceived their leaders to have high safety-specific transformational and high safety-specific passive characteristics compared with high transformational and low passive characteristics. Safety compliance is the act of following safety rules and regulations, whereas safety participation is the willingness to participate in safety (Neal, Griffin, & Hart, 2000). Therefore, Mullen et al. (2011) found that inconsistent leadership was a more reliable predictor of in-role, task-related than extra-role, citizenship-related safety performance. Overall, their claim that safety-related passive leadership attenuates the positive influence of safety-specific transformational leadership was supported.

Other researchers have also examined the concurrent effects of transformational and transactional leadership on safety outcomes. Safety climate strength was found to be positively associated with transformational leadership and negatively associated with passive leadership (Luria, 2008). A study conducted by Zohar (2002a) found that transformational and constructive leadership (i.e., contingent reward) were positively associated with leaders' preventative actions for safety. Furthermore, preventative actions mediated the relationship between leadership and injury rate. Laissez-faire and corrective (i.e., active and passive management-by-exception) leadership were negatively associated with leaders' prioritization of safety. While transformational leadership was related to lower injury rates, the three components of transactional leadership had differential influences on safety-related outcomes. Specifically, only contingent reward behaviors were directly related to injury rates, while laissez-faire and corrective leadership were negatively linked to prioritization of safety. However, before concluding that both active and passive management-by-exception were detrimental to safety, Zohar (2002a) did point out that there was a distinction between active and passive management-by-exception. Passive management-by-exception was significantly correlated with laissez-faire leadership. Subordinates perceived leaders who correct safety mistakes after they occur to be as incompetent as leaders who do nothing to promote safety. While active management-by-exception did not significantly correlate with other dimensions of leadership in Zohar's (2002a) study, meta-analytical findings showed that this specific type of transactional behavior associated more with transformational than laissez-faire leadership (Judge & Piccolo, 2004).

A recent survey similar to Zohar's (2002a) study came to a different conclusion regarding the role of active corrective leadership. Hoffmeister et al. (2014) discovered that active management-by-exception was a significant predictor of lower reported injuries in a sample of construction workers. Their study suggested that corrective leadership, specifically active management-by-exception, was better than no leadership at all. Furthermore, they also broke down transformational leadership into its four dimensions and found that only the idealized influence component was a significant predictor of safety participation and injury rates. Despite the contradictory results on active corrective leadership, Zohar (2002a) and Hoffmeister et al.'s (2014) studies illustrated that transformational leadership was consistently related to better proximal and distal safety outcomes.

Mixed findings on the role of active corrective leadership were resolved by a meta-analysis conducted by Clarke (2013). Clarke (2013) speculated that transactional leadership, particularly active management by exception, is valuable within a safety context because active monitoring may lead to higher adherence to rule-based safety compliance. Also, correcting errors before they occur may prevent future mistakes. Her meta-analysis revealed that transformational leadership was positively associated with safety participation, with safety climate partially mediating the relationship. Active transactional leadership was positively associated with safety compliance, and that relationship was also partially mediated by safety climate. Active transactional leadership's relationship to employee participation was fully mediated by safety climate. When the effect sizes were taken into consideration, transformational leadership was relatively more associated with safety extra-role citizenship-related behaviors (e.g., engagement in safety activities), and active transactional leadership was relatively more associated with safety in-role task-related behaviors (e.g., responsibilities concerning rules and regulations). After a decade of research, active transactional leadership finally established itself to be a positive influence on safety performance.

Empowering leadership

Despite the abundance of research on the Full Range Leadership Model, the generalizability of transformational leadership theory may not be ideal for certain safety critical industries. With regard to the nuclear safety industry, a group of researchers suggested that the empowering leadership model, rather than the transformational leadership model, is a better fit to the types of leaders' behaviors that promote safety (Martínez-Córcoles, Gracia, Tomás, & Peiró, 2011). Empowering leadership is based on the idea that a leader's primary goal is to generate the potential for self-management in their subordinates (Arnold, Arad, Rhoades, & Drasgow, 2000). Empowering leadership is about how the leaders treat their subordinates and how they communicate and carry out the understanding of task responsibilities and procedures in a manner that transfers power to the subordinates (Ford & Fottler, 1995). Empowering leadership is different from other leadership models because it is not only about the leaders having influence over their subordinates, but also passing on that ability of influence to their subordinates (Amundsen & Martinsen, 2014; Pearce et al., 2003). Indeed, empowering leadership was found to have incremental validity over transformational leadership in predicting psychological empowerment (Amundsen & Martinsen, 2014).

Martínez-Córcoles et al. (2011) developed a safety-related empowering leadership scale by adapting Arnold et al.'s (2000) measurement to reflect a safety context and used it to examine the impact of safety-specific empowering leadership on nuclear energy plant employees. According to Arnold et al.'s (2000) conceptualization of empowering leadership, five types of behaviors constitute empowering leaders: leading by example, participative decision-making, coaching, informing, and showing concern for their subordinates. In the context of safety (Martínez-Córcoles et al., 2011), leading by example can be demonstrated by the leaders' commitment to their safety goals. Safety-related participative decision-making is when leaders involve their subordinates in making safety-related decisions. Coaching refers to the ability of the leaders to motivate their subordinates to solve safety-related problems in a self-managed way. Informing is the leaders' ability to disseminate information and to provide feedback about safety on a regular basis. Finally, showing concern for their subordinates is when leaders provide emotional support or when they acknowledge and reward safety behaviors.

In Martínez-Córcoles et al.'s (2011) study, safety behaviors were assessed by a measurement that taps into the extent that the subordinates conform to safety norms, rules, and procedures (Mearns, Flin, Gordon, & Fleming, 2001); therefore, the outcome in this study was task-related and similar to the construct of safety compliance. Empowering leadership predicted better safety climate, which then predicted more safety behaviors. Interestingly, the positive relationship between empowering leadership and safety climate was stronger under weak safety culture, suggesting that empowering leadership compensated for a poor safety culture. Although in their first study Martínez-Córcoles and colleagues (2011) did not explore the central concept that empowering leadership facilitates self-management, there was some support for this in a follow-up study (Martínez-Córcoles, Schöbel, Gracia, Tomás, & Peiró, 2012). The second study was also conducted using a sample from a nuclear power plant, and empowering leadership was positively related to subordinates' safety participation. Most importantly, this relationship was mediated by collaborative team learning, which can be interpreted as empowering leadership fostering a stronger sense of independence in their subordinates.

For their third study on empowering leadership the researchers decided to conceptualize safety performance based on Rotundo and Sackett's (2002) tridimensional structure of job performance (Martínez-Córcoles, Gracia, Tomás, Peiró, & Schöbel, 2013). According to Routundo and Sackett (2002), there are three types of job performances: task-related, citizenship-related, and counterproductive behaviors. Task-related performance refers to carrying out the in-role responsibilities that are necessary to complete work. On the other hand, citizenship-related performance is a set of extra-role behaviors that are not explicitly required of employees but can enhance the overall organization effectiveness. Counter-productive behaviors are actions that have the intention to harm the organization. In terms of the commonly studied safety outcomes of safety participation and compliance, participation is a form of citizenship-related performance and compliance is a form of task-related performance (Neal et al., 2000). However, the lack of safety compliance and participation does not signify a presence of counterproductive safety behaviors. Thus, it is important to capture all three types of safety performance. Martínez-Córcoles et al. (2013) identified risky behaviors to be a type of counterproductive performance. Empowering leadership positively predicted both safety compliance and participation and negatively predicted risky behaviors in their third study.

Compared with the Full Range Leadership Model, empowering leadership is a relatively new area of research in safety, and because of that there are limited studies available on the topic. No research has been conducted yet on the empirical differences between em-powering, transformational, and transactional leadership, so the value that empowering leadership adds to the Full Range Leadership Model is to be determined.

Indirect Effects of Leadership

Knowing that leadership is important, the focus now shifts to why and under what cir-cumstances is leadership critical for safety performance. Supervisors are considered to have both direct and indirect influences on a variety of occupational factors that would affect subordinates' safety at work (Kelloway & Barling, 2010), which suggests that there are mediating factors underlying the mechanism of a leader's influence. Furthermore, Clarke (2013) concluded in her meta-analysis that the variability in the findings suggests the presence of moderators. Not only are the studies of mediation and moderation important for deepening our understanding of safety leadership, they are also critical for leadership training. Mediation identifies specifically what behaviors a good leader should carry out or enhance to obtain the desirable subordinates' outcomes. Moderation identifies the in-dividual and situational conditions that must be met for training to be successful. Having considered the direct effects of leadership on safety outcomes, we next turn our attention to indirect effects of leadership. We organize the indirect effects into whether they occur at the organizational or the individual level.

Organizational factors

Safety climate   Safety climate is defined as the shared perception among employees re-garding which procedures, practices, and behaviors are rewarded to support a specific performance of high-risk operations (Zohar, 2000). It is a commonly studied outcome of good leadership behaviors as demonstrated by research on transformational (e.g., Zohar & Tenne-Gazit, 2008), transactional (e.g., Zohar, 2002a), and empowering leadership (e.g., Martínez-Córcoles et al., 2011). Furthermore, safety climate plays an indirect role because it is considered to be a mediator of the relationship between transformational and transactional leadership styles and safety behaviors (Clarke, 2010, 2013; Zohar, 2000, 2002a). Safety climate also mediates the relationship between leadership attitudes and injuries (e.g., trust; Luria, 2010). Safety climate's role as a mediator can be broken down into more detailed steps. Safety consciousness (awareness of safety issues) was found to mediate the link between safety-specific transformational leadership and good safety climate, which was then associated with fewer safety violations and lower injury rate (Barling et al., 2002).

Aside from studying leadership styles, researchers also look into the quality of the interactions between a leader and their subordinate. These interactions are called leader–member exchange (Dansereau, Graen, & Haga, 1975). This assessment of leadership is considered to be relational as opposed to simply behavioral because it focuses on the dyad of the leader and a single subordinate. High-quality relationships are characterized by high mutual respect, trust, and obligation, whereas low-quality relationships are characterized by distrust, disrespect, and low obligation (Graen & Uhl-Bien, 1995; see also Conchie, Woodcock, & Taylor, Chapter 6, this volume). In an examination of truck drivers' safety behaviors, higher quality leader–member exchange between dispatcher and the driver positively predicted better trucking safety climate, which positively predicted driving safety behaviors, which subsequently negatively predicted hard braking behaviors electronically captured by the devices in the vehicles of the trucking company (Zohar, Huang, Lee, & Robertson, 2014). Regardless of how leadership is conceptualized, as a style, an attitude, or social exchanges, it affects subordinates' safety performance by creating a shared standard for safety at the workplace.

Safety climate also has a significant role as a moderator. The relationship between leadership and safety performance varies under conditions of good or poor safety climate (e.g., Kapp, 2012; Hofmann, Morgeson, & Gerras, 2003; Zohar & Luria, 2010). Under the condition of positive safety climate, high quality leader–member exchange predicted the likelihood of subordinates expanding their safety role beyond what was expected (Hofmann et al., 2003). Furthermore, there was no expansion of safety citizenship role when safety climate was poor regardless of quality of leader–member exchange. In a mixed sample of construction and manufacturing employees, transformational and contingent reward leadership were associated with higher safety compliance only when group safety climate was positive (Kapp, 2012). Zohar and Luria (2010) further differentiated between group level and organizational-wide safety climate and discovered that under a weak organizational safety climate, transformational leaders fostered a stronger sense of group safety climate (see also Luria, Chapter 16, this volume). The researchers attributed these contradictory findings to the idea that transformational leaders buffer the negative impact of poor organizational safety climate on subordinates. Consequently, the moderating role of safety climate depends on the type of safety climate and safety performance outcomes assessed, but overall the influence of leadership on subordinates' safety in-role and extra-role behaviors is more effective under a positively perceived safety climate.

Organizational support   There are organizational factors other than safety climate that mediate the relationship between leadership and safety outcomes. A leader's safety values may be a proxy for the organization's stance on safety because subordinates perceive their leader to represent upper management. Therefore, good safety leadership should be linked to higher levels of positive organizational factors and lower levels of negative organizational factors. In fact, Credo, Armenakis, Feild, and Young (2010) found evidence that subordinates' perceptions of management concern for safety positively predicted safety involvement and this pathway was mediated by perceived organizational support. Furthermore, the link between organizational support and safety involvement was mediated by perceived organizational ethics and leader–member exchange. Therefore, supportive organizations were seen as morally strong and less likely to weaken under organizational pressure (e.g., unethically hide or protect company image; Credo et al., 2010), and because of this subordinates were more willing to be involved in safety. In sum, a good safety leader can exert their influence on subordinates by enhancing the perception of organizational support.

Role stressors   Negative role stressors perceived by either the subordinates or their leaders can explain both parties' lack of adherence to safety at work. Qualitative interviews of leaders revealed that role overload and production pressure were recurring issues challenging leaders' own adherence to safety (Conchie, Moon, & Duncan, 2013). As well, in a sample of mixed industry blue-collar workers, subordinates' role stressors were found to mediate the relationship between quality of leader–member exchange and perceived injury risk (Muldoon, Matthews, & Foley, 2012). Employees who reported having a heavy workload were associated with a higher injury rate, regardless of leadership influence (Barling et al., 2002). Knowing that an overworked employee is an unsafe employee, a good safety leader should value safety over production and avoid giving too much work to their subordinates even at the risk of losing profits.

Individual factors

Trust   Aside from representing the values of upper management and the overall organization, leaders also exert their influences on safety by changing their subordinates' internal attitudes and beliefs. Trust has been identified as playing an important role in safety-related leadership because it is the foundation of a positive safety culture; trust promotes employee psychological safety for incident reporting (Clark & Payne, 2006; Conchie, Taylor, & Donald, 2012; Reason, 1997; see also Conchie, Woodcock, & Taylor, Chapter 6, this volume). Trust in leaders can be either affect-based or cognition-based, and while affect-based trust is the belief that leaders will act unselfishly in the good of their subordinates (Holmes & Rempel, 1989; McAllister, 1995), cognition-based trust is the belief that they can carry out their obligations and responsibilities (Cook & Wall, 1980). In a study of leader–subordinate dyads in the oil industry, safety-specific transformational leadership was positively associated with safety voice behaviors, and this was mediated by affect-based trust (Conchie et al., 2012). The relationship between affect-based trust and safety voice citizenship behaviors was further mediated by disclosure trust intention. Disclosure trust intention is the individuals' willingness to disclose sensitive information to another (Gillespie, 2003). A higher level of disclosure trust intention meant that trust in the leader outweighs the risk of negative consequences for speaking out about safety matters without worrying about repercussions from whistle-blowing (Conchie et al., 2012).

While affect-based trust was a mediator of safety voice behaviors, cognition-based trust was discovered to be more of a moderator (Conchie & Donald, 2009; Conchie et al., 2012). Transformational leadership associated with more safety citizenship behaviors only under high or moderate levels of cognitive trust (Conchie & Donald, 2009). Cognitive trust was also implied to play the role of a moderator in the Conchie et al. (2012) study. Cognitive trust predicted higher reliance trust intentions (i.e., the extent to which an individual relies on another), and the presence of these two trust variables facilitated a stronger positive relationship between disclosure trust and safety voice. In summary, affect-based trust is the mechanism by which safety leaders promote subordinate safety behaviors, and at least a moderate level of cognition-based trust is necessary for this association to thrive.

Motivation   According to the self-determination theory (Deci & Ryan, 1985), there are three main categories of motivation that fall on a continuum: amotivation (i.e., lack of motivation), extrinsic motivation (i.e., performance to attain an external outcome), and intrinsic motivation (i.e., performance driven by inherent satisfaction). An adapted version of the Situational Motivation Scale (Guay, Vallerand, & Blanchard, 2000) was used to assess safety-related motivation in a sample of construction workers (Conchie, 2013). Intrinsic motivation mediated the relationship between safety-specific transformational leadership and safety citizenship behaviors (i.e., whistle-blowing and safety voice behaviors). Additionally, extrinsic motivation mediated the relationship between safety-specific transformational leadership and safety compliance. These results support our understanding of self-determination theory because it validates that external rewards drive the task-related performance of safety compliance and intrinsic motivation drives extra-role behaviors that constitute safety participation. Furthermore, Conchie (2013) discovered that these relationships became statistically not significant when trust in the leader was low. Intrinsic motivation was a significant mediator of the relationship between safety-specific transformational leadership and safety citizenship behaviors only in subordinates with a high level of trust in their leaders. Trust in the leader is necessary for safety leadership to motivate safety behaviors.

Aside from motivation to engage in task and citizenship safety performance, leadership is also linked (negatively) to the motivation to behave counterproductively in regard to safety. In a sample of young workers, supervisory influence negatively predicted motivation to engage in risk-taking behaviors, which then predicted lower reports of work injury (Westaby & Lowe, 2005). Overall, different types of motivation are associated with task-related, citizenship-related, counterproductive safety performance and injury rate.

Measurement of Safety Leadership

Although we touched on some conceptual definitions of leadership, it is instructive to examine just how "safety leadership" has been operationalized in previous studies. The work on the Full Range Leadership Model (e.g., Barling et al., 2002) and empowering leadership (e.g., Martínez-Córcoles et al., 2011) used safety-specific measurements that were adapted directly from the general leadership scales. Accordingly, these modified versions do not deviate much from the original models. To date, there are three different groups of researchers who developed safety leadership measures that are not exact adaptations.

The first two groups of researchers intended to create safety leadership measures sensitive to Eastern cultural values, and they selected theoretical dimensions from pre-existing leadership models relevant to the national culture in which they conducted their studies. The Employee Safety Leadership Scale was created and tested by Wu (2008) with a sample of electrical engineering departments in universities across Taiwan. The scale consists of three dimensions: safety coaching, safety caring, and safety controlling. The first two dimensions relate to transformational leadership. Coaching refers to role modeling and engaging subordinates in decision-making, and caring refers to respect and concern for subordinates' needs. The safety-controlling dimension derives from transactional leadership theory and refers to the extent that safety is sustained under a rule-based system. When validating his scale, Wu (2008) found age, gender, and management hierarchy differences in subordinates' perceptions of leaders' safety behaviors. Direct leaders were perceived to care more about safety, and upper managers were more concerned about role-modeling and decision-making engagement. In universities with an absence of safety committees, therefore reflecting a low priority for safety, female leaders and younger leaders were rated lower in safety coaching, controlling, and caring behaviors. Although it cannot be determined if this was perceived as an inadequacy or an actual deficit in safety leadership, Wu's (2008) work raised legitimate concerns about how the leader's demographics such as age and gender can impact safety leadership.

Wu's research team continued his work with a study on safety leadership and safety culture within the Taiwanese telecommunication industry (Wu, Lin, & Shiau, 2010). They compared the Employee Safety Leadership Scale (Wu, 2008) to two other safety leadership measurements that they developed for the study. The first new scale was the Operations Manager Safety Leadership Scale (Wu et al., 2010), which assesses leaders' safety informing, safety decision-making, and safety interactions behaviors. The second new scale was the Safety Professional Safety Leadership Scale (Wu et al., 2010), which examines the role of the leader as an expert, a coordinator, and a regulator of safety. Four dimensions from these three scales were found to predict better safety culture: safety informing from the Operations Manager Safety Leadership Scale, safety caring from the Employee Safety Leadership Scale, safety coordination and safety regulation from the Safety Professional Safety Leadership Scale. Safety culture was measured using the researchers' own Safety Culture Scale (Wu et al., 2010) that assesses employee's safety participation, perceived risk, and emergency response. In summary, Wu and his colleagues identified that planning, monitoring, communicating about, and caring for safety were behaviors associated with positive safety culture. However, the ability of his safety leadership measures to predict subordinates' safety performance still needs to be examined.

Although Wu (2008) and Wu et al.'s (2010) scales have not been validated against subordinates' safety performance, another safety leadership scale developed by a different group of Taiwanese researchers has (Lu & Yang, 2010). This scale consists of three dimensions derived from the Full Range Leadership Model (Bass, 1985): safety motivation, safety policy, and safety concern (Lu & Yang, 2010). The safety motivation dimension involves rewarding and engaging subordinates in order to motivate them to perform safely. Rewards can have monetary value, or simply praise and recognition. Engaging activities can be participatory decision-making such as taking in subordinates' suggestions regarding safety. The safety policy dimension captures goal setting, responsibility delegation, and having a system for corrective actions. Lastly, the safety concern dimension is the extent to which the leader is a behavioral and attitudinal role model for safety. The researchers sampled workers from Taiwanese container terminal companies and found that safety motivation and concern positively associated with safety compliance and participation, and safety policy dimension positively associated with safety participation. Lu and Yang's (2010) study demonstrated that the predictive validity of transformational and transactional leadership was not confined to the measurement of the Multifactor Leadership Questionnaire, or to the Western cultural values from where the Full Range Leadership Model originated.

More recently, Australian researchers Griffin and Hu (2013) developed a scale of safety leadership based on theories entirely outside of the Full Range Leadership Model. Their critique for adapting from existing leadership theories was that these models are inherently style/trait-based, and a broad range of behaviors falls under each type of style rather than distinct behaviors. Also, they suggested that within these leadership styles, a specific behavior from one style may interact with a behavior from another, yet this possible augmentation is overlooked with the style/trait-based conceptualization. Using self-regulation and organizational learning theories, Griffin and Hu (2013) proposed three types of ideal safety leadership behaviors that promote self-regulation and learning with subordinates: safety inspiring, safety monitoring, and safety learning. According to Griffin and Hu (2013), safety inspiring provides meaning and value for subordinates to commit to safety, and because value increases interests in activities (Schunk & Ertmer, 2000), subordinates are more likely to participate in extra-role behaviors. Safety monitoring promotes subordinates' safety compliance because it allows them to be aware of and keep up with their adherence to safety (Dunlowski, Kubat-Silam, & Hertzog, 2003). Safety learning is proposed to be a moderator of the relationship between safety monitoring and safety participation; monitoring is positively related to extra-role behaviors when it is conducted in a non-threatening environment that encourages learning from mistakes (Griffin & Hu, 2013). Using a sample recruited from a research company, they found support for all three of their hypothesized relationships. In addition, for subordinates who rated their leaders to be low on safety learning behaviors, there was a negative relationship between monitoring and safety participation. Without an emphasis on learning, monitoring by itself was not an effective means of increasing extra-role safety behaviors. These findings showed that having a safety leadership measure derived independently of existing models can yield new knowledge; learning is not a component of the Full Range Leadership Model, and the monitoring items on the Multifactor Leadership Questionnaire have been critiqued as capturing controlling behaviors of monitoring instead of how leaders correct mistakes (Yukl, 1999).

The Five Core Safety Leadership Behaviors

Most leadership models examined in safety research have been modified from the general leadership literature (e.g., transformational leadership: Barling et al., 2002; empowering leadership: Martínez-Córcoles et al., 2011). As well, two groups of researchers successfully developed their own safety leadership measurements using selective dimensions from the Full Range Leadership Model to derive safety leadership measurements appropriate for Taiwan's cultural values (Lu & Yang, 2010; Wu, 2008; Wu et al., 2010). These findings speak to the generalizability of basic principles of leadership. At the same time, the general leadership models conceptualize leadership styles to encompass a wide range of behaviors rather than specific behaviors. Our experience in training and developing safety leaders also recognizes that the propositions of leadership theory may be too abstract for leaders. Griffin and Hu (2013) acknowledged this criticism and developed a safety leadership measurement that was based on the theories of self-regulation and organizational learning. We believe that these attempts to define safety leadership as concrete behaviors instead of broad styles have considerable value. Building on previous models and measurements of safety leadership, we have identified five specific core behaviors of good safety leaders. A good safety leader (1) speaks of safety, (2) acts safely at work, (3) focuses on maintaining safety standards, (4) engages others in safety initiatives, and (5) recognizes individuals who adhere to safety. Each of the five dimensions has empirical evidence supporting its influence on subordinates' safety performance independent of the safety research on leadership styles. We discuss each of the five core behaviors below.

Speaking about safety at work

Communication is a key component of safety leadership because it is the mechanism through which the leader's view and position on safety are shared with their employees. General workplace communication was found to be positively associated with safe working behaviors after controlling for organizational factors such as job autonomy, role overload, role conflict, supportive supervision, training adequacy, and job security (Parker,

Axtell, & Turner, 2001). Leaders themselves identify communication as a critical aspect of promoting safety leadership. Senior managers in the air traffic management industry indicated that a flatter organizational hierarchy fostered a stronger sense of leadership influence because it created a better flow of communication between leaders and subordinates (Fruhen, Mearns, Flin, & Kirwan, 2013). The managers also believed that one-way communication, such as reporting and providing data on safety performance, was important for workplace safety.

Communication may be mistaken for being identical to leader–member exchange. However, communication includes one-way verbal information dissemination from the leader to the subordinates, whereas leader–member exchange is always a dynamic interaction (verbal or physical) within the leader-subordinate dyad (Dansereau et al., 1975). When safety-specific communication was compared with leader–member exchange in examining their prediction of safety-related events, safety communication's effect was smaller and non-significant (Michael, Guo, Wiedenbeck, & Ray, 2006). Communication may then be one of the underlying mechanisms by which leader–member exchange influences followers' behaviors. Indeed, safety communication was demonstrated to mediate the relationship between leader–member exchange and safety commitment, and higher safety commitment was then linked to lower rates of accidents (Hofmann & Morgeson, 1999). Density of communication networks also mediated the relationship between transformational leadership and safety climate strength in a sample of infantry soldiers (Zohar & Tenne-Gazit, 2008). Overall, both quality and quantity of communication is important for workplace safety; a good safety leader needs to communicate meaningful information frequently.

The act of feedback is considered to be a form of communication because it is a one-way verbal dissemination of information about the subordinates' performance from the leader to the subordinates. Feedback is associated with better safety outcomes such as lower hazard frequencies (Sulzer-Azaroff & de Santamaria, 1980), and has been identified to be an important aspect of a correctly designed safety incentive system (Komaki, Barwick, & Scott, 1978). Feedback is especially important after a safety intervention. In particular, feedback in the form of written commitment strategies and group data has a positive impact on safety performance maintenance (Boyce & Geller, 2001). Feedback provided at least three times a week has been found to effectively maintain improved safety behaviors (Komaki, Heinzmann, & Lawson, 1980).

There are two intervention studies to date that aimed to improve safety performance by coaching leaders on how to communicate. Zohar (2002b) implemented a communication and feedback-based intervention to increase safety at work by training leaders in a machine repair and maintenance organization. His intervention involved teaching leaders how to communicate safety as a priority, as well as interview skills for giving their employees safety-related feedback. The intervention was successful; safety interactions were reported to be significantly higher in the experimental group. Minor injury rate, earplug use, and perceived safety climate were more stable over time for the experimental group than the control group. In another intervention study conducted with Danish construction foremen, coaching leaders on safety communication was found to improve safety outcomes as well (Kines et al., 2010). Pre- and post-test measures revealed that coaching was effective because it increased the number of verbal exchanges regarding safety between leaders and subordinates. Furthermore, coaching increased subordinates' attention to safety, and also the safety index of the work site. In summary, Zohar (2002b) and Kines et al.'s (2010) intervention studies demonstrated that safety communication and feedback facilitated better safety outcomes, and that those two behaviors were skills that can be successfully trained. Furthermore, earplug use (Zohar, 2002b) and safety index (Kines et al.,

2010) were objective evaluations of safety-related work performance by members of the research team blind to the intervention groups, thus reducing the likelihood of the findings being confounded by common method bias.

Acting safely at work

Despite communication being an important aspect of safety leaders, the physical visibility of their efforts to reinforce what they communicated is critical as well (Biggs, Banks, Davey, & Freeman, 2013; Luria, Zohar, & Erev, 2008). Leaders who state their support for organizational values but then behave in a manner that is incongruent are considered to be hypocrites (Cha & Edmondson, 2006). Within the context of safety, subordinates perceive hypocrisy behaviors as poor behavioral integrity toward safety (Leroy et al., 2012). Leader's behavioral integrity toward safety contributes to a safer workplace by establishing clear expectations for what types of behaviors are appropriate. Leaders high in behavioral integrity carry through with their actions and will not neglect to correct inappropriate behaviors because safety is a priority to them. This sends a clear message to subordinates, and their safety performance is improved either by being more involved because their sense of psychological safety is increased (Halbesleben et al., 2013; Leroy et al., 2012), or by being more compliant because in-role behavioral expectations are well established (Halbesleben et al., 2013). Indeed, priority of safety has been found to mediate the relationship between leader's behavioral integrity and reported treatment errors (Leroy at al., 2012). Team psychological safety moderated this relationship; when psychological safety was high, the negative association between safety priority and less reported treatment errors was stronger. Furthermore, cross-lagged analyses from a longitudinal study design demonstrated that psychological safety and safety compliance at Time 2 mediated the relationship between behavioral integrity of leaders at Time 1 and frequency and severity of injuries at Time 3 (Halbesleben et al., 2013).

Leader's behavioral integrity also enhances safety citizenship-related behaviors. Reporting mistakes, as opposed to ignoring them, is considered to be a characteristic of a healthy functioning workplace (Argyris, 1977). This is a type of extra-role behavior typical of subordinates who have a high sense of psychological safety because they believe that they will not be punished for speaking up (Edmondson, 1999). Findings from Halbesleben et al. (2013) and Leroy et al. (2012) confirmed this statement. Leader's behavioral integrity was positively associated with team psychological safety, which was then linked to more reported errors (Leroy et al., 2012). Psychological safety and safety compliance mediated the relationship between behavioral integrity of leaders and higher reporting ratio of injuries (Halbesleben et al., 2013). Therefore, it is important for leaders to practice what they preach because their behavioral integrity improves in-role and extra-role safety behaviors and distal safety outcomes by increasing subordinates' sense of psychological safety and safety priority.

Focusing on maintaining safety standards

Safety leaders must show commitment and perseverance in their safety behaviors over time. Leader's safety commitment is an important aspect of safety culture (Biggs et al., 2013) and has been found to predict subordinates' own perception of safety during organizational change (Lofquist, Greve, & Olsson, 2011). Perceptions of leaders' commitment to safety were related to lower perceived risk and more willingness from subordinates to participate in safety programs (Cree & Kelloway, 1997). The inability to adhere to safety standards consistently can be as detrimental as not even obliging to them in the first place (Mullen et al., 2011). Even when leaders identify commitment to safety to be vital, they point out that it can be a difficult behavior to maintain (Dea & Flin, 2001). An interview with a sample of offshore managers reported that consistently trying to upkeep safe practices was one of the top challenges of the job. Therefore, safety leaders need to recognize that they have to find means of keeping themselves motivated to maintain commitment to safety.

A concrete behavioral example of leaders' commitment to safety is the ability to recognize safety compliance issues and to be flexible enough to change their leadership strategies to adapt (Healy, 2012). In a sample of hospital workers in Australia, leaders who were responsive regulators and used multiple types of support strategies to improve safety compliance to surgery were considered to be most successful. These leaders began with persuasion and softer intervention strategies, and escalated to more forceful strategies if the compliance continued to be low. Another concrete example of a safety commitment behavior is monitoring, because leaders who are able to recognize problems at workplace are the ones who are constantly keeping track of their subordinates' safety performance. Consistent monitoring increases subordinates' safety behaviors because the act of monitoring enforces a clear standard for which safety behaviors are appropriate and which are not (Griffin & Hu, 2013). Likewise, Griffin and Hu (2013) found that safety-specific monitoring positively associated with safety compliance. An intervention study conducted by Zohar and Luria (2003) revealed that training leaders to monitor subordinates led to higher observer-rated frequency of safety behaviors and self-reported ratings of safety climate. Yet, as Griffin and Hu (2013) have pointed out, the work environment can contribute to whether monitoring behaviors are perceived as a threatening or as a positive act, which would subsequently have differential impacts on subordinates' safety performance. Given the right work environment, adaptive regulating and monitoring behaviors of the leaders keep subordinates focused on safety, while self-motivating behaviors keep the leaders themselves on track.

Engaging others in safety initiatives

Good safety leaders recognize that safety is a group effort and strive toward engaging their employees in important decisions and initiatives. Supervisory support was positively related to engagement and safety participatory behaviors of subordinates across industries in a meta-analysis (Nahrgang, Morgeson, & Hofmann, 2011). Engaging subordinates and encouraging their questions were considered to be important assets of a good leader in 97 percent of the respondents of a study conducted on offshore drill workers (Crichton, 2005). A comparison of successful and unsuccessful safety culture interventions identified engagement and empowerment to be a determining factor of intervention effectiveness (Hale, Guldenmund, van Loenhout, & Oh, 2010). Specifically, involving all employees in an environment where there were open discussions about safety issues and safety decisions (e.g., dangerous scenario reporting system, pre-operation checklist cards, e-learning forums) led to a significant improvement in safety performance.

The act of engaging subordinates manifests as specific leadership behaviors. One technique to engage subordinates is to have them partake in learning. Successful safety culture interventions engaged the organizations in a learning process (Hale et al., 2010). Empowering leadership was found to have a positive significant relationship with subordinates' safety participation, which was mediated by collaborative team learning (Martínez-Córcoles et al., 2012). A learning-friendly environment also fostered a positive relationship between monitoring behaviors and safety participation (Griffin & Hu, 2013). Showing care for subordinates is another way to engage them. People-oriented leadership is the employee's perception of how management cares about the workers and the manner that employees are treated; people-oriented leadership was found to be negatively associated with risk-taking behaviors (Størseth, 2004, 2006).

Good safety leaders do not only engage their subordinates in safety decisions, they also open up a two-way channel where safety issues can be brought up and addressed (e.g., Hale et al., 2010). Leaders' receptiveness to safety information was related to subordinates' willingness to raise safety issues (Mullen, 2005). Upward safety communication is a specific type of communication that happens when subordinates reach an adequate level of comfort to discuss safety issues with their leaders without the fear of being reprimanded (Hofmann & Stetzer, 1998). Upward communication occurs when there are high quality leader–member exchanges and high levels of perceived management support (Kath, Marks, & Ranney, 2010). In a sample of mixed industry blue-collar workers, upward safety communication mediated the relationship between the high quality of leader–member exchange and lower perceived injury risk (Muldoon et al., 2012). Overall, engagement behaviors in the form of facilitating learning, caring about subordinates, and creating a psychologically safe environment for subordinates to bring up safety issues are important for increasing extra-role safety behaviors and reducing counterproductive safety behaviors.

Recognizing safety performance

Aside from having a consistent feedback and monitoring system for correcting safety violations, a safety leader values and acknowledges subordinates who are safe in their everyday work. Recognition is considered to be a responsibility of a good safety leader. Barling et al.'s (2002) measurement of safety-specific transformational leadership contains two questions on contingent rewards because their factor analyses revealed that it consistently loaded on the dimensions of transformational leadership qualities. Contingent reward was related to leader effectiveness, and in some situations even more so than transformational leadership (i.e., field studies conducted in organizations compared with student and military samples; Judge & Piccolo, 2004). Behaviorism scientists have studied comprehensively the mechanisms by which reward and recognition influence behaviors. According to Skinner (1938), timely and consistent rewards reinforce social behaviors through a type of learning called operant conditioning. Therefore, to maximize the effectiveness of recognition, it should be given out as soon as possible after each accomplishment, and the definition of what types of accomplishments merit recognition should be consistent over time.

In a review of the efficiency of safety incentives and feedback on workplace safety performance, McAfee and Winn (1989) concluded that incentives enhanced safety and reduced accidents in the workplace over the short term. A properly designed safety-incentive program was identified to use social praise, recognition, tangible reinforcements, and non-monetary privileges to reinforce the reporting of hazards (Komaki et al., 1978). Such programs also recognize unsafe behaviors to target, ideally before the accident takes place, as a preventative measure rather than a reactive measure (Vredenburgh, 2002). A good safety leader does not necessarily need to reward safety accomplishments by monetary means. In an intervention study by Austin, Kessler, Riccobono, and Bailey (1996) the researchers found that monetary rewards were not necessary; rewarding employees with break times improved safety compliance. Non-monetary recognition in the form of feedback led to an improvement in observer-rated safety behaviors as well as self-rated safety climate in Zohar and Luria's (2003) intervention study. Also, Hale et al. (2010) identified prompt feedback after safety decisions or audits and inspections as one of the discriminating factors of successful and unsuccessful safety culture interventions.

However, safety rewards and incentives may be effective only under certain conditions and for certain groups of individuals in the organization. A study of work teams by Haines, Merrheim, and Roy (2001) revealed that safety incentives were more effective when supervisor–subordinate relationships were more positive, when the work team members were interdependent on each other (e.g., coordination is necessary for the team to function), and when the work team shared the same safety norms. Wilde (1994) pinpointed that rewards worked best when given for group and individual performance, and also when given to all levels of the organization, especially the front-line employees. The variability of the findings regarding reward and recognition suggest that many more undiscovered moderators may be at work. Nevertheless, recognition is a comparably cost-efficient form of reward that does not draw from company resources. Good safety leaders should use it to reinforce desirable subordinate safety behaviors.

Literature Overview

In summary, we covered leadership models that have been adapted to the occupational safety context. The Full Range Leadership Model is by far the most popular way to conceptualize safety leadership. Studies on the Full Range Leadership Model show that transformational leadership style is reliably linked to better safety performance, particularly citizenship-related behaviors such as safety participation (e.g., Mullen & Kelloway, 2009). The role of transactional leadership is critical as well, but in order to understand it fully we must break down transactional leadership into its four components. Contingent rewards (e.g., Zohar, 2002a) and active management-by-exception behaviors (e.g., Clarke, 2013) are associated with better task-related safety performance such as safety compliance. Passive management-by-exception and laissez-faire leadership styles are linked to poor safety outcomes (e.g., Zohar, 2002a). Furthermore, empowering leadership (e.g., Martínez-Córcoles et al., 2011) shows promise in predicting a wide range of safety performance outcomes, from task-related safety compliance, citizenship-related safety participation, to counterproductive risk-taking behaviors.

Since leadership has been empirically established to be critical for subordinates' safety behaviors, the research now focuses on mediators and moderators of this relationship. Numerous studies and meta-analyses assert that a good safety climate is not only a mediator but also a moderator for safety leadership. As well, safety leaders influence their subordinates' behaviors by changing their perception about the organization (i.e., support, workload) and attitudes within themselves (i.e., trust in leaders, motivation to be safe). Trust and safety culture also moderate the relationship between leadership and safety outcomes. For training purposes, it is valuable for the leaders to understand the importance of these mediating factors. Since these mediators are identified as a mechanism of influence on subordinates' safety performance, they should be the targets for change in order to capitalize on the benefits of the intervention. Also, the selection of leaders and organizations suitable for training should consider the level of trust subordinates have in their leaders and the safety climate and culture of those workplaces.

In addition to the safety leadership measurements that are modified from general leadership theories, several groups of researchers have developed their own measures.

In Taiwan, two separate groups of researchers created safety leadership scales for the engineering, telecommunication, and container terminal industries (Lu & Yang, 2010; Wu, 2008; Wu et al., 2010). However, these scales still draw from selective dimensions in the Full Range Leadership Model. The only safety leadership scale to date derived independently of existing leadership theories is the one by Griffin and Hu (2013), which assesses leaders' behaviors that promote self-regulation and learning in subordinates.

Building on these advances in research, we identified five core behaviors of a safety leader, which are (1) speaking of safety, (2) acting safely at work, (3) focusing on maintaining safety standards, (4) engaging others in safety initiatives, and (5) recognizing individuals who adhere to safety. Behaviors relating to speaking of safety are a one-way dissemination of information about safety. This can be data reporting, feedback, or simply verbal exchanges regarding safety. Acting safe is primarily the concept of behavioral integrity, which is the perceived alignment between the leaders' expectations and actions for safety. Focusing on safety involves using active monitoring and adaptive regulating methods to keep subordinates on track, as well as self-motivational skills to maintain leaders' own safety perseverance. Safety engaging behaviors include facilitating learning, caring about subordinates, and creating a psychologically safe environment to include others in safety initiatives. Lastly, non-monetary recognition is an act best conducted in a timely and appropriate manner to reinforce desirable safety performances.

Future Research and Practice: The S.A.F.E.R. Leadership Model

Based on the empirical literature and our own experiences in working with organizations around topics of safety leadership, we believe that safety leadership can be conceptualized as five specific core behaviors. We now present this as the S.A.F.E.R. Leadership Model. The model is explicitly developed to identify the key behaviors expected of safety leaders in the workplace, which are:

> Speaking about safety,
> Acting safely,
> Focusing on safety,
> Engaging others in safety initiatives, and
> Recognizing safe performance at work.

The S.A.F.E.R. Leadership Model is not meant to replace existing models of safety leadership. We see it as the manifestation of these existing models that illustrates the mechanism of influence because it specifically describes the safety-oriented tasks that are indicative of a good safety leader (Figure 5.1). Furthermore, the S.A.F.E.R. Leadership Model is not bound to existing models of safety leadership; we see it as being rooted in more general models of effective organizational leadership. We suggest that these refined dimensions make it easier to teach leaders the importance of, and skills involved in, safety-specific leadership. Using this framework, we provide ideas for future research that can address other limitations in the safety leadership literature. Specifically, we propose that industry, gender, and national culture values are possible moderators of safety leadership. We also discuss ways to raise the caliber of safety leadership research design.

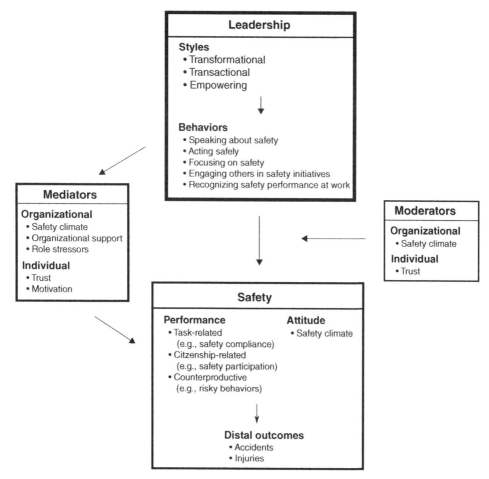

Figure 5.1 Outcomes, moderators, and mediators of safety leadership. The S.A.F.E.R. Leadership model describes specific behaviors that are qualities of a good safety leader.

Is safety leadership industry-specific?

Most of the studies on leadership and subordinates, safety outcomes were conducted in blue-collar safety critical populations, aside from a few university samples. Due to this, there is a possibility that differences between industries have an effect on the delivery and influence of safety leadership. In studies that tested their hypotheses over two different samples, findings cannot be replicated exactly – predictive relationships were found for different types of safety outcomes (e.g., Mullen et al., 2011), and the models that acquired best fit differed across samples (e.g., Barling et al., 2002). Also, Martínez-Córcoles et al. (2011) suggested that the nuclear industry is unique in that empowering leadership may be a better fit than transformational leadership to safety performance. These differences across industries raise the question of whether safety leadership is job-specific (e.g., tasks performed in offshore drilling versus health care) or is sensitive to inherent characteristics of the industry (e.g., proportionally more men working in offshore drilling, proportionally more females working in health care). Indeed, when Barling et al. (2002) replicated their predictive model of safety-specific transformational leadership and injuries from a sample of restaurant workers to young workers, an additional pathway in the model was added in the latter sample in order to achieve best fit. This implies that there is a potential difference between young and older workers in terms of safety leadership influence, or that may be a unique characteristic of the hospitality industry compared with a heterogeneous industry sample.

Consequently, industry differences should be explored in greater depth in future studies because these differences may impact whether or not safety leadership training programs can succeed. The S.A.F.E.R. Leadership Model can be utilized as a platform for investigating industry differences because it presents the concrete behaviors that can be susceptible to job or worker characteristics. For example, safety incentives are more effective when work team members are interdependent (Haines et al., 2001). Therefore, the act of recognizing and rewarding safety performances may be more highly associated with safety leadership competency for jobs that require team coordination in order to successfully complete work tasks than in jobs that require independent work.

Do women and men differ as safety leaders?

Although there is a large body of research on gender differences in leadership, no studies to date have examined the effect of gender on safety leadership competency. In the general leadership literature, women are perceived to be more transformational and less transactional than men (Eagly, Johannesen-Schmidt, & van Engen, 2003). Since our literature overview concluded that both safety transformational and transactional leadership behaviors are critical for subordinates' safety performance, the influence of gender on safety leadership may become apparent depending on the safety outcome of interest. Female safety leaders may be better at facilitating extra-role safety participation behaviors because they are perceived to be more transformational. Male safety leaders may be better at promoting in-role safety compliance behaviors because they are perceived to be more transactional.

However, men and women are perceived as an effective leader only if they are in a leadership role that reflects their gender (Eagly, Karau, & Makhijani, 1995). According to Eagly et al.'s (1995) definition of masculine or feminine leadership role, a masculine role is characterized by the leader's competency to direct and control people, whereas a feminine role is characterized by the leader's competency to cooperate and get along with other people. This raises the question of whether an ideal safety leader is perceived to be a "male," a "female," equally a "male" or a "female," or a gender-neutral role. The S.A.F.E.R. Leadership Model can be used as a starting point for generating research hypotheses by considering gender expectations and differences in the five specific core behaviors of safety leadership.

Given that certain safety critical workforces are male-dominant, there may exist a tendency to assume that a safety leader is a masculine role, even though this bias may simply be attributed to the higher proportion of men employed in these workplaces. This would suggest that regardless of the behaviors of a female safety leader, she is at a disadvantage compared with her male counterpart. This discrepancy in the distribution of gender in safety critical industries also poses difficulty in conducting research with female safety leaders because of their availability for recruitment. Knowing about gender differences in safety leadership can add value to the training of safety leaders and can also help bring into dispute the myths and beliefs around safety at work.

What is the role of cultural values?

National culture is defined as the collective core values of the members in a nation (Hofstede, 2001). These core values differ on the dimensions of power distance, uncertainty avoidance, individualism/collectivism, masculinity/femininity, and future orientation. Leadership researchers have long debated the generalizability of the Full Range Leadership Model across cultures. Having originated in the United States, there is a concern for transformational leadership theory to be applicable only in individualistic Western cultures and not collectivistic Eastern cultures. On the contrary, research by Jung, Bass, and Sosik (1995) conducted in East Asia showed that transformational leadership appears more readily in collectivistic rather than individualistic cultures. One possible explanation for this is that the moral obligation in a collectivistic culture enhances the reciprocation of positive behaviors between leaders and subordinates. For example, there is a mutual understanding that individual consideration is imbedded in the role of a leader in a collectivistic culture such as Japan (Yokochi, 1989). The leader is expected to mentor the subordinates, and in return the subordinates are resolutely obedient. Therefore, transformational leadership is a concept that is relevant in both Western and Eastern cultures.

While it is universal that transformational leadership is good leadership, transformational leadership does not encompass all types of good leadership behaviors (for review see Barling et al., 2010; Gelfand, Erez, & Aycan, 2007). Accordingly, Bass (1997) noted that the actual thoughts, understanding, and behaviors that manifest from transformational and transactional leaders differ across culture. Since the majority of research on safety leadership was carried out in societies with Western values (North America, Europe, Australia), the actual behaviors of a safety leader may not transfer over to Eastern cultures even though the ideology of leadership styles do. In fact, when Wu (2005) began his work on creating a safety leadership scale specifically for the Taiwanese population, he noted that he had to merge ideas from the transformational leadership theory with models of leadership developed by Asian researchers (Huang, 1997; Kang, Su, Jang, & Sheu, 2001) to reflect Eastern values. This demonstrates the importance of moving beyond leadership styles to studying concrete behaviors of safety leaders outlined in the S.A.F.E.R. Leadership Model. For example, Indonesian leaders are observed to be boastful about their competency to instill inspirational motivation, while Japanese leaders use different methods for inspiring their subordinates because bravado behavior is less socially acceptable in Japan (Bass, 1997). Therefore, the ideal safety leader in Japan may be one who provides private recognition as opposed to public praises and rewards.

Another related factor that may shape cultural values is the national legislation on safety. The standards for safety vary across countries depending on public policy, which is reflected in the countries' societal norms. Understanding how this influences the conceptualization of effective safety leadership behaviors is another area of future research. Safety leadership training can benefit from cross-cultural research because the knowledge can lead to customization of a training program that best suits the cultural audience, as well as provide insight on creating culturally appropriate safety leadership assessment tools.

How should safety leadership be measured and tested?

The context of safety is not immune to the limitations that general leadership researchers face. The most common issue is the over-reliance on using self-reported measurements to assess leadership behaviors. Leader-rated measurement only assesses leaders' perceptions of their competency, while subordinate-rated measurement introduces common method bias when safety outcomes are also reported by subordinate. This bias can be reduced if there are other forms of assessing safety leadership behaviors, such as having a third party rate the leadership behaviors by observation (e.g., performance appraisal, video recording observations), and measuring leadership as dyads or groups. Given that the nature of leadership is hierarchical in nature, collecting data in days or groups can enhance the power of the research design and analyses. Another important issue in research design is that the majority of the studies conducted on safety leadership are cross-sectional, and this research method does not demonstrate cause and effect. Future research in safety leadership should consider the rigid design of a longitudinal study, particularly a safety leader training intervention (e.g., Barling et al., 2002; Zohar & Luria, 2003). Not only does an intervention design allow for causal inferences, but it also highlights the applicability of safety leadership.

Conclusion

We suggest that the data are clear on the importance of leaders in creating safe working environments. The available research reveals that leaders' behaviors have a pervasive effect in changing working behaviors, changing perceptions of safety culture and, ultimately, enhancing safety outcomes. Based on these observations, we moved away from pre-defined leadership styles and turned to a consideration of what leaders actually do to facilitate safety performance. We proposed the S.A.F.E.R. model of safety leadership as a comprehensive identification of effective leadership behaviors. Although subject to operationalization and empirical validation, we believe that the S.A.F.E.R. model offers a platform for both research and practice in workplace safety.

References

Amundsen, S., & Martinsen, Ø. L. (2014). Empowering leadership: Construct clarification, conceptualization, and validation of a new scale. *Leadership Quarterly, 25*(3), 487–511. doi:10.1016/j.leaqua.2013.11.009

Argyris, C. (1977). Double loop learning in organizations: By uncovering their own hidden theories of action, managers can detect and correct errors. *Harvard Business Review, 55*, 115–126.

Arnold, J. A., Arad, S., Rhoades, J. A., & Drasgow, F. (2000). The empowering leadership questionnaire: The construction and validation of a new scale for measuring leader behaviors. *Journal of Organizational Behavior, 21*(3), 249–269. doi:10.2307/3100332

Austin, J., Kessler, M. L., Riccobono, J. E., & Bailey, J. S. (1996). Using feedback and reinforcement to improve the performance and safety of a roofing crew. *Journal of Organizational Behavior Management, 16*(2), 49–75. doi:10.1300/J075v16n02_04

Barling, J., Christie, A., & Hoption, C. (2010). Leadership. In S. Zedeck (Ed.), *APA handbook of industrial and organizational psychology* (pp. 183–240). Washington, DC: American Psychological Association.

Barling, J., Loughlin, C., & Kelloway, E. K. (2002). Development and test of a model linking safety-specific transformational leadership and occupational safety. *Journal of Applied Psychology, 87*(3), 488–496. doi:10.1037//0021-9010.87.3.488

Barling, J., Weber, T., & Kelloway, E. K. (1996). Effects of transformational leadership training on attitudinal and financial outcomes: A field experiment. *Journal of Applied Psychology, 81*(6), 827–832. doi:10.1037/0021-9010.81.6.827

Bass, B. M. (1985). *Leadership and performance beyond expectations.* New York, NY: Free Press.

Bass B. M. (1997). Does the transactional-transformational leadership paradigm transcend organizational and national boundaries? *American Psychologist, 52*(2), 130–139. doi:10.1037/0-003-066X.52.2.130

Bass, B. M., & Avolio, B. J. (1990). *Transformational leadership development: Manual for the Multifactor Leadership Questionnaire.* Palo Alto, CA: Consulting Psychologists Press.

Bass, B. M., & Avolio, B. J. (1994). *Improving organizational effectiveness through transformational leadership.* Thousand Oaks, CA: Sage.

Biggs, S. E., Banks, T. D., Davey, J. D., & Freeman, J. E. (2013). Safety leaders' perceptions of safety culture in a large Australasian construction organisation. *Safety Science, 52,* 3–12. doi:10.1016/j.ssci.2012.04.012

Boyce, T. E., & Geller, E. S. (2001). Applied behavior analysis and occupational safety: The challenge of response maintenance. *Journal of Organizational Behavior Management, 21*(1), 31–60. doi:10.1300/J075v21n01_03

Burke, C. S., Sims, D. E., Lazzara, E. H., & Salas, E. (2007). Trust in leadership: A multi-level review and integration. *Leadership Quarterly, 18*(6), 606–632. doi:10.1016/j.leaqua.2007.09.006

Cha, S. E., & Edmondson, A. C. (2006). When values backfire: Leadership, attribution, and disenchantment in a values-driven organization. *Leadership Quarterly, 17*(1), 57–78. doi:10.1016/j.leaqua.2005.10.006

Clark, M. C., & Payne, R. L. (2006). Character-based determinants of trust in leaders. *Risk Analysis, 26*(5), 1161–1173. doi: 10.1111/j.1539-6924.2006.00823.x

Clarke, S. (2010). An integrative model of safety climate: Linking psychological climate and work attitudes to individual safety outcomes using meta-analysis. *Journal of Occupational and Organizational Psychology, 83*(3), 553–578. doi:10.1348/096317909×452122

Clarke, S. (2013). Safety leadership: A meta-analytic review of transformational and transactional leadership styles as antecedents of safety behaviors. *Journal of Occupational and Organizational Psychology, 86*(1), 22–49. doi:10.1111/j.2044-8325.2012.02064.x

Conchie, S. M. (2013). Transformational leadership, intrinsic motivation, and trust: A moderated-mediated model of workplace safety. *Journal of Occupational Health Psychology, 18*(2), 198–210. doi:10.1037/a0031805

Conchie, S. M., & Donald, I. J. (2009). The moderating role of safety-specific trust on the relation between safety-specific leadership and safety citizenship behaviors. *Journal of Occupational Health Psychology, 14*(2), 137–147. doi:10.1037/a0014247

Conchie, S. M., Moon, S., & Duncan, M. (2013). Supervisors' engagement in safety leadership: Factors that help and hinder. *Safety Science, 51*(1), 109–117. doi:10.1016/j.ssci.2012.05.020

Conchie, S. M., Taylor, P. J., & Donald, I. J. (2012). Promoting safety voice with safety-specific transformational leadership: The mediating role of two dimensions of trust. *Journal of Occupational Health Psychology, 17*(1), 105–115. doi:10.1037/a0025101

Cook, J., & Wall, T. (1980). New work attitude measures of trust, organizational commitment and personal need non-fulfillment. *Journal of Occupational Psychology, 53*(1), 39–52. doi:10.1111/j.2044-8325.1980.tb00005.x

Credo, K. R., Armenakis, A. A., Feild, H. S., & Young, R. L. (2010). Organizational ethics, leader–member exchange, and organizational support: Relationships with workplace safety. *Journal of Leadership & Organizational Studies, 17*(4), 325–334. doi:10.1177/1548051810366712

Cree, T., & Kelloway, E. K. (1997). Responses to occupational hazards: Exit and participation. *Journal of Occupational Health Psychology, 2*(4), 304–311. doi:10.1037/1076-8998.2.4.304

Crichton, M. (2005). Attitudes to teamwork, leadership, and stress in oil industry drilling teams. *Safety Science, 43*(9), 679–696. doi:10.1016/j.ssci.2005.08.020

Dansereau, F., Graen, G., & Haga, W. J. (1975). A vertical dyad linkage approach to leadership within formal organizations. *Organizational Behavior and Human Performance, 13*(1), 46–78. doi:10.1016/0030-5073(75)90005-7

Dea, A. O., & Flin, R. (2001). Site managers and safety leadership in the off-shore oil and gas industry. *Safety Science, 37*(1), 39–57. doi:10.1016/S0925-7535(00)00049-7

Deci, E. L., & Ryan, R. M. (1985). *Intrinsic motivation and self-determination in human behavior.* New York, NY: Plenum Press.

Detert, J. R., & Burris, E. R. (2007). Leadership behavior and employee voice: Is the door really open? *Academy of Management Journal, 50*(4), 869–884. doi:10.5465/AMJ.2007.26279183

Eagly, A. H., Johannesen-Schmidt, M. C., & van Engen, M. L. (2003). Transformational, transactional, and laissez-faire leadership styles: A meta-analysis comparing women and men. *Psychological Bulletin, 129*(4), 569–591. doi:10.1037/0033-2909.129.4.569

Eagly, A. H., Karau, S. J., & Makhijani, M. G. (1995). Gender and the effectiveness of leaders: A meta-analysis. *Psychological Bulletin, 117*(1), 125–145. doi:10.1037/0033-2909.117.1.125

Edmondson, A. (1999). Psychological safety and learning behavior in work teams. *Administrative Science Quarterly, 44*(2), 350–383. doi:10.2307/2666999

Ford, R. C., & Fottler, M. D. (1995). Empowerment: A matter of degree. *Academy of Management Perspectives, 9*(3), 21–29. doi: 10.5465/AME.1995.9509210269

Fruhen, L. S., Mearns, K. J., Flin, R. H., & Kirwan, B. (2013). From the surface to the underlying meaning – an analysis of senior managers' safety culture perceptions. *Safety Science, 57*, 326–334. doi:10.1016/j.ssci.2013.03.006

Gelfand, M. J., Erez, M., & Aycan, Z. (2007). Cross-cultural organizational behavior. *Annual Review of Psychology, 58*, 479–514. doi:10.1146/annurev.psych.58.110405.085559

Gillespie, N. (2003). Measuring trust in working relationships: The behavioral trust inventory. Paper presented at the annual meeting of the Academy of Management Meeting, Seattle.

Graen, G. B., & Uhl-Bien, M. (1995). Relationship-based approach to leadership: Development of leader-member exchange (LMX) theory of leadership over 25 years: Applying a multi-level multi-domain perspective. *Leadership Quarterly, 6*(2), 219–247. doi:10.1016/1048-9843(95)90036-5

Griffin, M. A., & Hu, X. (2013). How leaders differentially motivate safety compliance and safety participation: The role of monitoring, inspiring, and learning. *Safety Science, 60*, 196–202. doi:10.1016/j.ssci.2013.07.019

Guay, F., Vallerand, R. J., & Blanchard, C. M. (2000). On the assessment of situational intrinsic and extrinsic motivation: The Situational Motivation Scale (SIMS). *Motivation and Emotion, 24*(3), 175–213. doi: 10.1023/A:1005614228250

Haccoun, R. R., & Saks, M. (1998). Training in the 21st century: Some lessons from the last one. *Canadian Psychology, 39*(2), 33–47. doi:10.1037/h0086793

Haines, V. Y., Merrheim, G., & Roy, M. (2001). Understanding reactions to safety incentives. *Journal of Safety Research, 32*(1), 17–30. doi:10.1016/S0022-4375(00)00051-7

Halbesleben, J. R. B., Leroy, H., Dierynck, B., Simons, T., Savage, G. T., McCaughey, D., & Leon, M. R. (2013). Living up to safety values in health care: The effect of leader behavioral integrity on occupational safety. *Journal of Occupational Health Psychology, 18*(4), 395–405. doi:10.1037/a0034086

Hale, A. R., Guldenmund, F. W., van Loenhout, P. L. C. H., & Oh, J. I. H. (2010). Evaluating safety management and culture interventions to improve safety: Effective intervention strategies. *Safety Science, 48*(8), 1026–1035. doi:10.1016/j.ssci.2009.05.006

Hater, J. J., & Bass, B. M. (1988). Superiors' evaluations and subordinates' perceptions of transformational and transactional leadership. *Journal of Applied Psychology, 73*(4), 695–702. doi:10.1037/0021-9010.73.4.695

Healy, J. M. (2012). How hospital leaders implemented a safe surgery protocol in Australian hospitals. *International Journal for Quality in Health Care, 24*(1), 88–94. doi:10.1093/intqhc/mzr078

Hoffmeister, K., Gibbons, A. M., Johnson, S. K., Cigularov, K. P., Chen, P. Y., & Rosecrance, J. C. (2014). The differential effects of transformational leadership facets on employee safety. *Safety Science, 62*, 68–78. doi:10.1016/j.ssci.2013.07.004

Hofmann, D. A., & Morgeson, F. P. (1999). Safety-related behavior as a social exchange: The role of perceived organizational support and leader-member exchange. *Journal of Applied Psychology, 84*(2), 286–296. doi:10.1037//0021-9010.84.2.286

Hofmann, D. A., Morgeson, F. P., & Gerras, S. J. (2003). Climate as a moderator of the relationship between leader-member exchange and content specific citizenship: Safety climate as an exemplar. *Journal of Applied Psychology, 88*(1), 170–178. doi:10.1037/0021-9010.88.1.170

Hofmann, D. A., & Stetzer, A. (1998). The role of safety climate and communication in accident interpretation: Implications for learning from negative events. *Academy of Management Journal, 41*(6), 644–657. doi:10.2307/256962

Hofstede, G. H. (2001). *Culture's consequences: Comparing values, behaviors, institutions and organizations across nations.* Thousand Oaks, CA: Sage.

Holmes, J. G., & Rempel, J. K. (1989). Trust in close relationships. In C. Hendrick (Ed.), *Close relationships* (pp. 187–220). Newbury Park, CA: Sage.

Howell, J. M., & Avolio, B. J. (1993). Transformational leadership, transactional leadership, locus of control, and support for innovation: Key predictors of consolidated-business-unit performance. *Journal of Applied Psychology, 78*(6), 891–902. doi:10.1037/0021-9010.78.6.891

Huang, N. Y. (1997). Interpretation and execution of leadership in school administration. *Shing-Da Humanity and Sociology Publication, 6,* 1–32.

Inness, M., Turner, N., Barling, J., & Stride, C. B. (2010). Transformational leadership and employee safety performance: A within-person, between-jobs design. *Journal of Occupational Health Psychology, 15*(3), 279–290. doi:10.1037/a0019380

Judge, T. A., & Bono, J. E. (2000). Five-factor model of personality and transformational leadership. *Journal of Applied Psychology, 85*(5), 751–765. doi:10.1037/0021-9010.85.5.751

Judge, T. A., & Piccolo, R. F. (2004). Transformational and transactional leadership: A meta-analytic test of their relative validity. *Journal of Applied Psychology, 89*(5), 755–768. doi:10.1037/0021-9010.89.5.755

Judge, T. A., Piccolo, R. F., & Ilies, R. (2004). The forgotten ones? The validity of consideration and initiating structure in leadership research. *Journal of Applied Psychology, 89*(1), 36–51. doi:10.1037/0021-9010.89.1.36

Jung, D. I., & Avolio, B. J. (2000). Opening the black box: An experimental investigation of the mediating effects of trust and value congruence on transformational and transactional leadership. *Journal of Organizational Behavior, 21*(8), 949–964. doi:10.1002/1099-1379 (200012)21:8<949::AID-JOB64>3.0.CO;2-F

Jung, D. I., Bass, B. M., & Sosik, J. (1995). Bridging leadership and culture: A theoretical consideration of transformational leadership and collectivistic cultures. *Journal of Leadership & Organizational Studies, 2*(4), 3–18. doi:10.1177/107179199500200402

Kang, T. L., Su, G. J., Jang, S. S., & Sheu, S. C. (2001). The development of leadership behavior scale for directors of technical and vocational schools in Taiwan. *Human Resource Management, 1*(3), 43–57.

Kapp, E. A. (2012). The influence of supervisor leadership practices and perceived group safety climate on employee safety performance. *Safety Science, 50*(4), 1119–1124. doi:10.1016/j. ssci.2011.11.011

Kath, L. M., Marks, K. M., & Ranney, J. (2010). Safety climate dimensions, leader–member exchange, and organizational support as predictors of upward safety communication in a sample of rail industry workers. *Safety Science, 48*(5), 643–650. doi:10.1016/j.ssci.2010.01.016

Kelloway, E. K., & Barling, J. (2010). Leadership development as an intervention in occupational health psychology. *Work & Stress, 24*(3), 260–279. doi:10.1080/02678373.2010.518441

Kelloway, E. K., Mullen, J., & Francis, L. (2006). Divergent effects of transformational and passive leadership on employee safety. *Journal of Occupational Health Psychology, 11*(1), 76–86. doi:10.1037/1076-8998.11.1.76

Kines, P., Andersen, L. P. S., Spangenberg, S., Mikkelsen, K. L., Dyreborg, J., & Zohar, D. (2010). Improving construction site safety through leader-based verbal safety communication. *Journal of Safety Research, 41*(5), 399–406. doi:10.1016/j.jsr.2010.06.005

Komaki, J., Barwick, K. D., & Scott, L. R. (1978). A behavioral approach to occupational safety: Pinpointing and reinforcing safe performance in a food manufacturing plant. *Journal of Applied Psychology, 63*(4), 434–445. doi:10.1037/0021-9010.63.4.434

Komaki, J., Heinzmann, A. T., & Lawson, L. (1980). Effect of training and feedback: Component analysis of a behavioral safety program. *Journal of Applied Psychology, 65*(3), 261–270. doi: 10.1037/0021-9010.65.3.261

Leroy, H., Dierynck, B., Anseel, F., Simons, T., Halbesleben, J. R. B., McCaughey, D., …, & Sels, L. (2012). Behavioral integrity for safety, priority of safety, psychological safety, and patient safety: A team-level study. *Journal of Applied Psychology, 97*(6), 1273–1281. doi:10.1037/ a0030076

Lofquist, E. A., Greve, A., & Olsson, U. H. (2011). Modeling attitudes and perceptions as predictors for changing safety margins during organizational change. *Safety Science, 49*(3), 531–541. doi:10.1016/j.ssci.2010.11.007

Lu, C. S., & Yang, C. S. (2010). Safety leadership and safety behavior in container terminal operations. *Safety Science, 48*(2), 123–134. doi:10.1016/j.ssci.2009.05.003

Luria, G. (2008). Climate strength – How leaders form consensus. *Leadership Quarterly, 19*(1), 42–53. doi:10.1016/j.leaqua.2007.12.004

Luria, G. (2010). The social aspects of safety management: Trust and safety climate. *Accident Analysis and Prevention, 42*(4), 1288–1295. doi:10.1016/j.aap.2010.02.006

Luria, G., Zohar, D., & Erev, I. (2008). The effect of workers' visibility on effectiveness of intervention programs: supervisory-based safety interventions. *Journal of Safety Research, 39*(3), 273–280. doi:10.1016/j.jsr.2007.12.003

Martínez-Córcoles, M., Gracia, F., Tomás, I., & Peiró, J. M. (2011). Leadership and employees' perceived safety behaviors in a nuclear power plant: A structural equation model. *Safety Science, 49*(8–9), 1118–1129. doi:10.1016/j.ssci.2011.03.002

Martínez-Córcoles, M., Gracia, F. J., Tomás, I., Peiró, J. M., & Schöbel, M. (2013). Empowering team leadership and safety performance in nuclear power plants: A multilevel approach. *Safety Science, 51*(1), 293–301. doi:10.1016/j.ssci.2012.08.001

Martínez-Córcoles, M., Schöbel, M., Gracia, F. J., Tomás, I., & Peiró, J. M. (2012). Linking empowering leadership to safety participation in nuclear power plants: A structural equation model. *Journal of Safety Research, 43*(3), 215–221. doi:10.1016/j.jsr.2012.07.002

McAfee, R. B., & Winn, A. R. (1989). The use of incentives/feedback to enhance work place safety: A critique of the literature. *Journal of Safety Research, 20*(1), 7–19. doi:10.1016/0022-4375 (89)90003-0

McAllister, D. J. (1995). Affect and cognition-based trust as foundations for interpersonal cooperation in organizations. *Academy of Management Journal, 38*(1), 24–59. doi:10.2307/256727

Mearns, K., Flin, R., Gordon, R., & Fleming, M. (2001). Human and organizational factors in offshore safety. *Work & Stress, 15*(12), 144–164. doi:10.1080/026783701102678370110066616

Michael, J. H., Guo, Z. G., Wiedenbeck, J. K., & Ray, C. D. (2006). Production supervisor impacts on subordinates' safety outcomes: An investigation of leader–member exchange and safety communication. *Journal of Safety Research, 37*(5), 469–477. doi:10.1016/j.jsr.2006.06.004

Morag, I., & Luria, G. (2013). A framework for performing workplace hazard and risk analysis: A participative ergonomics approach. *Ergonomics, 56*(7), 1086–1100. doi:10.1080/00140139.2013.790484

Muldoon, J., Matthews, R. A, & Foley, C. (2012). Mediated effects of physical risk factors, leader–member exchange and empowerment in predicting perceived injury risk. *Stress and Health, 28*(2), 149–162. doi:10.1002/smi.1415

Mullen, J. (2005). Testing a model of employee willingness to raise safety issues. *Canadian Journal of Behavioral Science, 37*(4), 273–282. doi:10.1037/h0087262

Mullen, J. E., & Kelloway, E. K. (2009). Safety leadership: A longitudinal study of the effects of transformational leadership on safety outcomes. *Journal of Occupational and Organizational Psychology, 82*(2), 253–272. doi:10.1348/096317908x325313

Mullen, J., Kelloway, E. K., & Teed, M. (2011). Inconsistent style of leadership as a predictor of safety behavior. *Work & Stress, 25*(1), 41–54. doi:10.1080/02678373.2011.569200

Nahrgang, J. D., Morgeson, F. P., & Hofmann, D. A. (2011). Safety at work: A meta-analytic investigation of the link between job demands, job resources, burnout, engagement, and safety outcomes. *Journal of Applied Psychology, 96*(1), 71–94. doi:10.1037/a0021484

Neal, A., Griffin, M., & Hart, P. (2000). The impact of organizational climate on safety climate and individual behavior. *Safety Science, 34*(1), 99–109. doi:10.1016/S0925-7535(00)00008-4

Northouse, P. G. (2012). *Leadership: Theory and practice* (6th edn.). Thousand Oaks, CA: Sage Publications.

Parker, S. K., Axtell, C., & Turner, N. A. (2001). Designing a safer workplace: Importance of job autonomy, communication quality, and supportive supervisors. *Journal of Occupational Health Psychology*, *6*(3), 211–228. doi:10.1037/1076-8998.6.3.211

Pearce, C. L., Sims Jr, H. P., Cox, J. F., Ball, G., Schnell, E., Smith, K. A., & Treviño, L. (2003). Transactors, transformers and beyond: A multi-method development of a theoretical typology of leadership. *Journal of Management Development*, *22*(4), 273–307. doi: 10.1108/02621710310467587

Reason, J. T. (1997). *Managing the risks of organizational accidents*. Aldershot, UK: Ashgate.

Rotundo, M., & Sackett, P. R. (2002). The relative importance of task, citizenship, and counterproductive performance to global ratings of job performance: A policy-capturing approach. *Journal of Applied Psychology*, *87*(1), 66–80. doi:10.1037/0021-9010.87.1.66

Schunk, D. H., & Ertmer, P. A. (2000). Self-regulation and academic learning: Self-efficacy enhancing interventions. In M. Boekaerts, P. R. Pintrich, M. Zeidner (Eds.), *Handbook of self-regulation* (pp. 631–649). San Diego, CA: Academic Press.

Skinner, B. F. (1938). *The behavior of organisms: An experimental analysis*. Oxford, UK: Appleton-Century.

Størseth, F. (2004). Maintaining work motivation during organizational change. *International Journal of Human Resources Development and Management*, *4*(3), 267–287.

Størseth, F. (2006). Changes at work and employee reactions: Organizational elements, job insecurity, and short-term stress as predictors for employee health and safety. *Scandinavian Journal of Psychology*, *47*(6), 541–550. doi:10.1111/j.1467-9450.2006.00548.x

Sulzer-Azaroff, B., & de Santamaria, M. (1980). Industrial safety hazard reduction through performance feedback. *Journal of Applied Behavior Analysis*, *13*(2), 287–295. doi:10.1901/jaba.1980.13–287

Vredenburgh, A. G. (2002). Organizational safety: Which management practices are most effective in reducing employee injury rates? *Journal of Safety Research*, *33*(2), 259–76. doi:10.1016/S0022-4375(02)00016-6

Westaby, J. D., & Lowe, J. K. (2005). Risk-taking orientation and injury among youth workers: Examining the social influence of supervisors, coworkers, and parents. *Journal of Applied Psychology*, *90*(5), 1027–1035. doi:10.1037/0021-9010.90.5.1027

Wilde, G. J. (1994). *Target risk*. Toronto, ON: PDE Publications.

Wu, T. C. (2005). The validity and reliability of safety leadership scale in universities of Taiwan. *International Journal of Technology and Engineering Education*, *2*(1), 27–42.

Wu, T. C. (2008). Safety leadership in the teaching laboratories of electrical and electronic engineering departments at Taiwanese universities. *Journal of Safety Research*, *39*(6), 599–607. doi:10.1016/j.jsr.2008.10.003

Wu, T. C., Lin, C. H., & Shiau, S. Y. (2010). Predicting safety culture: The roles of employer, operations manager and safety professional. *Journal of Safety Research*, *41*(5), 423–431. doi:10.1016/j.jsr.2010.06.006

Yokochi, N. (1989). Leadership styles of Japanese business executives and managers: Transformational and transactional. Unpublished doctoral dissertation, United States International University, San Diego, CA.

Yukl, G. (1999). An evaluation of conceptual weaknesses in transformational and charismatic leadership theories. *Leadership Quarterly*, *10*(2), 285–305. doi:10.1016/S1048-9843(99)00013-2

Zohar, D. (2000). A group-level model of safety climate: Testing the effect of group climate on micro-accidents in manufacturing jobs. *Journal of Applied Psychology*, *85*(4), 587–596. doi:10.1002/job.130

Zohar, D. (2002a). The effects of leadership dimensions, safety climate, and assigned priorities on minor injuries in work groups. *Journal of Organizational Behavior*, *23*(1), 75–92. doi:10.1002/job.130

Zohar, D. (2002b). Modifying supervisory practices to improve subunit safety: A leadership-based intervention model. *Journal of Applied Psychology*, *87*(1), 156–163. doi:10.1037//0021-9010.87.1.156

Zohar, D., & Luria, G. (2003). The use of supervisory practices as leverage to improve safety behavior: A cross-level intervention model. *Journal of Safety Research, 34*(5), 567–577. doi: 10.1016/j.jsr.2003.05.006

Zohar, D., & Luria, G. (2010). Group leaders as gatekeepers: Testing safety climate variations across levels of analysis. *Applied Psychology, 59*(4), 647–673. doi:10.1111/j.1464–0597.2010.00421.x

Zohar, D., Huang, Y., Lee, J., & Robertson, M. (2014). A mediation model linking dispatcher leadership and work ownership with safety climate as predictors of truck driver safety performance. *Accident Analysis and Prevention, 62*, 17–25. doi:10.1016/j.aap.2013.09.005

Zohar, D., & Tenne-Gazit, O. (2008). Transformational leadership and group interaction as climate antecedents: A social network analysis. *Journal of Applied Psychology, 93*(4), 744–757. doi:10.1037/0021-9010.93.4.744

6

Trust-Based Approaches to Safety and Productivity

Stacey M. Conchie, Helena E. Woodcock, and Paul J. Taylor

Introduction

> The importance of trust is often acknowledged but seldom examined, and scholars tend to mention it in passing, to allude to it as a fundamental ingredient or lubricant, an unavoidable dimension of social interaction, only to move on to deal with less intractable matters.
>
> (Gambetta, 1988; Foreword, p. 1)

Gambetta's observation about research on trust defined the status of the safety literature up until a decade ago. Historically, researchers were quick to observe that trust was an important precedent of open communication and a positive safety culture, and thus key to the success of an organization's safety initiatives. Yet, the claims of these researchers were rarely accompanied by empirical research demonstrating the presumed roles of trust. This evidence base has emerged only more recently as the field has matured. Over the last decade there has been a shift within the trust literature from proposing models, to testing hypotheses derived from these models and considering the role of trust among other organizational processes (e.g., Bstieler, 2006; Cote & Latham, 2006; Ferrin, Bligh, & Kohles, 2007; Jones & George, 1998; Kramer & Tyler, 1996; Lewicki, McAllister, & Bies, 1998; Mayer, Davis, & Schoorman, 1995; McAllister, 1995; Vlaar, Van Den Bosch, & Volberda, 2007). This chapter reviews this research and what we currently know about the role of trust in creating a safe, effective workplace.

We begin our chapter by defining trust and explaining how it develops at the interpersonal level. The basic research we review makes it clear that trust is a complex construct, which likely explains why it was not subject to empirical examination in early

The Wiley Blackwell Handbook of the Psychology of Occupational Safety and Workplace Health, First Edition. Edited by Sharon Clarke, Tahira M. Probst, Frank Guldenmund, and Jonathan Passmore. © 2016 John Wiley & Sons Ltd. Published 2020 by John Wiley & Sons Ltd.

writings. It is complex because, as Kramer (2010) notes, it is defined by a three-part relationship between the person investing trust (the "trustor"), the recipient of that trust (the "trustee"), and the context of organizational functioning in which trust takes place (i.e., a specific domain of expertise, such as safety). Each of these components plays a role in the emergence and consequence of trust, and each is interrelated with the others. It is a complex construct because it is latent; it cannot be observed directly and must instead be inferred from changes in a trustor's beliefs and behaviors toward the trustee.

This background informs our understanding of how trust operates in a safety framework and we explore these relationships in the remainder of the chapter. Specifically, the second section of this chapter considers how trust interacts with other factors (e.g., safety leadership) to influence employees' engagement in safety (see also Wong, Kelloway, & Makhan, Chapter 5, this volume). One critical area of progress has been in relation to examining the role of trust in shaping the relationship among management and employees. Consistent with early claims, this research links the existence of trust with greater employee engagement in safety, a greater willingness to comply with management requests, and a greater propensity to take the initiative. However, it also makes clear that too much trust may be detrimental to safety because a degree of creative mistrust (Hale, 2000) may help an organization maintain the vigilance necessary for good safety.

In addition to highlighting the importance of interpersonal trust for promoting safety, this latter discussion gives us further insight into some of the ways that trust develops between occupational groups. The final section of our chapter considers what occurs when trust breaks down and how this can be rectified to regain good safety practices. There are many potential circumstances when this might happen, such as when a supervisor incorrectly administers patient medication and tries to cover this up, or when a coworker takes a short cut to complete a job more quickly. We review emerging research in this area, arguing that management can take appropriate responses to begin to restore employees' confidence and, ultimately, regain some of the trust that was lost.

What does it mean to Trust?

The end of the twentieth century witnessed the start of a marked increase in attention given to trust within organizations (e.g., Bigley & Pearce, 1998; Kramer & Tyler, 1996; Lewicki, 1998; Mayer et al., 1995; McAllister, 1995; McEvily, Perrone, & Zaheer, 2003; Rousseau, Sitkin, Burt, & Cramerer, 1998; for reviews see Colquitt, Scott, & LePine, 2007; Dirks & Ferrin, 2002). With this attention came a plethora of definitions and conceptualizations of trust, which, although informative, muddied the waters somewhat in terms of what researchers should focus on in their empirical work (see Hosmer, 1995, for a similar conclusion about early trust research). However, central to most definitions of trust, both in the last decade and earlier, is the element of vulnerability (e.g., Boon & Holmes, 1991; Deutsch, 1958; Mayer et al., 1995; Rousseau et al., 1998; Zand, 1972). Investing trust in a trustee involves giving up control, which exposes the trustor to the risk that the trustee may act with negative intent and harm the trustor in some way. For example, consider an employee who reports an error or near-miss to their supervisor. In doing this, the employee is exposing him or herself to the risk that the information will be used negatively (e.g., to discipline people) rather than positively (e.g., to promote learning). In this case, and in all situations defined as one of trust, the trustor is allowing themselves to be *vulnerable* to the trustee, as the outcome of misplaced trust is often greater and more significant than the gains made from trusting.

A trustor's willingness to accept vulnerability develops from their positive expectations about the trustee. This is captured in the often cited definition provided by Rousseau et al. (1998), who suggest that trust is "a psychological state comprising an intention to accept vulnerability based upon positive expectations of the intentions or behaviour of another" (p. 395). This definition has two main parts: the antecedents of trust, which are a set of *beliefs* about a trustee, and the act of trusting, which is the *intention* to accept vulnerability. According to Mayer et al. (1995), it is the intention to act, and not the set of expectations, that we call trust.

Positive expectations about a trustee may originate from a number of sources. These include the trustee's personal qualities (e.g., behaviors and intentions), generalized assumptions held by the trustor about different groups, and the trustor's general disposition to trust. Of these sources, a trustee's personal qualities, or trustworthiness, is generally regarded as having the strongest influence on expectations (Hardin, 2002). In their integrative model of organizational trust, Mayer et al. (1995) categorized trustworthiness qualities into ability, integrity, and benevolence. *Ability* concerns a person's competence to complete tasks and their role safely. *Integrity* reflects a person's openness and honesty about safety, including the degree to which they hold safety as a personal value and show consistency between espoused values and safety behavior. Finally, *benevolence* relates to holding a genuine interest and concern for ensuring other people's welfare and safety (see Colquitt et al., 2007 for a review).

Each of these three sets of qualities has been shown to be important to positive expectations. Being competent in one's job can reduce the risk of errors and mistakes, and recent research by Fruhen, Mearns, and Flin (2014) shows that – when manifested as problem solving – it is related to safety commitment. Specifically, Fruhen et al. (2014) found that the number of issues and information sources that senior managers consider when seeking to understand problems and generate solutions can serve as a proxy of their commitment to safety, as measured through things such as the effects that their decision-making has on work conditions. Having integrity encourages, among other things, the free flow of open communication, which in turn encourages sharing of information that leads to fewer errors when carrying out safety-critical work tasks (Fox, Costie, & Pickering, 1992). Finally, benevolence is associated with participative decision-making (Dirks & Ferrin, 2002), which when enacted from leaders may result in employees being encouraged to engage in, and take greater ownership of, decision-making regarding safety. It may also be reasonable to assume that those concerned for others' welfare will prioritize safety over goals that have a more self-focused outcome, such as production.

The importance of integrity to trustworthiness judgments has been particularly noted in the general trust literature. Colquitt et al. (2007) carried out a meta-analysis and found that integrity was the strongest predictor of workers' trust in supervisors across studies carried out in different business sectors. Others have since shown similar findings in domains where safety is a paramount concern. For example, Lapidot, Kark, and Shamir (2007) found integrity was the most important determinant of cadets' trust in their leader. Similarly, Conchie and Donald (2008) found integrity to be the most cited predictor of offshore workers' trust in management with regard to their safety. Interestingly, studies on trust suggest that the stronger importance of integrity is perhaps restricted to situations where the trustee is a supervisor or leader. For example, Colquitt et al. (2007) found that trust in coworkers shared a stronger relationship with a trustor's beliefs in their ability. As they suggest, integrity likely features more dominantly in worker–supervisor/leader relationships because the power difference between parties means that issues of fairness, consistency, ethical values – essentially those qualities indicative of integrity – are more salient and relevant.

Although a trustee's personal qualities are prominent in determining trust expectations, the other two sources of influence do have an impact, particularly in novel contexts, or in first encounters with a potential trustee. In these situations they provide a trustor with information on which to make a judgment, where no history of experience with that actual person exists. For example, trust expectations may be assumption-based, such that a person confers trust on another based upon a generalized expectation that the other person is trustworthy (Kim, Dirks, & Cooper, 2009; Kramer, 2010). These expectations may develop from formal and informal rules around what is acceptable behavior (e.g., the organization's culture is such that it is normative to speak out about safety, therefore a person socialized into the culture may be trusted as they are likely to be open), role occupancy (e.g., managers are trained to be safe, and may therefore be trusted in this regard), group membership (e.g., those who are the same as me (electrician/surgeon) are open and honest), third party effects (e.g., my workmates trust my supervisor, therefore I can trust her), and transference effects (e.g., my previous supervisor was trustworthy, therefore I can trust this supervisor) (Brewer, 1996; Burt & Knez, 1995; Doney & Cannon, 1997; Foddy, Platow, & Yamagishi, 2009; Kramer, 2010). In all of these cases, the trustor invests trust in another based upon some form of heuristic rather than on direct experience with the trustee. This facilitates interaction between two parties, and over time expectations based on assumed trust are replaced with expectations based upon the trustee's actual behaviors.

Another form of generalized expectation that occurs early in a relationship originates from an individual's personality. Rotter (1967) argued that people with a high disposition to trust are more likely to trust another. Others have further argued that disposition to trust makes the person more or less susceptible to other trust cues, such as social influences (Lewis & Weigert, 1985). However, evidence in support of these ideas is mixed and often weak (Colquitt et al., 2007; Conchie, 2005; Schlenker, Helm, & Tedeschi, 1973). One explanation for this inconsistency may be the nature of the trusting relationships being examined across studies. Rotter argued that personality is important in new relationships where the trustor has no previous experience of the trustee's behavior. This is because it shapes first impressions where no other information exists. Where experience does exist, or when a person is relying on a different type of generalized expectation, personality has a weaker effect. Therefore, when personality is examined in established relationships, its effects may be minimal compared with when it is examined in contexts with unfamiliar partners (Bigley & Pearce, 1998).

In summary, research suggests that "to trust" refers to a person's willingness to engage in an act that may be damaging to them personally if trust is misplaced. Informing this intention is how trustworthy the trustee is believed to be. Within an organizational context, and specifically in the domain of safety, these beliefs draw heavily on the trustee's actual behaviors (Conchie, 2005) but they can be influenced by norms and individual personalities when relevant experience of the trustee's behavior is not available.

How does Trust Relate to Safety?

The notion that trust reflects an intention, which is informed by beliefs regarding another person's trustworthiness, overlaps with classic attitude theory (Ajzen, 1985; Ajzen & Fishbein, 1980; Fishbein & Ajzen, 1975; Weiss & Cropanzano, 1996). In brief, these theories propose that a person's behavior is predicted by their specific intentions to act. Intentions are, in turn, predicted by: (i) a person's attitude toward the behavior (i.e., their beliefs regarding the behavior to be enacted); (ii) the subjective norms for the situation (i.e., their beliefs regarding how people they care about view the behavior); and (iii) perceived behavioral control (i.e., beliefs about what is under their control). In addition to informing intentions to act, perceived behavioral control has a direct impact on actual behavior. Attitude models offer a useful framework for understanding both the direction of effect from trust beliefs to intentions, and also how these components link to actual behaviors. Essentially, a trustor believes another person to be trustworthy, which increases their intention to trust that person. These intentions manifest as relying on the person to act with positive intent, or disclosing sensitive information to the trustee (Gillespie, 2003; Mayer & Davis, 1999). As intentions increase, so do related behaviors (e.g., open communication). For this reason, trust becomes an important social commodity as it shapes behaviors that are difficult to reach through formal routes.

One example of this process in action concerns the determinants of safety engagement. Safety engagement is marked by acts of safety participation and safety citizenship (Didla, Mearns, & Flin, 2009; Griffin & Neal, 2000; Turner, Stride, Carter, McCaughey, & Carroll, 2012), which are behaviors that go beyond formal (transactional) role requirements (e.g., safety compliance) to promote social environments that support safety. These behaviors include helping others with safety (Flin, Mearns, O'Connor & Bryden, 2000), proactively responding to limitations in safety measures (Burt & Stevenson, 2009), raising suggestions for change (Conchie, Taylor, & Donald, 2012), and engaging in voluntary safety activities (Neal & Griffin, 2006). Two factors that have been shown to be successful in promoting these acts are good safety leadership and a positive safety climate (e.g., Barling, Loughlin, & Kelloway, 2002; Clarke, 2006, 2013; Clarke & Ward, 2006; Conchie & Donald, 2009; Griffin & Neal, 2000; Inness, Turner, Barling, & Stride, 2010; Mullen & Kelloway, 2009; Neal & Griffin, 2006). At the heart of these two factors, and which we discuss below, is interpersonal trust (e.g., Conchie, 2013; Conchie et al., 2012; Kath, Magley, & Marmet, 2010; Luria, 2010). The importance of safety leadership and climate are considered elsewhere in this volume, and so we offer only a limited coverage of this literature in our following discussion (see also Wong, Kelloway & Makhan, Chapter 5; Guediri & Griffin, Chapter 13; Luria, Chapter 16, this volume).

Trust and Safety Leadership

The importance of managerial leadership in the promotion of employees' engagement in safety is well established. It was first shown in early work on safety culture and climate, where management commitment to safety emerged as the strongest influence on employees' safety attitudes and behaviors (see Flin et al., 2000). It has since been shown more directly through studies that have focused on specific styles of leadership and their relationship to employees' safety engagement behaviors (e.g., Barling et al., 2002; Clarke & Ward, 2006; Hofmann, Morgeson, & Gerras, 2003; Kelloway, Mullen, & Francis, 2006; Mullen & Kelloway, 2009; O'Dea & Flin, 2001). Of the different styles of leadership, much attention has been given to transformational behaviors (see Clarke, 2013, for a meta-analysis of the safety leadership literature). Transformational leadership, or safety-specific transformational leadership as it is often referred (Barling et al., 2002; Conchie, 2013; Conchie & Donald, 2009), is defined by behaviors that inspire and motivate employees, provide vision and individualized support, and encourage employees to think of new ways of doing tasks. These behaviors are effective at promoting safety participation among employees (Clarke, 2006), and to a lesser extent their safety compliance.

One explanation for why transformational leadership is effective at promoting employees' engagement is that it increases trust among employees, and in turn, this increases employees' engagement in behaviors that are believed to be desired by the leader (e.g., Jung & Avolio, 2000; Pillai, Schriesheim, & Williams, 1999; Podsakoff, MacKenzie, Moorman, & Fetter, 1990). A more complete explanation of this process is given by a social exchange theory (Blau, 1964) account of how a series of interactions between two parties can give rise to certain behaviors. When a person enters into a relationship, a sense of obligation to reciprocate the other person's actions often develops (Cropanzano & Mitchell, 2005). The resulting reciprocal acts cannot be managed or bargained, and do not always equal the other's behavior in terms of quantity. For this reason, social exchanges rely on a degree of trust that the other person is going to reciprocate fairly. This trust strengthens over time as the social exchange obligations are met by each party. Importantly, social exchanges are distinct from economic exchanges, as the latter can be determined through a simple state of quid pro quo (Blau, 1964). For this reason, economic exchanges do not rest on trust, as the outcome is most often negotiated.

Applying the principles of social exchange to our discussion of safety leadership shows how the latter promotes employees' safety engagement through trust. Specifically, when a leader engages in transformational behaviors they confer some benefits on their followers. This may include an opportunity to engage in non-requisite training, to shape the safety system, or to use a resource as the team feels appropriate. When this occurs, employees not only trust their leader with safety, they also feel a sense of obligation to reciprocate their leader's actions. One way that employees may do this is by displaying safety engagement behaviors. For example, voicing concerns about safety in a constructive manner reciprocates the leader's actions, but it also benefits the leader by allowing for safer practices and a reduction in accidents and injury. When safety concerns relate to the leader, we may argue that the behaviors have arisen not because of trust, but because of an absence of trust.

Support for the importance of trust in safety leadership has been reported in several studies. Flin and Burns (2004) discussed the importance of trust in safety management and outlined how this may be enhanced among employees using the bases of ability, integrity, and benevolence. Watson, Scott, Bishop, and Turnbeaugh (2005) showed that trust in first line managers/supervisors influenced employees' perceptions of organizational safety and their subsequent actions to reduce injuries. Zacharatos, Barling, and Iverson (2005) showed that trust in management transmitted the effects of high-performance work systems (e.g., management systems that empower employees to take responsibility for safety through greater information flow and decision-latitude) on near-misses and minor injuries.

A direct test of the notion that trust acts as a mediator in the transformational leadership–employee safety engagement link was carried out in a number of studies by Conchie and colleagues (Conchie, 2013; Conchie & Donald, 2009; Conchie et al., 2012;). Conchie and Donald (2009) examined the role of trust as a mediator between safety-specific transformational leadership and workers' safety engagement behaviors within the construction industry. Their results showed no support for the proposal that trust mediates transformational leadership effects and instead found that trust interacted with leadership to enhance its effect. Specifically, their analysis showed that transformational leaders influenced employees' safety behaviors when employees held high levels of trust in the leader, but not when they reported lower levels of trust in the leader. They accounted for this finding with the suggestion that employees reported how trustworthy their leader was, based on their experience of past leaders. This is a particularly interesting finding because of the transient nature of the construction industry. When employees have brief relationships with their leaders, they may be forced to make judgments about leader trustworthiness based on their experiences of past leaders. If this is the case, Conchie and Donald's findings demonstrate how important it is for management to develop a "trust legacy," since the effectiveness of transformational leadership rests on the basic level of employee–management trust beyond the single leader.

A subsequent study by Conchie et al. (2012) sought to explore this further. They looked at a similar model to Conchie and Donald but used as their safety outcome measure the frequency of "safety voice" behaviors. They defined safety voice behaviors as those that challenge the status quo to bring about change, such as encouraging others to engage in safety, trying to change policies to make them safer, and telling new members to follow safety procedures. They extended the model to include a trust intention component, and broke trust beliefs down into two types: cognition-based and affect-based. As per early work (Cook & Wall, 1980; Costigan et al., 2007; McAllister, 1995), cognition-based trust referred to beliefs about a leader's competence or ability to carry out their obligations. Affect-based trust referred to the belief that the leader would show care and concern for employees' welfare. Conchie et al. proposed that affect-based trust mediated the effects of safety-specific leadership (consistent with work in organizations generally), as this was consistent with the type of exchange implicated in safety-specific transformational leadership. For example, Dirks and Ferrin's (2002) meta-analysis of the trust in leadership literature suggested that transformational leadership operated in a framework where trust was based on the quality of the relationship with the leader, and not on how competent they were believed to be. Yang, Mossholder, and Peng (2009) also noted that affect-based trust promoted the relational aspects of exchanges at work, which according to Blau (1964) implicates trust. Essentially, Conchie et al. proposed that their earlier study might have focused on the wrong type of trust. They also proposed that affect-based trust would inform trust intentions and that these would be the immediate precursor of safety voice behaviors. Consistent with their proposal, they found that safety-specific transformational leadership promoted affect-based trust in leaders, which increased disclosure trust intentions, and ultimately increased employees' safety voice behaviors.

As these studies illustrate, the focus of attention has been largely in the direction of employees' trust in leaders. However, the direct question of what it means to be trusted by one's management or organization remains relatively neglected in the literature, and is completely absent in the safety literature. This is unfortunate as the few studies that have examined this other direction of trust suggest that employees who feel trusted by management increase their work outcomes, and they do so over and above what occurs when they simply report trust in management (Lau & Lam, 2008; Lester & Brower, 2003; Salamon & Robinson, 2008). One reason that feeling trusted increases performance outcomes is because employees feel a sense of responsibility, which leads to a feeling of obligation to respond to an organization's targets. The more that responsibility is felt, the greater employees engage in their job (Pearce & Gregersen, 1991). Although no direct empirical evidence exists for this type of relationship within a safety context, it seems logical to assume that similar results would emerge. As Törner (2011) observed, a perception that management trusts employees with their safety should increase employees' felt obligation to contribute to good safety (e.g., assume responsibility for helping others), which in turn should translate into an increase in actual safety behavior by employees. Indirect support for this link comes from programs that try instilling feelings of responsibility for safety within employees through decentralized decision-making and other means of empowerment (e.g., employee-led safety committees). Indeed, empowering employees with safety may be argued to signal a sense of trust within employees to fulfill this role competently and with integrity.

Trust and Safety Climate

Safety climate reflects shared perceptions among organizational members about the priority given to procedures, policies, and practices concerning safety (Griffin & Neal, 2000). Given the facet-specific nature of these perceptions (i.e., their specificity to safety), they play a strong role in shaping safety behaviors. In a meta-analysis of the literature, Clarke (2006) showed that positive safety climates are related to greater safety participation, greater safety compliance and, to a weaker extent, fewer accidents. Safety climate perceptions shape behavior by informing employees' expectations about what is acceptable safety behavior and what will be rewarded by the organization (Schneider, 1990). In this way, safety climate offers an indication of how committed to safety employees believe management to be, and how much they should consider safety as central to their own role.

Some have suggested that trust is important to the development of a positive safety climate and, consequently, safety behaviors. Indirect support for this claim comes from research on the related construct of safety culture (see Guldenmund, Chapter 19, this volume). Safety culture reflects the shared attitudes and behaviors relating to hazards and risks, which manifest at a surface level through climate perceptions (Mearns, Flin, Gordon, & Fleming, 2001). As argued by Mearns et al. (2001), safety climate perceptions offer a real-time snapshot of the state of an organization's safety culture. Reason (1997) proposed that positive safety cultures comprise three separate, but interlinked, subcultures: an informed culture, a reporting culture, and a just culture. An informed culture facilitates organizational learning and encourages the proactive implementation of safety measures, but its existence depends on the presence of a reporting culture in which organizational members feel confident to report on safety issues. Similarly, an effective reporting culture depends on the existence of a just culture, defined by an atmosphere of trust whereby organizational members are not afraid to report on safety (see Dirks & Ferrin, 2002, for evidence in support of the link between justice and trust).

The basis of a just culture is knowledge about what is considered acceptable and unacceptable behavior, and which acts will be disciplined. In this way, just cultures may be argued to instill a sense of psychological safety (Edmondson, 1999) among employees. Psychological safety refers to the extent to which groups view their social climate as receptive to interpersonal risk, as defined by sharing views that others may disagree with but are not likely to retaliate against. As argued by Edmondson, trust lies at the foundation of this state. Thus, and as suggested by Reason, trust lies at the foundation of the three tiers of safety culture.

Evidence to support the central role of trust in shaping an organization's safety culture comes from several detailed case studies. In their case study of the nuclear industry, Cox, Jones, and Collinson (2006) found that efforts to promote a positive safety culture, through behavioral programs that promote open communication, effectively increased trust between occupational groups. This increase in trust resulted in greater ownership for, and commitment toward, safety and facilitated organizational learning. Conversely, in their case study of the offshore industry, Cox et al. (2006) found that the culture was defined by a lack of trust, which resulted in organizational members withholding important safety information concerning accidents and near-misses. As might be expected, this prevented learning but also perpetuated low trust relations.

Jeffcott, Pidgeon, Weyman, and Walls (2006) reported similar findings for the railway industry. Their study showed a number of factors within the industry that shaped the prevailing culture and also impacted on trust relations. These included overregulation and proceduralization, which promoted a "rule-based trust," or put simply, trust in another based on an understanding of the systems that govern appropriate behavior, and the expectation that people will adhere to these systems. Although this offered a confidence in others with safety, it prevented flexibility in thinking and discouraged people from using their professional judgment when something unexpected arose. They also found that overregulation hampered the development of trust based on foundations of integrity or benevolence. The outcome of not developing trust on these foundations mirrored what Cox et al. (2006) observed in the offshore industry, namely, a blunted communication that had a negative impact on safety. Thus, both studies highlight the importance of trust for open communication and organizational learning.

One limitation of Cox et al. (2006) and Jeffcott et al. (2006) is that they focus on safety culture and so offer only indirect evidence for the link between trust, safety climate and safety performance. As mentioned above (and discussed in Guldenmund, Chapter 19, this volume), an organization's safety culture reflects the shared attitudes and beliefs regarding safety, which are expressed though safety climate perceptions. Although the two are linked, culture comprises many more dimensions than climate, and is considered as being a more stable construct (Guldenmund, 2000). Recently, Luria (2010) examined this missing link between trust and safety climate within a military setting. He found that safety climate fully mediated the effects of trust in leaders on injury rates. As an explanation, Luria suggests that relationships defined by high trust should ensure leaders (supervisors in this study) create a safer environment for employees. Through these safety practices, employees will come to recognize the importance of safety for their leader, and will start to believe, and respond to, the safety information communicated to them by their leader. Both of these things will lead to positive safety climate perceptions, which other research shows to be negatively related to accidents and positively related to safety engagement.

Luria's study is interesting as it suggests that safety climate may be one route through which trust in transformational leadership shapes safety engagement. For example, if we piece together the research discussed thus far then we might reasonably argue for a model in which leadership influences employees' trust in the leader, which in turn shapes safety climate perceptions and consequently, safety behaviors. A model of this description has not been tested empirically, but it seems a logical ordering of the variables from the research findings that have been reported.

Incidents that Reduce Trust

The value of trust to an organization becomes most apparent when it is lost or broken. Research has identified a number of negative consequences associated with a lack of trust, which are typically discussed in relation to management. For example, a lack of trust in management has been associated with employees' spending large amounts of time and energy "covering their backs," which detracts from work performance (Mayer & Gavin, 2005), increases turnover (Roberts, Cooper, & Lawrence, 1999), reduces information sharing (Chua, Kaynak, & Foo, 2007), and hinders organizational learning about safety (Hale, 2000; O'Toole, 2002). There is even evidence that a lack of trust has a direct impact on safety because it leads to an increased rate of accidents and near-miss events (Conchie & Donald, 2006).

The relative ease by which trust may be broken, compared with the time it takes to build, has led several authors to describe it as a fragile entity (Slovic, 1993). Trust in another reduces following what is often referred to as a "trust violation." These violations are incidents that show a failure – intentional or not – to fulfill the trustor's expectations. A supervisor who fails to adhere to safety procedures is one such example. When these incidents occur, the trustor's beliefs and subsequent trust intentions toward the trustee are reduced (Kim et al., 2009). Crucially, such a reduction in trust may occur following a single incidence of untrustworthiness (Hansson, Jones, & Fletcher, 1990; Jones & Burdette, 1994) and it may even occur in situations where the incident is mere hearsay (Penrod & Cutler, 1995).

When trust reduces, the trustor finds himself or herself in a situation of trying to rebuild trust from a state of distrust. This is more complex than initial trust formation as the trustee must both show him or herself to be trustworthy and also address the salient negative expectations that may have developed about their character. Despite this complexity, the trustee may wish to engage in such efforts for a number of reasons. These include the fact that the trustee may be genuinely remorseful, they may perceive the reduced trust as unjustified (e.g., they responded to external pressures that the trustor may be unaware of), or that they want to access the social benefits that trust brings (e.g., cooperation, free flow of information) (Kim et al., 2009).

Ferrin, Dirks, and their colleagues have carried out a large body of empirical research on trust violations and trust repair within organizations. Their work has shown that trust violations fall into one of two broad categories: competence-based violations and integrity-based violations (Dirks & Ferrin, 2002; Ferrin, Kim, Cooper, & Dirks, 2007; Kim, Dirks, Cooper, & Ferrin, 2004, 2006). Competence-based violations are incidents that suggest a trustee lacks ability in some area, such as when a supervisor fails to identify all of the risks in a set task due to a lack of skill or qualification. Integrity-based violations are incidents that suggest the trustee is dishonest, secretive, or acting with selfish intent, such as when a supervisor openly announces the importance of safety, but then takes short cuts when carrying out tasks.

Of the two types of violation, those that breach integrity expectations have been shown to be most detrimental to trust. For example, Conchie and Donald (2008) interviewed offshore workers about their trust in a number of occupational groups. They found that workers reported the least trust in management, and attributed this belief to a lack of management integrity. Specifically, they reported acts of dishonesty, displays of behavioral inconsistency (e.g., stating that workers would not be disciplined following an event, but then issuing discipline), and a disregard for safety over career advancement – essentially, prioritizing production over safety – as predictive of their faltering trust. Within this study, Conchie and Donald found very few, if any, examples of a lack of competence being given as a reason for reduced trust in management.

Conchie, Taylor, and Charlton (2011) supported these findings in a later study carried out within the construction industry. Conchie et al. (2011) used a ranking exercise in which workers were asked to state which of two supervisors displaying different qualities (e.g., a lack of honesty or a lack of competence) they would trust the least with safety. Unlike the interviews carried out by Conchie and Donald (2008), which relied to some extent on free recall, the ranking exercise forced workers to consider qualities related to competence, and so made this as salient as those related to integrity and benevolence. Conchie et al. (2011) compared a total of eight specific qualities and paired all against each other. Their results showed that dishonesty and a lack of care and concern for others' safety and welfare were the most significant predictors of distrust. Consistent with Conchie and Donald, they found that qualities indicative of a lack of competence featured much lower, with a lack of expertise having the least diagnostic weight about supervisors' untrustworthiness with safety.

One way to understand the differential impact on trust of violations in competence and integrity is through Attribution Theory (Heider, 1958; Weiner, 1992). Attribution Theory concerns the way in which people make sense of another's actions by looking for causes for their behavior. According to Heider (1958), people make one of two attributions about another's actions: (i) external attributions, where the person's behavior is attributed to external events; and (ii) internal attributions, where the person's behavior is assumed to reflect their personality, character, or attitude. Competence-based violations are often attributed externally (i.e., the trustee's actions are due to some uncontrollable external event) (Maddux, Kim, Okumura, & Brett, 2011). As noted by Elangovan and Shapiro (1998), a lack of competence reflects a situation of "can't" rather than "won't." An example of this within industry is when employees are tasked with jobs that they are not skilled to deal with. In contrast, integrity-based violations are often attributed internally (i.e., the trustees' actions are volitional and thus reflects their character) as there often exists no obvious external cause for a lack of integrity.

To explain why internal attributions have a more damaging effect on trust, Kim et al. (2004) draw on Reeder and Brewer's (1979) schematic model of dispositional attribution. This theory proposes that people process positive and negative information about another's ability and integrity differently, and it is for this reason that integrity-based violations are more damaging on trust. Specifically, the theory suggests that positive information about another's competence holds strong diagnostic weight about another's trustworthiness, as only those highly skilled can perform at this level. However, as a lack of competence is not skill-dependent (i.e., both those high or low in competence can make mistakes), a single act of incompetence carries weak diagnostic information about another's trustworthiness. By contrast, integrity works in the opposite direction. Those with high integrity are assumed to act honestly across situations, regardless of any incentive to act otherwise. Those low on integrity, however, may act honestly or dishonestly, depending on the specific opportunity or motivation in front of them. For this reason, a single act of dishonesty is regarded as a strong indication that the person is untrustworthy. From a safety perspective this research suggests that acts displaying a lack of integrity are most damaging for trust, since they are taken as indicative of the person's character and volitional nature.

Ways to Rebuild Trust

What can be done to rebuild trust following the kinds of violations identified above? Although research to answer this question remains in its infancy, some early findings suggest that what occurs at the general organizational level transfers to the safety context. That is, strategies shown to be effective in repairing trust in non-safety contexts generally emerge as effective in high-risk domains. The starting point of much of this analysis is a distinction between non-substantive and substantive acts. We consider each in turn.

Non-substantive responses are verbal accounts that aim to repair trust through denial, excuse, justification, or apology (Cody & McLaughlin, 1990; Kim et al., 2004; Ohbuchi, Kameda, & Agarie, 1989; Tomlinson & Mayer, 2009). They affect trust by addressing the causal attribution that a trustor makes about a trustee's actions. That is, they encourage an external attribution by deflecting "blame" for the event to an external source, or they encourage an internal attribution by accepting responsibility for the event and conveying remorse. For example, a denial rejects responsibility for the event and provides a clear statement that the allegation is false in an attempt to encourage an external attribution for the event (Cody & McLaughlin, 1990; Tedeschi & Norman, 1985). Similarly, excuses and justifications point to external factors to weaken the causal links to the person's character and instead encourage the trustor to regard the act as necessary, or the result of good motive. In this way, verbal responses help to repair trust by allowing a person's actions to be accounted for by events outside of their control, thus making the trustee appear more favorable and trustworthy (Kelley & Michela, 1980; Pettersen, 1987; Sitkin & Bies, 1993;

Tomlinson & Mayer, 2009). In contrast, an apology signals acceptance of responsibility for a violation, but also communicates remorse for the act and a promise to reform. In this way, an apology is said to improve trust as it reduces the trustor's felt vulnerability of future risk.

The effectiveness of these strategies is evidenced by studies of trust repair in general organizational contexts. Crant and Bateman (1993; see also Kim et al., 2004; Wood & Mitchell, 1981) found that management offered less severe punishment to employees when an external account was given for their poor performance. Keltikangas-Jarvinen and Lindeman (1997) showed that acts of dishonesty were more readily perceived as being acceptable when the employee justified their action as being performed under duress or when provoked. However, justification following an act of betrayal is considered less acceptable when the trustee is regarded as being vindictive (Feldman & Cauffman, 1999) or acting for self-protective reasons (Peterson, Peterson, & Seeto, 1983). Finally, apology has been shown to result in more positive trust beliefs about the trustee and a greater willingness to trust the person, when compared with situations in which an external account for the event is offered (Gill, Thompson, Febbraro, & Barnes, 2010; Maddux et al., 2011; Tomlinson, Dineen, & Lewicki, 2004). Apology positively influences the interpretation of the trustee's intention behind their actions (Ferrin et al., 2007), and promotes reconciliation through favorable attributions about the trustee's actions (Kellerman, 2006; Tucker, Turner, Barling, Reid, & Elving, 2006).

Substantive responses concentrate on safeguarding against future transgressions by imposing some form of control or constraint on the person's actions to prevent reoccurrence of the behavior. They achieve this by either modifying the system in which employees operate or by directly modifying the person's behavior. A system-focused substantive response may be the introduction of a new procedure, which regulates how all employees approach a situation or a given task. An individual-focused substantive response may include monitoring the person, imposing some type of formal discipline such as suspension, or implementing some other form of penance (Dirks, Kim, Ferrin, & Cooper, 2011; Nakayachi & Watabe, 2005; Schweitzer & Ho, 2005; Slovic, 1993). As observed by Janowicz-Panjaitan and Krishnan (2009), substantive responses are akin to legalistic remedies that relate to formal mechanisms that regulate behavior, whereas non-substantive responses are akin to non-legalistic remedies that involve some form of social account that affect beliefs concerning the trustor.

Studies of substantive responses are limited, but there exists some support for their effectiveness. At an organizational level, Gillespie and Dietz (2012) reported a case study of a large engineering company that had been accused of systematic bribery and consequently suffered a breakdown in relationships with stakeholders, employees and the general public. The company implemented a system that detected and prevented unethical conduct following the event, which they found to result in an improvement in people's beliefs regarding the company's integrity. At an interpersonal level, Desmet, De Cremer, and van Dijk (2011) found that overcompensating another following an economic transgression (i.e., unfairly retaining more money than the other person) repaired trust when no negative intent was detected. Dirks et al. (2011) examined the effects of regulation (e.g., monitoring) and penance (e.g., giving some resource unfairly gained on a joint task to the other person) on the repair of trust in peer and employee–manager relationships. They found that both penance and regulation were effective in repairing trust, but only if these responses signaled repentance. Of the two, they found that regulation could be interpreted either way – as signaling repentance or not – and when the latter occurred, regulation had no effect on trust beliefs or intentions. The statement of repentance is important in this case as it offers a frame of reference in which to consider the substantive response. More specifically, it signals to the trustor that a recurrence in the behavior that violated trust is unlikely (Bottom, Gibson, Daniels, & Murnighan, 2002).

Substantive responses operate to repair trust by setting parameters around a person's behavior (Perrone, Zaheer, & McEvily, 2003; Shapiro, 1987), thus making their actions prototypical of somebody who is trustworthy (Gillespie & Dietz, 2009). This promotes positive trust beliefs within the trustor about the trustee (Kramer & Lewicki, 2010; McKnight, Cummings, & Chervany, 1998; Sitkin & Roth, 1993) and encourages a willingness to accept vulnerability and rely on the person in future situations (Nordgren, van Harreveld, & van der Pligt, 2009). Moreover, and as indicated by Dirks et al. (2011), the effectiveness of a substantive response is enhanced when combined with a non-substantive response (e.g., an apology) as together they offer more than what may simply be regarded as "cheap talk" (Lewicki, 2006).

When looking at the effectiveness of substantive and non-substantive repair strategies as a function of violation type, the picture becomes more complex. For example, in relation to non-substantive strategies, apologies have been shown to be most effective following a competence-based violation, but not following an integrity-based violation (Kim et al., 2004; Kim, Cooper, Dirks, & Ferrin, 2013). However, others have found that apologies are more effective than other verbal responses, irrespective of the type of violation (Gill et al., 2010). Similarly, while some research has shown the effectiveness of justifications for repairing trust, others have found that offering a justification promotes the perception that the person is deceptive, self-absorbed, unreliable, and has a flawed character (Schlenker, Pontari, & Christopher, 2001). Similarly, in relation to substantive strategies, the general suggestion from available work is that they are most effective when they show repentance and are implemented by the trustee (as they are seen as diagnostic of the trustees' commitment to refrain from future violations), and they are less effective when they occur indirectly through less personal means (Desmet et al., 2011; McCabe, Rigdon, & Vernon, 2003; Nakayachi & Watabe, 2005).

The mixed results reported for repair strategies are due to the complex nature of trust. Simply put, repairing trust – and more specifically deciding whether the person can be trusted – depends on a number of factors and the interplay between these factors. Kim et al. (2013) point toward two factors, suggesting that trust repair is the process of reconciling two competing views: the trustor's belief that the trustee is untrustworthy, and the trustee's belief that greater trust is deserved. In resolving this, the trustor may ask three questions: (i) is the trustee innocent or guilty of the violation; (ii) if guilty, is an internal or external attribution most appropriate; and (iii) if an internal attribution is appropriate, does the act reflect an enduring characteristic or something that can be changed? How the trustor answers these questions will dictate the effectiveness of a specific response. For example, an apology may be ineffective if the trustee is held accountable for the act, as in the case of an integrity violation, since the acceptance of guilt may suggest that the person is unpredictable and likely to repeat the behavior that violated trust. By contrast, when the violation is believed to be under minimal personal control, as in the case of a lapse in competence, an apology may be more effective.

Many of the empirical studies we have discussed in this section have focused on business contexts in which the trust violation relates to incorrect filing of tax forms, taking a larger bonus than promised, not fairly reciprocating a social exchange, and so on. Despite the obvious lack of personal risk, as measured through exposure to hazards, emerging research suggests that these findings still transfer to a safety context. For example, Woodcock and Conchie (2010) had participants read about a (fictitious) manager in two very different industries (pharmaceutical and nuclear) who failed to report unsafe equipment, either because of a poor understanding of the equipment (lapse in competence) or because reporting the problem would slow down production and prevent targets from being met (lapse in integrity). They found that public trust in the manager following the event was higher if the manager apologized following the competence-based violation rather than denied responsibility. This effect emerged in both contexts, despite the different hazards and potential implications of unsafe equipment, thus showing the power of an apology. Furthermore, they found that denying responsibility had no effect on trust in the risk manager, irrespective of the reason for the violation.

Woodcock and Conchie (in prep. a) developed this initial work by presenting employees with information about an event in which management breached safety to speed up production. They examined two levels of management: supervisors and managers, and manipulated information about the event to reflect low risk (no injury) or high risk (injury). Their results showed that when the breach in safety resulted in injury, an apology and preventative procedure (i.e., one that prohibited similar breaches to safety in the future) was necessary to repair employees' trust. Put simply, employees expressed more positive trust beliefs in management when these two things occurred together. Furthermore, they found that a procedure implemented voluntarily was more important when a manager violated safety than when a supervisor did so. In the latter case, the mere presence of the preventative procedure was enough to result in more trust from employees. It is likely that the combination of both an apology and a preventative procedure was regarded as matching the severity of the violation, thus increasing the likelihood of trust repair.

One limitation of the Woodcock and Conchie studies, as well as with previous non-safety-specific work, is a reliance on fictitious events whereby the participant is asked to imagine him or herself as a manager or employee faced with a situation. As the participant may have no experience of similar events, it is not possible to know how much their responses transfer to a real situation. To address this limitation, Woodcock and Conchie (in prep. b) recently conducted a field study in which employees at an energy plant were asked to state how often their manager and supervisor engaged in wrong-doing, what if any non-substantive and substantive response followed such a wrong-doing, and how this impacted the employees' own trust beliefs and intentions toward their manager/supervisor as a result. Within their analysis, they also controlled for employees' disposition to trust, the number of years they had worked in the industry and had been reporting to their current manager and supervisor, and their site of work.

Their findings revealed that the term "wrong-doing" was invariably linked to a breach in safety, and that these were mostly discussed in relation to integrity violations. Within this context, when a manager or supervisor committed a wrong-doing, substantive responses played a role in restoring employees' integrity beliefs and trust intentions, but had no effect on their beliefs regarding the manager's ability. To impact beliefs about ability, it was necessary for the manager to be seen as undergoing re-training (an act that also restored integrity beliefs). Furthermore, Woodcock and Conchie (in prep. b) found that integrity beliefs increased when a manager was disciplined, but that trust intentions reduced when the manager or supervisor was monitored. Indeed, across all outcome measures, they found that attributing the event to, or relying on, an external source (e.g., the event was out of their control) had a significant negative effect on trust. For example, employees regarded a supervisor as having less integrity if they blamed an external source.

Considered together, the results discussed in this section, in particular the Woodcock and Conchie studies, highlight a number of ways to rebuild trust. First, apologies have the strongest positive effect on trust repair when compared with other non-substantive responses. Second, attributing the event to an external source reduces trust. Third, monitoring, although regulating future behavior and reducing the recurrence of events, reduces trust in the person being monitored. One possible explanation for this latter finding is that employees regard monitoring as ineffective or unjust. Kramer (2010) suggested that effective monitoring, which is considered to be aligned to the wrong-doing and an effective deterrent, provides employees with confidence in the fairness of procedures, and offers a reassurance that it is safe to trust again. Instead of monitoring, we may tentatively conclude that a more effective response to monitoring, as suggested by this study, is to offer training to the person, or discipline them using some agreed on and fair method.

Future Research

Our discussion has highlighted several areas in which future work should focus to have the greatest impact. First, attention should be given to testing a model in which leadership, trust, and safety climate are sequentially linked to safety outcome behaviors. Support exists for the individual relationships within this model (e.g., leadership to trust) and so we would expect a model linking these together to also receive support. When exceptions and the relative strengths among model components are revealed, then it becomes possible to talk in more nuanced terms about the relationship between actors, their beliefs and intentions around trust, and their resulting behavior. Thus, testing such a model provides the basis for developing a more complete model of safety behaviors.

Second, attention should be given to testing the notion that feeling trusted by management is equally, if not more, important than trusting management for increasing employee engagement in safety. Establishing a sense of empowerment within employees is often striven for within organizations looking to promote safety, and the research cited here hints that one way to achieve this may be to entrust employees with safety. For example, while the specific acts that lead to feelings of being trusted with safety have not been established, we would expect such feelings to be positively related to acts such as dissolving decision-latitude to employees, asking for input on safety issues, and openly communicating both positive and negative safety information. Once these relationships have been demonstrated empirically, a second more interesting question is whether it is easier to establish employees' feelings of being trusted *by*, than employees' trust *in*, management. As we reviewed above, trust development is a slow process (Slovic, 1993), which may be compounded by a history of negative events, stereotypes, and skepticism when the trustee is management. If instilling feelings of being trusted is easier for an organization to achieve, and equally effective at generating safe behavior, then this represents a route for organizations to direct their energies to see quicker results in terms of improved safety.

Third, we introduced emerging research on trust repair and suggested that this is an important area of growth. This is especially so given that acts that violate trust (real or imagined) are relatively frequent within organizations and have the potential to damage social relations and productivity. The existing research has only scratched the surface with likely strategies that may prove effective in restoring social relations in these situations. Going beneath the surface will not only benefit safety research, but it will also enrich the organizational literature more generally because it forces us to consider relationships as dynamic, evolving entities within organizations that must be considered from a longitudinal perspective. The challenge for researchers in this regard is finding a method to study trust repair that takes us outside of the laboratory and away from relying on student data.

An additional area worthy of future research, which we did not cover in our discussion above, concerns implicit trust (Burns, Mearns, & McGeorge, 2006). Implicit trust refers to the beliefs that a person holds about another, which exist at a subconscious level (i.e., the person is not overtly aware of these attitudes). Research carried out in the gas industry (Burns et al., 2006) showed that employees' implicit trust toward another group (e.g., management) was not correlated with their explicit trust toward that group (explicit trust is the type of trust captured in the studies cited throughout this chapter). For example, employees reported explicit trust toward their workmates, supervisor, and plant leadership, but only reported implicit trust for their workmates. Drawing on the Motivation and Opportunity as Determinants Model of whether the attitude-to-behavior process is primarily spontaneous or deliberate, Burns et al. (2006) suggest that implicit trust may be a stronger determinant of automatic behaviors, which are essentially those acts that occur when there is insufficient time to allow for the pros and cons of a decision to be calculated. This link has not been tested empirically, but it has important practical implications if supported. Specifically, support for this link raises questions such as: what factors shape implicit trust? What level of implicit trust is optimal for safety, and at what level does implicit distrust become problematic? How robust are implicit attitudes to change? Some of these questions have received some attention (e.g., Burns & Conchie, 2014; Woodcock, 2013), but there is still much that we need to unpack about implicit trust when considered in a safety context.

Conclusion

Although the importance of trust has been long recognized, it is only recently that researchers have taken seriously the task of unpacking both the nature of this complex psychological construct and its relationship to external factors of significance, such as safety. Despite the infancy of this research, a number of key patterns are beginning to emerge. First, trust among employees and between employees and their management is both related directly to good safety, and indirectly related to good safety because of its positive impact on communication and safety engagement behaviors. Second, while trust is comprised of beliefs relating to the trustee's ability, benevolence, and integrity, it is both evidence of, and violation of, integrity beliefs that have the biggest impact on trust. This is because, in no small part, violations of integrity raise questions about the person's inner motives and make it difficult for the trustee to reliably evaluate the person's actions in the future. Third, it is possible to repair trust once it is lost through a number of mechanisms, but substantive actions that are implemented personally appear to be the most effective at reconciliation in most (but not all) scenarios.

References

Ajzen, I. (1985). From intentions to actions: A theory of planned behaviour. In J. Kuhl & J. Beckman (Eds.), *Action-control: From cognition to behaviour* (pp. 11–39). Heidelberg: Springer.

Ajzen, I., & Fishbein, M. (1980). *Understanding attitudes and predicting social behaviour.* Englewood Cliffs, NJ: Prentice-Hall.

Barling, J., Loughlin, C., & Kelloway, E. K. (2002). Development and test of a model linking safety-specific transformational leadership and occupational safety. *Journal of Applied Psychology, 87,* 488–496.

Bigley, G., & Pearce, J. (1998). Straining for shared meaning in organization science. Problems of trust and distrust. *Academy of Management Review, 23,* 405–421.

Blau, P. (1964). *Exchange and power in social life.* New York, NY: John Wiley & Sons, Inc.

Boon, S. D., & Holmes, J. G. (1991). The dynamics of interpersonal trust: Resolving uncertainty in face of risk. In R. A. Hinde & J. Groebel (Eds.), *Cooperation and pro-social behavior* (pp. 190–211). Cambridge, UK: Cambridge University Press.

Bottom, W. P., Gibson, K., Daniels, S., & Murnighan, J. K. (2002). When talk is not cheap: Substantive penance and expressions of intent in rebuilding cooperation. *Organization Science*, *13*, 497–513.

Brewer, M. B. (1996). In-group favoritism: The subtle side of intergroup discrimination. In D. M. Messick & A. Tenbrunsel (Eds.), *Codes of conduct: Behavioral research and business ethics* (pp. 160–171). New York, NY: Russell Sage Foundation.

Bstieler, L. (2006). Trust formation in collaborative new product development. *Journal of Product Innovation Management*, *23*, 56–72.

Burns, C., & Conchie, S. M. (2014). Implicit trust and automatic attitude activation. In F. Lyon (ed.), *Handbook of research methods on trust* (2nd edn., pp. 239–248). Cheltenham, UK: Edward Elgar.

Burns, C., Mearns, K., & McGeorge, P. (2006). Explicit and implicit trust within safety culture. *Risk Analysis*, *26*, 1139–1150.

Burt, D. B., & Stevenson, R. J. (2009). The relationship between recruitment processes, familiarity, trust, perceived risk and safety. *Journal of Safety Research*, *40*, 365–369.

Burt, R., & Knez, M. (1995). Kinds of third-party effects on trust. *Journal of Relational Sociology*, *7*, 255–292.

Chua, A. Y. K., Kaynak, S., & Foo, S. S. B. (2007). An analysis of the delayed response to Hurricane Katrina through the lens of knowledge management. *Journal of the American Society for Information Science and Technology*, *58*, 391–403.

Clarke, S. (2006). The relationship between safety climate and safety performance: A meta-analytic review. *Journal of Occupational Health Psychology*, *11*, 315–327.

Clarke, S. (2013). Safety leadership: A meta-analytic review of transformational and transactional leadership styles as antecedents of safety behaviours. *Journal of Occupational and Organizational Psychology*, *86*, 22–49.

Clarke, S., & Ward, K. (2006). The role of leader influence tactics and safety climate in engaging employees' safety participation. *Risk Analysis*, *26*, 1175–1185.

Cody, M. J., & McLaughlin, M. L. (1990). Interpersonal accounting. In H. Giles & W. P. Robinson (Eds.). *Handbook of language and psychology* (pp. 227–255). New York, NY: John Wiley & Sons, Inc.

Colquitt, J. A., Scott, B. A., & LePine, J. A. (2007). Trust, trustworthiness, and trust propensity: A meta-analytic test of their unique relationships with risk taking and job performance. *Journal of Applied Psychology*, *92*, 902–927.

Conchie, S. M. (2005). The role of trust in offshore safety: The development and empirical validation of a safety-specific trust tool. Unpublished doctoral thesis. University of Liverpool, UK.

Conchie, S. M. (2013). Transformational leadership, intrinsic motivation and trust: A moderated-mediated model of workplace safety. *Journal of Occupational Health Psychology*, *18*, 198–210.

Conchie, S. M., & Donald, I. J. (2006). The role of distrust in offshore safety performance. *Risk Analysis*, *26*, 1151–1159.

Conchie, S. M., & Donald, I. J. (2008). The functions and development of safety-specific trust and distrust. *Safety Science*, *46*, 92–103.

Conchie, S. M., & Donald, I. J. (2009). The moderating role of safety-specific trust in the relation between safety-specific transformational leadership and safety citizenship behaviours. *Journal of Occupational Health Psychology*, *14*, 137–147.

Conchie, S. M., Taylor, P. J., & Charlton, A. (2011). Trust and distrust in safety leadership: Mirror reflections? *Safety Science*, *49*, 1208–1214.

Conchie, S. M., Taylor, P. J., & Donald, I. J. (2012). Promoting safety voice with safety-specific transformational leadership: The mediator role of two dimensions of trust. *Journal of Occupational Health Psychology*, *17*, 105–115.

Cook, J., & Wall, T. (1980). New work attitude measures of trust, organizational commitment and personal need non-fulfillment. *Journal of Occupational Psychology*, *53*, 39–52.

Costigan, R. D., Insinga, R. C., Berman, J., Ilter, S. S., Kranas, G., & Kureshov, V. A. (2007). A cross-cultural study of supervisory trust. *International Journal of Manpower*, *27*, 764–787.

Cote, J., & Latham, C. K. (2006). Trust and commitment: Intangible drivers of interorganizational performance. *Advances in Management Accounting*, *15*, 293–325.

Cox, S., Jones, B., & Collinson, D. (2006). Trust relations in high-reliability organizations. *Risk Analysis, 26*, 1123–1138.

Crant J. M., & Bateman, T. S. (1993). Assignment of credit and blame for performance outcomes. *Academy of Management Journal, 36*, 7–27.

Cropanzano, R., & Mitchell, M. S. (2005). *Social exchange theory: An interdisciplinary review. Journal of Management, 31*, 874–900.

Desmet, P. T. M., De Cremer, D., & van Dijk, E. (2011). Trust recovery following voluntary or forced financial compensations in the trust game: The role of trait forgiveness. *Personality and Individual Differences, 51*, 267–273.

Deutsch, M. (1958). Trust and suspicion. *Journal of Conflict Resolution, 2*, 265–279.

Didla, S., Mearns, K., & Flin, R. (2009). Safety citizenship behaviour: A proactive approach to risk management. *Journal of Risk Research, 12*, 475–483.

Dirks, K. T., & Ferrin, D. L. (2002). Trust in leadership: Meta-analytic findings and implications for organizational research. *Journal of Applied Psychology, 87*, 611–628.

Dirks, K. T., Kim, P. H., Ferrin, D. L., & Cooper, C. D. (2011). Understanding the effects of substantive responses on trust following a transgression. *Organizational Behavior and Human Decision Processes, 114*, 87–103.

Doney, P. M., & Cannon, J. P. (1997). An examination of the nature of trust in buyer–seller relationships. *Journal of Marketing, 61*(2), 35–51.

Edmondson, A. C. (1999). Psychological safety and learning behavior in work teams. *Administrative Science Quarterly, 44*, 350–383.

Elangovan, A. R., & Shapiro, D. L. (1998). Betrayal of trust in organizations. *Academy of Management Review, 23*, 547–566.

Feldman, S., & Cauffman, E. (1999). Your cheating heart: Attitudes, behaviours, and correlates of sexual betrayal in late adolescents. *Journal of Research on Adolescence, 15*, 227–253.

Ferrin, D. L., Bligh, M. C., & Kohles, J. C. (2007). Can I trust you to trust me? A theory of trust, monitoring, and cooperation in international and intergroup relationships. *Group and Organization Management, 32*, 465–499.

Ferrin, D. L., Kim, P. H., Cooper, C. D., & Dirks, K. T. (2007). Silence speaks volumes: The effectiveness of reticence in comparison to apology and denial for responding to integrity- and competence-based trust violations. *Journal of Applied Psychology, 92*, 893–908.

Fishbein, M., & Ajzen, I. (1975). *Belief, attitude, intention, and behavior: An introduction to theory and research.* Reading, MA: Addison-Wesley.

Flin, R., & Burns, C. (2004). The role of trust in safety management. *Human Factors and Aerospace Safety, 4*, 275–288.

Flin, R., Mearns, K., O'Connor, P., & Bryden, R. (2000). Measuring safety climate: Identifying the common features. *Safety Science, 34*, 177–192.

Foddy, M., Platow, M. J., & Yamagishi, T. (2009). Group-based trust in strangers: The role of stereotypes and expectations. *Psychological Science, 20*, 419–422.

Fox, R. D., Costie, K. A., & Pickering, R. J. (1992). *Health professionals' expectations of physicians: Report of the survey of selected health professionals in Ontario.* Educating Future Physicians for Ontario (EFPO).

Fruhen, L. S., Mearns, K., & Flin, R. (2014). Skills, knowledge and senior managers' demonstrations of safety commitment. *Safety Science, 69*, 29–36.

Gambetta, D. (1988). *Trust, making and breaking cooperative relations.* Oxford, UK: Blackwell.

Gill, R., Thompson, M. M., Febbraro, A. R., & Barnes, M. (2010). *Trust restoration in international military missions.* Defence R&D Canada technical report, DRDC, Toronto.

Gillespie, N. (2003). *Measuring trust in working relationships: The behavioral trust inventory.* Paper presented at the Academy of Management annual meeting, Seattle, WA, USA.

Gillespie, N., & Dietz, G. (2009). Trust repair after organization-level failure. *Academy of Management Review, 34*, 127–145.

Gillespie, N., & Dietz, G. (2012). *The recovery of trust: Case studies of organisational failures and trust repair.* London, UK: Institute of Business Ethics.

Griffin, M. A., & Neal, A. (2000). Perceptions of safety at work: A framework for linking safety climate to safety performance, knowledge, and motivation. *Journal of Occupational Health Psychology, 5*, 347–358.

Guldenmund, F. W. (2000). The nature of safety culture: A review of theory and research. *Safety Science, 34*, 215–257.

Hale, A. R. (2000). Culture's confusions. *Safety Science, 34*, 1–14.

Hansson, R., Jones, W., & Fletcher, W. (1990). Troubled relationships in later life: Implications for support. *Journal of Social and Personal Relationships, 7*, 451–463.

Hardin, R., (2002). *Trust and trustworthiness.* New York, NY: Russell Sage Foundation.

Heider, F. (1958). *The psychology of interpersonal relations.* New York, NY: John Wiley & Sons, Inc.

Hofmann, D. A., Morgeson, F. P., & Gerras, S. (2003). Climate as a moderator of the relationship between LMX and content specific citizenship: Safety climate as an exemplar. *Journal of Applied Psychology, 88*, 170–178.

Hosmer, L. T. (1995). Trust: The connecting link between organizational theory and philosophical ethics. *Academy of Management Review, 20*, 379–403.

Inness, M., Turner, N., Barling, J., & Stride, C. (2010). Transformational leadership and employee safety performance. A within-person, between-jobs design. *Journal of Occupational Health Psychology, 15*, 267–278.

Janowicz-Panjaitan, M., & Krishnan, R. (2009). Measures for dealing with competence and integrity violations of interorganizational trust at the corporate and operating levels of organizational hierarchy. *Journal of Management Studies, 46*, 245–268.

Jeffcott, S., Pidgeon, N., Weyman, A., & Walls, J. (2006). Risk, trust and safety culture in U.K. train-operating companies. *Risk Analysis, 2*, 1105–1121.

Jones, W., & Burdette, M. P. (1994). Betrayal. In A. L. Weber & J. H. Harvey (Eds.), *Perspectives on close relationships* (pp. 243–262). Boston, MA: Allyn & Bacon.

Jones, G. R., & George, J. M. (1998). The experience and evolution of trust: Implications for cooperation and teamwork. *Academy of Management Review, 23*, 531–546.

Jung, D. I., & Avolio, B. J. (2000). Opening the black box: An experimental investigation of the mediating effects of trust and value congruence on transformational and transactional leadership. *Journal of Organizational Behavior, 21*, 949–964.

Kath, L. M., Magley, V. J., & Marmet, M. (2010). The role of organisational trust in safety climate's influence on organisational outcomes. *Accident Analysis and Prevention, 42*, 1488–1497.

Kellerman, B. (2006). When should a leader apologize – and when not? *Harvard Business Review, 84*, 72–81.

Kelley, H., & Michela, J. (1980). Attribution theory and research. *Annual Review of Psychology, 31*, 457–501.

Kelloway, E. K., Mullen, J., & Francis, L. (2006). Divergent effects of passive and transformational leadership on safety outcomes. *Journal of Occupational Health Psychology, 11*, 76–86.

Keltikangas-Jarvinen, L., & Lindeman, M. (1997). Evaluation of theft, lying, and fighting in adolescence. *Journal of Youth and Adolescence, 26*, 467–483.

Kim, P. H., Cooper, C. D., Dirks, K. T., & Ferrin, D. L. (2013). Repairing trust with individuals vs. groups. *Organizational Behavior and Human Decision Processes, 120*, 1–14.

Kim, P. H., Dirks, K. T., & Cooper, C. D. (2009). The repair of trust: A dynamic bilateral perspective and multilevel conceptualization. *Academy of Management Review, 34*, 401–422.

Kim, P. H., Dirks, K. T., Cooper, K. D., & Ferrin, D. L. (2004). Removing the shadow of suspicion: The effects of apology vs. denial for repairing ability vs. integrity based trust violation. *Journal of Applied Psychology, 89*, 104–118.

Kim, P. H., Dirks, K. T., Cooper, C. D., & Ferrin, D. L. (2006). When more blame is better than less: The implications of internal vs. external attributions for the repair of trust after a competence vs. integrity-based trust violation. *Organizational Behavior and Human Decision Processes, 99*, 49–65.

Kramer, R. M. (2010). Collective trust within organizations: Conceptual foundations and empirical insights. *Corporate Reputation Review, 13*, 82–97.

Kramer, R. M., & Lewicki, R. J. (2010). Repairing and enhancing trust: Approaches to reducing organizational trust deficits. *Academy of Management Annals, 4*, 245–277.

Kramer, R. M., & Tyler, T. R. (1996). *Trust in organizations.* Thousand Oaks, CA: Sage.

Lapidot, Y., Kark, R., & Shamir, B. (2007). The impact of situational vulnerability on the development and erosion of followers' trust in their leader. *Leadership Quarterly, 18*, 16–34.

Lau, D., & Lam, L. (2008). Effects of trusting and being trusted on team citizenship behaviours in chain stores. *Asian Journal of Social Psychology, 11*, 141–149.

Lester, S. W., & Brower, H. H. (2003). In the eyes of the beholder: The relationship between subordinates' felt trustworthiness and their work attitudes and behaviours. *Journal of Leadership and Organizational Studies, 10*, 17–33.

Lewicki, R. J. (1998). Trust and distrust: New relationships and realities. *Academy of Management Review, 23*, 438–458.

Lewicki, R. J. (2006). Trust, trust development and trust repair. In M. Deutsch, P. Coleman, & E. Marcus (Eds.), *The handbook of conflict resolution: Theory and practice* (2nd edn., pp. 92–119). Hoboken, NJ: John Wiley & Sons, Inc.

Lewicki, R. J., McAllister, D., & Bies, R. (1998). Trust and distrust: New relationships and realities. *Academy of Management Review, 23*, 438–458.

Lewis, J., & Weigert, A. (1985). Trust as social reality. *Social Forces, 63*, 967–985.

Luria, G. (2010). The social aspects of safety management: Trust and safety climate. *Accident Analysis and Prevention, 42*, 1288–1295.

Maddux, W. W., Kim, P. H., Okumura, T., & Brett, J. M. (2011). Cultural differences in the function and meaning of apologies. *International Negotiation, 16*, 405–425.

Mayer, R. C., & Davis, J. H. (1999). The effect of the performance appraisal system on trust for management: A field quasi-experiment. *Journal of Applied Psychology, 84*, 123–136.

Mayer, R. C., & Gavin, M. B. (2005). Trust in management and performance: Who minds the shop while the employees watch the boss? *Academy of Management Journal, 48*, 874–888.

Mayer, R., Davis, J., & Schoorman, D. (1995). An integrative model of organizational trust. *Academy of Management Review, 20*, 709–734.

McAllister, D. J. (1995). Affect- and cognition-based trust as foundations for interpersonal cooperation in organizations. *Academy of Management Journal, 38*, 24–59.

McCabe, K. A., Rigdon, M. L., & Smith, V. L. (2003). Positive reciprocity and intentions in trust games. *Journal of Economic Behavior & Organization, 52*, 267–275.

McEvily, B., Perrone, V., & Zaheer, A. (2003). Introduction to the special issue on trust in an organizational context. *Organization Science, 14*, 1–4.

McKnight, D. H., Cummings, L. L., & Chervany, N. L. (1998). Initial trust formation in new organizational relationships. *Academy of Management Review, 23*, 473–490.

Mearns, K., Flin, R., Gordon, R., & Fleming, M. (2001). Human and organizational factors in offshore safety. *Work & Stress, 15*, 144–160.

Mullen, J., & Kelloway, E. K. (2009). Safety leadership: A longitudinal study of the effects of transformational leadership on safety outcomes. *Journal of Occupational and Organisational Psychology, 82*, 253–272.

Nakayachi, K., & Watabe, M. (2005). Restoring trustworthiness after adverse events: The signaling effects of voluntary "Hostage Posting" on trust. *Organizational Behavior and Human Decision Processes, 97*, 1–17.

Neal, A., & Griffin, M. A. (2006). A longitudinal study of relationships among safety climate, safety motivation, safety behaviour, and accidents at the individual and group levels. *Journal of Applied Psychology, 91*, 946–953.

Nordgren, L. F., van Harreveld, F., & van der Pligt, J. (2009). The restraint bias: How the illusion of self-restraint promotes impulsive behavior. *Psychological Science, 20*, 1523–1528.

O'Toole, M. (2002). The relationship between employees' perceptions of safety and organizational culture. *Journal of Safety Research, 33*, 231–243.

O'Dea, A., & Flin, R. (2001). Site managers and safety leadership in the offshore oil and gas industry. *Safety Science, 37*, 39–57.

Ohbuchi, K., Kameda, M., & Agarie, N. (1989). Apology as aggression control: Its role in mediating appraisal of and response to harm. *Journal of Personality and Social Psychology, 56,* 219–227.

Pearce, J. L., & Gregersen, H. B. (1991). Task interdependence and extra-role behavior: A test of the mediating effects of felt responsibility. *Journal of Applied Psychology, 76,* 838–844.

Penrod, S., & Cutler, B. (1995). Witness confidence and witness accuracy: Assessing their forensic relation. *Psychology, Public Policy, and Law, 1,* 817–845.

Perrone, V., Zaheer, A., & McEvily, B. (2003). Free to be trusted? Organizational constraints on trust at the boundaries. *Organization Science, 14,* 422–439.

Peterson, C. C., Peterson, J. L., & Seeto, D. (1983). Developmental changes in ideas about lying. *Child Development, 54,* 1529–1535.

Pettersen, N. (1987). A conceptual difference between internal–locus external locus of control and causal attributions. *Psychological Reports, 60,* 203–209.

Pillai, R., Schriesheim, C., & Williams, E. (1999). Fairness perceptions and trust as mediators for transformational and transactional leadership: A two-sample study. *Journal of Management, 6,* 897–933.

Podsakoff, P. M., MacKenzie, S. B., Moorman, R. H., & Fetter, R. (1990). Transformational leader behaviors and their effects on followers' trust in leaders, satisfaction, and organizational citizenship behaviors. *Leadership Quarterly, 1,* 107–142.

Reason, J. (1997). *Managing the risks of organizational accidents.* Aldershot, UK: Ashgate.

Reeder. G. D., & Brewer, M. B. (1979). A schematic model of dispositional attribution in interpersonal perception. *Psychological Review, 86,* 61–79.

Roberts, J. A., Cooper, K., & Lawrence, B. C. (1999). Salesperson perceptions of equity and justice and their impact on organizational commitment and intent to turnover. *Journal of Marketing Theory and Practice, 7,* 1–16.

Rotter, J. B. (1967). A new scale for the measurement of interpersonal trust. *Journal of Personality, 35,* 651–665.

Rousseau, D. M., Sitkin, S. B., Burt, R. S., & Camerer, C. (1998). Not so different after all: A cross-discipline view of trust. *Academy of Management Review, 23,* 393–404.

Salamon, S. D., & Robinson, S. (2008). Trust that binds: The impact of collective felt trust on organizational performance. *Journal of Applied Psychology, 93,* 593–601.

Schlenker, B. R., Helm, B., & Tedeschi, J. T. (1973). The effects of personality and situational variables on behavioral trust. *Journal of Personality and Social Psychology, 25,* 419–427.

Schlenker, B. R., Pontari, B. A., & Christopher, A. N. (2001). Excuses and character: Personal and social implications of excuses. *Personality and Social Psychological Review, 5,* 15–32.

Schneider, B. (1990). The climate for service: An application of the climate construct. In B. Schneider (Ed.), *Organizational climate and culture* (pp. 383–412). San Francisco, CA: Jossey-Bass.

Schweitzer, M., & Ho, T. (2005). Trust but verify: Monitoring in interdependent relationships. *Experimental and Behavioral Economics, 13,* 87–106.

Shapiro, S. P. (1987). The social control of impersonal trust. *American Journal of Sociology, 93,* 623–658.

Sitkin, S. B., & Bies, R. J. (1993). Social accounts in conflict situations: Using explanations to manage conflict. *Human Relations, 46,* 349–370.

Sitkin, S. B., & Roth, N. L. (1993). Explaining the limited effectiveness of legalistic remedies for trust/distrust. *Organization Science, 4,* 367–392.

Slovic, P. (1993). Perceived risk, trust and democracy. *Risk Analysis, 13,* 675–682.

Tedeschi, J., & Norman, N. (1985). Social power, self-presentation, and the self. In B. Schlenker (Ed.), *The self and social life* (pp. 1–28). New York, NY: McGraw-Hill.

Tomlinson, E. C., & Mayer, R. C. (2009). The role of causal attribution dimensions in trust repair. *Academy of Management Review, 34,* 85–104.

Tomlinson, E. C., Dineen, B. R., & Lewicki, R. J. (2004). The road to reconciliation: antecedents of victim willingness to reconcile following a broken promise. *Journal of Management, 30,* 165–187.

Törner, M. (2011). The "social psychology" of safety. An integrative approach to understanding organisational psychological mechanisms behind safety performance. *Safety Science*, *49*, 1262–1296.

Tucker, S., Turner, N., Barling, J., Reid, E. M. & Elving, C. (2006). Apologies and transformational leadership. *Journal of Business Ethics*, *63*, 195–207.

Turner, N., Stride, C. B., Carter, A. J., McCaughey, D., & Carroll, A. E. (2012). Job demands–control–support model and employee safety performance. *Accident Analysis and Prevention*, *45*, 811–817.

Vlaar, P. W. L., Van Den Bosch, F. A. J., & Volberda, H. W. (2007). On the evolution of trust, distrust, and formal coordination and control in interorganizational relationships: Toward an integrative framework. *Group Organization Management*, *32*, 407–429.

Watson, G., Scott, D., Bishop, J., & Turnbeaugh, T. (2005). Dimensions of interpersonal relationships and safety in the steel industry. *Journal of Business and Psychology*, *19*, 303–318.

Weiner, B. (1992). *Human motivation: Metaphors, theories, and research*. Newbury Park, CA: Sage.

Weiss, H. M., & Cropanzano, R. (1996). Affective events theory: A theoretical discussion of the structure, causes and consequences of affective experiences at work. In B. M. Staw, & L. L. Cummings (Eds.), *Research in organizational behavior: An annual series of analytic essays and critical reviews* (Vol. 18, pp. 1–74). London: Elsevier.

Wood, R. E., & Mitchell, T. R. (1981). Manager behavior in a social context: The impact of impression management on attributions and disciplinary actions. *Organizational Behavior and Human Decision Processes*, *28*, 356–378.

Woodcock, H. E. (2013). The effectiveness of non-substantive and substantive responses in the repair of employee trust in management. Unpublished doctoral thesis. University of Liverpool, UK.

Woodcock, H. E. & Conchie, S. M. (July, 2010). *Trust repair in high-risk industries: The effectiveness of verbal response strategies*. Poster presented at the Second Biannual Institute of Work Psychology Conference, Sheffield, UK.

Woodcock, H. E., & Conchie, S. M. (in prep a). Boosting the effects of an apology in repairing employees' trust in management with safety: The importance of preventatives measures.

Woodcock, H. E., & Conchie, S. M. (in prep b). How leaders can retain trust in their followers following a wrong-doing concerning safety.

Yang, J., Mossholder, K. W., & Peng, T. K. (2009). Supervisory procedural justice effects: The mediating roles of cognitive and affective trust. *Leadership Quarterly*, *20*, 143–154.

Zacharatos, A., Barling, J., & Iverson, R. D. (2005). High-performance work systems and occupational safety. *Journal of Applied Psychology*, *90*, 77–93.

Zand, D. E. (1972). Trust and managerial problem solving. *Administrative Science Quarterly*, *17*, 229–239.

7

Jobs and Safety Behavior

Nik Chmiel and Isabelle Hansez

Introduction

A large number of studies of safety-related behaviors at work consider their relationships to job and organizational factors by invoking psychological processes to formulate and explain predictions about them. We use the general accident causation scenario proposed by Wagenaar and his colleagues (e.g., Wagenaar, Hudson, & Reason, 1990) to provide a framework for our discussion relating jobs to safety behaviors. Research has shown many organizationally related factors associate with accidents, and a number of conceptually distinct safety behaviors do likewise, but surprisingly there are relatively few studies that actually include measures of the psychological processes that may explain the mechanisms linking them. Many studies also use measures of safety outcomes without taking into account that different behaviors may have different antecedent psychological processes. In our view the time has come where we need to understand more about what type of psychological process leads to what type of violation, and what types of job-related phenomena lead to what types of psychological processes. Thus our objective in this chapter is to discuss the main psychological processes invoked to explain safety behaviors at work, and in so doing emphasize the position that many job-related organizational phenomena may invoke multiple psychological processes that bear on safety behaviors and hence accidents.

We first consider the extent of accidents at work and then the nature of accident-related safety behaviors, including types of cognitive error, violation, and discretionary safety activity in which we distinguish between errors that result from largely automatic cognitive processes and those that are more considered, and between violations that result from prioritizing personal goals from those that result from job and organizational constraints. We also discuss discretionary safety activities that predict violations. We then introduce the General Accident Causation Scenario that proposes organizational practices are linked to accidents through psychological processes that produce safety behaviors and give examples of the organizational and job factors linked to accidents.

The Wiley Blackwell Handbook of the Psychology of Occupational Safety and Workplace Health, First Edition.
Edited by Sharon Clarke, Tahira M. Probst, Frank Guldenmund, and Jonathan Passmore. © 2016 John Wiley & Sons Ltd. Published 2020 by John Wiley & Sons Ltd.

We consider five distinct psychological processes linked to safety behavior: mental processes involving cognitive energy related to job strain and burnout; motivational processes connected to work engagement and the willingness to do a job; motivational beliefs about the value or valence of safety; instrumental expectations (rewards and punishments) related to perceived management commitment to safety; and finally social exchange processes involving feeling obliged to reciprocate received benefits by behaving safely or participating in discretionary safety activities related to high quality leader–member exchange relationships and support from the organization and coworkers. In short we consider being exhausted, feeling engaged, valuing safety as important, feeling rewarded, and feeling obliged, as fundamental to predicting cognitive errors, violations, and participatory safety activities.

Accidents and Figures

A man returning early from a coffee break had mistaken which of two adjacent electrical transformers (each in a separate block) he had been working on earlier in the day. He then violated the procedure for safely opening a locked door guarding the transformer. The correct procedure involved walking back some way to an electrical switch that would open the door only if the power to the transformer had been turned off. Rather than walk back the operator opened the door by pushing his arm through a fence and opening the lock from the inside with a screwdriver, entering the block and touching a wire carrying 10,000 volts. Apparently operators regularly opened locked doors in this way, and the man was just able to say so before he died (Wagenaar et al., 1990).

The death of someone at work is a catastrophic event for family, friends, colleagues, and workplace. Whilst life is preserved, a major injury, such as fractures, amputation, dislocation of joints, and blindness is also traumatic. An "over-3-day" injury means, at the very least, the injured person is away from work or unable to do their full range of normal duties for more than three days, and so is a considerable disruption for the individual and the organization.

Figures for 2010 suggest that worldwide there were approximately 350,000 workplace fatalities, and over 313 million occupational accidents leading to more than three days away from work (ILO, 2014). Furthermore, there is a good chance official accident figures do not represent an accurate picture. Workplace accidents appear frequently to be underreported to the relevant authorities. Probst, Brubaker, and Barsotti (2008) reported on 38 contractor companies working on a large construction project in the USA and showed considerable underreporting by comparing injuries reported to the Occupational Safety and Health Administration (OSHA) and medical claims under an Owner-Controlled Insurance Program. Underreporting ranged from 81 percent to 47 percent of eligible injuries across companies. Chmiel (2005) reported that a comparison of formally recorded minor injuries in a chemical processing plant in the UK revealed a large discrepancy with those reported through an independent survey, a ratio of approximately 1:11. In follow-up interviews one reason offered to explain the underreporting was that bonuses would be affected by a poor safety record. Weddle (1996) reported that of hospital environmental service workers who recalled having been injured in the previous year, 39 percent had not reported one or more injuries, and that the most frequently cited reason for not reporting was that the injury had seemed too minor, even though roughly 64 percent of unreported injuries required medical care and 44 percent resulted in lost work time. The next most common reason involved not wanting a supervisor to think that the worker was careless. Other studies suggest underreporting because of the perceived reaction and negative attitude of managers (Clarke, 1998), and the fear of blame and punishment (Reason, 1997).

Accident-related Behaviors

It is possible to put forward many types of behavior that are involved in injuries to workers, for example tripping over and falling, and many organizations have accident report forms with categories like this. However such categories do not lend themselves to a ready understanding of the psychological aspects of accidents; the behaviors concerned are too specific to particular situations and contexts, including those related to reporting them (Sheehy & Chapman, 1987). In the above illustration, the man who died touching a wire carrying 10,000 volts made two types of error. First, he made an error of judgment: he thought he was choosing the transformer he had been working on before the coffee break whereas in fact he chose the wrong one. Maybe he had been distracted, or was under some time pressure to finish the job and didn't think enough about it. Whatever the reason, he made a mistake of inference, a cognitive error. Second he violated a basic safety rule, in place to protect him and his colleagues: he pushed his hand through the fence and opened the door with a screwdriver. He knowingly violated a safety rule rather than walk some distance to turn the power off, a motivational error. We want therefore a behavioral taxonomy that captures the kind of errors the transformer operator made, and which affords insight into generalizable psychological and organizational processes involved, and the most influential and well known has been provided by Reason (1990).

Reason (1990) proposed the classification of all unsafe behaviors into two broad categories within the framework of purposeful activity related to safety: *unintended acts* in relation to planned actions and their goal; and *intended acts*. Unintended actions are further broken down into slips and lapses, and intended actions into mistakes and violations. An attraction of Reason's conceptualization is that slips, lapses, and mistakes are explicitly related to cognitive functioning, and violations to the psychosocial work environment. These categories facilitate understanding of unsafe behaviors such as those involved in the transformer case and we discuss them next.

Cognitive Errors

Slips and lapses are defined as errors that result from some failure in the execution and/ or storage of an action sequence, regardless of whether the plan that guided them was adequate to achieve its objective. Mistakes, on the other hand, are defined as deficiencies or failures in the judgmental and/or inferential processes involved in the selection of an objective, or in how to achieve it, irrespective of whether the actions necessary to realize the objective run according to plan.

Reason further related errors to a hierarchy of performance levels developed by Rasmussen and colleagues (e.g., Rasmussen, 1986; Rasmussen & Jensen, 1974). Rasmussen studied workers engaged in fault-finding in electronic components using a verbal protocol technique, asking workers to explain what they were doing during their task. As a result Rasmussen classified activity relevant to industrial settings in terms of whether it was skill, rule, or knowledge-based. The activity levels reflect decreasing familiarity with the activity and situation. The skill-based level is concerned with routine actions in a highly familiar operating environment involving largely automatic cognitive (perceptual-motor) processing. At the other extreme, knowledge-based performance is required in novel situations and circumstances, and is dependent on effortful problem solving and reasoning to work out and decide on a course of action. Rule-based performance also involves problem solving but where a situation or set of circumstances has been encountered before, and where the action is governed by the selection and use of stored rules of the form IF(situation) THEN(action) rather than a direct automatic response. Slips and lapses are deemed errors at the skill-based level and are associated with attentional and memory failures. Mistakes are refined into two types: rule-based and knowledge-based. Rule-based errors are associated with problem solving activities involving the misapplication of good rules, for example misclassifying a situation as one demanding a certain well-rehearsed action plan, or the application of bad rules. Knowledge-based errors are associated with the limitations of human ability to solve problems and reason with new and unfamiliar circumstances.

Reason (1990) documented examples of slips, lapses, and mistakes from incidents in the nuclear power industry. For example, at the Davis-Besse plant in the USA, an operator, wanting to start the steam and feedwater rupture control system manually, inadvertently pressed the wrong two buttons on the control panel (a slip). At Three-Mile Island, again in the USA, a cooling system pressure relief valve had stuck open despite operators commanding it shut from the control panel. The belief that it was actually shut was a mistake. Wagenaar and Groeneweg (1987) analyzed Dutch shipping reports of 100 accidents at sea. The accidents all resulted from several behavioral events, frequently from two or more people, and had multiple causes. Nonetheless the authors could attribute in a principled way individual human error behavior in 93 percent of the accidents that involved failures of reasoning and cognitive rule following. Similarly Salminen and Tallberg (1996) found that human error could be implicated in a majority (more than 80 percent) of 99 serious accidents investigated in Finland. Retrospective analyses such as those just outlined support the idea that cognitive errors are a suitable basis for retrospective accident analysis, although questions of identification, analysis and measurement are raised by it. Rasmussen (1990) makes the point that any retrospective analysis is pragmatic and subjective in its search for causes, and is dependent on the purpose of the analysis; for example, whether to allocate blame or identify system improvements, and on the implicit theories of the analyst concerning accident causation.

Several self-report methods of assessing slips and lapses have been developed (Wilhelm, Witthöft, & Schipolowski, 2010), that can be used to investigate their association with accident outcomes, thus avoiding some of the issues raised in relation to retrospective analyses. The most well known is probably the cognitive failures questionnaire (CFQ) of Broadbent, Cooper, Fitzgerald, and Parkes (1982). The Short Inventory of Minor Lapses (SIML), too, was based on a similar approach to the CFQ, and these two measures have been reported to correlate strongly (Reason, 1993). Wallace and Chen (2005) developed a scale measuring work specific cognitive failures (Workplace Cognitive Failure Scale, WCFS), basing their conceptualization on the CFQ. Their conceptualization supposed that such failures were those of memory, attention, and action, and were unintended. Their results supported a three-factor solution, as well as their claim that the three factors related to a common second order factor.

Such measures have been found to associate with accident and injury outcomes. For example, Larson, Alderton, Neideffer, and Underhill (1997) found that the CFQ score was associated with what they called "composite mishaps," defined as an accident- or injury-caused hospitalization or serious fall. However, when these were split, there were CFQ differences between those involved in a fall or hospitalized, but not for accident involvement. More compelling evidence for a link between CFQ scores and accidents comes from Wallace and Vodanovich (2003), who showed a significant positive association between the CFQ and self-reported involvement in injuries requiring treatment but not time off work. Wallace and Chen (2005) also showed that the common factor from their WCFS scale predicted a similar measure of accident involvement. Simpson, Wadsworth, Moss, and Smith (2005) found a single item cognitive failures measure (previously shown to correlate .7 with CFQ scores) related to minor injuries as well as accidents.

Violations

Violations, in contrast to errors, are not seen as breakdowns in normal cognitive processing, but as deliberate flouting of safety procedures and rules.

> While errors may be defined in relation to the cognitive processes of the individual, violations can only be described with regard to a social context in which behavior is governed by operating procedures, codes of practice, rules and the like . . . violations can be defined as deliberate – but not necessarily reprehensible-deviations from those practices deemed necessary (by designers, managers and regulatory agencies) to maintain the safe operation of a potentially hazardous system. (Reason, 1990, p. 195)

Violations are therefore "knowing" departures from specified safety rules and procedures. It is possible of course to violate rules unwittingly through ignorance of the rules, and these have been called "unintentional violations" but "to all intents and purposes should be regarded as errors" (Reason, Parker, & Lawton, 1998, p. 293).

Intended violations of safety rules and procedures could include a range of behaviors, for example taking shortcuts rather than following procedures, or non-compliance with self-protective precautions, such as not wearing personal protective equipment like safety glasses or a hard hat. Reason (1990, pp. 195–196) identified as of greatest interest a category of "deliberate but non-malevolent infringements": *routinized violations* were "largely habitual, forming part of an individual's behavioural repertoire"; *exceptional violations* were "singular violations occurring in a particular set of circumstances."

Routinized violations

Reason et al. (1998) suggested three major categories of "routinized" violation had been distinguished: routine, optimizing, and situational. Routine violations typically involved corner-cutting – taking a path of least effort. Optimizing violations involved optimizing non-functional goals ahead of safety, for example the enjoyment of speeding when driving. These two categories were linked to the attainment of personal goals. Situational violations involved seeing violations as essential "to get the job done," for example, because of organizational failings related to the work environment or equipment, such as making personal protective equipment hard to access and use.

Consistent with Reason et al.'s (1998) analysis, Lawton (1998) found that out of 14 endorsed reasons for violations in shunting operations given by 36 UK railway personnel, the most common were to do with the violations being seen as a quicker way of working: due to time pressure; due to high workload; and due to inexperience. Least common were reasons connected to psychological gratification: that is, violations being seen as exciting or macho ways to work. Other reasons included management turning a blind eye, a belief that skill means a violation is still a safe way to work, a belief that the rule is impossible to work to, and the belief that violation was necessary due to design of the railway sidings where the railway personnel worked.

More recent psychometric analyses of self-reported safety behaviors reinforce the distinction between routine and situational violations made by Reason et al. (1998). In the UK chemical industry Chmiel (2005) found two dimensions through exploratory factor analysis consistent with their conceptualization, one relating to on-task procedures and corner-cutting, and one referring to task-related organizational requirements such as wearing protective clothing, using safety equipment, and reporting incidents. Routine violations were found to associate with increased odds of reporting being involved in an injury. Subsequent studies further support the distinction between routine and situational violations as separable constructs, also finding them to be associated with different psychological processes (Hansez & Chmiel, 2010). Clarke (2006a) summarized the situation with respect to the relationships between self-reported safety compliance (a composite of routine and situational violations) and accidents using meta-analysis. Although the effect sizes were small the relationships between safety compliance and accidents and injuries for the nine studies included were valid and generalizable.

Exceptional violations

Reason et al. (1998, p. 293) proposed also that "recognizing a situation as hazardous and/or a rule as inappropriate is likely to lead to the adoption of self-protective behaviour" and hence would lead to a violation under certain circumstances. We also though consider the situation where no precautions may be adopted. We consider first circumstances where a situation is perceived as both hazardous and established safety rules as inappropriate, before considering the case where rules are judged inappropriate per se.

Hazardous situations and judging rules to be inappropriate   In the hazardous case, and where existing rules are violated but other precautions are adopted, it may take extreme or unusual situations, those with strong and obvious threats to life and limb for example, to trigger a violation of this sort. A strong implication is that cognitive processes are central, possibly involving some sort of cost–benefit analysis. Moreover, it should be noted that these safety violations are not inherently "wrong" behaviors, as they may lead to future rule recommendations in line with self-protective behavior. Violations may also occur when an individual realizes that a system is in jeopardy and that saving the system requires actions that are outside of normal operation (Alper & Karsh, 2009). Thus in addition to self-protection in such situations, other motivations may be involved, for example, altruism. In both cases violations may not only improve safety, but can ultimately even become "best practice" in the situations that produced them.

In more normal situations judged hazardous but where a worker thinks their skill level mitigates any risk and where other precautions are not adopted, health belief models point to the importance to action of risk perception and personal susceptibility; that is, the belief that one will be personally affected by a perceived health hazard (e.g., Weinstein, 1988). A worker who believes they have the skill to mitigate any risk (cf. Lawton, 1998) is therefore likely to believe they are not personally susceptible, and so considers the rule redundant and that there is no need to follow it. It may also be they think a rule inappropriate and they may be at risk but are happy to accept a certain level of risk. Soane and Chmiel (2005) found that risk preferences in the work domain were predicted by lower conscientiousness, and higher openness and extraversion, but not a consideration of payoffs and costs.

Judging rules to be inappropriate   Interesting, however, is the case where there is no perception of threat but a rule is judged inappropriate. Since the analysis of many accidents at work suggests that conscious appraisal of risk is rarely undertaken (Wagenaar, 1992; Wagenaar & Groeneweg, 1987) this situation has the potential to be quite common unless mitigated by organizations requiring workers to address risk, for example, through "last minute risk analysis" (LMRA). In not following the prescribed rule a range of alternative self-protective actions could be chosen (as Reason et al., 1998, implied), however we could also choose to take no self-protective action, as was common in the accidents analyzed by Wagenaar and Groeneweg. The particular course of action is likely to depend on why we make the initial judgment.

In the first case, where the adoption of precautions is pursued, health belief models, as noted, include the involvement of risk perception and personal susceptibility, so it is unclear why one would choose to adopt precautions in this circumstance unless one had a general disposition to always protect oneself "just in case." This would be so if an employee were, say, to be generally risk averse and act in accordance with this predisposition, rather than as a result of an appraisal of the particular situation they were in. In these circumstances NOT adopting a precaution would be taking a risk. There is evidence that some people can be consistently risk averse across domains in their lives including work, and these individuals were distinguished by higher scores on Big Five personality dimensions of agreeableness and conscientiousness (Soane & Chmiel, 2005).

In the second case it would appear straightforward: no risk is perceived, no personal susceptibility assumed, therefore no need to take precautions, so none taken. However, Soane and Chmiel (1999) surveyed nuclear power workers and found that the perception of risk per se was not necessary for some people to intend to follow rules at work. This observation therefore still begs a question: why would some employees choose to ignore the rule and yet take no other precaution? Potential reasons could be to do with attitudes toward rules and regulations and/or authority.

Meta-analysis has shown that personality dimensions are associated with accidents (see Smith, Jordan & Wallace, Chapter 2; Foster & Nichols, Chapter 3, this volume). Clarke (2006b) contrasted perceptual, attitudinal, and dispositional approaches to accident involvement in the workplace. Although effect sizes were quite small her conclusions were that safety perceptions (i.e., the basis for safety climate) had greater predictive utility than attitudes, but that one aspect of personality (agreeableness) had greater utility than either. This aspect of the Big Five personality traits surfaces along with others as associated with accidents in subsequent meta-analyses (Clarke & Robertson, 2005, 2008). Although these meta-analyses are suggestive of the effects of general dispositions in accident involvement the mechanisms involved are not clear; for example, is personality a factor only for exceptional violations, and does a risk-averse approach extend to all types of compliance behavior?

A further problem in interpreting the relationship between personality (and indeed other factors) and accident involvement is that such analyses have not controlled for accident exposure or the opportunity to have an accident (see Chmiel & Taris, 2014 for discussion of this point). Thus it is entirely plausible that different types of people select themselves into different types of jobs; for example, sensation-seekers might prefer deep-sea diving rather than office work, and hence an association between personality characteristics and accidents may be observed because of it. Further research is needed to disentangle these effects (see also Smith, Jordan & Wallace, Chapter 2, this volume).

We have discussed exceptional violations more fully here rather than in the section on psychological processes below because there is a paucity of research exploring the possible processes involved. Therefore we will not be considering exceptional violations further in this chapter, but they remain an area ripe for future research.

Discretionary Safety-related Behaviors

Until now we have discussed behaviors (errors and violations) that have direct bearing on carrying out tasks safely. However there is another class of behaviors relevant to these behaviors within organizations, and these can be called *safety citizenship behaviors*. These behaviors are mostly discretionary and regarded as beyond an employee's usual job role. For example, Neal, Griffin, and Hart's (2000) items to measure "safety participation" encompassed: promotion of the safety program within the organization; extra effort to improve the safety of the workplace; helping coworkers when they are working under risky or hazardous conditions; and voluntarily carrying out tasks or activities that help to improve workplace safety. Given that these behaviors are discretionary why should we give them attention here? The answer is that safety citizenship/participation behaviors could have an important impact on job-related safety behaviors. First, because discretionary safety behaviors are also associated with the accidents and injuries associated with rule violations (e.g., Clarke, 2006a); second, because participation behaviors are positively correlated with task-related compliance with safety rules and procedures (e.g., Griffin & Neal, 2000); and third, because Neal and Griffin (2006) showed safety participation predicted future safety motivation and safety compliance, and Chmiel and Hansez (2013) showed that employees defining discretionary safety activities as more part of their job predicted less situational violations.

Active and Latent Failures

Reason (1990) suggested that the human contributions to complex system breakdowns and accidents were a function of active and latent failures, an idea that has been extremely influential and which is essentially an expansion of the notion that accidents result from unsafe behaviors and unsafe conditions. Active failures were unsafe acts, either cognitive errors or violations of safety rules. Latent failures consisted of several categories: fallible managerial decisions; line management deficiencies; psychological precursors to unsafe acts; and inadequate defenses (against unsafe acts). The key idea was that latent and active failures combined to contribute to major accidents, even though the precise nature of the failures was unique to each disaster.

A case study by Lawton and Ward (2005) illustrates how the interaction of active and latent failure can contribute to an accident, and how latent failures may be implicated in psychological precursors to unsafe acts. In 1999 two trains collided just outside Paddington Station, near Ladbroke Grove in London, UK. A total of 31 people were killed and more than 400 injured. The immediate "cause" was a Signal Passed at Danger (SPAD), that is, the driver of one train went through a red light. A report on the accident, several hundred pages long, was compiled in 2000 by Lord Cullen. Lawton and Ward used witness statements and the Cullen report in an analysis of contributory factors from a systems perspective. The main features of the disaster identified by Lawton and Ward were: driver cognitive error (it was likely the driver who went through the red light expected a green signal – a finding in other investigations of SPADs); the driver had only recently been trained and had no experience of the signal he went through; evidence suggested that the driver was unaware of his error, and could have misread the signal, that is, misclassifying the situation; there was a new track layout designed to allow more train throughput, leading to a very complex driving task; the signal itself was poorly sited, creating viewing problems; the signal had a history of being passed at danger (eight SPADs had been reported between 1993 and 1998) leading Lord Cullen to include in his report the calculation that there was an 86 percent chance in each year of a SPAD at this signal; drivers were not made aware of SPAD histories along their routes; training methods were considered suspect, especially with regard to route handling. A result of this and other train crashes led to 25 recommendations concerning safety leadership and management and 41 recommendations directed at training, skills, competence, and behavior.

General Accident Causation Scenario

Based on retrospective accident analyses and extending the idea of active and latent contributions to accident causation, Wagenaar et al. (1990) proposed a general accident causation scenario "which describes how all accidents originate" (1990: 274), with an emphasis on cognitive error. The last event in the scenario is the accident, and these are always caused by unsafe acts (which meant that whether the act was deliberate or not the accident could have been prevented by elimination of some preceding action). Defenses stand between unsafe acts and accidents. If an accident occurs the defenses must have been breached or were inadequate. Unsafe acts have their immediate origins in psychological precursors argued to be elicited by the physical and organizational environment. These influences were called general failure types (GFTs). GFTs are created by management decisions. Wagenaar et al. (1990) used the general accident causation scenario to analyze the example of the maintenance operator in a transformer station tragically killed by touching a wire carrying 10,000 volts. Defenses were inadequate: no alarm was triggered when a fence was opened with the power still on; and there was no automatic power shutdown. The unsafe acts were that the door was opened with a screwdriver, and the wire touched without a power check. Psychological precursors were confusion between the transformer cells, and the habitual response to violate procedures. GFTs comprised: labeling of cells that was ambiguous; a physical distance from cells to power switches that was too far; an alarm system wrongly designed; wrong habits not corrected by supervisors; and insufficient time to finish the job. Management decisions allowed an out-of-date design not to be replaced, and maintenance staff to be reduced.

General failure types

Similar organizational characteristics were in evidence, sufficient for Wagenaar et al. (1990) to define a limited number of general failure types (GFTs) based on features of an operation that have been wrong for some time, but remain unrecognized as problematic until implicated in an accident, and which promote cognitive precursors to unsafe acts. The types were defined "somewhat arbitrarily, but after reading and analyzing hundreds of accident scenarios" (1990: 287). The GFTs were grouped into three broad categories: *Physical Environment*, that included design failures, missing defenses, hardware defects, negligent housekeeping, and error-enforcing conditions (i.e., design takes no account of its use under extreme time pressure, or by unqualified personnel); *Human Behavior*, that included poor procedures (bad planning, insufficient control) and defective training (e.g., lack of training in specific expertise so people act as novices); and *Management*, that included organizational failures (e.g., safety not treated as an important goal), incompatible goals (e.g., production trade-offs with safety), and lack of communication (leading to absence of information). Wagenaar, Groeneweg, Hudson, and Reason (1994) refined the types to include failures in maintenance, giving 11 types where the "frequencies of occurrence of failures in the eleven classes are essentially independent" (1994: 2001).

Support for the idea that GFTs are implicated in accidents, and that the taxonomy proposed by Wagenaar et al. (1990) has some merit extending beyond cognitive error, has come from evidence gained through survey and interview methodologies that have produced associations between a variety of organizational procedures and accident and injury outcomes, including: management style and culture (including empowerment of the workforce and good relations between management and workforce); organizational philosophy on health and safety (including delegation of safety activities, training and an active role in health and safety of top management); good housekeeping and safety controls on machinery (Shannon, Mayr, & Haines, 1997); safety climate (Zohar, 1980); performance-based pay, training, and team-working (Kaminski, 2001); rewards for reporting safety hazards, safety training, selecting those with a good safety record, communication/feedback on incidents and unsafe behaviors, worker participation in safety decisions, and management commitment to safety (Vredenburgh, 2002); regularly scheduled safety meetings (Hoonakker et al., 2005); collective high-performance work system practices of employment security, selective hiring, extensive training, self-managed teams, and decentralized decision-making, reduced status distinctions, information sharing, compensation contingent on safe performance, transformational leadership, high-quality work, and measurement of management practices (Zacharatos, Barling, & Iverson, 2005); the need to save time and work to tight schedules (Salminen, Saari, Saarela, & Rasanen, 1993); extent of training received, task variety, and autonomy (Barling, Kelloway, & Iverson, 2003); hours per week worked (Dembe, Erickson, Delbos, & Banks, 2005; Kaminski, 2001; Lombardi, Folkard, Willets, & Smith, 2010); and supervisory and coworker support (Iverson & Erwin, 1997).

Melamed, Yekutieli, Froom, Kristal-Boneh, and Ribak (1999) examined the safety impact when exposed to unfavourable job conditions. They found that being exposed to noise increased the odds of being injured at work by 15–36 percent; climate problems increased this likelihood by 28–30 percent; lighting problems led to a risk increment of 7 percent; and excessive vibration increased the odds of being injured by 19 percent. We have the situation that a number of organizational and job factors relate to accidents and several types of safety behavior also relate to accidents. The General Accident Causation Scenario (GACS) proposes job and organizational factors relate to safety behaviors through promoting psychological processes that underlie those behaviors, yet which processes are promoted by which factors has not been analyzed with respect to the 11 GFTs within the GACS framework. That work remains to be done. In the following sections we discuss those psychological processes so far shown to be directly related to safety behaviors in the workplace and argued, as part of their founding conceptualization, to connect to particular organizational factors relevant to doing one's job.

Psychological Processes

Cognitive-energetical processes (feeling exhausted)

Demanding jobs lead to feelings of strain and burnout (Karasek, 1979; Demerouti, Bakker, Nachreiner, & Schaufeli, 2001). Bakker and Demerouti (2007) define job demands as "those physical, psychological, social, or organizational aspects of the job that require sustained physical and/or psychological (cognitive and emotional) effort or skills," and Schaufeli and Bakker (2004) theorize that job demands affect cognitive-energetical/effort-based processes that lead to the depletion of energy and burnout that is associated with poor work behaviors (see also Taris & Schaufeli, Chapter 8, this volume).

The extreme state of energy depletion represented by burnout is associated with increased cognitive failures (Van der Linden, Keijsers, Eling, & Van Schaijk, 2005). Even without reaching a "burned out" state effects of circadian rhythms and loss of sleep, conditions associated with shift-work, also lead to performance impairment (Campbell, 1992; Folkard & Monk, 1979; Williams, Lubin, & Goodnow, 1959). For example, Hobbs, Williamson, and Van Dongen (2010) observed a circadian rhythm in skill-based cognitive errors in aircraft maintenance workers, with a peak in errors occurring between 1 and 6 o'clock in the morning. Cognitive energy depletion due to fatigue can lead to failures of attention that underpin slips and lapses (Craig & Cooper, 1992) and an aversion to investing more mental effort into a task (Holding, 1983). In addition, characteristics of the physical work environment, stressors such as noise and temperature, affect cognitive processing efficiency and performance (e.g., Hockey, 1986; Ramsey & Morrisey, 1978). Interestingly, increasing demand or fatigue may not lead to an overall reduction in performance on all aspects of the job. Compensatory effort processes may allow priority to be given to performance on key aspects of a task (Chmiel, Totterdell, & Folkard, 1995; Hockey, 1997). In such circumstances maintaining production levels leads to less energy for other aspects of work or performance (Hockey & Earle, 2006). Hansez and Chmiel (2010) proposed this would affect routine rather than situational violations since the former are related to effort. Hansez and Chmiel (2010) provided evidence, in line with these expectations, that the effect of job demands on routine violations was mediated by job-related strain, but there was no mediation effect of job strain for situational violations. Consistent with this Li, Jiang, Yao, and Li (2013) showed emotional exhaustion (a dimension of burnout) did not mediate the relationship between job demands and a measure of safety compliance akin to Hansez and Chmiel's measure of situational violations, but rather mediated the relationship between job demands and injuries and near misses. Li et al. (2013) did not measure routine violations directly in their study. Additionally, job demands predict whether employees decide to view discretionary safety behaviors as part of their job. Turner, Chmiel, and Walls (2005) found that safety citizenship role definitions, reflecting the extent to which employees regarded discretionary safety activities as part of their job, were related to job demands and job control: job control had a positive relationship and job demands a negative relationship. Interestingly, the interaction between job control and demands was significant: low control and high demands were associated with lower safety-role definitions. Thus it is likely that effort-related processes are implicated in safety participation behaviors also because safety-role definitions predict involvement in discretionary safety activities (Hofmann, Morgeson, & Gerras, 2003). Finally, individual appraisals of job demands to determine whether they constitute hindrance or challenge stressors may moderate the effects of such demands on safety behaviors. Clarke (2012) provided evidence from a meta-analysis consistent with the notion that demands considered hindrance stressors affected both safety compliance and safety participation, whereas those considered challenge stressors did not. Further research utilizing direct measures of the effort-related processes related to such appraisals is needed to explore this idea.

Motivational processes (feeling engaged, believing safety is important)

Safety motivation has been defined as reflecting an individual's "willingness to exert effort to enact safety behaviors and the valence associated with those behaviors" (Neal & Griffin, 2006, p. 947). We discuss both aspects of motivation in turn, starting with willingness to exert effort, and then consider whether these two concepts should be further differentiated.

Motivational processes (feeling engaged and willingness to exert effort)

Work engagement has been defined as a psychological state characterized by absorption, vigor, and dedication (Schaufeli & Bakker, 2004). In explaining its role in the Job Demands-Resources (JD-R) model, Schaufeli and Bakker theorized that job resources are functional in achieving work goals and outcomes through work engagement because job resources foster employees' growth, learning, and development on the one hand, and the willingness to invest one's efforts and abilities to the work task on the other. Job resources promote greater work engagement and hence, for example, taking part in extra-role behaviors (Bakker, Demerouti, & Verbeke, 2004). The JD-R model proposes that job resources may also help reduce the psychological and physiological effects of job demands (Bakker & Demerouti, 2007). Note however that the conceptualization of engagement is subject to different perspectives (Macy & Schneider, 2008), and other authors have used the term to encompass behaviors such as worker participation in safety, communication, and information sharing in relation to job demands, resources, and safety (Nahrgang, Morgeson, & Hofmann, 2011). In the sense proposed by Schaufeli and Bakker (2004), engagement reflects the willingness part of motivation. Using the latter approach Hansez and Chmiel (2010) showed there was a positive association between engagement and both routine and situational violations, demonstrating that the effect of job resources on violations was partially mediated by engagement and hence that non-safety specific motivational processes are implicated in safety behaviors.

Motivational processes (believing safety to be important, safety valence)

Using a job performance framework (e.g., Motowidlo, Borman, & Schmit, 1997), Griffin and Neal (2000) and Neal et al. (2000) proposed immediate antecedents to safety compliance (their measure included items relating to both routine and situational violations) and participation included safety motivation and safety knowledge. Their measure of safety motivation asked about the importance of safety behaviors, so focused on valence rather than willingness to invest effort. Their modeling provided evidence that compliance and participation were predicted by safety valence, supporting their proposition. Christian, Bradley, Wallace, and Burke (2009) extended this approach proposing that situation-related factors, such as safety climate and leadership, and person-related factors, such as personality characteristics and job attitudes, are distal antecedents that act through the proximal factors of safety motivation and knowledge to influence safety compliance and safety participation, and hence accidents and injuries. Their model predicted stronger relationships with safety performance for proximal compared with distal factors, and meta-analysis of the effect sizes of the relationships predicted by their model tended to support it.

Differentiating motivational constructs   A question raised by the studies discussed in this section so far is whether we should treat all aspects of motivation as equivalent in their effect or whether different aspects of motivation may associate with different safety behaviors? Recent research suggests the latter for several reasons: first, using a longitudinal design, Neal and Griffin (2006) found, using their valence-based safety importance measure, a lagged effect of safety motivation on safety participation, but not on safety compliance. Second, when Griffin and Neal (2000) measured valence for compliance separately from valence for participation behaviors they found a significant path from participation valence to safety participation and, in contrast, significant paths from compliance valence to both safety participation and safety compliance. Third, using different forms of safety motivation derived from a Self-determination Theory perspective, Conchie (2013) found that the effect of transformational leadership on safety compliance was partially mediated by identified regulation (similar to safety valence) but not by intrinsic motivation (defined as promoting behavior because of its inherent satisfaction such that the activity is challenging, interesting, or enjoyable). Interestingly though, intrinsic motivation partially mediated the effect of transformational leadership on the discretionary behaviors of whistle-blowing and safety voice (termed challenge citizenship behaviors) whereas valence did not. Further, in a second study partial mediation by intrinsic motivation was replicated for challenge behaviors but not for helping (affiliative citizenship) behaviors. Fourth, Clarke (2013) found that transformational leadership had a direct effect on safety participation but not on safety compliance, whereas active transactional leadership had a direct effect on safety compliance but not on safety participation.

Thus the results from Neal and Griffin (2006), Conchie (2013), and Clarke (2013) suggest safety compliance and discretionary behaviors may have different motivational antecedents, which would be consistent with the view for task and contextual job performance expressed by Motowidlo et al. (1997). In addition though, Conchie's results suggest different forms of discretionary safety behaviors may have different antecedents too, a result that chimes with that found by Hansez and Chmiel (2010) for routine and situational violations.

Instrumental processes (feeling rewarded/punished)

Zohar (2003, 2008) proposed that perceptions of organizational safety phenomena alter behavior-outcome expectancies, thereby affecting safety behavior. Individual employee perceptions of key aspects of the organizational environment that are evaluated to affect personal well-being have been defined as psychological climate perceptions (James et al., 2008). Perceptions by individuals will be affected by their own idiosyncratic worldviews, perceptual biases and experiences which can lead to different employee interpretations of the same organizational phenomena and so differentially affect individual behavior-outcome expectancies, a supportive climate reinforces safe behavior whereas an unsupportive one does not (Beus, Payne, Bergman, & Arthur, 2010).

Organizational dimensions for safety climate perceptions were identified by Zohar (1980): the importance of safety training programs; management attitudes to safety; effects of safe conduct on promotion; level of risk in the workplace; pace of work demands related to safety; status of the safety officer; the effects of safe conduct on social status; and the status of the safety committee. Subsequent research on the number and nature of the dimensions has supported differing views of the dimensions involved (Brown & Holmes, 1986; Cooper & Philips, 2004; Dedobbeleer & Béland, 1991; Griffin & Neal, 2000; Shannon & Geoffrey, 2009). A core dimension that has emerged is management commitment to safety, and this incorporates perceptions of management attitudes and behaviors in relation to safety (Flin, Mearns, O'Connor, & Bryden, 2000). Other labels such as "perceived safety climate" have also been used for what appear similar conceptualizations of individual perceptions of management's approach to safety based on Zohar's original work (e.g., Barling, Loughlin, & Kelloway, 2002; Clarke, 2013) and we use these terms interchangeably here (see also Guediri & Griffin, Chapter 13, this volume).

Hansez and Chmiel (2010), in addition to the observations noted above for cognitive-energetical and engagement processes related to the JD-R framework, found that perceived management commitment to safety predicted both routine and situational violations, and explained additional variance in them. Thus cognitive-energetical, motivational/engagement and instrumental processes all contributed separately to violations. This finding supports the view that safety climate perceptions give rise to processes separable from general motivational and cognitive-energetical effort related processes, but surprisingly we have not been able to find empirical studies relating such perceptions to measures of employees' behavioral-outcome expectancies and hence safety behaviors. One interview-based study does provide some evidence consistent with this view. Didla, Mearns, and Flin (2009) found that one of the reasons given by employees for being involved in safety citizenship behaviors was that they felt it was expected of them by management. In addition some circumstantial evidence is reported in two recent studies. Conchie (2013) found that although transformational leadership was linked to other motivational processes it was not associated with an instrumental (external regulation) measure, even though that measure linked to safety com*pliance. Consistent with this, and as noted above, Clarke (2013) found that transformational leadership had a direct effect on safety participation but not on safety compliance, whereas active transactional leadership (i.e., leadership more associated with instrumental processes) had a direct effect on safety compliance but not on safety participation. Furthermore Clarke's model incorporated a mediating role for perceived safety climate, but consistent with the idea that perceived safety climate is largely instrumental, in effect there was no significant mediation between transformational leadership and safety compliance, whereas there was between active transactional leadership and safety participation, a result consistent with Didla et al.'s (2009) observation. Earlier work showing an initially puzzling mediating role for perceived safety climate between transformational leadership and other safety outcomes (e.g., Barling et al., 2002; Kelloway, Mullen, & Francis, 2006) could be accounted for because the measure of leadership used included contingent reward items, and contingent reward is a transactional leadership dimension.

In sum, involvement of behavioral-outcome expectancies as a result of safety climate perceptions is taken as a given more based on the theoretical derivation entailed in the concept of climate than empirical studies in the safety domain but we can say it involves processes separable from cognitive-energetical and engagement processes.

Job resources, job demands, and perceived management commitment to safety

Now we turn to the question whether there is any connection between job resources, job demands, and safety-climate perceptions? Neal et al. (2000) proposed, for example, if employees perceive that the organization is supportive of their general welfare and well-being, they will be more likely to perceive that the organization values the safety of employees. Neal et al. (2000) found a composite construct that included role clarity, supportive leadership, participative decision-making, professional growth, professional interaction, appraisal and recognition, and goal congruency predicted employees' perceptions of their management's commitment to safety, which in turn predicted safety knowledge and the importance with which employees regarded safety, which in turn predicted safety compliance. Similarly, Larsson, Pousette, and Torner (2008) found a composite construct that included, inter alia, measures of role clarity, feedback, social support, and quality of leadership, predicted safety motivation and knowledge, that in turn related to safety compliance behavior. A number of the dimensions in these composite constructs relate to job resources, but others do not, so a question is whether job resources per se predict perceived management commitment to safety and hence violations. Hansez and Chmiel (2010) provide evidence that this is the case. They reported a significant path from job resources to perceived management commitment to safety.

A second question then is whether job demands affect safety climate perceptions? It could be, for example, that by increasing an employee's workload management is signaling that safety is less important and hence expectations about behaviors should be adjusted accordingly. Some evidence supports this line of reasoning. Barling et al. (2002) found perceptions of role overload predicted perceived safety climate. In contrast, Hansez and Chmiel (2010) found the path between job demands and perceived management commitment to safety was non-significant. At the moment therefore we can conclude job resources and possibly job demands may have some of their effect on safety behaviors through safety-specific instrumental processes in addition to more general motivational and cognitive-energetical ones.

Social exchange processes (feeling obliged)

Social exchange theory proposes that a range of material and non-material goods can be exchanged at work: task-related behaviors, loyalty, and liking, advice, workflow, and friendship (Liden & Maslyn, 1998). A core aspect of social exchange theory is "felt obligation" that leads to exchanges being reciprocated (Blau, 1964; Gouldner, 1960). Thus, for example, perceived organizational support is associated with increased commitment to the organization based on the norm of reciprocity (Rhoades & Eisenberger, 2002). In line with previous theorizing Hofmann and Morgeson (1999) showed among workgroup leaders in a manufacturing plant that both perceived organizational support and high quality leader–member exchange (LMX) associated with more upward communication about safety, and LMX associated also with commitment to safety that involved taking responsibility for the organization's safety record; concern with the safety of their work group's performance; and trying to get their work group to meet or exceed safety standards. A key observation Hofmann and Morgeson (1999) made about their results is that they conformed to a theoretical view that obligations are reciprocated in a targeted way. Thus perceived organizational support leads to employees reciprocating to benefit the organization, whereas high-quality leader–member exchange leads to reciprocating activities designed to benefit the supervisor in the eyes of the organization. Results from Hofmann et al. (2003) showed that expanded safety citizenship role definitions (treating discretionary safety activities such as volunteering for a safety committee as part of one's job) were predicted by high quality LMX relationships when there was a positive safety context. The study further showed that such "safety citizenship role definitions" predicted corresponding discretionary safety citizenship behaviors, suggesting that employees will reciprocate implied obligations by expanding their role and behaving consistently with contextual behavioral expectations. Chmiel and Hansez (2013) have shown further that "safety citizenship role definitions" predict situational safety violations consistent with the view that participating in contextual safety activities enables employees to change organizational constraints that provoke such violations, for example by making personal protective equipment easier to access.

In line with social exchange theory, Mearns and Reader (2008) found perceived support from the organization and from workmates and supervisors predicted a range of safety citizenship behaviors. Tucker, Chmiel, Turner, Hershcovis, and Stride (2008) found the effect of perceived organizational support for safety on employee safety voice (i.e., the willingness to speak out about safety to management) to be mediated by perceived coworker support for safety, implying that such discretionary activity could involve reciprocation to coworkers rather than the organization itself. Interestingly Turner, Stride, Carter, McCaughey, and Carroll (2012) found the interaction between social support and job control predicted safety participation, leading the authors to conclude that "having the opportunity (job control) in combination with a supportive work environment (social support) is likely to result in a heightened propensity to undertake activities that promote workplace safety (safety participation)" (p. 816). In addition, social support was positively related to higher safety compliance (a composite of situational and routine violations).

Bakker and Demerouti (2007), in explaining the JD-R model, proposed that job resources may be located at the level of the organization at large (e.g., job security), in interpersonal and social relations (e.g., supervisor support), in the organization of work (e.g., participation in decision-making), and at the level of the task (e.g., autonomy). Following our discussion of support as implying exchange processes and obligation-based psychological processes, it is likely that at least some job resources may entail both motivational and obligation processes in their effects on safety behaviors. This view is consistent with evidence from Turner et al. (2005) showing that safety citizenship role definitions were negatively associated with job demands but that this effect was moderated by job control.

Future Research

Although a number of studies have provided insights into the psychological processes involved in safety behaviors as they are related to the jobs employees do, we need a more comprehensive picture of which psychological processes influence which safety behaviors, and in turn which organizational phenomena invoke which psychological processes. We know, too, very little about how the processes discussed in this chapter operate together. Do they make largely independent contributions, or not? And we are unclear whether there are any organizational phenomena that produce a single psychological reaction, or whether, as is more likely, they produce several psychological reactions that are differentially relevant to different safety behaviors. Thus identifying psychological processes is a key step in understanding the reasons for unsafe behaviors and why particular organizational phenomena influence them, and we argue there should be more studies that include direct measures of the putative psychological processes involved.

One obvious case in point would be to consider the processes ensuing from leadership. For example, your supervisor may have a positive attitude to safety and value it highly as demonstrated through his or her actions, so you know what to expect by way of approval or disapproval if you behave accordingly. But also your supervisor may inspire and motivate you through his or her leadership style leading you to value safety, and have a high quality exchange relationship with you leading you to feel obliged to reciprocate, but a high quality exchange may mean also you are more privileged with regard to job resources and therefore more engaged with your job. By way of illustration, Inness, Turner, Barling, and Stride (2010) found transformational leadership predicted safety participation behaviors, and Clarke and Ward (2006) found some leadership tactics (rational persuasion and consultation) had direct effects on safety participation and also indirect effects through perceived actions and expectations of supervisors. Further Clarke (2013) found that there was a direct effect on safety participation of safety-specific transformational leadership as well as an effect through perceived safety climate. Thus processes separable from instrumental processes appear to be involved in safety-specific transformational leadership and Clarke and Ward suggested these may involve trust. However we need further information on the psychological processes involved to understand such results. Conchie observes her findings suggest that "safety-specific transformational leadership affects the various forms of safety citizenship behaviors in different ways" (2013, p. 205).

Further, the psychological processes we have discussed may be differentially moderated in their effect by other variables, such as the personality of employees, or the trust they place in their supervisors and management, or the appraisals they make of stressors in their work environment, and research on these variables may shed further light on the operation and nature of the processes we have discussed. For example, Conchie and Donald (2009) showed safety-specific trust moderated the effect of safety-specific transformational leadership on safety citizenship behaviors, and Conchie (2013) argued for such trust as a moderator between transformational leadership and safety voice when mediated by intrinsic motivation. Conchie, Taylor, and Donald (2012) argued on the other hand that the affective dimension of trust should have a mediating role in the effect of transformational leadership on safety voice. Other authors have suggested trust is implicated in social exchanges and thereby related to safety outcomes (Kath, Magley, & Marmet, 2010). Including direct measures of the psychological processes involved in the constructs in question could lead to a better understanding of their relationships to the processes involved and associated safety behaviors (see also Conchie, Woodcock, & Taylor, Chapter 6, this volume).

We also do not know very much about the interplay between cognitive errors and violations. Do errors lead to violations for example, or vice versa, and under what circumstances and what are the psychological processes involved? And under what circumstances is it likely for both an error and a violation to occur independently but together? This area deserves further research too.

Conclusion

We have focused in this chapter on types of safety behaviors related to accidents, and associated psychological processes and organizational phenomena important in employees doing their jobs. Although set within a framework based on case study analysis of accidents and cognitive error, much of the research we have drawn upon to elucidate the fundamental psychological processes involved is questionnaire-based, with attendant limitations. Nonetheless such research suggests important psychological precursors appear to be both safety-specific, and more general, involving: instrumental processes; mental strain and burnout; engagement and safety-specific motivational/valence processes; and feelings of obligation and reciprocation. A number of organizational aspects contribute to these psychological processes and states including: the working environment; job demands; job resources; and leaders' commitment to safety and leadership style. However, we know relatively little about how these phenomena produce psychological processes that interact to predict unsafe behaviors, and how they may be influenced by other psychological factors such as trust, personality and cognitive appraisal. What is clear, though, is that different types of error and violation are related to different psychological processes and a proper understanding of safety behavior at work needs to take both into account.

References

Alper, S. J., & Karsh, B. T. (2009). A systematic review of safety violations in industry. *Accident Analysis and Prevention, 41*, 739–754.

Bakker, A. B., & Demerouti, E. (2007). The job demands-resources model: State of the art. *Journal of Managerial Psychology, 22*, 309–328.

Bakker, A. B., Demerouti, E., & Verbeke, W. (2004). Using the job demands-resources model to predict burnout and performance. *Human Resource Management, 43*, 83–104.

Barling, J., Kelloway, E. K., & Iverson, R. D. (2003). High-quality work, job satisfaction, and occupational injuries. *Journal of Applied Psychology, 88*, 276–283.

Barling, J., Loughlin, C., & Kelloway, E. K. (2002). Development and test of a model linking safety specific transformational leadership and occupational safety. *Journal of Applied Psychology, 87*, 488–496.

Beus, J. M., Payne, S. C., Bergman, M. E., & Arthur, W. (2010). Safety climate and injuries: An examination of theoretical and empirical relationships. *Journal of Applied Psychology, 93*, 713–727.

Blau, P. M. (1964). *Exchange and power in social life.* New York, NY: John Wiley & Sons, Inc.

Broadbent, D. E., Cooper, P. J., Fitzgerald, P. F., & Parkes, K. R. (1982). The cognitive failures questionnaire (CFQ) and its correlates. *British Journal of Clinical Psychology, 21*, 1–16.

Brown, R. L., & Holmes, H. (1986). The use of a factor-analytic procedure for assessing the validity of an employee safety climate model. *Accident Analysis & Prevention, 18*, 445–470.

Campbell, S. (1992). Effects of sleep and circadian rhythms on performance. In A. P. Smith & D. Jones (Eds.), *Handbook of human performance* (vol. 3. pp. 195–216). London, UK; San Diego, CA: Academic Press.

Chmiel, N. (2005). Promoting healthy work: Self-reported minor injuries, work characteristics, and safety behaviour. In C. Korunka & P. Hoffman (Eds.), *Change and quality in human service work* (pp. 277–288). Munich and Mering, Germany: Rainer Hampp Verlag.

Chmiel, N., & Hansez, I. (2013). Safety citizenship role definitions and safety violations. Proceedings of the Sixteenth European Congress of Work and Organizational Psychology, Munster, Germany.

Chmiel, N., & Taris, T. (2014). Safety at work. In J. de Jonge, M. Peeters, & T. Taris (Eds.), *Work psychology* (pp. 342–366). Chichester, UK: John Wiley & Sons, Ltd.

Chmiel, N., Totterdell, P., & Folkard, S. (1995). On adaptive control, sleep loss and fatigue. *Applied Cognitive Psychology, 9*, S39–S53.

Christian, M. S., Bradley, J. C., Wallace, J. C., & Burke, M. J. (2009). Workplace safety: A meta-analysis of the roles of person and situation factors. *Journal of Applied Psychology, 94*, 1103–1127.

Clarke, S. (1998). Organizational factors affecting the incident reporting of train drivers. *Work & Stress, 12*, 6–16.

Clarke, S. (2006a). The relationship between safety climate and safety performance: A meta-analytic review. *Journal of Occupational Health Psychology, 11*, 315–327.

Clarke, S. (2006b). Contrasting perceptual, attitudinal and dispositional approaches to accident involvement in the workplace. *Safety Science, 44*, 537–550.

Clarke, S. (2012). The effect of challenge and hindrance stressors on safety behavior and safety outcomes: A meta-analysis. *Journal of Occupational Health Psychology, 17*, 387–397.

Clarke, S. (2013). Safety leadership: A meta-analytic review of transformational and transactional leadership styles as antecedents of safety behaviours. *Journal of Occupational and Organizational Psychology, 86*, 22–49.

Clarke, S., & Robertson, I. T. (2005). A meta-analytic review of the big five personality factors and accident involvement in occupational and non-occupational settings. *Journal of Occupational and Organizational Psychology, 78*, 355–376.

Clarke, S., & Robertson, I. T. (2008). An examination of the role of personality in work accidents using meta-analysis. *Applied Psychology: An International Review, 57*, 94–108.

Clarke, S., & Ward, K. (2006). The role of leader influence tactics and safety climate in engaging employee safety participation. *Risk Analysis, 26*, 1175–1186.

Cooper, M. D., & Phillips, R. A. (2004). Exploratory analysis of the safety climate and safety behavior relationship. *Journal of Safety Research, 35*, 497–512.

Conchie, S. M. (2013). Transformational leadership, intrinsic motivation, and trust: a moderated-mediated model of workplace safety. *Journal of Occupational Health Psychology, 18*, 198–210.

Conchie, S. M., & Donald, I. J. (2009). The moderating role of safety-specific trust in the relation between safety-specific leadership and safety citizenship behaviors. *Journal of Occupational Health Psychology, 14*, 137–147.

Conchie, S. M., Taylor, P. J., & Donald, I. J. (2012). Promoting safety voice through safety-specific transformational leadership: The mediator role of two dimensions of trust. *Journal of Occupational Health Psychology, 17*, 105–115.

Craig, A., & Cooper, R. (1992). Symptoms of acute and chronic fatigue. In A. P. Smith & D. Jones (Eds.), *Handbook of human performance* (vol. 3, pp. 289–340). London, UK; San Diego, CA: Academic Press.

Dedobbeleer, N. & Béland, F. (1991). A safety climate measure for construction sites. *Journal of Safety Research, 22*, 97–103.

Dembe, A. E., Erickson, J. B., Delbos, R. G., & Banks, S. M. (2005). The impact of overtime and long work hours on occupational injuries and illnesses: New evidence from the United States. *Occupational and Environmental Medicine, 62*, 588–597.

Demerouti, E., Bakker, A. B., Nachreiner, F., & Schaufeli, W. B. (2001). The job demands–resources model of burnout. *Journal of Applied Psychology, 86*, 499–512.

Didla, S., Mearns, K., & Flin, R. (2009). Safety citizenship behaviour: A proactive approach to risk management. *Journal of Risk Management, 12*, 475–483.

Flin, R., Mearns, K., O'Connor, P., & Bryden, R. (2000). Measuring safety climate: Identifying the common features. *Safety Science, 34*, 177–192.

Folkard, S., & Monk, T (1979). Shiftwork and performance. *Human Factors, 21*, 483–492.

Gouldner, A. W. (1960). The norm of reciprocity: A preliminary statement. *American Sociological Review, 25*, 161–178.

Griffin, M. A., & Neal, N. (2000). Perceptions of safety at work: A framework for linking safety climate to safety performance, knowledge, and motivation. *Journal of Occupational Health Psychology, 5*, 347–358.

Hansez, I., & Chmiel, N. (2010). Safety behavior: Job demands, job resources and perceived management commitment to safety. *Journal of Occupational Health Psychology, 15*, 267–278.

Hobbs, A., Williamson, A., & Van Dongen, H. P. A. (2010). A circadian rhythm in skill-based errors in aviation maintenance. *Chronobiology International, 27*, 1304–1316.

Hockey, G. R. J. (1986). Changes in operator efficiency as a function of effects of environmental stress, fatigue and circadian rhythm. In K. Boff, L. Kaufman, & J. P. Thomas (Eds.), *Handbook of perception and human performance, Vol. 2: Cognitive processes and performance* (ch. 44, pp. 1–49). New York, NY: John Wiley & Sons, Inc.

Hockey, G. R. J. (1997). Compensatory control in the regulation of human performance under stress and high workload: A cognitive-energetical framework. *Biological Psychology, 45*, 73–93.

Hockey, G. R. J., & Earle, F. (2006). Control over the scheduling of simulated office work reduces the impact of workload on mental fatigue and task performance. *Journal of Experimental Psychology: Applied, 12*, 50–65.

Hofmann, D., & Morgeson, F. P. (1999). Safety-related behaviour as a social exchange: The role of perceived organizational support and leader–member exchange. *Journal of Applied Psychology, 84*, 286–296.

Hofmann, D. A., Morgeson, F. P., & Gerras, S. J. (2003). Climate as a moderator of the relationship between leader–member exchange and content specific citizenship: Safety climate as an exemplar. *Journal of Applied Psychology, 88*, 170–178.

Holding, D. H. (1983). Fatigue. In G. R. J. Hockey (Ed.), *Stress and fatigue in human performance* (pp. 145–168). New York, NY: John Wiley & Sons, Inc.

Hoonakker, P., Loushine, T., Carayon, P., Kallman, J., Kapp, A., & Smith, M. J. (2005). The effect of safety initiatives on safety performance: A longitudinal study. *Applied Ergonomics, 36*, 461–469.

Inness, M., Turner, N., Barling, J., & Stride, C. B. (2010). Transformational leadership and employee safety performance: A within-person, between-jobs design. *Journal of Occupational Health Psychology, 15*, 279–290.

International Labour Organization (2014). *Safety and health at work: A vision for sustainable prevention.* http://www.ilo.org/safework/info/publications/WCMS_301214/lang-ja/index.htm (accessed May 14, 2015).

Iverson, R. D., & Erwin, P. J. (1997). Predicting occupational injury: The role of affectivity. *Journal of Occupational and Organizational Psychology, 70*, 113–128.

James, L. R., Choi, C. C., Ko, C. E., McNeil, P. K., Minton, M. K., Wright, A., & Kim, K. (2008). Organizational and psychological climate: A review of theory and research. *European Journal of Work and Organizational Psychology, 17*, 5–32.

Kaminski, M. (2001). Unintended consequences: Organizational practices and their impact on workplace safety and productivity. *Journal of Occupational Health Psychology, 6*, 127–138.

Karasek, R. A. (1979). Job demands, job decision latitude, and mental strain: Implications for job redesign. *Administrative Science Quarterly, 24*, 285–307.

Kath, L. M., Magley, V. J., & Marmet, M. (2010). The role of organizational trust in safety climate's influence on organizational outcomes. *Accident Analysis & Prevention, 42*, 1488–1497.

Kelloway, E. K., Mullen, J., & Francis, L. (2006). Divergent effects of transformational and passive leadership on employee safety. *Journal of Occupational Health Psychology, 11*, 76–86.

Larson, G. E., Alderton, D. L., Neideffer, M., & Underhill, E. (1997). Further evidence on the dimensionality and correlates of the Cognitive Failures Questionnaire. *British Journal of Psychology, 88*, 29–38.

Larsson, S., Pousette, A., & Torner, M. (2008). Psychological climate and safety in the construction industry-mediated influence on safety behavior. *Safety Science, 46*, 405–412.

Lawton, R. (1998). Not working to rule: Understanding procedural violations at work. *Safety Science, 28*, 77–95.

Lawton, R., & Ward, N. J. (2005). A systems analysis of the Ladbroke Grove rail crash. *Accident Analysis and Prevention, 37*, 235–244.

Li, F., Jiang, L., Yao, X., & Li, Y. (2013). Job demands, job resources and safety outcomes: The roles of emotional exhaustion and safety compliance. *Accident Analysis and Prevention, 51*, 243–251.

Liden, R. C., & Maslyn, J. M. (1998). Multidimensionality of leader–member exchange: An empirical assessment through scale development. *Journal of Management, 24*, 43–72.

Lombardi, D. A., Folkard, S., Willetts, J. L., & Smith, G. S. (2010). Daily sleep, weekly working hours, and risk of work-related injury: US National Health Interview Survey (2004–2008). *Chronobiology International, 27*, 1013–1030.

Macey, W. H., & Schneider, B. (2008). The meaning of employee engagement. *Industrial and Organizational Psychology, 1*, 3–30.

Mearns, K. J., & Reader, T. (2008). Organizational support and safety outcomes: An un-investigated relationship? *Safety Science, 46*, 388–397.

Melamed, S., Yekutieli, D., Froom, P., Kristal-Boneh, E., & Ribak, J. (1999). Adverse work and environmental conditions predict occupational injuries: The Israeli Cardiovascular Occupational Risk Factors Determination in Israel (CORDIS) Study. *American Journal of Epidemiology, 150*, 18–26.

Motowidlo, S. J., Borman, W. C., & Schmit, M. J. (1997). A theory of individual differences in task and contextual performance. *Human Performance, 10*, 71–83.

Nahrgang, J. D., Morgeson, F. P., & Hofmann, D. A. (2011). Safety at work: A meta-analytic investigation of the link between job demands, job resources, burnout, engagement, and safety outcomes. *Journal of Applied Psychology, 96*, 71–94.

Neal, A., & Griffin, M. A. (2006) A study of the lagged relationships among safety climate, safety motivation, safety behavior, and accidents at the individual and group levels. *Journal of Applied Psychology, 91*, 946–953.

Neal, A., Griffin, M. A., & Hart. (2000). The impact of organizational climate on safety climate and individual behaviour. *Safety Science, 34*, 99–109.

Probst, T. M., Brubaker, T. L., & Barsotti, A. (2008). Organizational injury rate underreporting: The moderating effect of organizational safety climate. *Journal of Applied Psychology, 93*, 1147–1154.

Ramsey, J. and Morrisey, S. (1978). Isodecrement curves for task performance in hot environments. *Applied Ergonomics, 9*, 66–72.

Rasmussen, J. (1986). *Human information processing and human machine interaction*. Amsterdam, The Netherlands: North-Holland.

Rasmussen, J. (1990). Human error and the problem of causality in analysis of accidents. *Philosophical Transactions of the Royal Society London B, 327*, 449–462.

Rasmussen, J. & Jensen, A. (1974). Mental procedures in real-life tasks: A case study of electronic trouble-shooting. *Ergonomics, 17*, 293–307.

Reason, J. T. (1990). *Human error*. Cambridge, MA: Cambridge University Press.

Reason, J. T. (1993). Self-report questionnaires in cognitive psychology: Have they delivered the goods? In A. Baddeley & L. Weiskrantz (Eds.), *Attention: Selection, awareness, and control – A tribute to Donald Broadbent* (pp. 406–423). Oxford, UK: Oxford University Press.

Reason, J. T. (1997). *Managing the risks of organizational accidents*. Aldershot, UK: Ashgate.

Reason, J. T., Parker, D., & Lawton, R. (1998). Organizational controls and safety: The varieties of rule-related behaviour. *Journal of Occupational and Organizational Psychology, 71*, 289–304.

Rhoades, L., & Eisenberger, R. (2002). Perceived organizational support: A review of the literature. *Journal of Applied Psychology, 87*, 698–714.

Salminen, S., Saari, J., Saarela, K. L., & Rasanen, T. (1993). Organizational factors influencing occupational accidents. *Scandinavian Journal of Work, Environment & Health, 19*, 352–357.

Salminen, S., & Tallberg, T. (1996). Human errors in fatal and serious occupational accidents in Finland. *Ergonomics, 39*, 980–988.

Schaufeli, W. B., & Bakker, A. B. (2004). Job demands, job resources, and their relationship with burnout and engagement: A multi-sample study. *Journal of Organizational Behavior, 25*, 293–315.

Shannon, H. S. & Geoffrey, R. (2009). Deriving the factor structure of safety climate scales. *Safety Science, 47*, 327–329.

Shannon, H. S., Mayr, J., & Haines, T. (1997). Overview of the relationship between organizational and workplace factors and injury rates. *Safety Science, 26*, 201–217.

Sheehy, N., & Chapman, A. (1987). Industrial accidents. In C. L. Cooper & I. T. Robertson (Eds.), *International review of industrial and organizational psychology* (pp. 201–227). Oxford, UK: Blackwell.

Simpson, S. A., Wadsworth, E. J. K., Moss, S. C., & Smith, A. P. (2005). Minor injuries, cognitive failures and accidents at work: Incidence and associated features. *Occupational Medicine, 55*, 99–108.

Soane, E., & Chmiel, N. (1999). Emotional risk communication and the adoption of safety precautions in a safety-critical workplace. Proceedings of the British Psychological Society Annual Psychology Conference, Belfast, Northern Ireland.

Soane, E., & Chmiel, N. (2005). Are risk preferences consistent? The influence of decision domain and personality. *Personality & Individual Differences, 38*, 1781–1791.

Tucker, S., Chmiel, N., Turner, N., Hershcovis, M. S., & Stride, C. (2008). Perceived organizational support for safety and employee safety voice: The mediating role of coworker support for safety. *Journal of Occupational Health Psychology, 13*, 319–330.

Turner, N., Chmiel, N., & Walls, M. (2005). Railing for safety: Job demands, job control, and safety citizenship role definitions. *Journal of Occupational Health Psychology, 10*, 504–512.

Turner, N., Stride, C. B., Carter, A. J., McCaughey, D., & Carroll, A. E. (2012). Job Demands-Control-Support model and employee safety performance. *Accident Analysis & Prevention, 45*, 811–817.

Van Der Linden, D., Keijsers, G. P. J., Eling, P., & Van Schaijk, R. (2005). Work stress and attentional difficulties: An initial study on burnout and cognitive failures. *Work & Stress, 19*, 23–36.

Vredenburgh, A. G. (2002). Organizational safety: Which management practices are most effective in reducing employee injury rates? *Journal of Safety Research, 33*, 259–276.

Wagenaar, W. A. (1992). Risk taking and accident causation. In J. F. Yates (Ed.), *Risk-taking behavior* (pp. 257–281). Chichester, UK: John Wiley & Sons, Ltd.

Wagenaar, W. A., & Groeneweg, J. (1987). Accidents at sea: Multiple causes and impossible consequences. *International Journal of Man–Machine Studies, 27*, 587–598.

Wagenaar, W. A., Groeneweg, J., Hudson, P. T. W., & Reason, J. T. (1994). Promoting safety in the oil industry. *Ergonomics, 37*, 1999–2013.

Wagenaar, W. A., Hudson, P. T. W., & Reason, J. T. (1990). Cognitive failures and accidents. *Applied Cognitive Psychology, 4*, 273–294.

Wallace, J. C., & Chen, G. (2005). Development and validation of a work-specific measure of cognitive failure: Implications for occupational safety. *Journal of Occupational and Organizational Psychology, 78*, 615–632.

Wallace, J. C., & Vodanovich, S. J. (2003). Workplace safety performance: Conscientiousness, cognitive failure, and their interaction. *Journal of Occupational Health Psychology, 8,* 316–327.

Weddle, M. G., (1996). Reporting occupational injuries: The first step. *Journal of Safety Research, 27,* 217–233.

Weinstein, N. D. (1988). The precaution adoption process. *Health Psychology, 7,* 355–386.

Wilhelm, O., Witthoft, M., & Schipolowski, S. (2010). Self-reported cognitive failures: Competing measurement models and self-report correlates. *Journal of Individual Differences, 31,* 1–14.

Williams, H., Lubin, A. and Goodnow, J. (1959). Impaired performance with acute sleep loss. *Psychological Monographs, 73,* 1–26.

Zacharatos, A., Barling, J., & Iverson, R. D. (2005). High-performance work systems and occupational safety. *Journal of Applied Psychology, 90,* 77–93.

Zohar, D. (1980). Safety climate in industrial organisations: Theoretical and applied implications. *Journal of Applied Psychology, 65,* 96–102.

Zohar, D. (2003). Safety climate: Conceptual and measurement issues. In J. Quick & L. Tetrick (Eds.), *Handbook of occupational health psychology.* Washington, DC: American Psychological Association.

Zohar, D. (2008). Safety climate and beyond: A multi-level multi-climate framework. *Safety Science, 46,* 376–387.

Part II

Workplace Health and Well-Being

8

The Job Demands-Resources Model

Toon W. Taris and Wilmar B. Schaufeli

Introduction

One of the currently most popular models in occupational health psychology is the Job Demands-Resources (JD-R) model (Demerouti, Bakker, Nachreiner, & Schaufeli, 2001). The JD-R model describes the relations between work characteristics, work outcomes (i.e., health, well-being, and performance), and personal characteristics. The present version of the model holds that high job demands lead to high levels of stress and health issues (the *health impairment process*), whereas the presence of high levels of job resources results in high levels of motivation and excellent job performance (the *motivational process*). Since the model was first published in 2001, it has attracted much attention from both researchers and practitioners. For example, according to *Google Scholar* the three most significant papers on the JD-R model (Bakker & Demerouti, 2007; Demerouti et al., 2001; Schaufeli & Bakker, 2004) had been cited nearly 7,000 times as of January 2015.

Schaufeli and Taris (2013, 2014) argue that one likely reason for this apparent popularity is the fact that the JD-R model builds on established models such as Karasek's Job Demand-Control (-Support) model (DCS model; Karasek, 1979; Karasek & Theorell, 1990) and Siegrist's (1996) Effort-Reward Imbalance (ERI) model. For example, the JD-R's central tenet that work outcomes are the result of negative (demands) and positive (resources) work characteristics parallels the assumption of the DCS that the adverse effects of high job demands can be offset by the presence of high support and high control. Similarly, the ERI model proposed that the harmful effects of "high effort" can be compensated by the presence of sufficient "rewards." The terms "job demands" and "job resources," referring to broad and open categories in which a wide range of very different job characteristics could be placed, had earlier been coined in an influential meta-analysis of the antecedents of job burnout

The Wiley Blackwell Handbook of the Psychology of Occupational Safety and Workplace Health, First Edition. Edited by Sharon Clarke, Tahira M. Probst, Frank Guldenmund, and Jonathan Passmore. © 2016 John Wiley & Sons Ltd. Published 2020 by John Wiley & Sons Ltd.

by Lee and Ashforth (1996; cf. Taris, Schreurs, & Schaufeli, 1999). Finally, the JD-R model proposes that the two central processes linking work characteristics and work outcomes involve *motivation* and *health impairment*; these processes bear more than a superficial similarity to the *motivation/active learning* and *stress* hypotheses in the DCS model, respectively (Karasek & Theorell, 1990). Apparently, then-current models and ideas had already prepared the minds for the JD-R model.

The major innovation in the JD-R model is the fact that it combines Lee and Ashforth's (1996) conceptualization of demands and resources with earlier notions about the effects of demands and resources on worker health and well-being. Rather than confining itself to a limited set of particular job demands and job resources as most earlier models had done, it proposes that *any* job demand and *any* job resource can affect worker health and well-being. Indeed, the JD-R model assumes that relevant demands and resources can vary across jobs, thus enhancing the flexibility and scope of the model (Bakker & Demerouti, 2007). In effect, building on familiar, tried-and-tested notions, the JD-R model provides a simple, yet comprehensive heuristic framework for relating a wide variety of job characteristics to a broad range of work outcomes – something that at the time of its inception very few of the models then used in the emerging discipline of occupational health psychology could offer.

Since its first publication in the early 2000's, the JD-R model has been modified and extended considerably. Whereas an early version of the model focused on burnout as the primary outcome variable, later versions incorporate more diverse outcomes and more antecedents, including both work-related and personal resources. Below these models are discussed and reviewed in further detail.

The Jobs Demands-Resources Model of Burnout

In their seminal (2001) publication in the *Journal of Applied Psychology*, Demerouti et al. attempted to account for the antecedents of burnout, defined in terms of exhaustion/fatigue and disengagement/withdrawal (the two key dimensions of burnout; Schaufeli & Taris, 2005). At the heart of the model was Lee and Ashforth's (1996) distinction between job demands and job resources, combined with the *structural model of burnout* proposed by Maslach, Jackson, and Leiter (1996, p. 36).

The model

Demerouti et al. (2001) defined job demands as "those physical, social, or organizational aspects of the job that require sustained physical or mental effort and are therefore associated with certain physiological and psychological costs" (Demerouti et al., 2001, p. 501). This conceptualization is broad enough to encompass concepts such as Karasek's (1979) job demands and Siegrist's (1996) effort (which is measured in terms of obligations and task interruptions). Demerouti et al. defined job resources analogously as "those physical, social or organizational aspects of the job that may do any of the following: (a) be functional in achieving work goals; (b) reduce job demands and the associated physiological and psychological costs; (c) stimulate personal growth and development" (p. 501). Again, concepts such as Karasek and Theorell's (1990) job control and social support, and Siegrist's (1996) financial rewards, esteem, job security, and career opportunities fit well with this conceptualization of job resources.

The JD-R model of burnout argued that demands and resources could affect the two burnout components in two ways. First, following Hockey (1997), the model assumed that dealing adequately with high job demands requires high levels of energy. Chronic high effort expenditure due to high job demands leads to physiological and psychological costs, including high levels of fatigue. Recovery from this state of exhaustion can be achieved by taking breaks, by switching to other tasks, or by working more slowly. However, when there is little opportunity for such recovery-promoting strategies, for instance when performance standards are high, employees will enter a state of *sustained activation* (Knardahl & Ursin, 1985) that can ultimately lead to physical and psychological exhaustion – the energetic component of burnout (Maslach, Schaufeli, & Leiter, 2001). Second, the JD-R model proposed that resources help employees cope with the negative influences of the work environment (e.g., high demands) and are conducive in achieving their goals. A lack of resources will instill a self-protective process in which reduced motivation and withdrawal from the job (i.e., the motivational component of burnout: Maslach et al., 2001) prevents possible negative effects resulting from the future frustration of not obtaining work-related goals. Although Demerouti et al. acknowledged that this reasoning implies that a statistical interaction of demands and resources is central to the development of burnout (p. 502), on the basis of previous research on the absence of such interactions in Karasek's (1979) Demand-Control model they argued that demands-resource interactions would rarely occur. Therefore, the JD-R model of burnout proposed that exhaustion is primarily linked to high demands, and that disengagement/withdrawal primarily results from lack of resources.

Evidence for the JD-R model of burnout

Research employing the JD-R model of burnout has provided much, although not fully consistent, support for the main effects of job demands and job resources on burnout, with high job demands being associated with high levels of fatigue and exhaustion, and lack of resources being associated with withdrawal (Bakker, Demerouti, & Euwema, 2005; Bakker, Demerouti, Taris, Schaufeli, & Schreurs, 2003; Bakker, Demerouti, & Verbeke, 2004; Crawford, LePine, & Rich, 2010; Demerouti et al., 2001; Hansen, Sverke, & Näswall, 2009; Huyn, Winefield, Xanthopoulou, & Metzer, 2012; Li, Jiang, Yao, & Li, 2012; Lizano & Mor Barak, 2012; Van Riet & Bakker, 2004; Xanthopoulou, Bakker, Dollard, et al., 2007; see Alarcon, 2011, for a review). Interestingly, in spite of the fact that in the seminal publication on the JD-R model of burnout the importance of demands × resource interactions was downplayed (Demerouti et al., 2001), later research did examine this interaction. For example, Bakker et al. (2003) showed that demands and resources interacted statistically in predicting the two burnout components. As expected, they found that high levels of resources mitigated the adverse effects of high job demands on exhaustion, and that the positive effect of resources on withdrawal/cynicism was weaker when demands were high. Follow-up research by Bakker et al. (2005) and Xanthopoulou et al. (2007) revealed that about 60 percent of all possible interactions between job demands and job resources were significant and in the expected direction; none of these interactions ran counter to the predictions. Hansen et al. (2009) replicated these findings in the context of three hospitals, adding credence to these findings. As regards the outcomes of high levels of burnout, Van Riet and Bakker (2004) showed that high levels of cynicism were associated with lower sales performance of teams (with cynicism mediating the association between job resources and sales performance). Similarly, Bakker et al. (2004) reported that high levels of cynicism and exhaustion were associated with lower levels of objectively measured in- and extra-role performance.

Conclusions: The JD-Resources model of burnout

While previous research has largely confirmed the assumptions of the JD-R model of burnout, it is important to note that the large majority of the studies cited above draw upon self-report cross-sectional data sets. For example, in a two-sample longitudinal study, Diestel and Schmidt (2012) found little support for the idea that demands and resources would predict later burnout. Moreover, the evidence for the main effects of job demands and job resources on the outcome variables is considerably stronger than that for statistical interactions, but this is not uncommon in the area of job stress research (cf. Taris, 2006). One possible reason for this lack of demand × resource interaction effects is that interactions are especially likely when job demands, job resources, and job-related outcomes refer to qualitatively identical dimensions, e.g., *emotional* demands, *emotional* support, and *emotional* exhaustion, respectively. There is some support for this reasoning (among others, De Jonge & Dormann, 2006; De Jonge, Dormann, & Van den Tooren, 2008; Feuerhahn, Bellingrath, & Kudielka, 2013; Van de Ven & Vlerick, 2013), which goes against Demerouti et al.'s (2001) implicit assumption that the qualitative differences among different demands (or resources) can be neglected, since these demands (resources) would all trigger the same underlying processes.

The Revised Job Demands-Resources Model

Three years after the publication of the JD-R model of burnout, Schaufeli and Bakker (2004) presented an extended and revised version of the model that included not only burnout but also job engagement (Figure 8.1). Engagement is a positive, fulfilling, work-related state of mind that is characterized by vigor (i.e., high levels of energy and resilience), dedication (experiencing a sense of significance, pride, and challenge) and absorption (being fully concentrated and happily engrossed in one's work) (cf. Schaufeli & Bakker, 2010). The revised model included two main hypotheses, referring to two distinct underlying processes:

1   The first hypothesis is that strain mediates the associations between job demands and health problems (or, more generally, negative outcomes). Similar to the JD-R model of burnout, the revised model assumes that strain results from experiencing high levels of (stress-inducing) demands and low levels of resources. However, contrary to the JD-R model of burnout, the revised JD-R model construes strain as a concept that can have multiple indicators, including – but not limited to – the two core dimensions of burnout (i.e., exhaustion and withdrawal/cynicism). Although this presents a conceptual shift as compared with the JD-R model of burnout (in which these two dimensions were treated as theoretically distinct concepts, each with a different set of antecedents), it should be acknowledged that both indicators of burnout are empirically usually strongly related (e.g., Taris, Le Blanc, Schaufeli, & Schreurs, 2005). To account for the fact that previous research on the JD-R of burnout had shown that job resources were related to withdrawal, the revised model also included a direct effect of resources on strain. Further, consistent with previous research (Melamed, Shirom, Toker, Berliner, & Shapira, 2006), it was assumed that strain could lead to health problems such as depression, cardiovascular complaints, and psychosomatic complaints. Thus, this part of the model proposes that the presence of high demands and low resources leads to a gradual decrease of mental energy (burnout), which in turn could trigger the development of other health and well-being issues. This was termed the *energetic* or *health impairment process*.

2   The second main hypothesis is that engagement mediates the association between job resources and positive outcomes (such as low turnover and high performance). The revised JD-R model emphasizes the fact that some job characteristics (resources) have inherently motivational qualities (e.g., Bakker, Demerouti, & Sanz-Vergel, 2014). Drawing on Meijman and Mulder's (1998) Effort-Recovery Model, the revised JD-R model proposes that the presence of job resources activates workers' willingness to devote their efforts and abilities to their tasks at work. That is, job resources increase workers' levels of extrinsic motivation since they increase their willingness to spend compensatory effort in order to reach work goals. However, job resources such as high levels of autonomy, support, and feedback could also increase workers' levels of intrinsic motivation, since they serve to satisfy the basic human needs for autonomy, affiliation, and competence (cf. Deci & Ryan, 2000; Van den Broeck, Vansteenkiste, De Witte, & Lens, 2008). For example, high levels of autonomy and feedback could promote learning behavior, which would, in turn, lead to increased levels of perceived competence (Taris, Kompier, Geurts, Houtman, & Van den Heuvel, 2010). This implies that job resources lead to higher levels of engagement through two motivational paths: an extrinsic path (through reaching one's work goals) and an intrinsic path (through satisfaction of basic human needs). In turn, work engagement is presumed to increase the level of positive work outcomes, including work performance. Thus, job resources increase motivation and work engagement, which, in turn, leads to higher performance. This part of the model is referred to as the *motivational process*.

A further refinement of the revised JD-R model was made in 2007 by Bakker and Demerouti, who explicitly acknowledged the fact that job demands and job resources could interact in affecting job strain and motivation. Drawing on previous findings obtained for Karasek's (1979) Demand-Control model (where the demand × control interaction takes a central place) and on Diener and Fujita (1995) (who found that many different types of resources could facilitate the achievement of particular goals), Bakker and Demerouti argued that "the JD-R model proposes that the interaction between job

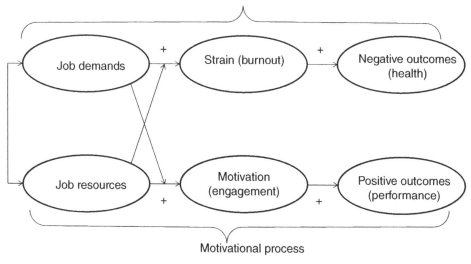

Figure 8.1   The revised Job Demands-Resources model.

demands and job resources is important for the development of job strain and motivation as well" (2007, p. 217), and that "different types of job demands and job resources may interact in predicting job strain" (p. 217).

Interestingly, counter to the idea that job resources trigger *one specific motivational process* that explains why various resources are associated with higher levels of motivation (work engagement) and performance, Bakker and Demerouti (2007, p. 315) argued that the reason why job resources can act as buffers may vary across – and even within – resources. For example, a worker's high-quality relationship with their supervisor may alleviate the adverse effects of high demands on job strain, since their supervisor's appreciation and support puts demands in a different perspective. It could also help the worker in coping with his or her job demands, facilitate performance, or protect against ill-health. Thus, whereas the main effects of job demands and job resources on strain and motivation are interpreted in terms of two separate and unambiguous processes (health impairment and motivation), this does not apply to the possible demand × control interactions: here a multitude of specific explanations may apply. Although this somewhat spoils the attractive simplicity of the revised JD-R model, it probably does justice to the fact that real-life processes may be too complex to be represented adequately by the two relatively straightforward processes proposed in models such as the JD-R model.

Evidence for the revised JD-R model

During the last decade or so, the revised JD-R model has constituted the theoretical basis for a large body of research. On the one hand, this research intended to test the model's assumptions; on the other, it was also used as a framework in which other concepts and phenomena were studied. Both types of research can be used to examine the degree to which the model is supported empirically.

Cross-sectional evidence   The first studies employing the revised JD-R model were conducted in the Netherlands among call center employees (Bakker, Demerouti, & Schaufeli, 2003), industrial workers (Bakker, Demerouti, De Boer, & Schaufeli, 2003) and administrative staff and health care employees (Schaufeli & Bakker, 2004). These studies supported the model's hypotheses regarding the main effects of demands and resources on strain and motivation, respectively, and were replicated internationally as well as in other occupations, for example, among Finnish dentists (Hakanen, Bakker, & Schaufeli, 2006), Australian volunteers (Lewig, Xanthopoulou, Bakker, Dollard, & Metzer, 2007), employees of Chinese family-owned businesses (Hu & Schaufeli, 2011), Dutch interns and temporary workers (Akkermans, Schaufeli, Brenninkmeijer, & Blonk, 2013), and blue- and white-collar workers in Austria (Korunka, Kubicek, Schaufeli, & Hoonakker, 2009), Belgium (Hansez & Chmiel, 2010), Spain (Llorens, Bakker, Schaufeli, & Salanova, 2006), South Africa (De Beer, Rothmann, & Pienaar, 2012), and China (Hu, Schaufeli, & Taris, 2011). A similar study among Italian call center agents (Consiglio, Borgogni, Alessandri, & Schaufeli, 2013) showed that at the individual level, higher job demands were associated with higher burnout; the effect of resources on burnout was not statistically reliable. At the team level, higher demands and lower resources were associated with higher burnout. Finally, Kinnunen, Feldt, Siltaloppi, and Sonnentag (2011) showed that the associations between job demands and fatigue/strain, and between job resources and engagement, were partly mediated through the degree to which workers were able to detach from work. High demands were both directly and indirectly (through low detachment) associated with low engagement; high resources were directly associated with low strain, and both directly and indirectly (through high detachment) with high engagement.

A much smaller number of studies have not only examined the main effects of demands and resources, but also their statistical interaction. For example, a study among Finnish teachers found that high job resources, such as a positive school climate, social support, and appreciation by the supervisor, were especially strongly related to high levels of engagement when job demands were high (Bakker, Hakanen, Demerouti, & Xanthopoulou, 2007). Hu et al. (2011) reported for one of their samples that the adverse effects of high job demands on burnout decreased in the presence of high job resources. However, this interaction effect accounted for little variance in burnout beyond what was already accounted for by the main effects of demands and resources. In two samples, one from Australia and one from China, and each including more than 4,000 participants, Brough et al. (2013) found that out of the eight interactions of job demands and various forms of social support tested in this study, two were statistically significant and in the correct direction. Interestingly, two other demand × support interactions were also significant, but went against the model's predictions. Finally, in a study among more than 12,000 Dutch workers, Bakker, Van Veldhoven, and Xanthopoulou (2010) found that 28 out of the 32 tested demand × resource interactions were statistically significant and in the expected direction, although it should be noted that on average these interactions accounted for only 0.5 percent of the variance (mode = 0.1 percent) in this study's outcome variables (i.e., task enjoyment and organizational commitment).

All in all, from the evidence discussed above it can be concluded that there is strong cross-sectional evidence for the main effects of job demands and job resources on outcome variables such as strain (especially burnout) and motivation (especially work engagement). Tests of demands × resources interaction effects have been published much less frequently. Overall, the available evidence on interactions suggests that the adverse effects of job demands on work outcomes may be mitigated or even be turned into positive effects when participants possess high levels of resources, which confirms the predictions of the JD-R model and is consistent with earlier work on demands × control interaction effects in Karasek's (1979) Demand-Control model (see Häusser, Mojzisch, Niesel, & Schulz-Hardt, 2010, and Taris & Kompier, 2004, for reviews). However, similar to previous findings on interaction effects in the Demand-Control model (e.g., Taris, 2006), the current evidence on demand × resource interaction effects shows that, even if significant, the practical relevance of such interactions tends to be low.

Longitudinal evidence   Correlation does not imply causation: cross-sectional associations – even if these are in accordance with a particular theory – present only weak evidence for the causal assumptions of that theory. Fortunately, a number of studies on the revised JD-R model have employed a longitudinal design, allowing us to examine the evidence for the causal relations proposed in the JD-R model more appropriately. Several of these studies provide longitudinal support for the JD-R. For example, a three-year study among Finnish dentists (Hakanen, Schaufeli, & Ahola, 2008) showed that job resources predicted the degree of later job engagement, which was in turn related to dentists' work engagement. Further, this study showed that high demands predicted later levels of burnout, which was in turn related to depression. Similarly, a study among Dutch managers showed that an increase of job demands and a decrease of job resources across one year were associated with an increase of burnout complaints during that same year (Schaufeli, Bakker, & Van Rhenen, 2009). As expected, an increase of job resources was associated with an increase in job engagement. This study also revealed that burnout was associated with the *duration* of sickness absence (an indicator of health), whereas engagement was associated with sickness absence *frequency* (an indicator of motivation). Further, Akkermans, Brenninkmeijer, Van den Bossche, Blonk, and Schaufeli (2013) found in two statistically independent samples (of low and high-education young employees, respectively) that higher resources at the start of the study were associated with higher later dedication and lower later exhaustion, and that higher demands were associated with higher later exhaustion. No reversed effects (from dedication and exhaustion on job demands/resources) were found. In a three-wave study, Barbier, Hansez, Chmiel, and Demerouti (2013) reported that an increase in opportunities for development predicted higher concurrent (i.e., within-wave) and later work engagement; for the second resource included in this study, social support, only concurrent support was found. Finally, in a ten-year study among Finnish firefighters, Airila et al. (2014) showed that the initial level of job resources predicted later work engagement and work ability, which is also consistent with the motivational predictions of the JD-R. However, this study did not include a measure of initial work ability, meaning that it is unclear whether the effect of job resources on later work ability can be interpreted causally.

These positive findings for the longitudinal predictions of the JD-R model are counterbalanced by the results of other longitudinal studies. In a one-year study among Dutch university employees, Ouweneel, Le Blanc, and Schaufeli (2012) found no evidence for lagged effects of job resources on work engagement: apparently, these effects were "overwhelmed" by the high temporal stability of engagement. Similarly, contrary to the JD-R's expectations, a three-wave study among Swiss workers (Brauchli, Schaufeli, Jenny, Füllemann, & Bauer, 2013) found no evidence for lagged effects of demands and resources on job burnout or engagement; however, *within* the three study waves cross-sectional evidence for the expected associations was obtained. This study suggested that job resources were more stable across time than job demands, but provided no longitudinal evidence for the causal processes proposed in the JD-R. In a seven-year three-wave study among Finnish dentists, Seppälä et al. (2014) found that work engagement and job resources were largely stable across time, and that it was unclear whether job resources and job engagement were causally related. In a prospective cohort study with a one-year follow-up among Norwegian nurses, Roelen et al. (2014) showed that high initial job demands and low initial social support (a resource) were associated with later sickness absence. No main effects of job control (another resource) or demand × resource interactions were statistically significant. Finally, in a two-nation longitudinal study among 1,600 Chinese and Australian workers, Brough et al. (2013) found no lagged main effects of job demands on the outcome variables in their study (strain and engagement), whereas only one out of eight lagged main effects of two forms of support (from supervisor and coworker) on these outcomes was statistically reliable and in the expected direction. Moreover, inclusion of the interactions between demands and supervisor and coworker support did not account for any additional variance in strain or engagement. Apparently somewhat disappointed, Brough et al. (2013) conclude that their "results are (…) markedly different from the proportions of significant job demands × job resources interaction terms reported elsewhere" (p. 1326), and that "the theoretical associations between the job demands and job resources variables in the prediction of psychological strain and work engagement may be more transient than has been previously identified" (p. 1330).

Conclusions: The revised JD-R model

All in all, it seems fair to say that the findings discussed above provide compelling cross-sectional evidence for the main effects of job demands on strain/exhaustion, and of job resources on motivation/engagement. The longitudinal evidence for these associations is less convincing, with the number of studies supporting the expected associations being matched by a similar number of studies finding no or reversed effects. As for the

JD-R model of burnout, the evidence for demands × resources interaction effects in the revised JD-R model is weak, which might – again – be due to the fact that it is possible that interactions are especially likely when demands, resources, and outcomes refer to qualitatively similar dimensions (De Jonge & Dormann, 2006; Van de Ven & Vlerick, 2013). Another possibility is that the associations between demands and resources on the one hand, and outcomes such as strain/burnout and motivation/engagement are contingent upon other variables or that they are sample specific. In the next section we discuss a line of research that examines the role of personal resources in the job demands-resources model.

Extension of the Jobs Demands-Resources Model: Personal Resources

When these models were introduced, neither the JD-R model of burnout nor its revision considered factors other than characteristics of the job and the work environment. However, psychological theories usually emphasize that human behavior results from the interaction of environmental factors (such as work characteristics) and personal factors (such as personality). Therefore, it is hardly surprising that such personal factors have been incorporated in the JD-R model as well. Bearing a strong analogy to job resources, personal resources are defined as "positive self-evaluations that are linked to resiliency and refer to individuals' sense of their ability to control and impact upon their environment successfully (…) [and] (a) are functional in achieving goals, (b) protect from threats and the associated physiological and psychological costs, and (c) stimulate personal growth and development" (Xanthopoulou, Bakker, Demerouti, & Schaufeli, 2009, p. 236).

Personal resources strongly resemble job resources in that they are instrumental in achieving the same goals as job resources (cf. Demerouti et al., 2001). However, this strong resemblance of job and personal resources does not imply that both categories of resources take a similar place in the JD-R model. Whereas job resources are usually considered antecedents of especially motivation and (sometimes) strain (perhaps in interaction with job demands), up until now personal resources have been included in at least five different ways in the JD-R model (Schaufeli & Taris, 2014).

Firstly, one natural way of including personal resources is to consider them as *antecedents of strain and motivation,* just like job resources and job demands. Since personal resources are defined in terms of resilience, they should be associated with higher levels of engagement/motivation and lower levels of strain/burnout. Consistent with this reasoning, a longitudinal study among Spanish teachers, Llorente, Salanova, Martinez, and Schaufeli (2008) found that higher levels of mental and emotional competencies at the start of the academic year were related to lower levels of burnout and higher levels of engagement at the end of the year, independent of job demands and job resources. Similarly, in an 18-month longitudinal study, Xanthopoulou et al. (2009) showed that the initial level of personal resources (measured as optimism, self-efficacy, and organizational-based self-esteem) predicted higher later levels of engagement. Moreover, engagement as measured at the start of the study predicted future higher levels of job and personal resources. This suggests that so-called *gain* and *loss spirals* may occur (cf. Hobfoll, 2002), in which the presence (absence) of resources leads to higher (lower) levels of engagement, in turn leading to even higher (lower) levels of resources, etc. (Salanova, Schaufeli, Xanthopoulou, & Bakker, 2010, and Taris & Kompier, 2014, for more thorough discussions of this subject).

A second way of including personal resources in the JD-R model is to consider them as *moderators of the associations between job characteristics and work outcomes*. The definition of personal resources suggests that they could affect the magnitude of the associations between job demands/resources on the one hand, and outcomes on the other. Theoretically, the adverse effects of high job demands on strain should be mitigated by high levels of personal resources, whereas the already positive effects of high resources on motivation could be enhanced further by high personal resources. Consistent with this idea, Van den Broeck, Van Ruysseveldt, Smulders, and De Witte (2011) showed that high levels of intrinsic motivation reduced the adverse effects of lack of learning opportunities on exhaustion, and strengthened the positive effect of job control on job engagement. Similarly, Brenninkmeijer, Demerouti, Le Blanc, and Van Emmerik (2010) reported that the adverse effects of high job demands and conflicts at work on exhaustion were stronger among prevention-oriented workers (i.e., those who focus on safety, obligations, and avoidance of loss).

Thirdly, personal resources could *mediate the relations between job characteristics and outcomes*. For example, workers in high-resource work environments are often expected to experience higher levels of self-efficacy and optimism. These could in turn lead to higher levels of work engagement. So far, four cross-sectional studies have tested and confirmed the mediating role of personal resources, focusing on self-esteem/optimism and self-efficacy (Xanthopoulou et al., 2007), psychological capital (PsyCap: self-efficacy, optimism, hope, and resilience; Vink, Ouweneel, & Le Blanc, 2011), creativity (Bakker & Xanthopoulou, 2013), and psychological need fulfillment (for competence, affiliation, and autonomy; Van den Broeck et al., 2008) as mediators, respectively. Two further longitudinal studies showed that self-efficacy mediated the association between job resources and engagement over time (Llorens, Salanova, Schaufeli, & Bakker, 2007; Simbula, Guglielmi, & Schaufeli, 2011).

A fourth way of incorporating personal resources into the JD-R model is to consider them as possible *antecedents of work characteristics*. In the past, it has been proposed that personal resources could affect the work environment, either factually or by altering workers' perceptions of that environment. For example, Bandura's (1997) social-cognitive theory proposes that a person's subjectively perceived competence determines their perception of and their reactions to their environment. Similarly, Judge, Bono, and Locke (2000) argued that an employee's core self-evaluation (CSE; an amalgamate of self-esteem, generalized self-efficacy, locus of control, and neuroticism) affects their perception of the work environment, which, in turn affects job satisfaction and work performance. Consistent with these ideas, Xanthopoulou, Bakker, Demerouti, and Schaufeli (2007) reported that job resources mediated the association between personal resources (i.e., self-efficacy, optimism, and self-esteem) and engagement.

Finally, personal resources could act as a *confounder of the associations among job demands, job resources, and work outcomes*. That is, if it is correct that personal resources affect both work characteristics as well as work outcomes (see above), failing to control for personal resources could bias the associations between work characteristics and work outcomes. For example, Bakker, Boyd, Dollard, et al. (2010) found that the level of extraversion of Australian academics partly accounted for the associations between job resources and engagement.

In summary, the findings discussed above show that: (i) a wide range of personal resources can fruitfully be integrated into the JD-R model, (ii) their effects can be substantial, but (iii) it is unclear which place they should take in the model. It can be presumed that there is no single "correct" place, since findings may vary across different types of personal resources. For example, relatively stable personal characteristics such as personality traits are probably better conceptualized as possible antecedents of job characteristics and/or work outcomes, rather than as mediators of the relations in the JD-R model. Conversely, relatively malleable personal characteristics (e.g., psychological capital) could well be studied as mediators (cf. Van der Heijden, Van Dam, Xanthopoulou, & De Lange, 2014). Apparently, additional research on the role of personal resources would seem desirable.

Applications and Extensions of the Job Demands-Resources Model

Since the publication of the JD-R model, it has been applied in various contexts and with different goals. In this section we briefly discuss how the model can be used in practice and how it can be extended.

Examining the relations between work characteristics and work outcomes

The most obvious application of the JD-R model is to examine the work-related antecedents of a particular type of outcome, perhaps in conjunction with personal characteristics. As the review above indicated, initially the outcome to be studied was burnout or its sub-dimensions (exhaustion and depersonalization, later complemented with engagement in the revised JD-R model). Moreover, since strain (burnout) and affect/motivation (engagement) were presumed to be linked to positive and negative outcomes, concepts such as in-role and extra-role performance (Bakker et al., 2004, 2010), commitment (Bakker et al., 2010), turnover, safety behavior (Hansez & Chmiel, 2010; see also Chmiel & Hansez, Chapter 7, this volume), sickness absence (Schaufeli et al., 2009), and health issues such as depression (Hakanen et al., 2008) have all been studied in this research. The main purpose of much of this research was to test and further validate various aspects of the JD-R model, yielding evidence as to the robustness of the model as well as regarding the antecedents of the outcomes that were involved.

Mapping work characteristics as a basis for interventions

JD-R based research may also have a strong practical component, that is, when the antecedents of a particular phenomenon (such as burnout or work engagement) have been mapped, a logical next step is to design and implement interventions in order to address possible issues and concerns. The JD-R model fits well in a cyclical process that starts with a particular practical question or even a problem: *problem definition*, e.g., (1) "how do this company's employees experience their jobs?"; (2) "how can the experienced levels of exhaustion and cynicism in this organization be reduced?"; (3) "how can levels of work engagement be increased?"; or (4) "how can we reduce levels of sickness absence in this department?" The JD-R model offers a clear conceptual framework to study such questions, in that it focuses on two important indicators of employee well-being (strain/burnout and motivation/engagement) which is relevant to question 1, indicates how employee scores on these concepts are related to possible work-related and personal antecedents (addressing questions 2 and 3), and suggests what can be expected – e.g., in terms of sickness absence – if adverse scores on these antecedents are addressed (question 4). In addition, the rationale behind the JD-R model is straightforward and therefore relatively easy to communicate, also to HR and occupational health practitioners as well as to executives, managers, and employees.

One often-applied approach in JD-R based intervention studies is to identify the job demands, personal and job resources, indicators of well-being, motivation and health (usually including burnout and engagement), and outcomes that are most significant for the organization, profession or jobs under study. According to the JD-R model these demands, resources and outcomes may vary across organizations and professions, but the basic JD-R model and its assumptions remain the same (cf. Bakker & Demerouti, 2007). Deciding which demands, resources and outcomes are relevant in a specific situation may require the input of key agents such as HR officers, the company management, occupational physicians, and so on (Schaufeli & Taris, 2014).

On the basis of these insights, the next step (*diagnosis*) involves an empirical (survey) study in which participants complete a questionnaire tapping the study's central concepts. After the data collection phase is concluded, the data can be analyzed and fed back into the organization. For example, it is often helpful to compare the average scores on the study concepts across departments, jobs, various types of workers (e.g., age and gender) and – if applicable – organizations, since this allows for identifying possible issues. One JD-R-based study among 1,500 Dutch police officers revealed that especially supervisory and management staff reported high levels of engagement and low levels of burnout and correspondingly favorable scores on the job demands and resources included in this study, whereas especially police patrol officers obtained considerably less favorable scores in these respects (Van Beek, Taris, & Schaufeli, 2013). This knowledge on the one hand suggests where possible issues are located and, on the other hand, indicates which interventions – if any – may be suitable.

Based on these findings, interventions may be selected and implemented (*intervention phase*). Interventions may be directed at specific demands and/or resources and be implemented in the organization as a whole or be targeted toward specific groups (e.g., older workers or workers in a particular occupation). They may take on different forms, ranging from job redesign and training programs to cultural change. In the final step the results of the intervention may be evaluated (*evaluation*). It is often useful to conduct a follow-up to the initial survey study in which the same concepts are measured again. Comparison of the findings of this follow-up study to the initial study provides an indication of the effects of the intervention and whether possible problems have been resolved.

Example: Job stress interventions in the Dutch domiciliary care sector   In an early application of the JD-R model of burnout, Taris et al. (2003) reported on the effects of various types of job stress interventions in the Dutch domiciliary care sector. Organizations in this sector (i.e., the care agencies) offer short- and long-term services to people who need help or attendance with regard to housekeeping, care, or nursing, such as elderly or chronically ill people. Levels of burnout are traditionally high in this sector (cf. Taris, Stoffelsen, Bakker, Schaufeli, & Van Dierendonck, 2005). In order to address this issue, a large-scale intervention program was conducted.

In the first step (*diagnosis*), a survey was devised that incorporated outcomes (job stress, measured in terms of emotional exhaustion), job demands, and job resources. These demands and resources were selected on the basis of discussions with work council members, members of employer and employee organizations, government representatives, and researchers in this area. At the first wave of the study (1999–2000), all employees of 105 participating home care organizations received the survey. Based on these data, detailed reports were compiled for and discussed with each participating organization in which the scores on all resources and exhaustion were compared across specific target groups, both within the organization – revealing which groups of workers were better off than others in terms of demands, resources, and outcomes – and across organizations –

that is, organizations could compare themselves with other, similar organizations (a *benchmarking* approach).

On the basis of these reports, organizations could individually decide which interventions they wanted to implement to address possible issues that had been identified (*intervention*). Two years later a follow-up study was conducted among employees of the participating organizations (*evaluation*), using the same format as the initial study. Comparison of the levels of work stress, job demands, and job resources indicated that working conditions had improved during the study period. At the follow-up study, the workers reported lower levels of exhaustion and job demands, and higher levels of skill discretion, decision latitude, and social support.

Moreover, all organizations that had participated in both waves of the study received a questionnaire listing 80 interventions that they might have implemented since the first wave of the study. Most organizations (72 percent) indicated that they had implemented at least one intervention during the study period. Organizations with favorable scores on job demands, job resources and/or job stress at the first study wave implemented significantly fewer interventions than other organizations: apparently, organizations used the information they had received in the diagnostic phase to decide whether they should implement any interventions. Organizations implemented different types of interventions, ranging from interventions that focused on factual changes in the work content and/or relations at work (e.g., job redesign and restructuring, ergonomic improvements) to person-directed interventions that focused on changing personal characteristics without the explicit aim to improve employee functioning at work (e.g., promoting exercise, employee assistance programs, relaxation training). Interestingly, further analysis revealed that *only* the work-directed intervention programs affected the central concepts in this study. All in all, this example shows that: (i) a JD-R-based survey study can help in diagnosing problematic issues in an organization, (ii) organizations tend to respond to information about possible work-related risks in their organization, (iii) implementing measures that directly address work-related issues is more effective than taking other measures, and (iv) such interventions affect job stress (exhaustion) in ways predicted by the JD-R model.

Job crafting Interventions are usually instigated by organizations. That is, the management of organizations decides more or less top-down whether there is a need for change. However, employees may also spontaneously and on an individual basis (i.e., bottom-up) apply strategies that optimize their work conditions and could therefore lead to higher well-being, motivation, and performance at work. In the literature this phenomenon is referred to as content innovation (Feij, Whitely, Peiro, & Taris, 1995; Schein, 1971) or, more recently, job crafting (Wrzesniewski & Dutton, 2001). Whereas in both cases work characteristics are the main drivers of employee proactive behavior, the difference is that content innovation is usually examined as a direct precursor of performance improvement (focusing on worker's attempts to increase their skills, knowledge, and performance). Conversely, job crafting is primarily examined as an antecedent of meaningful work, well-being, and motivation, focusing on workers' efforts to make their work more interesting and enjoyable, and less demanding (cf. Berg, Dutton, & Wrzesniewski, 2013; Petrou, Demerouti, Peeters, Schaufeli, & Hetland, 2010; Wrzesniewski & Dutton, 2001). Job crafting is defined as a personal strategy to change the content of the job – or its cognitive representation – in such a way that it fits better to one's competencies, preferences, and values.

The JD-R model fits well with both traditions, in that the JD-R model encompasses both well-being and motivation (in the form of strain/burnout and engagement) and performance (as an outcome thereof). Two recent questionnaires tapping job crafting behavior were fully based on the JD-R model, distinguishing between strategies to increase job resources, increase challenging demands, and decrease hindering and/or stressful job demands (Nielsen & Abildgaard, 2012; Tims, Bakker, & Derks, 2012). In practice, such JD-R based job crafting questionnaires can be used to examine whether employee job crafting behaviors lead to the desired outcomes, both for the employees (e.g., in terms of reducing hindering job demands and maximizing job resources) and for the organization (e.g., in terms of performance).

In an interesting application, De Groot, Van den Heuvel, Demerouti, and Peeters (2012) examined whether a JD-R based job crafting training among 39 police officers resulted in improved well-being. Participants in the intervention condition completed a four-week, four-session training program in which they wrote a personal job crafting plan that specified how they could increase their job resources (weeks 1 and 4), reduce hindering job demands (week 2), and increase challenging demands (week 3). Pre- and post-test comparisons with a non-intervention control group showed that participants in the intervention condition reported improved well-being (i.e., lower levels of negative emotions, higher levels of self-efficacy), increases in the opportunities for development, and better supervisor relations. Apparently, the training program was more effective in increasing job resources (i.e., opportunism for development and supervisor relations) than in reducing job demands.

Conclusions: Application of the JD-R model

Intuitively appealing as the JD-R may be, the proof of the pudding lies in the eating. That is, can the JD-R model be used to change the work context in such a way that well-being, health, motivation, and performance are improved? The examples provided in this section suggest that this is the case. In previous research the JD-R model has been used as a means to map relevant characteristics of the work environment, resulting in practical and effective organizational interventions to reduce work stress. Moreover, it offers some potential to design and examine job crafting behaviors – as a spontaneous, individual-level type of intervention – as well. Clearly, the JD-R model is not just an analytical framework that is primarily relevant to academics; rather, one of its great attractions is probably that the findings generated by the model can easily be translated into practical applications and interventions (cf. Schaufeli & Taris, 2013).

The Range of the Job Demands-Resources Model

Scientifically and practically attractive as the JD-R model might be, it is not without limitations. Two main limitations are discussed below.

Flexibility of the JD-R: Can the JD-R be falsified?

One important advantage of the JD-R model is that it is extremely flexible, one of its main assumptions being that relevant demands and resources can vary across work contexts (e.g., Demerouti & Bakker, 2011). For example, a particular job demand may be relevant in occupation A, but not in occupation B; in the context of the JD-R model, such diverging findings are not necessarily problematic, since they only reflect the fact that not all demands are equally relevant across all job contexts (which would also be interpreted as supporting the model). However, this poses the ontological problem that the model itself cannot be falsified, which is – according to Popperian logic (Popper, 1963) – the hallmark of truly scientific theories. This issue does not only apply at the operational level (i.e., the specific choice of demands and resources to be included in a study), but also at the level of the associations among the basic study concepts (i.e., the associations between demands, resources, stress, and motivation/well-being, respectively). That is, if a particular set of demands (resources) is unrelated to stress (motivation/well-being), this could simply be accounted for by stating that this signifies that the demands (resources) were not salient in this particular profession. Indeed, this issue is already present in the definition of demands as "those … aspects of the job that … are … associated with certain … costs" (Demerouti et al., 2001, p. 501) – that is, if a particular "job demand" would in a particular application *not* result in such "costs" (i.e., high levels of strain or exhaustion), this job characteristic would not be a demand, at least not in the population under study – *and this would not discredit the JD-R model in any way*. The same remark applies to Demerouti et al.'s (2001, p. 501) definition of resources. Apparently there is a certain circularity in the model that makes it difficult to decide which set of findings would falsify the model.

Interpreting the relations in the JD-R model/ heterogeneity of demands/resources?

On a higher level, the model holds that "motivation" and "health impairment" are the fundamental processes that link work characteristics to outcomes. However, there are many different processes that could account for the relations between work characteristics and work outcomes. Even within the two fundamental types of work characteristics (demands vs. resources), the processes underlying the relations between specific work characteristics and outcomes may differ strongly. For example, the effects of instrumental support on engagement are often interpreted differently than the effects of emotional support on engagement, and "motivation" may not be the most plausible process that links these forms of support to engagement. Similarly, the effect of job control/autonomy on work outcomes draws on a different underlying process than the effect of support (and, again, "motivation" is not necessarily a relevant factor here). Apparently, it is not immediately clear how the relations between demands/resources on work outcomes should be interpreted, and it is unclear whether health impairment/motivation are indeed the most relevant processes accounting for these relations. This suggests that the JD-R model is better construed as a heuristic framework that conveniently summarizes previous findings on the associations between job characteristics and work outcomes than as a theoretical model on its own. Note that this issue can easily be resolved, since theories relating specific work characteristics to work outcomes are readily available (cf. Schaufeli & Taris, 2014).

Further, given the conceptual heterogeneity of the characteristics within the two clusters of job characteristics, it is not immediately clear *why* these factors should covary. For example, empirically it is often found that all sorts of theoretically heterogeneous "resources" tend to cluster in a single, latent "resources"factor. This might be due to the fact that some resources actually affect the scores on other resources (e.g., high levels of autonomy could allow workers to seek and find social support), job design processes in relation to organizational labor market policies (jobs may be designed to be attractive in terms of the presence of resources, in order to allow organizations to attract the best staff, cf. Wagenaar et al., 2012), methodological issues (job characteristics are often measured using self-reports, meaning that halo-effects or common method variance may be an issue), and even conscious post-hoc selection of demands/resources on the basis of empirical findings (relating to the issue of whether the JD-R can be falsified). In this sense, one could maintain that what is gained by using the JD-R model in terms of generality (all sorts of concepts can be included in the model), is lost in terms of specificity (i.e., insightful theoretical distinctions as to how particular work characteristics would affect the outcomes are lost).

Summarizing, in spite of the apparent popularity of the JD-R model, the model is not without its limitations. As a catch-all model, from a theoretical point of view the value of the JD-R model is perhaps not so much the fact that it encompasses all sorts of different concepts and provides an account for the relationships among these concepts, but rather that it serves as a heuristic classification scheme that describes how particular broad categories are empirically related to each other. The model describes clearly *which* concepts are related to each other and *how* they are related to each other, but does not convincingly specify *why* they are related. However, this issue can be resolved by drawing on complementary, more specific and often well-established theories.

Future Research

The JD-R model has generated a considerable body of research since its inception, and much of this research has been summarized in this chapter. As we have seen, the main assumptions of the model have been tried and tested across many occupational and na-tional/cultural contexts. These tests have often confirmed its assumptions, at least in cross-sectional research: longitudinal support is apparently considerably scarcer, but in this respect the JD-R model does not differ from other job stress models such as Karasek's (1979) Demand-Control model. At present there seems little need for additional research on the basic relationships proposed by the JD-R model, as these have already been estab-lished firmly in cross-sectional and (to a lesser degree) in longitudinal studies. What, then, are the most pressing issues that need to be addressed in future research? We believe there are at least three such issues.

1 *The nature of demands and resources.* One basic assumption in the JD-R model is that many (if not most) work characteristics can be neatly divided across two broad categories: demands and resources, respectively. However, one important issue with this assumption is that the difference between these two categories is less clear than it would seem. On the one hand, having to deal with a structural lack of a particular resource might be construed as a demand, since it fits the definition of a demand as an aspect of the job that requires "sustained physical or mental effort" and will therefore be "associated with certain physi-ological and psychological costs" (Demerouti et al., 2001, p. 501). For example, lack of resources at work will imply that workers must work harder to achieve their work goals. This suggests that a lack of resources is equivalent with high demands. Indeed, previous research using Karasek and Theorell's (1990) Demand-Control-Support model has fre-quently shown that the absence of support and autonomy (two "resources") are associ-ated with adverse health outcomes (see De Lange, Taris, Kompier, Houtman, & Bongers, 2003, for a review of high-quality longitudinal studies). Similarly, excessively high job demands could well be considered as a lack of resources, since this would surely be *dys-functional* in achieving work goals and would *hinder* personal growth and development (cf. Demerouti et al., 2001).

On the other hand, it has been suggested that not all demands are created equal. Drawing on the distinction between challenge demands and hindrance demands (LePine, LePine, & Jackson, 2004; LePine, Podsakoff, & LePine, 2005), Van den Broeck and colleagues showed that high levels of hindrance demands (i.e., threatening demands that impede employees' control, cannot easily be overcome and elicit an emotion-focused coping response) were associated with higher exhaustion and lower vigor, whereas challenging demands (i.e., demands that do not just require effort to deal with, but are also stimulating, elicit a problem-focused coping response and contribute to the achievement of work goals) related positively to vigor (but not to exhaustion) (Van den Broeck, De Cuyper, De Witte, & Vansteenkiste, 2010). These findings were largely confirmed in Crawford et al.'s (2010) meta-analysis.

Apparently, the distinction between demands and resources that was posed in early formulations of the JD-R model is not as unambiguous as initially thought. Future research should address this issue, distinguishing between different types of demands (and, perhaps, resources) and preferably across different types of jobs (Demerouti & Bakker, 2011; Schaufeli & Taris, 2013).

2 *Demand × resource interactions.* Another recurrent issue in discussions on Karasek's (1979) Demand-Control (DC) model refers to the presumed interaction between job demands and job control. Although such an interaction is the central tenet of the DC model, empirical research rarely confirmed this interaction (Taris, 2006). History seems to repeat itself: the interaction between demands and resources is central to the JD-R model (Demerouti & Bakker, 2011), yet the evidence for this interaction effect is considerably weaker than that for both main effects of demands and resources. Moreover, even if interactions are found, the practical relevance of these interactions is small, as evidenced by small effect sizes (e.g., Bakker, Van Veldhoven, & Xanthopoulou, 2010). What is important is perhaps not so much that interactions are rare and usually small, but rather the issue as to when interactions are most likely to occur. Bakker and Demerouti's (2007) idea that "different types of job demands and job resources may interact in predicting job strain" (p. 217) was challenged by De Jonge and colleagues, arguing that the likelihood of finding interactions between demands and resources varies with the degree to which these job characteristics and the outcome under study refer to qualitatively identical domains (e.g., De Jonge & Dormann, 2006; De Jonge, Demerouti, & Dormann, 2014). Although they do not deny that qualitatively different types of demands and resources may interact, interactions between qualitatively non-matching demands and resources would be considerably less frequent and practically less important than when demands, resources, and outcomes have a qualitatively strong match.

Since – insofar as interactions have been reported in the literature – both Bakker and Demerouti (2007) and De Jonge and Dormann's (2006) ideas have been confirmed, at present it is by no means clear which of these sets of assumptions has received the strongest support, or, alternatively, under which circumstances which type of interactions – if any – can be expected. This issue is not just of academic interest: from a practical point of view it is important to know whether high levels of a particular demand can indeed be mitigated by high levels of resources, and whether it matters which type of resource is offered.

3 *Gain and loss cycles/reciprocal effects.* As discussed above, much JD-R based research shows that the presence of job resources and the absence of excessively high job demands tends to lead to higher levels of well-being. Interestingly, building on Fredrickson's (2001) Broaden-and-Build theory, it can be expected that high levels of well-being (engagement) can also lead to higher levels of resources (Salanova et al., 2010, for an overview). This research suggests that high-resource workers tend to become more engaged over time

and that engaged workers tend to collect more resources in their job, which in turn leads to even higher levels of engagement (the so-called gain spiral), whereas low-engagement and/or burned-out workers tend to lose job resources, leading to even lower levels of engagement (the loss spiral) – findings that find an analog in Merton's (1968) well-known Matthew effect, stating that: *For unto everyone that has shall be given, and he shall have abundance: but from him that has not shall be taken away even that which he has* (Matthew 25:29). However, how do these findings translate into practice – if they have any practical value at all, that is? Although research has frequently demonstrated longitudinal reciprocal effects between job resources and job engagement, it is not entirely clear how a gain (or loss) spiral would develop, or even whether such a spiral actually exists. That is, gain and loss spirals refer to changes in the *level* of engagement and resources, but the evidence available today draws on correlational studies, referring to the correspondence of the *order* of the study participants on the variables of interest. Since information on the order of participants on the study variables tells us nothing about the stability or change in terms of the actual level of the participants' scores on these variables (Mortimer, Finch, & Kumka, 1982, for a discussion), the currently available evidence hardly supports any claims regarding the existence of gain and loss spirals. In order to examine such spirals properly, researchers should examine the across-time development of mean levels of engagement (and resources) for low- and high-resources (engagement) groups (cf. Salanova et al., 2010), rather than to look only at suggestive – but largely irrelevant – patterns of lagged regression effects. Clearly, more – well-designed and correctly analyzed – research on this intriguing issue is needed.

Conclusion

In this chapter, we have: (i) provided an overview of the development and conceptual bases of the JD-R model, drawing parallels with earlier job stress models such as Siegrist's (1996) Effort-Reward Imbalance model and Karasek and Theorell's (1990) Demand-Control-Support model; (ii) discussed the empirical support from cross-sectional and longitudinal studies for the various versions of the model; (iii) addressed some applications and extensions of the model; (iv) discussed several important limitations of the model; and, (v) suggested a number of venues for future research on the JD-R model.

Our overview showed that the major innovation of the JD-R model was that it extended the notion forwarded in earlier job stress models that particular positive and negative work characteristics could affect workers' motivation and well-being with the idea that these job characteristics could be assigned to two broad categories: job demands and job resources, respectively (Lee & Ashforth, 1996). Later on, the model was extended with a third category: personal resources. A considerable body of research – covering a wide range of occupations and nations/cultures – supported the model; although most evidence was obtained in cross-sectional research, several longitudinal studies also reported support for the model's assumptions. The currently available evidence on the presumed interactions between demands and resources is relatively sparse, often weak, and cannot always unequivocally be interpreted. As regards the application of the model, we have indicated how the JD-R model can be used to guide practical interventions. Moreover, we have shown how the current body of research on job crafting could be framed in the terms of the JD-R model. The fact that the model has several important limitations (relating to its epistemological status, the interpretation of the specific relations included in the model, and the nature of demands and resources) suggests that the JD-R model is perhaps better considered a heuristic framework that integrates all sorts of findings and approaches, rather than a well-developed theory on its own. Finally, we identified a number of important issues to be addressed in future research, including clarification of the nature of demands and resources, the interaction between demands and resources, and the existence of gain/loss cycles. All in all, the present overview illustrates that the JD-R model sparked quite some research in the area of occupational health psychology and that it has the potential to continue to do so.

References

Airila, A., Hakanen, J. J., Schaufeli, W. B., Luukkonen, R., Punokallio, A., & Lusa, S. (2014). Are job and personal resources associated with work ability 10 years later? *Work & Stress, 28*, 87–105.

Akkermans, J., Brenninkmeijer, V., Van den Bossche, S. N. J., Blonk, R. W. B., & Schaufeli, W. B. (2013). Young and going strong? A longitudinal study on occupational health among young employees of different educational levels. *Career Development International, 18*, 416–435.

Akkermans, J. Schaufeli, W. B., Brenninkmeijer, V., & Blonk, R. W. B. (2013). The role of career competencies in the Job Demands-Resources model. *Journal of Vocational Behavior, 83*, 356–366.

Alarcon, G. M. (2011). A meta-analysis of burnout with job demands, resources, and attitudes. *Journal of Vocational Behavior, 79*, 549–562.

Bakker, A. B., Boyd, C. M., Dollard, M., Gillespie, N., Winefield, A. H., & Stough, C. (2010). The role of personality in the Job Demands-Resources model. *Career Development International, 15*, 622–636.

Bakker, A. B., & Demerouti, E. (2007). The Job Demands-Resources model: State of the art. *Journal of Managerial Psychology, 22*, 309–328.

Bakker, A. B., Demerouti, E., De Boer, E., & Schaufeli, W. (2003). Job demands and job resources as predictors of absence duration and frequency. *Journal of Vocational Behavior, 62*, 341–356.

Bakker, A. B., Demerouti, E., & Euwema, M. C. (2005). Job resources buffer the impact of job demands on burnout. *Journal of Occupational Health Psychology, 10*, 170–180.

Bakker, A. B., Demerouti, E., & Sanz-Vergel, A. I. (2014). Burnout and work engagement: The JD-R approach. *Annual Review of Organizational Psychology and Organizational Behavior, 1*, 389–411.

Bakker, A. B., Demerouti, E., & Schaufeli, W. B. (2003). Dual processes at work in a call center: An application of the Job Demands-Resources model. *European Journal of Work and Organizational Psychology, 12*, 393–417.

Bakker, A. B., Demerouti, E., Taris, T. W., Schaufeli, W. B., & Schreurs, P. J. G. (2003). A multigroup analysis of the Job Demands-Resources Model in four home care organizations. *International Journal of Stress Management, 10*, 16–38.

Bakker, A. B., Demerouti, E., & Verbeke, W. (2004). Using the Job Demands-Resources model to predict burnout and performance. *Human Resource Management, 43*, 83–104.

Bakker, A. B., Hakanen, J. J., Demerouti, E., & Xanthopoulou, D. (2007). Job resources boost work engagement particularly when job demands are high. *Journal of Educational Psychology, 99*, 274–284.

Bakker, A.B., Van Veldhoven, M., & Xanthopoulou, D. (2010). Beyond the Demand-Control model: Thriving on high job demands and resources. *Journal of Personnel Psychology, 9*, 3–16.

Bakker, A. B., & Xanthopoulou, D. (2013). Creativity and charisma among female leaders: The role of resources and work engagement. *International Journal of Human Resource Management, 24*, 2760–2779.

Bandura, A. (1997). *Self-efficacy: The exercise of control*. New York, NY: Freeman.

Barbier, M., Hansez, I., Chmiel, N., & Demerouti, E. (2013). Performance expectations, personal resources, and job resources: How do they predict work engagement? *European Journal of Work and Organizational Psychology, 22*, 750–762.

Berg, J. M., Dutton, J. E., & Wrzesniewski, A. (2013). Job crafting and meaningful work. In B. J. Dik, Z. S. Byrne, & M. F. Steger (Eds.), *Purpose and meaning in the workplace* (pp. 81–104). Washington, DC: American Psychological Association.

Brauchli, R., Schaufeli, W. B., Jenny, G. J., Füllemann, D., & Bauer, G. F. (2013). Disentangling stability and change in job resources, job demands, and employee well-being: A three-wave study on the job demands-resources model. *Journal of Vocational Behavior, 83*, 117–129.

Brenninkmeijer, V., Demerouti, E., Le Blanc, P., & Van Emmerik, H. (2010). Regulatory focus at work: The moderating role of regulatory focus in the Job Demands-Resources model. *Career Development International, 15*, 708–728.

Brough, P. M., Timms, C., Siu, Q., Kalliath, T., O'Driscoll, M. P., Sit, C. H. P., Lo, D., & Lu, C. (2013). Validation of the job demands-resources model in cross-national samples: Cross-sectional and longitudinal predictions of psychological strain and work engagement. *Human Relations, 66*, 1311–1335.

Consiglio, C., Borgogni, L., Alessandri, G., & Schaufeli, W. B. (2013). Does self-efficacy matter for burnout and sickness absenteeism? The mediating role of demands and resources at the individual and team levels. *Work & Stress, 27*, 22–42.

Crawford, E. R., LePine, J. A., & Rich, B. L. (2010). Linking job demands and resources to employee engagement and burnout: A theoretical extension and meta-analytic test. *Journal of Applied Psychology, 95*, 834–848.

De Beer, L., Rothmann, S., & Pienaar, J. (2012). A confirmatory investigation of a job demands-resources model using a categorical estimator. *Psychological Reports, 111*, 528–544.

De Groot, K., Van den Heuvel, M., Demerouti, E., & Peeters, M. (2012). *Succesvol job craften door middel van een groepstraining* [in Dutch]. In J. de Jonge, M. Peeters, S. Sjollema, & M. de Zeeuw (Eds.), *Scherp in werk: Vijf routes naar optimale inzetbaarheid* (pp. 27–52). Assen, The Netherlands: Van Gorcum.

De Jonge, J., Demerouti, E., & Dormann, C. (2014). Current theoretical perspectives in work psychology. In M. C. W. Peeters, J. de Jonge, & T. W. Taris (Eds.), *An introduction to contemporary work psychology* (pp. 89–113). Oxford: Wiley-Blackwell.

De Jonge, J., & Dormann, C. (2006). Stressors, resources, and strain at work: A longitudinal test of the triple-match principle. *Journal of Applied Psychology, 91*, 1359–1374.

De Jonge, J., Dormann, C., & Van den Tooren, M. (2008). The Demand-Induced Strain Compensation model: Renewed theoretical considerations and empirical evidence. In K. Naswall, J. Hellgren, & M. Sverke (Eds.), *The individual in the changing working life* (pp. 67–87). Cambridge, UK: Cambridge University Press.

De Lange, A. H., Taris, T. W., Kompier, M. A. J., Houtman, I. L. D., & Bongers, P. M. (2003). The very best of the millennium: Longitudinal research and the Demand-Control(-Support) model. *Journal of Occupational Health Psychology, 8*, 282–305.

Deci, E. L. & Ryan, R. M. (2000). The "what" and "why" of goal pursuits: Human needs and the self-determination of behavior. *Psychological Inquiry, 11*, 319–338.

Demerouti, E., & Bakker, A. B. (2011). The Job Demands-Resources model: Challenges for future research. *South-African Journal of Industrial Psychology, 37*, doi:10.4102/sajip.v37i2.974

Demerouti, E., Bakker, A. B., Nachreiner, F., & Schaufeli, W. B. (2001). The Job Demands-Resources model of burnout. *Journal of Applied Psychology, 86*, 499–512.

Diener, E., & Fujita, F. (1995). Resources, personal strivings, and subjective well-being: A nomothetic and idiographic approach. *Journal of Personality and Social Psychology, 68*, 926–935.

Diestel, S., & Schmidt, K.-H. (2012). Lagged mediator effects of self-control demands on psychological strain and absenteeism. *Journal of Occupational and Organizational Psychology, 85*, 556–578.

Feij, J. A., Whitely, W. T., Peiro, J. M., & Taris, T. W. (1995). The development of career-enhancing strategies and content innovation: A longitudinal study of new workers. *Journal of Vocational Behavior, 46*, 231–256.

Feuerhahn, N., Bellingrath, S., & Kudielka, B. M. (2013). The interplay of matching and non-matching job demands and resources on emotional exhaustion among teachers. *Applied Psychology: Health and Well-being, 5*, 171–192.

Fredrickson, B. L. (2001). The role of positive emotions in positive psychology: The broaden-and-build theory of positive emotions. *American Psychologist, 56,* 218–226.

Hakanen, J., Bakker, A. B., & Schaufeli, W. B. (2006). Burnout and work engagement among teachers. *Journal of School Psychology, 43,* 495–513.

Hakanen, J. J., Schaufeli, W. B., & Ahola, K. (2008). The Job Demands-Resources model: A three-year cross-lagged study of burnout, depression, commitment, and work engagement. *Work & Stress, 22,* 224–241.

Hansen, N., Sverke, M., & Naswall, K. (2009). Predicting nurse burnout from demands and resources in three acute care hospitals under different forms of ownership: A cross-sectional questionnaire survey. *International Journal of Nursing Studies, 46,* 95–106.

Hansez, I., & Chmiel, N. (2010). Safety behavior: Job demands, job resources, and perceived management commitment to safety. *Journal of Occupational Health Psychology, 15,* 267–278.

Häusser, J. A., Mojzisch, A., Niesel, M., & Schulz-Hardt, S. (2010). Ten years on: A review of recent research on the job demand-control (-support) model and psychological well-being. *Work & Stress, 24,* 1–35.

Hobfoll, S. E. (2002). Social and psychological resources and adaptation. *Review of General Psychology, 6,* 307–324.

Hockey, G. R. J. (1997). Compensatory control in the regulation of human performance under stress and high workload: A cognitive energetical framework. *Biological Psychology, 45,* 73–93.

Hu, Q. & Schaufeli, W. B. (2011). Job insecurity and remuneration in Chinese family-owned business workers. *Career Development International, 16,* 6–19.

Hu, Q., Schaufeli, W. B., & Taris, T. W. (2011). The Job Demands-Resources Model: An analysis of additive and joint effects of demands and resources. *Journal of Vocational Behavior, 79,* 181–190.

Huyn, J.-Y., Winefield, A. H., Xanthopoulou, D., & Metzer, J. C. (2012). Burnout and connectedness in the Job Demands-Resources model: Studying palliative care volunteers and their families. *American Journal of Hospice and Palliative Medicine, 29,* 462–475.

Judge, T. A., Bono, J. E., & Locke, E. A. (2000). Personality and job satisfaction: The mediating role of job characteristics. *Journal of Applied Psychology, 85,* 237–249.

Karasek, R. (1979). Job demands, job decision latitude and mental strain: Implications for job redesign. *Administrative Science Quarterly, 24,* 285–306.

Karasek, R. A., & Theorell, T. (1990). *Healthy work: Stress, productivity, and the reconstruction of working life.* New York, NY: Basic Books.

Kinnunen, U., Feldt, T., Siltaloppi, M., & Sonnentag, S. (2011). Job demands-resources model in the context of recovery: Testing recovery experiences as mediators. *European Journal of Work and Organizational Psychology, 20,* 805–832.

Knardahl, S., & Ursin, H. (1985). Sustained activation and the pathophysiology of hypertension and coronary heart disease. In J. F. Orlebeke, G. Mulder, & L. J. P. van Doornen (Eds.), *Psychophysiology of cardiovascular control: Models, methods, and data* (pp. 151–167). New York, NY: Plenum.

Korunka, C., Kubicek, B., Schaufeli, W., & Hoonakker, P. L. T. (2009). Burnout and work engagement: Do age, gender, or occupation level matter? Testing the robustness of the Job Demands-Resources Model. *Positive Psychology, 4,* 243–255.

Lee, R. T., & Ashforth, B. E. (1996). A meta-analytic examination of the correlates of the three dimensions of job burnout. *Journal of Applied Psychology, 81,* 123–133.

LePine, J. A., LePine, M. A., & Jackson, C. (2004). Challenge and hindrance stress: Relationships with exhaustion, motivation to learn, and learning performance. *Journal of Applied Psychology, 89,* 883–891.

LePine, J. A., Podsakoff, N. P., & LePine, M. A. (2005). A meta-analytic test of the challenge stressor-hindrance stressor framework: An explanation for inconsistent relationships among stressors and performance. *Academy of Management Journal, 48,* 764–775.

Lewig, K. A., Xanthopoulou, D., Bakker, A. B., Dollard, M., & Metzer, J. C. (2007). Burnout and connectedness among Australian volunteers: A test of the Job Demands-Resources model. *Journal of Vocational Behavior, 71,* 429–445.

Li, F., Jiang, L., Yao, X., & Li, Y. (2012). Job demands, job resources and safety outcomes: The roles of emotional exhaustion and safety compliance. *Accident Analysis and Prevention, 51*, 243–251.

Lizano, E. L., & Mor Barak, M. E. (2012). Workplace demands and resources as antecedents of job burnout among public child welfare workers: A longitudinal study. *Children and Youth Services Review, 34*, 1769–1776.

Llorens, S., Bakker, A. B., Schaufeli, W. B., & Salanova, M. (2006). Testing the robustness of the Job Demands-Resources model. *International Journal of Stress Management, 13*, 378–391.

Llorens, S., Salanova, M., Schaufeli, W. B., & Bakker, A. (2007). Does a positive gain spiral of resources, efficacy beliefs and engagement exist? *Computers in Human Behavior, 23*, 825–841.

Llorente, L., Salanova, M., Martinez, I., & Schaufeli, W. B. (2008). Extension of the Job Demands-Resources model in the prediction of burnout and engagement among teachers over time. *Psicotema, 20*, 354–360.

Maslach, C., Jackson, S. E., & Leiter, M. (1996). *Maslach Burnout Inventory* (3rd edn.). Palo Alto, CA: Consulting Psychologists Press.

Maslach, C., Schaufeli, W. B., & Leiter, M. P. (2001). Job burnout. *Annual Review of Psychology, 52*, 397–422.

Meijman, T. F., & Mulder, G. (1998). Psychological aspects of workload. In P. J. D. Drenth, H. Thierry, & C. J. de Wolff (Eds.), *Handbook of work and organizational psychology* (pp. 5–33). Hove, UK: Psychology Press.

Melamed, A., Shirom, A., Toker, S., Berliner, S., & Shapira, I. (2006). Burnout and risk of cardiovascular disease: Evidence, possible causal paths, and promising research directions. *Psychological Bulletin, 132*, 327–353.

Merton, R. K. (1968). The Matthew effect in science. *Science, 159*, 56–63.

Mortimer, J. T., Finch, M. D., & Kumka, D. (1982). Persistence and change in development: The multidimensional self-concept. In P. B. Baltes & O. G. Brim, Jr. (Eds.), *Life span development and behavior* (Vol. 4, pp. 263–313). New York, NY: Academic Press.

Nielsen, K., & Abildgaard, J. S. (2012). The development and validation of a job crafting measure for use with blue-collar workers. *Work & Stress, 26*, 365–384.

Ouweneel, E., Le Blanc, P. M., & Schaufeli, W. B. (2012). Don't leave your heart at home: Gain cycles of positive emotions, resources, and engagement at work. *Career Development International, 17*, 537–556.

Petrou, P., Demerouti, E., Peeters, M. C. W., Schaufeli, W. B., & Hetland, J. (2010). Crafting a job on a daily basis: Contextual correlates and the link to work engagement. *Journal of Organizational Behavior, 33*, 1120–1141.

Popper, K. R. (1963). *Conjectures and refutations: The growth of scientific knowledge*. London, UK: Routledge.

Roelen, C., Van Rhenen, W., Schaufeli, W., Van der Klink, J., Mageroy, N., Moen, B., Bjorvatn, B., & Pallesen, S. (2014). Mental and physical health-related functioning mediates between psychological job demands and sickness absence among nurses. *Journal of Advanced Nursing, 70*, 1780–1792.

Salanova, M., Schaufeli, W. B., Xanthopoulou, D., & Bakker, A. B. (2010). Gain spirals of resources and work engagement. In A. B. Bakker & M. P. Leiter (Eds.), *Work engagement: A handbook of essential theory and research* (pp. 118–131). New York, NY: Psychology Press.

Schaufeli, W. B., & Bakker, A. B. (2004). Job demands, job resources, and their relationship with burnout and engagement: A multi-sample study. *Journal of Organizational Behavior, 25*, 293–315.

Schaufeli, W. B., & Bakker, A. B. (2010). The conceptualization and measurement of work engagement. In A. B. Bakker & M. P. Leiter (Eds.), *Work engagement: A handbook of essential theory and research* (pp. 10–24). New York, NY: Psychology Press.

Schaufeli, W. B., Bakker, A. B., & Van Rhenen, W. (2009). How changes in job demands and resources predict burnout, work engagement, and sickness absenteeism. *Journal of Organizational Behavior, 30*, 893–917.

Schaufeli, W. B., & Taris, T. W. (2005). The conceptualization and measurement of burnout: Common ground and worlds apart. *Work & Stress, 19*, 256–262.

Schaufeli, W. B., & Taris, T. W. (2013). Het job demands-resources model: Een kritische beschouwing. *Gedrag & Organisatie, 26*, 182–204.

Schaufeli, W. B., & Taris, T. W. (2014). A critical review of the job demands-resources model: Implications for improving work and health. In G. F. Bauer & O. Hämmig (Eds.), *Bridging occupational, organizational and public health: A transdisciplinary approach* (pp. 43–68). Dordrecht, The Netherlands: Springer.

Schein, E. (1971). Occupational socialization in the professions: The case of the role innovator. *Journal of Psychiatric Research, 8*, 521–530.

Seppälä, P., Hakanen, J., Mauno, S., Perhoniemi, R., Tolvanen, A., & Schaufeli, W. B. (2014). Stability and change model of job resources and job engagement: A seven-year, three-wave follow-up study. *European Journal of Work and Organizational Psychology, 24*, 360–375.

Siegrist, J. (1996). Adverse health effects of high-effort/low-reward conditions. *Journal of Occupational Health Psychology, 1*, 27–41.

Simbula, S., Guglielmi, D., & Schaufeli, W. B. (2011). A three-wave study on job resources, self-efficacy and work engagement among Italian school teachers. *European Journal of Work and Organizational Psychology, 20*, 285–305.

Taris, T. W. (2006). Bricks without clay: On urban myths in occupational health psychology. *Work & Stress, 20*, 99–104.

Taris, T. W., & Kompier, M. A. J. (2004). Job characteristics and learning behavior: Review and psychological mechanisms. In P. L. Perrewé & D. C. Ganster (Eds.), *Research in occupational health and well-being* (Vol. 4, pp. 127–166). Oxford, UK: Elsevier.

Taris, T. W., & Kompier, M. A. J. (2014). Cause and effect: Optimizing the designs of longitudinal studies in occupational health psychology. *Work & Stress, 28*, 1–8.

Taris, T. W., Kompier, M. A. J., Geurts, S. A. E., Houtman, I. L. D., & Van den Heuvel, F. F. M. (2010). Professional efficacy, exhaustion, and work characteristics among police officers: A longitudinal test of the learning-related predictions of the demand-control model. *Journal of Occupational and Organizational Psychology, 83*, 455–474.

Taris, T. W., Kompier, M. A. J., Geurts, S. A. E., Schaufeli, W. B., De Boer, E., Sepmeijer, K. J., & Wattez, C. (2003). Stress management interventions in the Dutch domiciliary care sector: Findings from 81 organizations. *International Journal of Stress Management, 10*, 297–325.

Taris, T. W., Le Blanc, P. M., Schaufeli, W. B., & Schreurs, P. J. G. (2005). Are there causal relationships between the dimensions of the Maslach Burnout Inventory? A review and two longitudinal tests. *Work & Stress, 19*, 238–255.

Taris, T. W., Schreurs, P. J. G., & Schaufeli, W. B. (1999). Construct validity of the Maslach Burnout Inventory–General Survey: A two-sample examination of its factor structure and correlates. *Work & Stress, 13*, 323–237.

Taris, T. W., Stoffelsen, J., Bakker, A. B., Schaufeli, W. B., & Van Dierendonck, D. (2005). Job control and burnout levels across occupations. *Psychological Reports, 97*, 955–961.

Tims, M., Bakker, A. B., & Derks, D. (2012). Development and validation of the job crafting scale. *Journal of Vocational Behavior, 80*, 173–186.

Van Beek, I., Taris, T. W., & Schaufeli, W. B. (2013). *Psychosocial health of police officers* [in Dutch]. The Hague, The Netherlands: WODC.

Van de Ven, B., & Vlerick, P. (2013). Testing the triple-match principle among technology employees. *European Journal of Work and Organizational Psychology, 22*, 658–669.

Van den Broeck, A., De Cuyper, N., De Witte, H., & Vansteenkiste, M. (2010). Not all demands are equal: Differentiating job hindrances and job challenges in the Job Demands-Resources model. *European Journal of Work and Organizational Psychology, 19*, 735–759.

Van den Broeck, A., Van Ruysseveldt, J., Smulders, P., & De Witte, H. (2011). Does intrinsic value orientation strengthen the impact of job resources? A perspective from the Job Demands-Resources model. *European Journal of Work and Organizational Psychology, 20*, 581–609.

Van den Broeck, A., Vansteenkiste, M., De Witte, H., & Lens, W. (2008). Explaining the relationships between job characteristics, burnout, and engagement: The role of basic psychological need satisfaction. *Work & Stress, 22*, 277–294.

Van der Heijden, B., Van Dam, K., Xanthopoulou, D., & De Lange, A. H. (2014). Individual characteristics and work-related outcomes. In M. C. W. Peeters, J. de Jonge, & T. W. Taris (Eds.), *An introduction to contemporary work psychology* (pp. 243–265). Oxford, UK: Wiley-Blackwell.

Van Riet, P., & Bakker, A. B. (2004). Financiële omzet als een functie van werkstressoren en energiebronnen (financial performance as a function of work stressors and energy sources). *Gedrag & Organisatie, 17,* 487–504.

Vink, J., Ouweneel, A., & Le Blanc, P. (2011). Psychologische energiebronnen voor bevlogen werknemers: Psychologisch kapitaal in het Job Demands-Resources model. *Gedrag & Organisatie, 24,* 101–120.

Wagenaar, A. F., Taris, T. W., Houtman, I. L. D., Van den Bossche, S., Smulders, P., & Kompier, M. A. J. (2012). Labour contracts in the European Union, 2000–2005: Differences among demographic groups and implications for the quality of working life and work satisfaction. *European Journal of Work and Organizational Psychology, 21,* 169–194.

Wrzesniewski, A., & Dutton, J. E. (2001). Crafting a job: Revisioning employees as active crafters of their work. *Academy of Management Review, 26,* 179–201.

Xanthopoulou, D., Bakker, A. B., Demerouti, E., & Schaufeli, W. B. (2007). The role of personal resources in the job demands-resources model. *International Journal of Stress Management, 14,* 121–141.

Xanthopoulou, D., Bakker, A. B., Demerouti, E., & Schaufeli, W. B. (2009). Work engagement and financial returns: A diary study on the role of job and personal resources. *Journal of Organizational and Occupational Psychology, 82,* 183–200.

Xanthopoulou, D., Bakker, A. B., Dollard, M. F., Demerouti, E., Schaufeli, W. B., Taris, T. W., & Schreurs, P. J. G. (2007). When do job demands particularly predict burnout? The moderating role of job resources. *Journal of Managerial Psychology, 22,* 766–785.

9

Working Hours, Health, and Well-Being

Michael P. O'Driscoll and Maree Roche

Introduction

Physical health and psychological well-being can be influenced by an array of factors, some of which are dispositional (such as personality variables) whereas others may be external to the individual (e.g., their home or work environment) (see Taris & Schaufeli, Chapter 8; Nielsen et al., Chapter 10; Cangiano & Parker, Chapter 11, this volume). The aim of this chapter is to overview research on one issue which has received considerable attention in the work stress literature – the hours invested by people in their paid employment. In previous eras, work hours were more tightly circumscribed and were (by and large) constrained to time spent at the work site or office. In these days of more flexible technologies, however, many people work both "non-standard" hours and not necessarily in an office or specific setting. Technologies such as the internet and smartphones have enabled people to be "on the job" even when not physically in their designated work setting.

At first glance it may seem apparent that spending more time at work or on work-related activities would be disadvantageous to an individual's health and well-being, both physical and psychological. However, the relationships between work time and well-being are more complex than this, and there are several factors which can either mitigate or exacerbate these relationships. In this chapter, we will discuss some of the more salient contributors to the relationship between work hours and well-being (both physical and psychological). These factors are covered in no specific order of importance or relevance, and the list is not exclusive – there are certainly other factors which can have a bearing on the link between work hours and well-being, but given the constraints of this chapter, plus the content of other chapters, we have selected these as being prominent issues. We begin with a general discussion of the meaning of "long" work hours, followed by an overview of the literature on long working hours and (a) physical health and (b) psychological well-being, following which we discuss some specific issues that are related to working long hours. Our

The Wiley Blackwell Handbook of the Psychology of Occupational Safety and Workplace Health, First Edition. Edited by Sharon Clarke, Tahira M. Probst, Frank Guldenmund, and Jonathan Passmore. © 2016 John Wiley & Sons Ltd. Published 2020 by John Wiley & Sons Ltd.

chapter concludes with some implications of the research findings, in respect of personal and organizational actions to address the problems inherent in long working hours.

Background

The relationship between time spent working and individuals' well-being is complex. Recent changes demonstrate wide variations in the typical patterns of working hours across countries. For example, Jacobs and Gerson (2004) reported a marked decline in the proportion of employees in the USA working a traditional 40-hour work week, and increases in the proportion of employees reporting either relatively short work weeks (less than 30 hours) or relatively long work weeks (50 hours or more). Similar trends have been documented in Australia (Drago, Wooden, & Black, 2009; Wooden & Drago, 2007), Canada (Sheridan, Sunter, & Diverty, 2001), Japan (Japanese Ministry of Health, Labour, and Welfare, 2004), New Zealand (Callister, 2005), and Norway (Wagstaff & Lie, 2011).

Kirkcaldy, Furnham, and Shephard (2009) have provided an informative overview of different patterns of working hours in the UK and Europe, noting variations in normal weekly work hours across different countries. In addition, they discuss some cultural differences (e.g., in work values and the relative importance of work–life balance) which can impact upon the number of hours devoted to work. *Average* work week statistics can be somewhat misleading, as they can mask considerable variations between people in a single country. For instance, Kirkcaldy et al. (2009) observed that in Britain around 10 percent of the population worked more than 50 hours per week and a further 10 percent worked less than 16 hours per week. It is more informative, therefore, to examine patterns of work hours rather than simply aggregated averages. Another useful distinction drawn by Kirkcaldy and his colleagues is between "voluntary" and "involuntary" work hours. That is, some people may choose to work longer hours (for instance, >50 hours per week), whereas other people have no choice, either because their job requires them to work a certain number of hours, or they need to work longer hours to obtain sufficient funding to support themselves and their family. Choice (or control) over work hours can make a substantial difference to the effects of having to work longer hours. We will discuss this construct a bit later, as a potential buffer (moderator) of the relationship between working hours and well-being.

Virtanen and Kivimaki (2012) discussed the concept of "too much work." That is, what exactly is meant by excessive work hours? Various definitions have been posited in the research literature. Frequently 40 hours per week are treated as the norm, but in some studies 50 hours (or more) are considered "normal." Others have examined "overtime," meaning work hours exceeding beyond the expected normal hours (subjectively defined), and yet others have referred to "irregular" or "non-standard" hours or "precarious employment," where work hours are changeable and unpredictable. This variability in definition and measurement creates uncertainty and difficulty in terms of comparing findings across studies.

Generally, the proportion of workers who report having to work longer hours appears to have increased over the past 25–30 years (Grosch, Caruso, Rosa, & Sauter, 2006). For instance, it would seem that American workers are now working longer hours than do people in most European countries. Park, Yi, and Kim (2010) investigated the impact of longer working hours on the reported stress complaints of Korean workers, where the standard work week is 40 hours. They divided their sample of Korean workers into three categories: those who worked 40–47 hours per week, those who worked 48–59 hours per week, and those working 60 or more hours per week. One interesting comparison in this study was that approximately 40 percent of the sample worked 40–47 hours per week, 28 percent worked 48–59 hours per week and 20 percent worked more than 60 hours per week. Consistent with findings from other studies, workers in this final category were significantly more prone to stress-related complaints, especially males, although the incidence of anxiety and depression was reported to be very low. Niedhammer and colleagues (Niedhammer, Sultan-Taieb, Chastang, Vermeylen, & Parent-Thirion, 2012) examined working hours across European countries (n = 31), with samples of approximately 15,000 males and 15,000 females. In this study, 27 percent of men and 12 percent of women reported work weeks of >48 hours per week. Men reported high demands, low support, and longer working hours than did women.

Another factor to consider is *how* work is undertaken. Traditionally, people "went to work" (e.g., an office, factory, or some other work site), but with the greater availability of sophisticated technologies (especially computers), many individuals now engage in *teleworking*, where they work at home or some other off-site location. The numerous advantages of teleworking (for both employers and employees) have been well-documented in the literature, along with some of the constraints and limitations. One issue which has not been discussed in great depth, however, is the impact of teleworking on the actual number of working hours. Although teleworking can have some significant benefits for individuals (e.g., enabling them to manage the work–family interface more effectively), potentially it can also increase the number of "unofficial" work hours which people engage in and do not record formally. As teleworking and other forms of alternative work arrangements (such as contingent working, compressed working weeks, flexitime, and shift working) become more prevalent, this issue will need to be addressed more directly. We will provide an overview of this relatively recent change later in the chapter.

Kirkcaldy and colleagues (2009) also discussed the impact of travel time on the total number of hours devoted to work. Often commuting time is not factored into calculations of working hours, although in some cases it can add considerably to the number of hours spent on work-related activity. For instance, if there are nominally 40 work hours per week but the person spends two hours each day commuting to and from their workplace, this equates with an actual work week of 50 hours. Kirkcaldy et al. (2009) noted that, despite the increase in teleworking (as discussed above), many workers are now spending much more time traveling to their workplace, given the increasing size of cities and the high cost of inner-city living, which forces many individuals to live farther away from their city office. Some countries (such as Finland and Canada) have begun to examine the potential impact of long commuting time on people's quality of life and, ultimately, their well-being, but there has been surprisingly little direct investigation of this issue.

Although this chapter is not directly concerned with retirement from work and its effects on well-being, the changes people make in their work hours as they make the transition to retirement are relevant in the present context. For younger people who are developing their careers, long hours of work and commuting to work may not be a major issue but for older workers approaching retirement, scaling back the number of work hours may be a significant consideration. That is, the impact of longer working hours may vary depending on a person's age, career stage, and their plans and intentions relating to work. As observed by several researchers (e.g., Flynn, 2010), engaging in part-time work as a transition from full-time employment to retirement provides some significant benefits for many people. Preferred work hours may become more salient for these individuals, and we discuss preferences later.

While extended work hours may imply movement away from a 40-hour working week, research tends to be divergent in the definition of "longer" working hours. Sometimes the term "overtime" is used to characterize work for more than 10–11 hours per day, although expressions such as "irregular work hours" and "non-standard work hours" are also used. Weekly work hours are similarly difficult to define (ranging from more than 40 hours to more than 65 hours) (Virtanen & Kivimaki, 2012). Regardless, long work hours entail extended time in work, and the trend to do so appears to be increasing globally. For example, Hewlett and Luce (2006) reported a growing trend for people to work 70 hours or more per week.

Below we summarize the extensive research which has been conducted on the effects of long work hours on both physical health and psychological well-being (cf. Burke & Fiksenbaum, 2008, for an additional comprehensive review). We begin with an overview of the relationship between working hours and physical health.

Physical Health

The notion that long working hours have the potential to induce or exacerbate physical ill-health has raised the interest of researchers within organizational psychology and health related fields. As early as 1991, Uehata discussed the Japanese phenomenon of *karoshi* (death from overwork) and examined the relationship between long working hours and cardiovascular disease, while Ono, Watanabe, Kaneko, Matsumoto, and Miyako (1991) found links between long working hours, alternative shift work, and fatigue among Japanese flight attendants. Research is emerging on the differences between working hours and work intensification, or work effort (Burke, Singh, & Fiksenbaum, 2010), and their impact on physical well-being. Work intensity, such as a faster work pace, includes job demands and job complexity, which are discussed in Taris and Shaufeli, Chapter 8 of the present volume. Here the focus is on extended working hours and alternative work hours.

Generally, the issue for people working longer hours is that they are likely to be exposed to increased job demands and stressors, as well as having reduced time available for recovery, and less time to undertake healthy lifestyle activities such as physical fitness and healthy eating. Similarly, those working non-traditional hours may experience physical fatigue due to physiological demands induced by changes in sleep patterns when working night shifts or unsociable hours. Vila and Moore (2008) discussed the prevalence and effects of long working hours among police officers in the USA. They noted that in many cases the work times of police personnel are not only long, but also erratic and unpredictable. Fatigue is one major consequence and the physical and psychological concerns which arise from long work hours are due mainly to fatigue rather than the length of the workday itself.

While differences exist in the literature regarding the extent and actual number of working hours that are detrimental to physical health, this topic – working hours and its relationship to physical well-being – has been the focus of meta-analyses (see Sparks, Cooper, Fried, & Shirom, 1997; Van der Hulst, 2003; Virtanen et al., 2012). Similarly, the effects of working "alternative" hours on physical health remain an important issue (Benavides, Benach, Diez-Roux, & Roman, 2000).

In one meta-analysis of work hours and physical health, Sparks et al. (1997) found a consistent and significant positive trend of increased health symptoms with greater hours of work. Härmä (2003) reviewed studies and found that the number of work hours was associated with adverse health, in particular cardiovascular disease, self-reported measures of poor health and exhaustion. The most thought-provoking studies show that working more than 11 hours a day is associated with a three times higher risk of cardiovascular disease, and a four times higher risk of type 2 diabetes, than working a "normal" workday.

The relationship between long working hours and coronary heart disease was investigated via a meta-analysis by Virtanen and colleagues (2012). They reviewed studies that included over 22,000 participants, finding that extended work hours had a positive association with heart disease. Indeed, the results across the studies suggest an approximate level of 40 percent risk of cardiovascular disease in employees working long hours. While the underlying mechanisms which link long work hours and cardiovascular disease are less known, two potential contributors are, firstly, that longer hours generate exposure to heightened cortisol levels and elevated blood pressure, and secondly, long work hours leave decreased time for proper nutrition, physical activity, and sleep. These factors – heightened cortisol levels, elevated blood pressure, poorer nutrition, and re- duced exercise – are markers of heart disease. Similarly, Tayama and Munakata (2014), in researching diabetes risk factors in China, found that men who were working over 55 hours per week had twice the number of risk factors associated with diabetes. This study controlled for lifestyle behaviors (such as alcohol and smoking), and for occupation status, however these factors (i.e., occupation and alcohol) failed to explain the likelihood of diabetes, over and above extended working hours.

The association between long work hours and sleep deprivation is also a significant factor in the decline in physical health. Härmä (2003) found that sleeping hours are remarkably shortened among those who work more than 50 hours a week, while Chatzitheochari and Arber (2009) observed that managers experienced greater risk of insufficient sleep when working long hours. Although lack of sleep may be due to insufficient time to wind down or recover after work, the relationship between extended work time, sleep, and heart disease is interesting. Indeed, sleeping between four to six hours a day (compared with seven to eight hours per day) is known to be associated with an increased risk of coronary heart disease. Insufficient sleep can increase the activity of the sympathetic nervous system and lead to an increase in blood pressure and heart rate. When combined with long work hours, insufficient sleep has been found to result in the highest risk of myocardial infarction (heart attack) in employees (Härmä, 2003; Virtanen et al., 2012). Parks et al. (2011), drawing on developments in human telomere length and longevity, found that this marker of cellular aging and disease risks is detrimentally influenced by long work hours, particularly in women (Parks et al., 2011). Although in its infancy, medical research into physical health and work time provides avenues for the development into objective health data (i.e., actual telomere length) that is needed to move beyond the preponder- ance of self-report data that dominates research (Sparks et al., 1997).

In summary, there is consistent evidence that longer hours of work are associated with several physical health risks and problems, although these may be offset by other factors (buffering variables) which can alleviate the negative impact of long work hours. We return to these buffering variables later in this chapter.

Psychological Well-being

New technologies do offer more flexibility in both the form and place of work, but on the other hand they can create greater expectations that people will be available to attend to work-related tasks even when they are not officially "at work." Numerous empirical studies have demonstrated that employees who are expected to work very long hours (for instance, >60 hours per week) frequently suffer from stress, anxiety, and depression. Hewlett and Luce (2006) referred to "extreme jobs," where job incumbents worked 70 hours per week or more. Although these jobs are often highly paid, there are several nega- tive consequences, including fast-paced work, tight deadlines, high levels of responsibility for other people's work, availability to clients 24/7, and even a physical presence in the workplace for many hours each day. Although people occupying these jobs indicated that they had high job satisfaction and engagement in their work, they also reported higher work–family conflict (WFC) and pressure (leading to distress). Burke and Fiksenbaum

(2008) also noted a combination of both positive and negative experiences among people who work extra-long hours. They observed, similar to studies outlined in the introduction that Japanese studies of *karoshi* (death from overwork) reflect extreme psychological and physiological responses to excessive work hours, accompanied by significant pressure from work. In other countries, however, there is also evidence that longer working hours are associated with a range of psychological and physical symptoms. Along with other authors, Burke and Fiksenbaum (2008) emphasized the importance of control over work time as a crucial buffering variable, along with social support from one's family, colleagues, and friends.

Several theoretical models have been proposed to explain the effects of long work hours on people's psychological well-being. One prominent theory is the Job Demands-Control model (discussed in Taris & Schaufeli, Chapter 8) originally developed by Karasek (1979) to describe the impact of work demands on stress (psychological strain). A more recent theoretical perspective is the Effort–Recovery model (Binnewies & Sonnentag, 2008). Van der Hulst, Veldhoven, and Beckers (2006) examined these two theoretical models in research on Dutch office workers. They were especially interested in the need for recovery, which has been described as a major contributor to both physical health and psychological well-being. Among these personnel in the Netherlands, working overtime was not directly related to the need for recovery, but in high strain jobs (those with high demands and low control) there was a greater need for recovery and these workers were "especially vulnerable to negative effects of long working hours" (p. 17). Different reasons for working overtime were also implicated as predictors of the negative effects of overtime on employee health and well-being. For instance, where workers have considerable personal control over their work hours, they are more likely to work overtime because they enjoy their work and are engaged in it. On the other hand, workers with little control may see long working hours as a burden that they have to endure, hence the psychological impact may be greater for them.

A study of Japanese physicians was reported by Tomioka, Morita, Saeki, Okamoto, and Kurumatani (2011), who used the Effort–Reward Imbalance model (Siegrist, 1988) to test predictions about the effects of working hours on depression. These researchers noted that physicians typically have longer than average working weeks, and that 50–70 hour work weeks are not uncommon in this profession. In their study, the average work week was reported as 62.8 hours, with men working somewhat longer hours than women. Their sample was divided into three groups, low hours (<54 hours per week), medium hours (54–70 hours) and long work hours (>70 hours). Only in the medium and long work hours groups was there an association between effort–reward ratio and depression scores. Tomioka et al. (2011) also found some evidence that social support from family and friends can buffer the negative effects of longer work hours. They concluded that overall their study illustrated that "the total number of working hours is a not decisive factor influencing depression among physicians" (p. 167). One difficulty, however, is that their cross-sectional design did not enable them to explore longer-term effects, and they did not include assessment of the level of control which physicians felt they had over their work hours.

A study of working hours and well-being among managers in 15 countries was conducted by Spector and his colleagues (2004), who found that, despite marked differences in the number of work hours reported across countries, there was a consistent negative relationship between length of the work week and well-being. Managers in countries classified as individualistic (defined by Spector et al., 2004, as Anglo countries) were more likely to show a negative relationship than managers in more collectivistic countries (Chinese and Latin American countries). The authors reasoned that longer work hours are more likely to be viewed as an intrusion on their family life by individualistic managers, whereas collectivists may see congruence between their work commitments and family responsibilities. As noted by Tomioka et al. (2011), availability of extended family support may also serve to alleviate some of the negative effects of working long hours in collectivistic countries.

Shirangi, Fritschi, Holman, and Morrison (2013) examined mental health and stress levels among female veterinarians in Australia. Their results illustrated that the number of reported work hours was associated with perceived job stress in this sample, although the correlation (r =.11) was very modest. Veterinarians who worked >45 hours per week scored <35 hours per week. Shirangi et al. (2013) noted that the objective number of work hours per se might not be a major contributor to increased stress, but rather whether this number of hours and demands in the job are considered satisfactory or favourable by workers. This is an important issue, analogous to the person's control over their work hours and preference for working hours, which we discuss later.

As we have already noted, there has been widespread concern that (a) working hours are increasing in various countries and that (b) these increases are associated with reductions in health and well-being. For instance, Ng and Feldman (2008) conducted a meta-analysis of 199 journal articles published prior to 2007; 93 percent of the studies were conducted on US samples. Their findings illustrated that longer work hours were associated with increased job stress and psychological strain, and higher levels of work to family conflict.

Another way of conceptualizing long work hours is the notion of "overtime," which typically means working beyond the number of hours specified in one's job description or contract. A study by Kleppa, Sanne, and Tell (2008) of Norwegian men and women, referred to as the Hordaland Health Study, examined the relationship of overtime working with anxiety and depression, and identified several possible reasons for this positive relationship. One plausible explanation is that long working hours generate maladaptive coping behaviors, including cigarette smoking, less engagement in physical activity and, in general terms, less adaptive lifestyles. There may also be less opportunity for physical (and perhaps psychological) recovery from work demands.

Another exploration of working overtime was conducted by Grosch et al. (2006) in the USA. They found that "overtime" (working beyond regulated hours) was associated with increased stress, feelings of overload, greater fatigue, and reduced well-being, especially when the total number of work hours exceeded 70 hours per week. Greater WFC was also found among individuals working overtime. However, the negative effects for people working less than 70 hours per week were not always significant. This raises a question of whether there is some nominal "cut-off" point, beyond which long working hours have more extensive negative effects on people's lives off the job. This issue has not been fully resolved, however, as different studies have operationalized long working hours in different ways.

"Precarious employment" is another expression used in the literature on working time. La-Montagne and his colleagues (2012) explored this notion in relation to the psychosocial work conditions of "casual" workers in one state of Australia. Based on the Job Demand-Control model and the Effort–Reward Imbalance model (Siegrist, 1988), the researchers considered the effects of both work hours and holding multiple jobs on the extent of skill discretion and decision authority reported by workers, along with their effort–reward ratio. Employees working 50+ hours per week reported higher effort–reward ratios than other categories of worker, and this was also related to greater strain (high job demands, low control). Comparison of work types is relevant in that it demonstrates that different work contracts may lead to varying outcomes for workers, and that precarious employment (especially casual, part-time work) is associated with greater difficulties and more strain for individuals.

Not all studies, however, have obtained negative effects from working long hours, and some have found no significant relationship between working hours and various well-being variables, suggesting that certain moderator variables (such as gender and work-time control) may be important to explore. A multi-country study (across 24 European countries) was recently reported by Pereira and Coelho (2013), who found that, although there were significant direct relationships between working hours and overall life satisfaction, which is one indicator of subjective well-being, these effects were substantially moderated by demographic factors, including gender (women suffered more than men) and age (older workers suffered more than younger workers). Another important variable was the person's social connections and availability of social support; those with more connections and support were less likely to experience a decline in their subjective well-being as a result of having to work long hours. In addition, control (autonomy) over work hours also moderated the relationship between number of working hours and life satisfaction. However, these authors assessed the extent of control individuals felt that they had over how their daily work was organized, rather than control over the number of hours of work, which may be another moderating factor. In addition, as we discuss later, people's preferences for working hours need to be considered.

Using Karasek's Job Demand-Control model as a theoretical framework, Karhula et al. (2013) studied the relationship between shift work and mental and physical workload among nurses in Finland. To test their assumptions, the researchers divided the sample into "high job strain" (high demands, low control) and "low job strain" (low demands, high control) conditions, but found no significant difference between these groups on the total number of hours worked. However, in line with the researchers' expectations, there were significant differences between these groups in respect of mental workload and recovery. These differences were attributed to shift work arrangements rather than work hours per se. As with some other studies, the results of the Karhula et al. (2013) research appear to demonstrate that there is no simple association between work hours and psychosocial well-being.

Finally, Gray, Qu, Stanton, and Weston (2004) examined the work hours of fathers in Australia and the effects of long hours on themselves and their families. They grouped respondents into four categories: 35–40 hours per week, 42–48 hours, 49–59 hours, and 60+ hours. Their findings indicated that long working hours are not necessarily associated with reduced well-being. In their study, of 13 criterion variables assessed, only three showed significant differences between work hour categories. These were the person's satisfaction with their relationship with their partner/spouse, WFC, and vitality. Other more general variables (including overall health and well-being) showed little difference between the four categories. There were two exceptions. Fathers who worked more than 48 hours per week reported lower "vitality" and more negative effects on their family life. These findings are consistent with the notion that longer working hours have negative effects on people's lives. Interestingly, however, fathers working more than 60 hours per week reported slightly higher satisfaction with their relationships with their spouse/partner, compared with fathers working "standard" hours. It would seem that there is no simple relationship between working hours and overall well-being, and that other factors need to be taken into consideration, especially the person's preferences for working hours, which we discuss later in this chapter.

Work–Home Interference

One very important dimension of people's lives is their family life. Over the past 30 years or so there has been considerable research on the interface between work and family life. Much of this research has focused on interference between work and family, typically referred to as *work–family conflict* (WFC). Several studies have examined the impact of long work hours on this form of conflict. Steinmetz, Frese, and Schmidt (2008), for instance, investigated this relationship among a large sample of German workers. One strength of their research was its longitudinal design, with data collection at two time points separated by a 12-month interval. Working hours at time 1 were significantly associated with work–home interference at both time 1 and time 2 and also with depression at time 2 (but not at time 1). These findings indicate that the negative effects of long work hours may not be immediately apparent, but may emerge over a longer time period. The effects of work hours on motivation to leave the job were mediated by work–home interference, supporting the criticality of this variable in terms of people's reactions to excessive work hours.

In an Australian study, Robinson and colleagues (Robinson, Magee, & Caputi, 2014) examined the effects of work hours on employed solo and partnered mothers, who are likely to experience "time poverty, that is, a lack of time to meet their work and family obligations" (p. 20). These authors noted that time spent at work can result in a lack of time available for family-related responsibilities, which is one potential explanation for the negative link between working hours and well-being among mothers in particular. Robinson et al. utilized data from a large Australian survey which included 200 solo mothers and almost 800 mothers who had spouses/partners. Interestingly, in this study the effects of longer working hours were not uniformly negative. Solo mothers who worked >40 hours per week in fact reported higher levels of physical health than all other categories. Robinson et al. (2014) posited that this may be due to greater income earned by these mothers, which can enhance health and well-being. On the other hand, lack of resources can have a significant impact on people's health and well-being, and solo mothers often have lower levels of social support (and other relevant resources) than do partnered mothers. These findings suggest that research should focus not simply on the number of hours worked, but also on other factors which can have a substantial effect on health and well-being, including financial resources and social support for employed parents.

A longitudinal Finnish study (Rantanen, Kinnunen, Pulkinnen, & Kokko, 2012) examined the relationship between working hours and both work-to-family (WTF) conflict and family-to-work (FTW) conflict in mid-life individuals. Participants in this study completed an interview and questionnaire at ages 36, 42, and 50, which enabled the researchers to explore patterns over time. Rantanen et al. (2012) found that individuals whose working hours did not depart substantially from 38 hours per week experienced least WTF conflict and FTW conflict, illustrating that 38 hours per week might be optimal in terms of maintaining good work–family balance. One implication of these findings is that having sufficient time to recover from work demands and stress may be crucial for maintaining good psychological health.

In the Ng and Feldman (2008) meta-analysis referred to earlier, the number of work hours was positively (albeit weakly) associated with job autonomy and opportunities for learning, as well as with job stress and mental strain. Curvilinear relationships were observed between working hours and well-being, indicating that there may be an optimal number of working hours. One relatively substantial correlation in this meta-analysis was between work hours and WTF conflict ($r = .26$). However, contrary to their predictions and to "common wisdom," the number of work hours was not significantly related to family-to-work (FTW) conflict, marital satisfaction, family satisfaction, and family cohesion. Ng and Feldman (2008) commented that "some individuals with high family identity will work longer hours because they are committed to providing a higher standard of living for their spouses and children" (p. 871). This suggests that the potential negative effects of work hours on variables such as WTF and satisfaction with family roles and commitments may be offset by the belief that longer work hours will bring significant benefits (e.g., greater income to be spent on family necessities).

Cousins and Tang (2004) explored the notion of "irregular" work hours in three countries (the UK, the Netherlands, and Sweden). Again flexibility in working time was demonstrated to yield positive outcomes, enabling individuals to reconcile their work and family commitments. In the UK and the Netherlands, men tended to report higher levels of WFC than did women. Interestingly, in Sweden, where there are established work–family policies and an emphasis on gender equality, higher proportions of both males and females reported WFC than in the UK or in the Netherlands. This somewhat paradoxical outcome requires further probing. That is, we might expect that in countries such as Sweden there would be lower, rather than higher, levels of WFC, but in fact more conflict was reported by people, especially women. It may be that there is a trade-off. In the UK and the Netherlands, women in particular may reduce their working hours in order to achieve greater work–life balance, whereas in Sweden there are longer working hours per week, which leads to greater conflict. As with other researchers, Cousins and Tang advocated greater flexibility and the need to accommodate family responsibilities when determining optimal work hours.

One work context in which long hours appear to be the norm is call centers, and several studies have examined the impact of long work hours on the stress and well-being of call center workers. Bohle, Willaby, Quinlan, and McNamara (2011), for instance, distributed a questionnaire to marketing and customer service operators in call centers in Australia, and observed that a combination of work intensity (demands) and working longer hours was linked with greater work–family conflict, which in turn was associated with chronic fatigue and psychological strain. However, control over work schedules served as a buffering variable, reducing the impact of long hours on individuals' dissatisfaction with their work hours. Bohle et al. suggested that call center organizations should institute policies and practices, such as flexibility and control over work hours, which may help to diminish the negative impacts of long and variable hours.

Overall, the evidence indicates that long working hours are associated with more WFC and related outcomes, but that this relationship is by no means a simple linear one. Several factors can function as moderators or buffers of the negative effects of work hours on WTF conflict, including flexibility (of work times), control over working hours, and social support (from both family members and work colleagues).

Alternative Work Schedules

Research has illustrated that it is not just the number of work hours that can exert a negative impact on health and well-being, but also the distribution and variability of these work hours. Not everyone works a "standard" week (typically viewed as approximately 40 hours per week) and many individuals are engaged in shift work (that is, irregular or changing patterns of work hours), compressed work weeks, irregular work hours and, as mentioned in the introduction, "precarious employment," where work hours are changeable and unpredictable. These alternative work schedules have been found to exert an effect on people's well-being, both physical and psychological. It has long been established, for instance, that shift work can have significant harmful effects on WFC and both physical and psychological well-being. A full discussion of the impact of shift work is beyond the scope of this chapter, but we will summarize the overall influence of non-standard working hours. Other researchers have observed that shift direction, that is "forward" versus "backward" rotation can have a significant bearing on employees' work attitudes and well-being, with forward (morning→afternoon→evening) rotation typically being less damaging to people's health and well-being than backward (evening→afternoon→morning) rotation (see, for example, Barnett, 2006; Kirkcaldy et al., 2009)

Barnett (2006) summarized empirical research on the impact of work hours in the USA, with a particular focus on couples and their management of the work–family interface. She questioned the assumption that working long hours inevitably leads to negative outcomes, and argued that it is more relevant to consider the distribution of working hours. One gap in the research literature, however, is the relative paucity of longitudinal investigations of the impact of work hours and work schedules.

Sleep deprivation is an issue in alternative work schedules and night work (Benavides, et al., 2000). Shift work, and particularly night time shift work, has been associated with a number of physical ailments. Shift work is associated with the disruption of circadian rhythms leading to sleep disruption and deprivation. Research has also found that it is associated with the de-synchronization of clock genes (caused by changes in work patterns at night) and cancer in long-term shift workers (see the meta-analysis by Wang, Armstrong, Cairns, Key, & Travis, 2011). Possible physiological antecedents of this association are the relationship between light at night and melatonin, since night light suppresses the secretion of endogenous melatonin associated with drowsiness and lowering of body temperature (required for sleep). While further research is needed in the area, shift work has also been hypothesized to contribute to the development of cardiac risk factors, and other metabolic disorders, including elevated blood pressure, elevated triglycerides, and elevated glucose, all of which result in illnesses such as heart disease, diabetes, and strokes (Wang et al., 2011).

Benavides et al. (2000) concluded that employees with irregular working hours and working compressed working weeks reported significantly more problems in respect of subjective health, well-being, and quality of sleep, compared ith those working more standard hours. They examined a range of health issues (including fatigue, stress, backache, and muscular pain) associated with working time (full time versus part time) and work permanency (fixed-term employment, full- and part-time temporary employment). Across 15 European countries, these researchers found that employees in non-conventional working time arrangements had higher rates of job dissatisfaction, fatigue, backache, and muscular pains than those in traditional and/or permanent employment.

While most research has focused only on certain health outcomes, in particular mental health and cardiovascular disorders (Sparks et al., 1997), medical research has produced some interesting findings. Shift work and particularly night-time shift work has been associated with cancer in long-term shift workers (see Wang et al., 2011). Although in its infancy, medical research into physical health and work time provides avenues for the investigation of objective health data (e.g., actual telomere length) that is needed to move beyond the reliance solely on self-report data (Sparks, et al., 1997).

Preference for Work Hours

Another issue that needs to be considered is people's preferences. Some people may prefer to work longer hours or to work "irregular" hours, and this will strongly influence their reactions to the number of hours worked. Although preferences and control (or discretion) over work hours are related variables, they are not synonymous and they should be treated as distinct predictors of reactions to work hours. Golden, Henly, and Lambert (2013) examined data from the US General Social Survey (GSS) in 2002 and 2006, which included a quality of life module. Results from this survey illustrated that people's preferences for work hours were more salient contributors to their overall happiness than the duration of working time per se.

In most European countries employees spend more hours at work than they would prefer. Stier and Lewin-Epstein (2003) found that a large number of individuals in 22 European countries were dissatisfied with their working time, and would prefer to either increase *or* decrease the time they invest at work. Indeed, even when a reduction in income is taken into account, a large proportion of the working population would prefer to work fewer hours than the actual length of their working week (Böheim & Taylor, 2004). At a country level, Stier and Lewin-Epstein found that those countries with a higher standard of living, as measured by Gross Domestic Product (GDP), generally preferred to work fewer hours, while those countries that recorded lower levels of wealth, preferred to work more.

However, although macro-economic forces may influence working time preferences, within-country also needs to be evaluated. For instance, Fagan (2001) found that employees in part-time work who had a preference for greater working time were disadvantaged in terms of well-being. Wooden, Warren, and Drago (2009) found that where part-time hours are consistent with workers' preferences, their well-being was generally no different from that of full-time workers. Similarly, Barnett (1998) found that long hours that were consistent with individual preferences did not affect well-being. Indeed, what Wooden and colleagues (2009) found is that average life and job satisfaction are lower for those who report a mismatch between working time and working time preferences. In summary, both over- and under-employment are detrimental to job and life satisfaction, if work preference time is mismatched. Thus, rather than the absolute number of hours of work being an indicator of well-being, it is the autonomy to be able to match actual working time with work time preferences, that explains where long hours can be meaningfully viewed as undesirable overwork, or short hours as undesirable under work.

Technology and Working Hours

The world of work is not only a physical space, but increasingly work is being performed in virtual and/or mixed settings, as well as spanning geographical places and time zones (Misra & Stokols, 2012). Employees are able to remain connected 24/7 with cell phones, internet, Skype, and social media sites, allowing connectivity at any time and from (almost) anywhere in the world. These new patterns of working time and space have created a growing reliance on computerized technology, and there is a trend toward even greater reliance on and increased use of computer-based technology at work (Hoch & Kozlowski, 2012).

Moreover, what we view as the workplace is broadening, with interconnectivity between home and work, and even geographic boundaries and time zones, having implications for the health and well-being of workers. Using technology, people are working from home while attending international meetings within varied time zones. Employees are working in alternative spaces such as cafes, which may have previously been reserved for socializing (Stokols, Misra, Runnerstorm, & Hipp, 2009). These issues create demands on employees, while also offering advantages such as increased flexibility and autonomy. In this section we consider some of the complex issues that technology brings in terms of working time and well-being. We consider the changes to work methods, the changing use of technology, and the move from individual performance to virtual teams in a technology-driven world of work.

Technology has allowed for greater worker autonomy such as working from home, working flexible hours, and for those who face long commutes teleworking (working from remote worksites) has created an efficient use of time, for both employers and employees. Telework has been associated with fewer absences, fewer interruptions, and greater control over task accomplishment (Diaz, Chiaburu, Zimmerman, & Boswell, 2012). Although the benefits of technology have been recognized, Fenner and Renn (2010) suggested that technology acts as supplemental work time, whereby employees are now engaged in the growing reality of the "24/7" work world. Constant reminders of work, such as checking emails or receiving texts, can increase both stress and guilt felt by employees, as they continue to work even during non-work hours. Technology can thus become an "electronic leash," allowing less time for recovery and rest from work, while enhancing the tie to the workplace (Diaz et al., 2012).

While the vast majority of workplace studies focus on the use of technologies outside of normal working hours, in general these studies conclude that the use of technology results in the blurring of work and non-work hours, allowing work to be more easily carried out during non-work time. Earlier we discussed the concept of work–family conflict, which is one potential outcome of such blurring of boundaries. Does this matter in terms of employee well-being? Overwhelmingly the answer is – it's complicated! For example, O'Driscoll et al. (2010) discussed how employee use of technology has both benefits and undesirable consequences. Although technology can be a constant work companion and an electronic leash, it can also enhance employee autonomy and engagement. Diaz et al. (2012) found evidence of technology facilitating this double-edged effect. Technology increases work satisfaction, perhaps by enabling the employee to stay on top of work demands, but it is also related to work–life conflict. In this research, use of computer technology generated greater work satisfaction, but also was associated with more conflict of work with family and personal life demands.

Another line of research has examined how employees manage technology, and how the blurring of the boundaries between working time and non-working time can be managed by individuals (Hislop & Axtell, 2011). Bittman, Brown, and Wajcman (2009) examined mobile phone use among Australian households and found that employees exerted control over *which* calls they let invade their personal time. Cousins and Robey (2005) emphasized that workers can play an active role in using a range of mobile technologies to manage the work/non-work boundary to their benefit. Thus, some research suggests that the work-related use of technologies does not inevitably produce the negative blurring of the work/non-work boundaries, and also that some workers may actually prefer to have blurred boundaries (Cousins & Robey, 2005).

As outlined in the introduction, teleworkers represent yet another dynamic. Teleworkers are largely hidden from the main workforce and may feel isolated from the workplace and lack social support (Golden, 2008). Koehne, Shih, and Olson (2012) found that lone teleworkers (that is, people working alone) often felt isolated and the lack of social interaction posed a serious issue for remote workers. Moreover, if teleworkers were not able to successfully adapt to a remote work style, they often suffered reduced work performance and a heightened sense of isolation. Finally, as these workers are only visible via technology, this also creates an additional issue of "tele-presence" that is, only connected via electronic media. Some may rely on "over communication" to avoid the appearance of being unreachable, which may create additional stress due to trying to live up to the unrealistic 24/7 expectations of employee reachability.

Overall, at an individual level, technology does enable 24/7 connectivity with work but this can aid autonomy, work satisfaction, and boundary management. However, this obviously allows less time for employees to switch off and engage in recovery activities such as family and leisure associated with health and well-being, which we discussed above.

While the above research has focused on individual experiences, the growth in virtual teams and supporting virtual team functioning is mushrooming. Virtual teams can work together over various time zones and distances, and communicate via electronic media to achieve a common goal. In one study, over 65 percent of small companies stated that their reliance on virtual teams will grow substantially in the future, with large companies projecting the use of virtual teams to be 80 percent (Hoch & Kozlowski, 2012). Thus the role of technology in teams is set to rise exponentially.

Virtual teams offer the benefit of being able to work with like-minded experts from other cultures and dispersed geographical areas. However, virtual team members also demonstrate lower levels of trust, work satisfaction, conflict, and team cohesion, with all of these outcomes having implications for workers' well-being (Hertel, Geister, & Konradt, 2005; Geister, Konradt, & Hertel, 2006). Finally, the diversity in time zones for team members can mean that there are major challenges for them in managing work-time meetings. These often impinge on sleeping, personal, or family time. Time zone issues present a major challenge for all virtual workers and result in many adjustments of their typical work, life, recovery from work and sleeping rhythms. Overall the issues of time, technology, and virtual team satisfaction over various time zones, geographical and cultural differences, create challenges for employee well-being that as yet remain under-investigated (Bergiel, Bergiel, & Balsmeier, 2008).

Finally, for virtual teams, teleworkers or work that is enabled by technology, a growing issue is the need for specialized computer/technology support, coupled with frustration when technology is not working (Coovert, Walvoord, Stilson, & Prewett, 2009). The issue of technological support, as well as the quality of technological devices in understanding the antecedents of *technostress*, have not been covered widely in research (Ragu-Nathan, Tarafdar, Ragu-Nathan, & Tu, 2008). Techno-stressors generally are viewed as factors that produce strain for users. Technostress covers techno-overload, techno-complexity, techno-insecurity, techno-uncertainty, and techno-invasion, and results in a variety of issues such as role stress, decreased job satisfaction, and job insecurity (Tarafdar, Pullins, & Ragu-Nathan, 2014). However, mitigating factors have been found in terms of organization support for technological literacy and technical support (Tarafdar et al., 2014). Technostress is likely to become an increasingly prominent issue as the reliance on complex technologies becomes more prevalent.

In conclusion, use of sophisticated technology at work has both positive and negative implications. Research demonstrating the average time taken to respond to text and email messages is declining, with the expectation of an almost immediate response to messages increasing (Rosen, Carrier, & Cheever, 2013), highlights the prominence and "immediacy" of technology in people's work lives. Rosen et al. suggested that the number of technologies, felt pressure to respond, time available to respond, and priority of intrusion (for instance, from family, work, friends) all create psychological demands and competition for attention, which can impact on productivity and well-being in the longer term. Simultaneously, increases in the number and range of technologies (i.e., email, text, Skype), the pervasiveness of technology (24/7 reachability), as well as the reliance on technology as a form of organizational structure (virtual teams), all add to the growing concern of researchers interested in technology, working time, and well-being. Furthermore, as future generations who are technology "natives" enter the workforce, the intensified use of technology will be evident. This cohort who, in some reports, are unable to go more than ten minutes without checking emails, texts, and Facebook, who are logged into a number of technologies simultaneously, and switched technologies every two minutes (Rosen et al., 2013) ensures that this field of inquiry is set to grow. Thus the 24/7 presence of workplace technology, stressors that result from technology, and the personal preference in technology use in the emerging workforce, is set to continue in research emphasis and workplace dominance. We might anticipate that "work time" and "non-work time" might in future become less discrete components of people's lives.

Moderator (Buffering) Variables

As we have noted above, the relationship between the number of hours worked per week and people's psychological well-being and physical health is by no means simple or straightforward. Although there is evidence that longer working hours can have detrimental effects on health and well-being, these effects can be buffered (alleviated) by an array of variables, some situational and others personal. Here we will focus on a small number of factors which have been consistently found to moderate the link between working hours and well-being.

A very salient moderator (buffering) variable is the extent of *control* which people can exert over their work hours. Much of the research on this issue is founded on the Job Demands-Control model of work stress developed by Karasek (1979). For instance, in a study of service workers in the USA, Valcour (2007) explored the moderating effects of personal control (over work time) on the relationship between work hours and work–family balance. As expected, longer working hours was associated with more dissatisfaction with work–family balance, but control over working time functioned as a buffer of this relationship. That is, the positive relationship between work hours and dissatisfaction was significant only for workers who had low levels of control over their work time. Similar to findings reported by Van der Hulst and her colleagues (Van der Hulst et al., 2006) in the Netherlands, Valcour's (2007) results illustrate the importance of having some degree of control over working time. In their study of workers in 24 European countries, Pereira and Coelho (2013) also found that autonomy (which leads to greater feelings of control) moderated the relationship between number of work hours and life satisfaction.

Johnson and Lipscomb (2006) reviewed potential similarities and differences between US, European, and Japanese workers. One issue that features in their discussion is that hours of work per se may not be the main contributor to reduced health and well-being. Rather, the extent to which individuals can exercise personal control (and have discretion) over their work hours and the regularity of hours appear to be more substantial determinants of psychosocial health and well-being. Johnson and Lipscomb noted that the "24/7 economy" can have significant effects in creating greater demand for jobs which have non-standard (irregular) work hours, and that this may impinge upon workers' off-the-job lives and overall well-being. Managerial and professional jobs are often touted as falling into this category, and workers in these professions are more likely to work extended and non-standard hours. They are also more prone to suffer from physical and emotional exhaustion, experience more family difficulties, and lower general health. On the other hand, these workers also tend to have greater control over their work hours, which can help to offset the negative impact of longer hours. Johnson and his colleagues suggested that these comparisons have several implications for organizational and governmental policies concerning working hours, including the need for more systematic consideration of the ideal number of work hours.

Hewlett and Luce (2006) studied work hours and work–life balance in a sample of Irish entrepreneurs. Theoretically, one might anticipate that entrepreneurs have a considerable degree of influence over their work time. However, they also may need to invest a considerable amount of time in developing their business, and they have no obvious work time boundaries. As noted by Hewlett and Luce, long working hours are commonly expected in this occupational group; the overall average in their study was 55 hours per week. These entrepreneurs reported that their working hours had clear effects on their family life and relationships with their spouse/partner, as well as their overall lifestyle.

Another study to examine the buffering effects of control over work time was conducted by Hughes and Parkes (2007), who investigated public-sector female workers in the United Kingdom. Hughes and Parkes observed that the total number of work hours would impact upon WFC, which in turn led to psychological distress and reduced family satisfaction. That is, employees working longer hours reported greater negative spill-over from work to their home life, which created more dissatisfaction with their family life. In this study, the direct relationship between working hours and psychological strain (distress) was not significant. Furthermore, control over work time moderated the relationship between work hours and WFC, such that the negative impact of work hours was attenuated when control was high, again illustrating the relevance of control over work time as a critical buffering variable.

As mentioned above, McNamara, Bohle, and Quinlan (2011) used the expression "precarious employment" to describe work that is characterized by insecurity (about job continuation), lack of control over work processes, and lack of benefits that are normally part and parcel of secure employment. Their focus was specifically on the ability to control one's work hours. They conducted a study of hotel workers in Sydney, Australia, differentiating between full-time and part-time/casual employees. Their findings indicated that frequency of working excessive hours mediated the relationship between employment status (part-time versus full-time) and both work intensity and work–life conflict. In turn, work intensity mediated the relationship between excessive hours and work–life conflict. People who reported low control over their work hours also reported other negative outcomes, including interpersonal conflict and even violence at work. This may be because these workers are likely to be working undesirable or unsocial shifts. These results are of interest in that they illustrate that the impact of working long hours may be both direct and indirect. They also suggest that simplistic assumptions about the negative impact of longer working hours may be unsubstantiated, and that researchers need to explore the dynamics of relationships between work hours and psychosocial outcomes.

A series of studies by Costa and his associates (Costa et al., 2004; Costa & Sartori, 2005; Costa, Sartori, & Åkerstedt, 2006) has also confirmed the importance of flexibility in working hours for enhancing people's overall health and well-being. Their research focused on varying numbers of European countries, noting that there has been increased diversification over time. They noted that working overtime can lead to negative consequences for health and well-being, but that these negative effects can be offset (to some extent) by having flexible work hours. Again a key issue appears to be whether the individual person has any say (discretion) and control over their work hours (that is, individual-oriented flexibility), or whether flexibility is enforced by the organization (company-oriented flexibility). If individuals' needs and preferences are not taken into consideration when implementing flexible work hours, the presumed benefits of flexibility may not eventuate.

Another potential moderator of the association between working hours and well-being is gender, which has been a subject of considerable debate. The fundamental question is whether the effects of long working hours differ between males and females. Some commentators have suggested that longer work hours are more likely to have a negative effect on women, as these hours will impact on family activities and commitments, which (at least traditionally) have been more the responsibility of women. Evidence on gender differences is, however, very inconsistent, which calls into question the validity of this assumption.

Gender comparisons were conducted by Nemoto (2013) in a study of Japanese workers in financial and cosmetic companies. Nemoto observed that Japan has a cultural norm of long work hours and that this has been linked with certain ill-effects, including *karoshi* (death from overwork). Furthermore, there are marked gender differences in expectations concerning the roles of men and women in Japanese society. Nemoto argued that the long work hours culture is disadvantageous to women especially, because it leads to gender discrimination and reinforcement of gender stereotypes. For instance, although many Japanese companies are now actively encouraging the promotion of women into managerial roles, expectations to work long hours make it difficult for mothers to flourish in these conditions, particularly as it is expected that managers will prioritize work time over family responsibilities and personal concerns. Although this paper did not directly examine the impact of long work hours on personal well-being, it highlights the need to consider the sociopolitical context when exploring the effects of work hours.

Another study which examined gender differences in the effects of working hours was reported by Artozcoz et al. (2013). They sampled workers from 25 European Union member states who were working 30–60 hours per week. Interestingly, they deliberately excluded individuals who reported working extremely long hours (>60 hours per week), who represented 1.5 percent of the overall sample. Marked between-country differences were observed in the number of hours devoted to work. In Anglo-Saxon countries (Ireland and the UK), the relationship between long working hours and stress was stronger for men. In Eastern European countries, the relationship was stronger for women, and in Nordic countries there were no significant gender differences in the link between working hours and health outcomes. The authors concluded that, overall, working moderately long hours was associated with poorer health (as indicated by reported stress) and that gender differences depended on the type of welfare state program which existed in different countries. Countries which were characterized as operating on a male bread-winner ideology were more likely to display gender differences. In general, working 41–60 hours per week was linked with poorer occupational health. As noted, the exclusion of people who worked more than 60 hours per week meant that the authors were unable to compare this sample with others.

Not all studies, however, have obtained significant gender differences. For example, in her investigation of US workers, Valcour (2007) found that, contrary to expectations, gender did not moderate relationships between work hours and satisfaction with work–family balance, which suggests that work hours were associated with dissatisfaction among both men and women. On the other hand, Pereira and Coelho (2013) observed that women suffered more than men from the negative effects of long work hours. Overall, it would seem that both genders experience the pressures of higher workloads, but there may be cross-country variability in the differential effects on males and females.

Coping with the Effects of Work Hours

To complete this chapter, we briefly discuss some ways in which individuals might cope with the potentially negative impact of work hours. These suggestions are not exhaustive, but they do illustrate some issues that warrant ongoing consideration at both the individual and organizational levels, and ultimately at the societal level.

One topic which has come to the fore recently is the notion of *job crafting*, which refers to modifying one's job to improve the fit between job demands or requirements and the person's own needs, abilities, and preferences. Job crafting explicitly focuses on employee job redesign and represents an upward influence on one's job and design (Wrzesniewski &

Dutton, 2001), thus it is also strongly linked to proactive employees (Berg, Wrzesniewski, & Dutton, 2010; see also Cangiano & Parker, Chapter 11, this volume). Job crafting can take many forms. Employees may modify their job by engaging in more (or fewer) tasks of interest, or change how tasks are performed. Job crafting can involve changing relationships at work and interactions with others. Originally, Wrzesniewski and Dutton (2001) also suggested it could involve cognitive changes and altering how one perceives the value of their role. However, empirical research on this aspect of job crafting has been scant.

While research to date has been mostly qualitative, recently Tims, Bakker, and Derks (2012, 2013) found that job crafting was positively related to employee engagement, job satisfaction and negatively related to burnout in professional workers, while Nielsen and Abildgaard (2012) found that job crafting for blue-collar workers was similarly effective in terms of well-being and managing the demands (and resources) at work, to their benefit. Therefore, future research should examine the role of job crafting in relation to the impact of working hours on employee well-being.

Mindfulness: Attention to and Awareness of the Task at Hand

Although working hours that match personal preferences and being able to adapt work to suit interests and abilities aid well-being, the concept of mindfulness adds another dimension to understanding working time and well-being. Mindfulness is defined as moment to moment attention to and awareness of the current task or situation. Thus, rather than a focus on the hours of work, or the job content, mindfulness focuses attention on the current situation at hand. Mindfulness describes a state of consciousness in which individuals attend to ongoing events and experiences in a receptive and non-judgmental way (Brown & Ryan, 2003). This state of moment-to-moment consciousness in itself facilitates well-being, and the field of mindfulness is gaining prominence in workplace studies.

Research on mindfulness suggests that it is an inner resource that supports beneficial psychological functioning that facilitates well-being (Brown & Ryan, 2003). In particular, mindfulness has been found to be important in "disengaging individuals from unhealthy thoughts, habits, and unhealthy behavioural patterns" (Brown & Ryan, 2003, p. 823). While the benefits of mindfulness have amassed in the clinical literature, recently it has been examined with regard to the beneficial effects on employee well-being at work (Roche, Haar, & Luthans, 2014; Ryan & Deci, 2008).

Brown and Ryan (2003) observed that mindfulness is positively related to relationship satisfaction, clarity of emotional states, enhanced mood repair, and negatively associated with rumination, social anxiety, and psychological distress (see also Chambers, Gullone, & Allen, 2009; Dekeyser, Raes, Leijssen, Leysen, & Dewulf, 2008). In terms of the potential beneficial effects for those working long hours, studies using the Mindfulness Awareness and Attention Scale (MAAS) have found that individuals with higher mindfulness are more resistant to stress as they cope more effectively with such events (Weinstein & Ryan, 2011). Similar positive relationships were also found in leaders' well-being. While the leadership role is associated with increasing work hours and stress (Brett & Stroh, 2003), mindful leaders report less negative affect, anxiety, depression, emotional exhaustion, and cynicism (Roche et al., 2014). Furthermore, mindfulness has been associated positively with work–family balance and sleep quality for working parents (Allen & Kiburz, 2011). As we mentioned earlier, both work–family balance and sleep quality are disturbed when employees are working long hours.

While there is evidence of direct effects of mindfulness, mindfulness also can play a mediating role; for example, Leroy, Anseel, Dimitrova, and Sels (2013) found that mindfulness had a positive impact in enhancing employees' receptivity toward authentic functioning, which in turn benefited employee engagement. Other researchers (e.g., Allen & Kiburz, 2011; Roche et al., 2014; Schutte & Malouff, 2011) found that mindfulness enhanced subjects' receptivity toward more proximal psychological and physiological constructs such as emotional intelligence and psychological capital. Hülsheger, Alberts, Feinholdt, and Lang (2013) found mindfulness, and meditation as an intervention, were positively related to service workers' well-being, confirming the benefits of mindfulness not only in leaders and professional employees (Roche et al., 2014), but blue-collar workers as well.

Future Research

Our discussion above has highlighted several issues that complexify the relationship between the number of hours devoted to work and people's psychosocial well-being. We noted earlier that the simplistic assumption that working longer hours will necessarily be linked with poorer psychological and physical health has not been borne out in research. There is certainly a relationship between these variables, but this relationship is neither simple nor linear. More comprehensive research designs are needed to explore the complexity of relationships between work experiences, including working hours, and well-being. Below we offer a few suggestions for future research on this topic.

Two variables which have figured prominently in our discussion above, and in empirical research, are the person's *preferences* for working hours and the extent of *control* they believe they have over both the number of hours they work and the timing of their work. These are related, albeit distinct, constructs. Preferences refer to desires and control refers to perceptions of autonomy. Both are important, but are infrequently explored by researchers in this field. Based on the self-determination theory of positive health and well-being (for a recent discussion of this theory, see Milyavskaya & Koestner, 2011), we recommend that both individuals' preferences for and perceived control over work hours be incorporated into research designs, which preferably should be longitudinal rather than cross-sectional (measurement at a single time only).

In addition, almost all research to date has examined individuals' experiences, in isolation from the experiences of their significant others, such as their spouse/partner and other close family members. Given that a person's experience of issues such as work–family conflict can impinge not only on their own well-being but also the well-being of family members, research needs to explore these interconnected outcomes. For instance, there has been very little research on the effects that an individual's long working hours can exert on their spouse/partner's quality of life and psychological well-being (Ng & Feldman, 2008; Robinson et al., 2014), even though the close link between these issues is well-known.

There is clear evidence that the nature of work is changing considerably, especially with the advancement of more sophisticated technologies which enable people to work "anytime, anywhere" (McMillan & O'Driscoll, 2008). For example, the increasing utilization of teleworking is evidence that technological changes offer opportunities for diversity in terms of work time and workplace (Kirkcaldy, Furnham, & Shephard, 2009). The flexibility provided by these technologies (such as smart phone, tablets, and similar devices) can be of substantial benefit to both individuals and organizations, but there are potential drawbacks, including increased "accesssibility" of the individual to work demands. More research is needed on strategies for managing the work–non-work interface so that individuals (and their families) can engage productively in their work *and* have fulfilling and satisfying lives outside of their job.

Finally, research on potential moderating (buffering) variables has been relatively sparse. Although there has been discussion of the role of demographic variables such as gender, age, and occupational status, these variables have infrequently been examined as possible moderators of relationships between working hours and well-being. As noted above, this relationship is not a simple one, and it is likely that it will vary depending on the person's demographic status, as well as their preference for and control over working hours, as we noted above. Another potential contributing factor is the degree of flexibility available to the person in terms of their work time and place. There is substantial evidence that this can have a very positive impact on work–life balance and overall well-being (Shockley & Allen, 2007).

Conclusions

In conclusion, in this chapter we have overviewed findings from research on the effects of working hours on physical health and psychological well-being, as well as exploring other relevant issues, including variables which may moderate the negative association between work hours and well-being, such as control over one's work hours and preferences. We completed the chapter with a brief discussion of how approaches such as job crafting and mindfulness may alleviate the negative effects of long work hours, and therefore enhance people's well-being. Similarly, as we have already commented, it is important to investigate potential moderator variables, including demographic factors but also resources available to individuals which may reduce some of the negative impacts of long and variable working hours.

References

Allen, T. D., & Kiburz, K. M. (2011). Trait mindfulness and work–family balance among working parents: The mediating effects of vitality and sleep quality. *Journal of Vocational Behavior*, *98*(2), 310–325.

Artozcoz, L., Cortes, I., Escriba-Aguir, V., Bartoli, X., Basart, H., & Borrell, C. (2013). Long working hours and health status among employees in Europe: Between-country differences. *Scandinavian Journal of Work Environment and Health*, *39*(4), 369–378.

Barnett, R. C. (1998). Towards a review and reconceptualization of the work/family literature. *Genetic Social and General Psychology Monographs*, *124*(2), 125–184.

Barnett, R. C. (2006). Relationship of the number and distribution of work hours to health and quality-of-life (QOL) outcomes. *Research in Occupational Stress and Well-Being*, *5*, 99–138.

Benavides, F. G., Benach, J., Diez-Roux, A. V., & Roman, C. (2000). How do types of employment relate to health indicators? Findings from the second European survey on working conditions. *Journal of Epidemiology Community Health*, *54*(7), 494–501.

Berg, J. M., Wrzesniewski, A., & Dutton, J. E. (2010). Perceiving and responding to challenges in job crafting at different ranks: When proactivity requires adaptivity. *Journal of Organizational Behavior*, *31*(2–3), 158–186.

Bergiel, B. J., Bergiel, E. B., & Balsmeier, P. W. (2008). Nature of virtual teams: A summary of their advantages and disadvantages. *Management Research News*, *31*(2), 99–110.

Binnewies, C., & Sonnentag, S. (2008). Recovery after work: Unwinding from daily job stress. In R. J. Burke & C. L. Cooper (Eds.), *The long work hours culture* (pp. 275–293). Bingley, UK: Emerald Group.

Bittman, M., Brown, J. E., & Wajcman, J. (2009). The mobile phone, perpetual contact and time pressure. *Work, Employment & Society*, *23*(4), 673–691.

Böheim, R., & Taylor, M. P. (2004). Actual and preferred working hours. *British Journal of Industrial Relations*, *41*(1), 149–166.

Bohle, P., Willaby, H., Quinlan, M., & McNamara, M. (2011). Flexible work in call centres: Working hours, work–life conflict and health. *Applied Ergonomics, 42*(2), 219–224.

Brett, J. M., and Stroh, L. K. (2003). Working 61 plus hours per week: Why do managers do it? *Journal of Applied Psychology, 88*(1), 67–78.

Brown, K. W., & Ryan, R. M. (2003). The benefits of being present: Mindfulness and its role in psychological wellbeing. *Journal of Personality and Social Psychology, 84*(4), 822–848.

Burke, R. J., & Fiksenbaum, L. (2008). Work hours, work intensity and work addiction: Costs and benefits. In R. J. Burke & C. L. Cooper (Eds.), *The long work hours culture* (pp. 3–36). Bingley, UK: Emerald Group.

Burke, R. J., Singh, P., & Fiksenbaum, L. (2010). Work intensity: Potential antecedents and consequences. *Personnel Review, 39*(3), 347–360.

Callister, P. (2005). Overworked families? Changes in the paid working hours of families with young children, 1986 to 2001. *Social Policy Journal of New Zealand, 24*, 160–184.

Chambers, R., Gullone, E., & Allen, N. B. (2009). Mindful emotion regulation: An integrative review. *Clinical Psychology Review, 29*(6), 560–572.

Chatzitheochari, S., & Arber, S. (2009). Lack of sleep, work and the long hours culture: Evidence from the UK Time Use Survey. *Work, Employment and Society, 23*(1), 30–48.

Coovert, M. D., Walvoord, A. G., Stilson, F. R., & Prewett, M. S. (2009). Technology and health. In S. Cartwright & C. L. Cooper (Ed.), *The Oxford handbook of organizational well-being.* Oxford, UK: Oxford University Press.

Costa, G., Åkerstedt, T., Nachreiner, F., Baltieri, F., José, C., Folkard, S., . . . Jorge, S. (2004). Flexible working hours, health, and well-being in Europe: Some considerations from a SALTSA project. *Chronobiology International, 21*(6), 831–844. doi:10.1081/CBI-200035935

Costa, G., & Sartori, S. (2005). Flexible work hours, ageing and well-being. *International Congress Series, 1280*, 23–28.

Costa, G., Sartori, S., & Åkerstedt, T. (2006). Influence of flexibility and variability of working hours on health and well-being. *Chronobiology International, 23*(6), 1125–1137. doi:10.1080/07420520601087491

Cousins, C. R., & Tang, N. (2004). Working time and work and family conflict in the Netherlands, Sweden and the UK. *Work, Employment and Society, 18*(3), 531–549.

Cousins, K. C., & Robey, D. (2005). The social shaping of electronic metals exchanges: An institutional theory perspective. *Information Technology & People, 18*(3), 212–229.

Diaz, I., Chiaburu, D. S., Zimmerman, R. D., & Boswell, W. R. (2012). Communication technology: Pros and cons of constant connection to work, *Journal of Vocational Behavior, 80*(2), 500–508.

Dekeyser, M., Raes, F., Leijssen, M., Leysen, S., & Dewulf, D. (2008). Mindfulness skills and interpersonal behavior. *Personality and Individual Differences, 44*(5), 1235–1245.

Drago, R., Wooden, M., & Black, D. (2009). Long work hours: Volunteers and conscripts. *British Journal of Industrial Relations, 47*(3), 571–600.

Fagan, C. (2001). Time, money and the gender order: Work orientations and working-time preferences in Britain. *Gender, Work & Organization, 8*(3), 239–266.

Fenner, G. H., & Renn, R. W. (2010). Technology-assisted supplemental work and work-to-family conflict: The role of instrumentality beliefs, organizational expectations and time management. *Human Relations, 63*(1), 63–82.

Flynn, M. (2010). Who would delay retirement? Typologies of older workers. *Personnel Review, 39*(3), 308–324.

Geister, S., Konradt, U., & Hertel, G. (2006). Effects of process feedback on motivation, satisfaction, and performance in virtual teams. *Small Group Research, 37*(5), 459–489.

Golden, L. (2008). Limited access: Disparities in flexible work schedules and work-at-home. *Journal of Family and Economic Issues, 29*(1), 86–109.

Golden, L., Henly, J. R., & Lambert, S. (2013). Work schedule flexibility: A contributor to happiness? *Journal of Social Research & Policy, 4*(2), 107–135.

Gray, M., Qu, L., Stanton, D., & Weston, R. (2004). Long work hours and the wellbeing of fathers and their families. *Australian Journal of Labour Economics, 7*(2), 255–273.

Grosch, J. W., Caruso, C. C., Rosa, R. R., & Sauter, S. L. (2006). Long hours of work in the U.S.: Associations with demographic and organizational characteristics, psychosocial working conditions and health. *American Journal of Industrial Medicine, 49*(11), 943–952.

Härmä, M. (2003). Are long workhours a health risk? *Scandinavian Journal of Work, Environment & Health, 29*(3), 167–169

Hertel, G., Geister, S., & Konradt, U. (2005). Managing virtual teams: A review of current empirical research. *Human Resource Management Review, 15*(1), 69–95.

Hewlett, S., & Luce, C. (2006). Extreme jobs: The dangerous allure of the 70-hour work week. *Harvard Business Review,* December, 49–59.

Hislop, D., & Axtell, C. (2011). Mobile phones during work and non-work time: A case study of mobile, non-managerial workers. *Information and Organization, 21*(1), 41–56.

Hoch, J. E., & Kozlowski, S. W. (2012). Leading virtual teams: Hierarchical leadership, structural supports, and shared team leadership. *Journal of Applied Psychology, 99*(3), 390–403

Hughes, E. L., & Parkes, K. R. (2007). Work hours and well-being: The roles of work-time control and work–family interference. *Work and Stress, 21*(3), 264–278.

Hülsheger U. R., Alberts H. J. E. M., Feinholdt, A., & Lang J. (2013). Benefits of mindfulness at work: The role of mindfulness in emotion regulation, emotional exhaustion, and job satisfaction. *Journal of Applied Psychology, 98*(2), 310–325

Jacobs, J. A., & Gerson, K. (2004). *The time divide: Work, family, and gender inequality.* Cambridge, MA: Harvard University Press.

Johnson, J. V., & Lipscomb, J. (2006). Long working hours, occupational health and the changing nature of work organization. *American Journal of Industrial Medicine, 49*(11), 921–929.

Japanese Ministry of Health, Labour and Welfare (2004). White paper on the labour economy 2004. http://www.mhlw.go.jp/english/wp/l-economy/2004/index.html (accessed May 15, 2015).

Karasek, R. A. (1979). Job demands, job decision latitude and mental strain: Implications for job redesign. *Administrative Science Quarterly, 24*(2), 285–308.

Karhula, K., Harma, M., Sallinen, M., Hublin, C., Virkhala, J., Kivimaki, M., . . . Puttonen, S. (2013). Association of job strain with working hours, shift-dependent perceived workload, sleepiness and recovery. *Ergonomics, 56*(11), 1640–1651.

Kirkcaldy, B., Furnham, A., & Shephard, R. (2009). The impact of working hours and working patterns on physical and psychological health. In S. Cartwright & C. L. Cooper (Eds.), *The Oxford handbook of organizational well-being* (pp. 303–330). Oxford, UK: Oxford University Press.

Kleppa, E., Sanne, B., & Tell, G. S. (2008). Working overtime is associated with anxiety and depression: The Hordaland health study. *Journal of Occupational and Environmental Medicine, 50*(6), 658–666.

Koehne, B., Shih, P. C., & Olson, J. S. (2012). Remote and alone: Coping with being the remote member on the team. In *Proceedings of the ACM 2012 Conference on Computer Supported Cooperative Work* (pp. 1257–1266). ACM.

LaMontagne, A. D., Smith, P. M., Louie, A. M., Quinlan, M., Ostry, A. S., & Shoveller, J. (2012). Psychosocial and other working conditions: Variation by employment arrangement in a sample of working Australians. *American Journal of Industrial Medicine, 55*(2), 93–106.

Leroy, H., Anseel, F., Dimitrova, N. G., & Sels, L. (2013). Mindfulness, authentic functioning, and work engagement: A growth modeling approach. *Journal of Vocational Behavior, 82*(3), 238–247

McMillan, L. H., & O'Driscoll, M. P. (2008). The wellsprings of workaholism: A comparative analysis of the explanatory theories. In R. J. Burke & C. L. Cooper (Eds.), *The long work hours culture: Causes, consequences and choices* (pp. 85–111). Bingley, UK: Emerald Publishing.

McNamara, M., Bohle, P., & Quinlan, M. (2011). Precarious employment, working hours, work–life conflict and health in hotel work. *Applied Ergonomics, 42*(2), 225–232.

Milyavskaya, M., & Koestner, R. (2011). Psychological needs, motivation, and well-being: A test of self-determination theory across multiple domains. *Personality and Individual Differences, 50*(3), 387–391.

Misra, S., & Stokols, D. (2012). A typology of people–environment relationships in the Digital Age. *Technology in Society, 34*(4), 311–325.

Nemoto, K. (2013). Long working hours and the corporate gender divide in Japan. *Gender, Work and Organization, 20*(5), 512–527.

Ng, T. W., & Feldman, D. C. (2008). Long work hours: A social identity perspective on meta-analysis data. *Journal of Organizational Behavior, 29*(7), 853–880.

Niedhammer, I., Sultan-Taieb, H., Chastang, J.-F., Vermeylen, G., & Parent-Thirion, A. (2012). Exposure to psychosocial work factors in 31 European countries. *Occupational Medicine, 62*(3), 196–202.

Nielsen, K., & Abildgaard, J. S. (2012). The development and validation of a job crafting measure for use with blue-collar workers. *Work & Stress, 26*(4), 365–384.

O'Driscoll, M. P., Brough, P., Timms, C., & Sawang, S. (2010). Engagement with information and communication technology and psychological well-being. In P. L. Perrewé, & D. C. Ganster (Eds.), *New developments in theoretical and conceptual approaches to job stress: Research in occupational stress and well-being* (vol. 8, pp. 269–316). London, UK: Emerald Publishing

Ono, Y., Watanabe, S., Kaneko, S., Matsumoto, K., & Miyako, M. (1991). Working hours and fatigue of Japanese flight attends. *Journal of Human Ergology, 20*(2), 155–164.

Park, J., Yi, Y., & Kim, Y. (2010). Weekly work hours and stress complaints of workers in Korea. *American Journal of Industrial Medicine, 53*(11), 1135–1141.

Parks, C. G., DeRoo, L. A., Miller, D. B., McCanlies, E. C., Cawthon, R. M., & Sandler, D. P. (2011). Employment and work schedule are related to telomere length in women. *Occupational and Environmental Medicine, 68*(8), 582–589.

Pereira, M. C., & Coelho, F. (2013). Work hours and well-being: An investigation of moderator effects. *Social Indicators Research, 111*(1), 235–253.

Ragu-Nathan, T., Tarafdar, M., Ragu-Nathan, B. S., & Tu, Q. (2008). The consequences of technostress for end users in organizations: Conceptual development and empirical validation. *Information Systems Research, 19*(4), 417–433.

Rantanen, J., Kinnunen, U., Pulkinnen, L., & Kokko, K. (2012). Developmental trajectories of work–family conflict for Finnish workers in midlife. *Journal of Occupational Health Psychology, 17*(3), 290–303.

Robinson, L. D., Magee, C. A., & Caputi, P. (2014). Social support, work hours and health: A comparative study of sole and partnered Australian mothers. *Women's Studies International Forum, 42*(1), 19–27.

Roche, M. A., Haar, J. M., & Luthans, F. (2014). The role of mindfulness and psychological capital on the well-being of leaders. *Journal of Occupational Health Psychology.* doi:10.1037/a0037183

Rosen, L. D., Carrier, L., & Cheever, N. A. (2013). Facebook and texting made me do it: Media-induced task-switching while studying. *Computers in Human Behavior, 29*(3), 948–958.

Ryan, R. M., & Deci, E. L. (2008). A self-determination theory approach to psychotherapy: The motivational basis for effective change. *Canadian Psychology, 49*(3), 186–193.

Schutte, N. S., & Malouff, J. M. (2011). Emotional intelligence mediates the relationship between mindfulness and subjective well-being. *Personality and Individual Differences, 50*(7), 1116–1119.

Sheridan, M., Sunter, D., & Diverty, B. (2001). The changing workweek. In G. Wong and G. Picot (Eds.), *Working time in comparative perspective, Volume I: Patterns, trends, and policy implications of earnings inequality and unemployment* (pp. 13–44). Kalamazoo, MI: W. E. Upjohn Institute.

Shirangi, A., Fritschi, L., Holman, C. D., & Morrison, D. (2013). Mental health in female veterinarians: Effects of working long hours and having children. *Australian Veterinary Journal, 91*(4), 123–130.

Shockley, K. M., & Allen, T. D. (2007). When flexibility helps: Another look at the availability of flexible work arrangements and work–family conflict. *Journal of Vocational Behavior, 71*(3), 479–493.

Siegrist, J. (1988). Adverse health effects of effort–reward imbalance at work. In C. L. Cooper (Ed.), *Theories of organizational stress.* Oxford, UK: Oxford University Press.

Sparks, K., Cooper, C., Fried, Y., & Shirom, A. (1997). The effects of hours of work on health: A meta-analytic review. *Journal of Occupational and Organizational Psychology, 70*(4), 391–408.

Spector, P. E., Cooper, C. L., Poelmans, S. A., Allen, T. D., O'Driscoll, M. P., Sanchez, J. I., . . . Yu, S. (2004). A cross-national comparative study of work–family stressors, working hours and well-being: China and Latin America versus the Anglo world. *Personnel Psychology, 57*(1), 119–142.

Steinmetz, H., Frese, M., & Schmidt, P. (2008). A longitudinal panel study on antecedents and outcomes of work–home interference. *Journal of Vocational Behavior, 73*(2), 231–241.

Stokols, D., Misra, S., Runnerstrom, M. G., & Hipp, J. A. (2009). Psychology in an age of ecological crisis: From personal angst to collective action. *American Psychologist, 64*(3), 181.

Stier, H., & Lewin-Epstein, N. (2003). Time to work: A comparative analysis of preferences for working hours. *Work and Occupations, 30*(3), 302–326.

Tarafdar, M., Pullins, E. B., & Ragu-Nathan, T. S. (2014). Technostress: Negative effect on performance and possible mitigations. *Information Systems Journal, 25*(2). doi:10.1111/isj.12042

Tayama, J., Li, J., & Munakata, M. (2014). Working long hours is associated with higher prevalence of diabetes in urban male Chinese workers: The rosai karoshi study. *Stress and Health*. Advance online publication. doi:10.1002/smi.2580

Tims, M., Bakker, A. B., & Derks, D. (2012). Development and validation of the job crafting scale. *Journal of Vocational Behavior, 80*(1), 173–186.

Tims, M., Bakker, A. B., & Derks, D. (2013). The impact of job crafting on job demands, job resources, and well-being. *Journal of Occupational Health Psychology, 18*(2), 230.

Tomioka, K., Morita, K., Saeki, K., Okamoto, N., & Kurumatani, N. (2011). Working hours, occupational stress and depression among physicians. *Occupational Medicine, 61*(3), 163–170.

Uehata, T. (1991). Long working hours and occupational stress-related cardiovascular attacks among middle-aged workers in Japan. *Journal of Human Ergonomics, 20*(2), 147–153.

Valcour, M. (2007). Work-based resources as moderators of the relationship between work hours and satisfaction with work–family balance. *Journal of Applied Psychology, 92*(6), 1512–1523.

Van der Hulst, M. (2003). Long workhours and health. *Scandinavian Journal of Work, Environment & Health, 29*(3), 171–188.

Van der Hulst, M., Veldhoven, M., & Beckers, D. (2006). Overtime and need for recovery in relation to job demands and job control. *Journal of Occupational Health, 48*(1), 11–19.

Vila, B., & Moore, J. M. (2008). Police long work hours: Causes, consequences and alternatives. In R. J. Burke & C. L. Cooper (Eds.), *The long work hours culture* (pp. 183–201). Bingley, UK: Emerald Publishing.

Virtanen, M., Heikkilä, K., Jokela, M., Ferrie, J. E., Batty, G. D., Vahtera, J., & Kivimäki, M. (2012). Long working hours and coronary heart disease: A systematic review and meta-analysis. *American Journal of Epidemiology, 176*(7), 586–596.

Virtanen, M., & Kivimaki, M. (2012). Saved by the bell: Does working too much increase the likelihood of depression? *Expert Reviews, 12*(5), 497–499.

Wagstaff, A. S., & Lie, J. A. S. (2011). Shift and night work and long working hours: A systematic review of safety implications. *Scandinavian Journal of Work, Environment & Health, 37*(3), 173–185.

Wang, X. S., Armstrong, M. E. G., Cairns, B. J., Key, T. J., & Travis, R. C. (2011). Shift work and chronic disease: The epidemiological evidence. *Occupational Medicine, 61*(2), 78–89.

Weinstein, N., & Ryan, R. M. (2011). A self-determination theory approach to understanding stress incursion and response. *Stress and Health, 27*(1), 4–17.

Wooden, M., & Drago, R. (2007). The changing distribution of working hours in Australia. Melbourne Institute Working Paper Series no. 19/07. Melbourne, Australia: Melbourne Institute of Applied Economic and Social Research, University of Melbourne.

Wooden, M., Warren, D., & Drago, R. (2009). Working time mismatch and subjective well-being. *British Journal of Industrial Relations, 47*(1), 147–179.

Wrzesniewski, A., & Dutton, J. E. (2001). Crafting a job: Revisioning employees as active crafters of their work. *Academy of Management Review, 26*(2), 179–201.

10

Exposure to Aggression in the Workplace

Morten Birkeland Nielsen, Helge Hoel,
Dieter Zapf, and Ståle Einarsen

Introduction

As the average worker spends much of his or her waking time at the workplace, work represents a significant area in life for most employees. While work in itself has many positive features and can fulfill many human needs such as affiliation needs, need for control, or self-actualization (Bradley, McColl-Kennedy, Sparks, Jimmieson, & Zapf, 2010; Jahoda, 1981), going to work may not always be enjoyable. It has been estimated that 41.4 percent of American employees experience psychological aggression, whereas 6 percent experience physical aggression, at their workplace every year (Schat, Frone, & Kelloway, 2006). In the representative sample of the Fifth European Working Conditions Survey (Eurofound, 2012), 11 percent of workers reported that they experienced verbal abuse in the previous month and 2 percent said that they were exposed to physical violence in the last year. Considering the impact satisfaction with work has on our satisfaction with life in general it is not surprising that exposure to aggression from leaders, coworkers, subordinates, or clients is assumed to have profound negative consequences for the health and well-being of the targeted employee.

During the last few decades there has been a remarkable growth in the amount of research conducted to investigate the potential detrimental consequences of workplace aggression and related constructs such as workplace mistreatment, incivility, abuse, harassment, bullying, and victimization. In this chapter we will summarize the current knowledge about the consequences of workplace aggression by reviewing the existing research literature. The chapter has several goals. First, we will define workplace aggression and briefly discuss similarities and differences between different forms of aggression. In doing so, we will highlight workplace bullying as an especially detrimental form of workplace

The Wiley Blackwell Handbook of the Psychology of Occupational Safety and Workplace Health, First Edition.
Edited by Sharon Clarke, Tahira M. Probst, Frank Guldenmund, and Jonathan Passmore. © 2016 John Wiley & Sons Ltd. Published 2020 by John Wiley & Sons Ltd.

aggression. Second, we will present research findings on the direct, indirect, and conditional impact of aggression on health and well-being and thereby show what we know, and what we do not know, about the consequences of exposure to aggression at work. Third, we will discuss some methodological characteristics of existing research with regard to measurement, sampling, and research design and explain how these characteristics may limit our understanding of how aggression is related to health and well-being. Finally, building on the reviewed literature, we will provide some suggestions for future research on the consequences of workplace aggression. While workplace aggression is a multidimensional construct in that it consists of an interpersonal dimension (i.e., aggression targeted at a person in the organization), and an organizational dimension (i.e., aggression targeted at the organization itself) (Hershcovis, 2011), it should be noted that this review will be limited to the former and as seen from the victim's perspective.

Defining Workplace Aggression

Although there are many definitions of aggression, most seem to build on the Frustration–Aggression hypothesis by Dollard and colleagues where aggression was referred to as any sequence of behavior whose goal-response is injury to the person toward whom it is directed (Dollard, Doob, Miller, Mowrer, & Sears, 1939). For instance, Neuman and Baron (2005) define aggression as "*any form of behavior directed toward the goal of harming or injuring another living being who is motivated to avoid such treatment*" (p. 16). As for workplace specific aggression, Schat and Kelloway (2005) conceptualize workplace aggression as "*behavior by an individual or individuals within or outside an organization that is intended to physically or psychologically harm a worker or workers and occurs in a work-related context*" (p. 189). According to Schat and Kelloway, this definition is (i) consistent with definitions used in the general human aggression literature, (ii) sufficiently general to include a wide range of physical and nonphysical behaviors that comprise workplace aggression, and (iii) encompasses aggressive behaviors enacted by a variety of sources within and outside of the organization.

From the perspective of evolutionary psychology, aggression is not a singular or unitary phenomenon. Rather, it represents a collection of behaviors or strategies that will manifest themselves under highly specific contextual conditions (Buss & Shackelford, 1997). According to Buss (1961), aggressive behavior can be classified in terms of three different dichotomies: verbal–physical, direct–indirect, and active–passive. Verbal forms of aggression involve harm to others through words rather than deeds, whereas physical forms of aggression involve overt actions. Direct forms of aggression are reflected through behaviors delivered directly to the victim, while indirect forms involve actions of other agents or through assaults on persons or objects valued by the victim. Finally, active aggression produces harm through the performance of behavior while passive aggression delivers harm through the withholding of behavior. Findings on prevalence of aggression show that verbal and passive forms of aggression, often labeled as psychological aggression, are rated as more frequent by participants than physical and active forms of aggression (Baron & Neuman, 1996; Schat et al., 2006).

Although the above definitions emphasize the role of intention as a feature of workplace aggression, there seems to be some disagreement between scholars about whether intentionality actually is a necessary component of workplace aggression. One of the arguments against including intention is that it is difficult to prove intent, and in some cases it may be that the target attributes intent to the perpetrator, which may not correspond with the alleged perpetrator's perception of the situation. Moreover, unskilled social behavior might harm somebody, for example, in the case of a supervisor who publicly criticizes one of his subordinates. Even if there was no intent to harm and even if this is recognized by the target person the target person may nevertheless suffer from the loss of reputation. Furthermore, intent is difficult to measure. Empirically, most studies on aggression and related concepts use measures consisting of lists of experienced or enacted negative behaviors. Explicit reference to intention usually does not take place. In fact, we know little about intentional vs. non-intentional negative behaviors and their effects on health.

In the scientific literature, exposure to psychological aggression at the workplace has been conceptualized with a variety of labels such as abusive supervision (Tepper, 2007), incivility (Cortina, Magley, Williams, & Langhout, 2001), bullying/mobbing (Einarsen, Hoel, Zapf, & Cooper, 2011), victimization (Aquino & Thau, 2009), interpersonal deviance (Berry, Ones, & Sackett, 2007), emotional abuse (Keashly, 1998), ostracism (Williams, 2007), and social undermining (Duffy, Ganster, & Pagon, 2002). It has been argued that this proliferation of constructs has led to a confusing state of affairs in which many scholars are studying virtually identical forms of mistreatment of subordinates and fellow workers, but with different terminology (Hershcovis, 2011; Neuman & Baron, 2005). Yet, others have argued that most of the construct labels researchers regularly employ capture meaningful theoretical differences (Tepper & Henle, 2011) and that the use of aggression as a uniform construct will make scholars overlook important distinctions among the individual forms of mistreatment. It is beyond the scope of this review to provide a detailed elaboration of the theoretical differences between the various forms of workplace aggression. Yet, the main differences between the constructs are related to the nature, frequency and duration of the experienced aggression, the source of aggression, and the formal power relationship between the involved parties. For instance, while concepts such as incivility, interpersonal deviance, abusive supervision, and social undermining may refer to occasionally occurring incidences, workplace bullying (Einarsen et al., 2011) and emotional abuse (Keashly, 1998) are by definition systematic and long-lasting forms of aggression. Similarly, while the concept of abusive supervision identifies managers as the specific source of aggression, other forms of aggression may also be perpetrated by colleagues, subordinates, customers, and clients.

Of the different forms of workplace aggression, it can be claimed that bullying, sometimes labeled as mobbing, represents an especially important and detrimental form of aggression due to the emphasis on repetition and persistency of the aggressive behavior, as well as the inclusion of a real or perceived power imbalance between target and perpetrator as a defining characteristic. Formally, workplace bullying is defined as a situation in which one or several individuals persistently and over a period of time, perceive themselves to be on the receiving end of negative actions from superiors or coworkers and where the target of the bullying finds it difficult to defend him- or herself against these actions (Einarsen et al., 2011; Einarsen & Skogstad, 1996; Olweus, 1993). This definition suggests that there are three main characteristics of workplace bullying. First, an employee becomes the target of systematic negative and unwanted social behaviors in the workplace. Secondly, the exposure occurs over a long time period often with ever more escalating intensity and frequency in the attacks. Thirdly, the target experiences that he or she cannot easily escape the situation, nor stop the unwanted treatment. It is this latter characteristic, that is, the feeling of being victimized by the harassment, which distinguishes bullying from other forms of mistreatment in the workplace (Einarsen et al., 2011). According to the above definition, workplace bullying comprises a two-step process. The first step includes exposure to systematic bullying behavior over time, whereas the second step comprises a subjective interpretation of being victimized by these bullying behaviors (Nielsen & Knardahl, 2014). This means that, compared with the exposure to aggressive behavior alone, the potential consequences of workplace bullying are influenced not only by the mere nature of the behavior, but also by the persistent and long-term exposure to aggression as well as a perception of not being able to avoid or stand up to this mistreatment. Hence, this form of exposure to aggression resembles the learned helplessness phenomenon which is the experience of being in a position in which there is no way to escape from harm or pain and in which an overall fatalism and resignation make one believe that there is no point in trying to improve the situation (Peterson & Seligman, 1984). It is firmly established in the research literature that clinical depression and other mental illnesses may result from such a perceived absence of control over the outcome of a situation (Abramson, Alloy, & Metalsky, 1989; Abramson, Garber, & Seligman, 1980).

Implications for Health and Well-being

The relationships between workplace aggression and health

Due to the quality and nature of the specific acts which constitute workplace aggression, it was early on assumed that exposure to aggression at work would have a substantial negative impact on the health and well-being of targets (Brodsky, 1976; Leymann, 1990). In order to verify this assumption, a range of empirical studies has been conducted on the potential health outcomes of workplace aggression during the last decades. As depicted in Figure 10.1, the relationship between aggression and health is assumed to be relatively complex and influenced by both moderating and mediating factors. In the upcoming sections we will present the theoretical foundation for this figure and present empirical findings that substantiate the model.

Linking concepts of workplace aggression and health is usually done with reference to Lazarus' transactional stress model which assumes a variety of stressors that are appraised by the person of how stressful they are, what means for coping with the stressors are available, and what kinds of coping strategies can be applied (Lazarus & Folkman, 1984). This results in a short-term stress response including stress emotions and may lead to ill-health in the long run (Kahn & Byosiere, 1992; Zapf & Einarsen, 2005). This process is additionally affected by internal and external resources, the most important external resources being control and social support (Semmer & Beehr, 2014). Internal resources

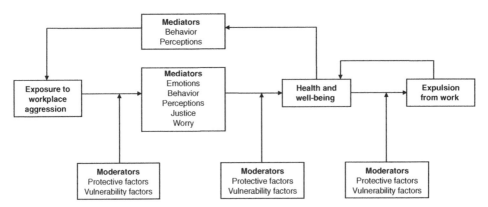

Figure 10.1 A theoretical model for the relationship between workplace bullying and health.

are coping competences or social or occupational competencies (Semmer & Meier, 2009). It should be noted that most theories on aggression in general (Anderson & Bushman, 2002; Geen, 2001) and also workplace aggression theories specifically (Neuman & Baron, 2005; Spector & Fox, 2005) focus on why and how aggression develops. A variety of situational and personal factors are discussed that may contribute to the development of aggression. Yet, a detailed presentation of these factors is beyond the scope of our chapter.

Many aggression theories assume that aggression is elicited by negative events (Anderson & Bushman, 2002; Spector & Fox, 2005), especially when these negative events go along with anger and frustration. Frustration typically occurs when goal attainment is impeded. Hindering goal attainment is part of many stressor concepts, for example role ambiguity and role conflicts (Kahn & Byosiere, 1992), organizational constraints (Spector & Jex, 1998), or regulation problems (Frese & Zapf, 1994). Anger occurs when one feels unfairly treated and when one's self-esteem is threatened (Barling, Dupré, & Kelloway, 2009; Neuman & Baron, 2011; Tedeschi & Felson, 1994). Because of these reasons, stressors at work that are related to anger and frustration are seen as triggers of workplace aggression (Chen & Spector, 1992; Neuman & Baron, 2005), workplace bullying (the work environment hypothesis; Salin & Hoel, 2011) or counterproductive work behavior (Spector & Fox, 2005). Looking at aggression as a dependent variable in the context of stress, aggression as an immediate response can either be classified as a short-term stress response or as a (maladaptive) coping strategy (Carver, Scheier, & Weintraub, 1989; note that affective reactions to stress and emotional coping are sometimes difficult to differentiate; see Semmer & Meier, 1989). In line with this enacted aggression often occurs as a response to being exposed to aggression from others (Geen, 2001), and can thus be seen as a maladaptive coping strategy (Semmer & Meier, 2009). As aggression often leads to anger and frustration and, thus, aggression of the interaction partner, similar levels of aggressive behavior can often be found within groups (Escartin, Ullrich, Zapf, Schluter, & van Dick, 2013). Also aggressive acts of perpetrators and targets are positively correlated (Escartin, Ceja, Navarro, & Zapf, 2013; Glomb & Liao, 2003; Lee & Brotheridge, 2006).

In the remaining parts of this chapter we will focus on the relationship between aggression and health and well-being. Only a few empirical studies have studied models that come close to the model presented in Figure 10.1. We will therefore structure our review of existing research in this field by moving from simple to more complex analyses of how work stressors, in our case aggression, can be related to stress outcomes (see Frone, 1999): (1) simple cause and effect analyses, (2) mediation analyses, (3) moderation analyses, and (4) moderated mediation analyses. While the number of longitudinal studies is steadily increasing, the most common research design within the field of workplace aggression is still the cross-sectional survey design with all variables measured at a single time-point. Unless a study is explicitly labeled as longitudinal, the studies reviewed below are cross-sectional.

Cause-effect analyses   Research based on simple cause-effect analyses attempts to document an overall relationship between exposure to workplace aggression and various outcomes. In most such studies, associations between aggression and indicators of health and well-being are usually adjusted for basic demographic variables such as age, gender, educational level, and occupation. Taken together, the findings from existing cross-sectional studies provide firm support for a relationship between aggression and health outcomes. Specifically, exposure to aggression has been found to be significantly associated with health problems in the form of anxiety (e.g., Baruch, 2005; Björkqvist, Österman, & Hjeltbäck, 1994; Mikkelsen & Einarsen, 2002b), depression (e.g., Hansen et al., 2006; Hauge, Skogstad, & Einarsen, 2010; Quine, 1999), psychosomatic symptoms (Zapf, Knorz, & Kulla, 1996); musculoskeletal problems (e.g., Kivimäki et al., 2004; Vie, Glasø,

& Einarsen, 2012), and symptoms of post-traumatic stress (e.g., Balducci, Alfano, & Fraccaroli, 2009; Leymann & Gustafsson, 1996; Mikkelsen & Einarsen, 2002a). Cause–effect relationships between exposure to aggression and outcomes such as sleep problems (Niedhammer et al., 2009; Rodríguez-Muñoz, Notelaers, & Moreno-Jiménez, 2011), chronic fatigue (Høgh, Borg, & Mikkelsen, 2003), burnout (Deery, Walsh, & Guest, 2011; Einarsen, Matthiesen, & Skogstad, 1998; Winstanley & Whittington, 2002), and anger (Aquino, Douglas, & Martinko, 2004; Vie, Glasø, & Einarsen, 2010) have also been documented in some cross-sectional studies.

Summarizing the cross-sectional evidence on associations between workplace harassment, a form of aggression which was defined as interpersonal behavior aimed at intentionally harming another employee in the workplace, and individual-level outcomes in a meta-analysis which included 90 samples, Bowling and Beehr (2006) found that exposure to harassment was positively associated with generic strain (corrected correlation: .35), anxiety (.31), depression (.34), burnout (.39), frustration (.40), negative emotions (.46), physical symptoms (.31), counterproductive work behavior (.37), and turnover intentions (.35). Significantly negative relationships were found between harassment and factors such as positive emotions at work (−.25), self-esteem (−.21), life satisfaction (−.21), job satisfaction (−.39), organizational commitment (−.36), and perceptions of justice (−.35). Similarly, in a meta-analysis of the outcomes of workplace bullying which comprised 66 independent samples and 77,721 respondents, Nielsen and Einarsen (2012) established average weighted correlations in the range of .23 to .37 between exposure to bullying and different psychological and somatic health outcomes. The findings showed that bullying was most strongly associated with psychological health in the form of post-traumatic stress symptoms, depression, and anxiety. Exposure to bullying was also associated with work-related outcomes such as intent to leave, lack of commitment, job dissatisfaction, and absenteeism, while no relationships were found with regard to sleep problems, core-self evaluations, and productivity.

A pending question within the literature on workplace aggression is whether the different forms of aggression vary with regard to potential consequences. In a meta-analysis of the consequences of incivility, abusive supervision, workplace bullying, and interpersonal conflict, Hershcovis (2011) found that only seven of 25 possible comparisons provided statistically significant differences between the different forms of aggression. Hence, the findings indicate that the investigated types of aggression do not differ with regard to their outcomes. While this finding may be due to conceptual similarities, there are also methodological problems. For instance, the Workplace Incivility Scale (Cortina et al., 2001), which is the most frequently used indicator of incivility, has many overlaps with the most frequently used indicator of workplace bullying, (i.e., the Negative Acts Questionnaire (NAQ); (Einarsen, Hoel, & Notelaers, 2009; Einarsen & Raknes, 1997), it is not surprising that these constructs correlate equally with other variables. The problem is that most instruments in this area consist of items that measure various kinds of negative social behavior, something which is the common factor for most constructs within the field. However, they often do not measure what distinguishes them (Tepper & Henle, 2011). The incivility items do not ask or include whether the behavior was unintended or whether there was an ambiguous intent. Items of bullying scales like the NAQ do not include inferiority or difficulties of self-defense. However, studies on bullying which have utilized a single item self-labeling question based on a formal definition of bullying typically demonstrate that the health consequences of bullying are on average much more severe than the consequences of other kinds of workplace aggression. For example, in the study by Zapf, Knorz, and Kulla (1996) mean scores for psychosomatic complaints, irritation, and depression of bullying victim samples were more than one standard deviation above the means of other samples. Schwickerath (2009) compared bullying victims receiving inpatient treatment with a representative control sample and found that physical symptoms of victims were two standard deviations (SDs) above the control group (although note that correlation or regression coefficients may not always be an adequate means for comparing effects). Repeated physical violence, for example, is relatively seldom in organizational contexts (cf. the 2 percent reported by Eurofound, 2012). Thus, there are considerable variance restrictions for this variable making high correlations impossible.

In recent years, the simple cause–effect model of aggression and well-being has been substantiated by an increasing number of longitudinal findings, and especially by findings on the time-lagged associations between workplace bullying and health problems. Taken together, the studies have established that exposure to, and victimization from, workplace aggression have a long-term negative impact on mental health (e.g., Finne, Knardahl, & Lau, 2011; Hoobler, Rospenda, Lemmon, & Rosa, 2010; Rugulies et al., 2012), headache (Tynes, Johannessen, & Sterud, 2013), chronic neck pain (Määriä, Laaksonen, Rahkonen, Lahelma, & Leino-Arjaas, 2012), fibromyalgia (Kivimäki et al., 2004), sleep difficulties (Hansen, Høgh, Garde, & Persson, 2014), work-related strain (Hoobler et al., 2010), job insecurity and intent to leave (Glambek, Matthiesen, Hetland, & Einarsen, 2014), turnover (Høgh, Hoel, & Carneiro, 2011), registered sickness absence (Ortega, Christensen, Høgh, Rugulies, & Borg, 2011; Suadicani, Olesen, Bonde, & Gyntelberg, 2014), and disability pension (Berthelsen, Skogstad, Lau, & Einarsen, 2011).

The association between bullying and subsequent mental health problems seems especially robust as it has been replicated in both general and occupation specific samples, as well as in different countries and cultures. Furthermore, the different time-lags between baseline and follow-up measurements used in the existing studies show that bullying is significantly related to subsequent health problems over relatively short (e.g., 6 months; Nielsen, Tvedt, & Matthiesen, 2012) and long time periods (e.g., 5–7 years; Einarsen & Nielsen, 2014; Lahelma, Lallukka, Laaksonen, Saastamoinen, & Rahkonen, 2012).

A reoccurring finding in many longitudinal studies on the cause–effect associations between psychological aggression and mental health problems that ought to be mentioned is that mental health problems at baseline is a strong predictor of later exposure to aggression. In a meta-analysis on time-lagged relationship between workplace bullying and health, Nielsen, Magerøy, Gjerstad, and Einarsen (2014) found that workplace bullying predicted subsequent mental health problems with an average odds ratio of 1.68 (95% C.I.=1.35–2.09) across 14 studies, whereas existing mental health problems also were significantly related to later exposure to bullying (odds ratio=1.74; 95% C.I.=1.44–2.12; K=7). According to Nielsen and Einarsen (2012), there are two different theoretical explanations for how health and well-being can influence subsequent risk of being exposed to aggression. The first explanation is based on the "gloomy perception" mechanism (de Lange, Taris, Kompier, Houtman, & Bongers, 2005), and suggests that employees with already reduced well-being and health have lower tolerance for exposure to aggression and, consequently, also have a lower threshold for interpreting certain behavior as aggressive. The second explanation is in line with a social interactionist perspective on aggression and suggests that employees with impaired health and/or low well-being can violate expectations, annoy others, and even violate social norms of polite and friendly interaction (Einarsen, 2000; Felson, 1992) and thus trigger aggressive behavior in others. When comparing these two explanations the main difference is that the former includes perceptions, whereas the latter includes actual behavior as the mediating variables that explain how health and well-being are related to aggression. Although the explanations emphasize different intervening variables in the relationship between health/well-being and exposure to aggression, the explanations are not mutually exclusive. A vicious circle of events may also exist where both parties are aggressive leading to a never-ending circle of "perpetration–becoming a target–developing negative health outcomes–becoming a perpetrator oneself– etc."

While the findings of mutual associations between exposure to aggression and indicators of health and well-being indicate a reciprocal causal relationship between the variables, and maybe even a self-reinforcing vicious circle in which the problems escalate over time, it must be emphasized that the two-wave prospective survey design does not provide information about whether the established associations between exposure to aggression and health start with aggression or mental health problems. Based on existing prospective findings it is therefore not possible to determine whether it is most likely that aggression causes mental health problems or whether it is more likely that mental health problems increase the risk of being exposed to aggression at a later stage. Yet, a study by Einarsen and Nielsen (2014) employing a five-year time-lag, indicated that the process starts with exposure to negative behavior while at work and not with mental health problems.

Further evidence on the aggression–health relationship can be found in research on social ostracism, which has been based on experimental designs. A considerable number of studies have assessed both self-reported and physiological reactions to ostracism, either during or immediately after an ostracism episode where the focal person experienced being excluded from a social interaction (e.g., while playing a video-game; van Beest & Williams, 2006; Williams & Jarvis, 2006). As for self-reported outcomes, the findings show that even brief ostracism episodes result in sadness and anger and threaten fundamental needs (Williams, 2007). With regard to physiological outcomes, evidence from a study examining the neural correlates of social exclusion through the use of functional magnetic resonance brain imaging (fMRI) showed that social pain actually activates similar brain bases to those of physical pain (Eisenberger, Lieberman, & Williams, 2003). The underlying mechanisms which are used to explain the consequences of social exclusion is based on social psychological theories where social exclusion or rejection from important social relationships is claimed to threaten a range of basic social needs, including the need to belong, the need for a worthy self, and the need to perceive the world as predictable and controllable (Williams, 2007; Williams & Sommer, 1997). Exposure to aggression is assumed to profoundly question the focal person's sense of being a capable and worthy individual, again reminding them of their fragile existence, hence constituting a severe source of social pain and even symbolizing a kind of "social death" (Mikkelsen & Einarsen, 2002a; Williams, 1997).

Mediation analyses   Some studies on workplace aggression have included a number of mediating variables which may explain how exposure to aggression influences health and well-being. For instance, in a comprehensive model of the causes and consequences of workplace harassment, Bowling and Beehr (2006) propose that individual outcomes of harassment are mediated by attributional processes in that the most aversive reactions occur when victims attribute blame for the harassment to themselves. Einarsen et al. (2011) suggest that the health consequences of workplace bullying are mediated by behavioral and emotional reactions. Using a stress perspective on workplace bullying, Zapf and Einarsen (2005) proposed that frequent exposure to bullying has an indirect effect on health outcomes through an appraisal process in which the individual evaluates how negatively he or she experiences the stressor and how well he or she can cope with it. Actual coping behaviors exhibited by the victim may also mediate the consequences of exposure to bullying. Finally, in a theoretical model on incivility at the workplace, Lim, Cortina, and Magely (2008) suggest that the effect of incivility on physical health is explained through a causal chain which involves job satisfaction and mental health as mediators.

Potential mediating variables have been tested in several studies on workplace aggression, of which the vast majority are based on cross-sectional research designs. Of the different mediators included in these studies, emotional reactions in the form of positive and negative affect seem to be the most frequently investigated (e.g., Hoobler & Hu, 2013). The lion's share of these cross-sectional studies has found support for negative affect as an intervening variable. For example, Djurkovic, McCormack, and Casimir (2004) found that exposure to bullying was positively associated with negative affect which in turn was related to somatic health problems. Similarly, in a study by Mikkelsen and Einarsen (2002b) results were consistent with state-negative affect as a mediator of relationships between exposure to bullying behaviors and both psychological health complaints and psychosomatic complaints. Furthermore, Hansen and colleagues (2006) established that negative affect acted as a partial mediator of the relationships between being bullied and health outcomes. In a study by Vie and colleagues (2012), the results pointed to both positive and negative emotions as mediators of the relationship between exposure to bullying and musculoskeletal complaints. Yet, in a study on workplace bullying and symptoms of post-traumatic stress among 102 victims of bullying, no mediator effects were found between bullying, positive/negative affect, and traumatic stress reactions (Matthiesen & Einarsen, 2004). This indicates that the impact of affect as a mediator may be dependent upon the outcome in question. However, as no longitudinal studies have examined emotions as mediators of the aggression–health relationship, more research is needed in order to establish this form of process.

Cognitive processes among targets have also been established as a potential mediator in the aggression–health relationship. In a cross-sectional study on the association between bullying and sleep problems, support was found for an indirect effect in which need for recovery and worry mediated the relationship between workplace bullying and sleep problems (Rodríguez-Muñoz et al., 2011). The cognitive evaluation of whether or not one perceives oneself as a victim of workplace aggression may also explain how bullying is related to health. In a cross-sectional study, Vie, Glasø, and Einarsen (2011) showed that self-labeled victimization partially mediated the relationship between exposure to bullying behaviors and the targets' health complaints. This finding was substantiated in a later prospective study based on a representative sample of Norwegian employees where the findings indicated that levels of exposure to workplace bullying behaviors was positively related to the cognitive evaluation of being a victim of bullying. This cognitive evaluation was, in turn, positively related to subsequent psychological distress two years later (Nielsen, Hetland, Matthiesen, & Einarsen, 2012).

A dominant theme in the management literature concerns organizational justice, that is, employees' evaluative assessments of fairness (Tepper, 2001). Research on justice in the workplace has established that associations between perceived injustice and mental health require that *both* unjust treatment and procedural injustice in the form of inadequate intervention by the employer are experienced (Cropanzano, Stein, & Nadisic, 2010). This suggests that perceptions of justice may be an important intervening variable in the association between bullying and health problems in that experienced health problems are attributable to a combination of exposure to bullying and unsatisfactory handling of the conflict situation at the management level. Testing this assumption, Tepper (2000) found that organizational justice fully mediated associations between experiences of abusive supervision and outcomes such as job satisfaction, life satisfaction, organizational commitment, and depression, whereas justice perceptions partially mediated relationships with anxiety and emotional exhaustion. While these findings indicate that justice is an important mediator with regard to outcomes of aggression, there is still a need of further studies which can substantiate the importance of justice perception as an intervening variable.

In addition to being an outcome of aggression, health and well-being may also mediate relationships between workplace aggression and other outcomes, such as job performance, absenteeism, and turnover (Nielsen & Einarsen, 2012). For instance, in a study based on data from a national probability sample, that is a representative sample, of US workers (N=2376) it was found that psychological aggression at work negatively predicted both task performance and contextual performance, and that these relations were explained by decrements in job attitudes (i.e., job satisfaction and organizational commitment) and health associated with exposure to psychological aggression at work (Schat & Frone, 2011). Taking into consideration that health problems may be a predictor of exposure to aggression, the findings of the above study indicate that the relationships between exposure to aggression, health, and well-being is complex and that many different causal associations are possible.

Moderation analyses   Although many employees are exposed to behaviors that may be perceived as aggression, it is unlikely that all react to this exposure in the same manner. Following most perspectives on stress, it is far more probable that the effects of workplace aggression on health are dependent upon a range of personal and organizational characteristics such as individual dispositions and resilience, coping behaviors, social support, and leadership. *Moderation models* explicitly include variables that moderate the relationship between exposure to aggression and outcomes. The basic premise for these models is that the strength of the relation between workplace aggression and outcomes differs as a function of moderator variables (see Figure 10.1). Thus, moderation models explain *when* and *under what conditions* workplace aggression is related to health and well-being. Most moderation models are in line with the transactional model of stress (Lazarus & Folkman, 1984) which proposes that the nature and severity of reactions following exposure to a given stressor are functions of a dynamic interplay between event characteristics and individual appraisal and coping processes. Hence, following this framework, both individual and situational factors may explain when workplace aggression is related to different outcomes. In the upcoming sections, we will present an overview of different individual and organizational factors which have been examined as potential moderators of effects of workplace aggression.

In studies which have examined individual characteristics of the targets of aggression as potential moderators, demographic characteristics, personality dispositions, and coping strategies are recurring themes. As for demographic characteristics, both age and gender have been found to moderate associations between exposure to workplace aggression and outcomes (Einarsen & Nielsen, 2014; Hitlan, Cliffton, & DeSoto, 2006; Hoel, Faragher, & Cooper, 2004). With regard to gender, findings seem to be somewhat contradictory in that some studies have found relationships between aggression and outcomes to be stronger among men than women, whereas other studies have found the opposite results (Aquino & Thau, 2009). These mixed results indicate that there may be other, unobserved, factors which may influence the potential impact of gender. For instance, following Hofstede's (2001) cultural dimensions theory, the role and impact of gender vary between masculine and feminine cultures and some of the inconsistency in the above findings may thereby be explained by cultural factors.

Several studies have examined how personality characteristics influence the potential consequences of aggression. For example, in a study of 183 targets of bullying it was shown that social anxiety and assertiveness moderated the bullying–health relationship (Moreno-Jiménez, Rodríguez-Muñoz, Moreno, & Carrosa, 2007). More specifically, the findings showed that exposure to bullying was most strongly related to health problems among targets who reported low levels of assertiveness and high levels of social anxiety. In one of the few longitudinal studies which have examined moderating factors, Tepper, Duffy, and Shaw (2001) found that the time-lagged relationship between abusive supervision and subordinates' dysfunctional resistance was stronger among subordinates who were lower in conscientiousness than among subordinates who were higher in conscientiousness, but this effect emerged only for subordinates who were also lower in agreeableness. The relationship between abusive supervision and subordinates' constructive resistance was stronger among subordinates who were higher in conscientiousness than among subordinates who were lower in conscientiousness.

It has been suggested that the specific personality dispositions which constitute core-self evaluations in the form of self-esteem, locus of control, neuroticism, and self-efficacy (Judge, Locke, Durham, & Kluger, 1998), may serve as a protective mechanism when exposed to workplace aggression. Supporting this view, Mikkelsen and Einarsen (2002b) reported that generalized self-efficacy acted as a moderator of the relationship between exposure to bullying behaviors and psychological health complaints. However, in a study of workplace bullying among workers in the offshore petroleum industry, Nielsen and colleagues (2013) found no evidence for a protective effect of self-esteem with regard to the association between bullying and mental health. Similarly, some findings on the interactive effect of negative affectivity, which is considered as a facet of neuroticism, show that this trait does not interact with measures of aggression with regard to variance in distress and symptoms of post-traumatic stress (Matthiesen & Einarsen, 2004). Yet, the impact of core-self evaluations, and especially the emotional facets may be dependent on type of aggression or specific outcomes, as other studies have found evidence for negative affectivity as a moderator of relationships between exposure to aggression and outcomes such as workplace deviance (Mitchell & Ambrose, 2007), counterproductive behavior (Penney & Spector, 2005), strain and turnover intentions (Harvey, Stoner, Hochwarter, & Kacmar, 2007). While there is little research on the impact of locus of control, the available research findings question the importance of this factor with regard to outcomes of aggression. In a two-sample study of the impact of perceived control on the outcomes of workplace aggression, the results of a series of moderated regression analyses suggested that perceived control did not moderate the relationships between physical aggression and fear or between fear and emotional well-being, somatic health, or neglect (Schat & Kelloway, 2000). Taken together, the evidence on personality dispositions as moderators of the association between aggression and health is mixed and some dispositions, for example conscientiousness, seem to be more important than others. Still, as there is a clear shortage of prospective studies which include moderating variables, more research is needed to further establish the moderating effect of personality.

Coping strategies have also been suggested to have a buffering impact on the outcomes of workplace aggression (Zapf & Gross, 2001). In a review of the literature, Aquino and Thau (2009) conclude that the coping strategy that appears to consistently produce a significant improvement in a victim's current circumstances is finding a way to avoid the perpetrator(s) or to leave the situation. Strategies that involve an active response to the perpetrator (e.g., fighting back with similar means, talking to the bullies) often make the situation significantly worse by the escalating conflict.

Following a job demands-resources perspective (Bakker & Demerouti, 2006) in which exposure to aggression is considered as an extreme form of job demands, organizational factors such as leadership and social support may serve as protective resources which moderate the impact of aggression on health related outcomes (see Taris & Schaufeli, Chapter 8, this volume). This perspective is substantiated by recent research findings. For instance, in an Australian study it was shown that psychosocial safety climate, that is, shared perceptions of organizational policies, practices, and procedures for the protection of worker psychological health and safety, had a buffering effect on the relationship between work-place bullying and post-traumatic stress symptoms (Bond, Tuckey, & Dollard, 2010; see also Zadow & Dollard, Chapter 18, this volume). Similarly, in another Australian study it was established that psychosocial safety climate moderated the positive relationship between bullying and psychological health problems (Law, Dollard, Tuckey, & Dormann, 2011).

The importance of social support has been substantiated in several studies. For instance, Schat and Kelloway (2003) examined the buffering effects of organizational support on the relationships between workplace aggression and both personal and organizational outcomes. Based on data from employees in a health care setting, the findings indicated that organizational support moderated the effects of physical violence, vicariously expe-rienced violence, and psychological aggression on emotional well-being, somatic health, and job-related affect, but not on fear of future workplace violence and job neglect. Simi-larly, Djurkovic, McCormack, and Casimir (2008) revealed that the effects of workplace bullying on intention to leave were significant with lower levels of organizational support but were non-significant with higher levels of organizational support.

A noteworthy finding from some studies which have tested moderation models is that the interactive effect of various moderators is dependent upon the intensity of the bully-ing. For example, in a study which examined sense of coherence as a protective mecha-nism among targets of workplace bullying, it was shown that sense of coherence offered the most protective benefits with regard to health among targets exposed to low levels of bullying, whereas the benefits of sense of coherence diminished among targets exposed to high levels of bullying (Nielsen, Matthiesen, & Einarsen, 2008). Similarly, Vie and colleagues (2011) found that self-labeling as a victim of bullying influenced the impact of exposure to bullying on the targets' health in cases of low exposure to bullying behaviors. When facing intense bullying behaviors, however, self-labeling did not make a difference regarding the targets' levels of health complaints. Taken together, these results suggest that highly intense workplace bullying is a traumatic experience for those exposed to it, regardless of the target's available coping resources.

Moderated mediation analyses   A moderated mediation model combines the features of the mediation and the moderation models. That is, by including both intervening and interactive factors, the moderated mediation models go beyond the models described above by simultaneously trying to explain *how*, as well as *when*, workplace aggression is re-lated to health and well-being (Hayes, 2013). Hence, moderated mediation models sug-gest that exposure to aggression has an indirect effect on health and well-being through specific intervening factors, and that the strength of the indirect effect is conditioned by characteristics of one or more moderating variables. Methodologically, it is the best rep-resentation of theoretical models like the one presented in Figure 10.1.

A moderated mediation framework can be found in several theoretical models on the consequences of workplace aggression (e.g., Djurkovic, McCormack, & Casimir, 2006; Einarsen et al., 2011; Zapf & Einarsen, 2005). Although moderated mediation relation-ships have been included in many theoretical models, there are only a handful of studies on workplace aggression which have explicitly empirically tested a full moderated mediation relationship (e.g., Burton & Hoobler, 2011; Law et al., 2011; Tepper, Duffy, Henle, & Lambert, 2006). In the following, we will highlight findings from studies on conditional processes where health and well-being are included as relevant factors.

Building on the psychosomatic model of workplace bullying in a cross-sectional sample of Ugandan and Australia employees, Casimir, McCormack, Djurkovic, and Nsubuga-Kyobe (2012) found that the relationship between bullying and physical health symptoms was mediated by negative affect, but that the association between bullying and negative affect was stronger in the Australian sample than in the Ugandan sample. Hence, the find-ings indicate that the magnitude of the indirect effect of aggression on health is depend-ent upon cross-cultural characteristics among those exposed. Attempting to explain the consequences of incivility, Miner-Rubino and Reed (2010) were able to show that trust mediated the relationship between incivility and work outcomes, and that regard for the workgroup moderated this process. Employees with lower group regard reported less organizational trust when they experienced incivility within their workgroup; lower trust, in turn, related to lower job satisfaction, especially for those with low group regard. In a study on abusive supervision and workplace deviance which included 283 employee–supervisor dyads, Want, Mao, Wu, and Liu (2012) revealed that the perception of inter-actional justice mediated the link between abusive supervision and workplace deviance and that abusive supervision had a stronger negative relationship with the perception of interactional justice for employees low in power distance than for employees high in power distance.

Illustrating the complex nature of relationships between aggression and other variables, Wheeler, Halbesleben, and Whitman (2013) tested a model in which emotional exhaus-tion was expected to mediate the association between abusive supervision and coworker abuse, but where the direct association between abusive supervision and emotional exhaus-tion was moderated by psychological entitlement. Using multilevel-moderated mediation analysis to analyze day-level survey data from a lagged panel design across five working days from 132 working adults and their coworkers across multiple industries, the authors found support for their hypothesized model.

Methodological characteristics of the existing literature

While existing research has contributed significantly to our understanding of the implica-tions of workplace aggression on health and well-being, there are some methodological characteristics of the research which should be taken into consideration in the interpreta-tion of the findings. First, although there are experimental and qualitative studies which have provided valuable insight in the phenomenon, the vast majority of studies have relied on survey data and quantitative data analysis techniques (Neall & Tuckey, 2014). Hence, our knowledge about the nature, causes, and consequences of workplace bullying is by far rooted in the advantages and disadvantages of the traditional questionnaire survey approach. For instance, as most surveys of workplace aggression are based on self-reported data, there is a high risk of reporting biases in the data such as common method variance and response set tendencies.

Another limitation of previous research is that there has been an overuse of cross-sectional research design (Neall & Tuckey, 2014). While the cross-sectional approach can be used to assess prevalence estimates of aggression and establish associations with correlates, it does not provide information about causality or directionality between vari-ables (Zapf, Dormann, & Frese, 1996). According to Hershcovis and Reich (2013), the reliance of cross-sectional design has led to a confusion about whether key correlates are predictors, consequences, or both, of workplace aggression. Adding to an understanding of the directionality between variables, there has been a steady increase in studies with prospective designs during the last years. Still, as most of these studies are limited to only two measurement points with an average time-lag between one to two years, little is known about both short- and long-term dynamics between aggression and outcomes. In order to add to the understanding of dynamics, longitudinal studies with three or more time-points and diary studies may be appropriate approaches. Illustrating the usefulness of diary studies, Tuckey and Neall (2014) found that weekly emotional exhaustion partially mediated the negative effects of weekly workplace bullying on both optimism and self-efficacy over a six-week period. Similarly, in a diary study of 130 security employees over a four-week period, Beattie and Griffin (2014) showed that participants had higher levels of stress on the days when they experienced more incivility, and that high supervisor support reduced this effect. In addition, a negative relationship between incivility and daily engagement was only significant for those with low core self-evaluation. Taken together these studies show how a diary study approach can provide information about the effects of aggression on outcomes over different time-periods, while they also allow for detecting potential moderators and mediators of the relationships.

In survey research, sampling is concerned with the selection of a subset of individuals from within a statistical population to estimate characteristics of the whole population. In order to achieve a valid and representative selection of individuals, an important assumption is therefore that respondents are selected through some sort of randomization mechanism. Yet, in addition to being cross-sectional, the majority of samples used in the aggression research are based on convenience sampling techniques, something which increases the risk of achieving a biased and non-random sample and where it is not possible to generalize the findings to a larger population (Nielsen & Einarsen, 2008).

It should also be noted that workplace aggression has been assessed with a range of different methods and measurement instruments. Meta-analyses show that findings on prevalence rates of aggression as well as associations between aggression and correlates vary between measurement methods (Nielsen & Einarsen, 2012; Nielsen, Matthiesen, & Einarsen, 2010). Consequently, findings on aggression should be interpreted according to how the phenomenon is measured, and it is necessary to exercise caution when comparing findings when different methods have been used.

Future Research

Although the number of studies on the outcomes of workplace aggression is steadily increasing and the methodological quality of the research is becoming more and more sophisticated, our understanding of the phenomenon will benefit from further studies with more refined research designs. This review of the literature on workplace aggression, health, and well-being shows that most studies have assessed the simple cause and effect relationships between variables. However, both theoretical models and results summarized in this chapter clearly demonstrate that the relation between the variables is complex and that more attention should be devoted to identifying and testing plausible mediating and moderating variables, as well as reversed associations between variables.

When testing these kinds of relationship, researchers should aim at using more advanced methods and refined research designs with high internal and external validity and where it is possible to determine directionality between variables. As discussed above, diary studies seem to be especially beneficial. Yet, other time-lagged designs are also valuable in that they provide indications of causal direction between variables and thereby allow for the detection of reversed relationships between aggression and health and well-being (Zapf, Dormann, & Frese, 1996). Building on the seminal research on social exclusion, researchers within the field should also consider the potential of an experimental approach. While there are clear ethical boundaries which limit the manipulated levels of exposure in experiments on aggression, it has been shown that "milder" forms of psychological aggression can be included without risking long-term harm to the subjects (Eisenberger et al., 2003; Williams, 2007).

As established both in this review as well as in previous meta-analyses (Bowling & Beehr, 2006; Hershcovis, 2011; Nielsen & Einarsen, 2012), we know that exposure to workplace aggression is related to factors such as mental health, physical health, job satisfaction, intent to leave, and organizational commitment. There are, however, other outcomes which have received less attention. For instance, following the associations between aggression and health problems, one could expect a relatively clear association between bullying and absenteeism. However, based on the existing literature on the association, it is still questionable whether aggression is related to absenteeism. In their meta-analysis of outcomes of harassment, Bowling and Beehr (2006) found a non-significant correlation of .06 between harassment and absenteeism. Similarly, Nielsen and Einarsen (2012) found an average correlation of .11 between bullying and absenteeism across nine cross-sectional studies, whereas a correlation of .12 between bullying at baseline and absenteeism at follow-up was established across six prospective studies. Taken together, these findings clearly suggest a weak association between the variables. Still, in a study which examined associations between a range of psychosocial work factors and sickness absence in 31 European countries, workplace bullying was established as the strongest and most consistent predictor of absence (Niedhammer, Chastang, Sultan-Taieb, Vermeylen, & Parent-Thirion, 2013). In a prospective study comprising 925 female health and social workers in Norway, Aagestad and colleagues (2014) found that violence and threats of violence were the most important predictors of doctor-certified long-term sick leave, whereas exposure to workplace bullying had no impact on sick–leave. Hence, findings are mixed and more studies are needed in order to understand the relationship between exposure to aggression and absenteeism, preferably using register data on sick leave rather than self-report data in order to achieve objective assessments.

Conclusions

Despite some variations in their manifestations, the literature on various forms of workplace aggression, including workplace bullying which here has been given particular attention, establishes beyond doubt that a very considerable association exists between exposure to workplace aggression and negative outcomes for victims' health and well-being and their organizational functioning. However, as has been emphasized in this chapter, our current levels of insight and knowledge are based on a variety of research designs, each offering its own strengths and limitations. Above all, these approaches, whether considered on their own or in combination, demonstrate the complexity of the relationship between a variety of causal variables, workplace aggression and outcomes, acknowledging the presence of a number of plausible intervening variables, each of which potentially may mediate or moderate these relationships.

As observed in the literature, and welcomed by us, there appears to be a move away from an over-reliance on cross-sectional survey data and related problems associated with self-report biases, to a growing focus on, and drive to undertake prospective studies. Offering the prospect of helping disentangle the causal relationship between variables and their directionality, such studies can also assist us in better understanding issues associated with the intensity and duration of the experience of workplace aggression, on the one hand, and outcomes, on the other, including revealing new insights about possible reverse relationships between variables, by the use of repeated measurements and greater time-lag between measurement. In terms of individual outcomes of workplace aggression, we have emphasized the impact of self-labeling, thus revealing the importance of cognitive processes therein. In this respect and to better explain the complexity of the processes involved, we have repeatedly returned to the transactional model of stress, with its emphasis on the dynamics of individual cognition, the individual's coping resources and the organizational responses involved, including the role of social support.

To take our knowledge, and thus, implicitly, our ability to respond proactively to the problem of workplace aggression further, we particularly would like to advocate the application of a moderation–mediation framework whose research design allows us to test simultaneously "the why and when" of situations where workplace aggression is related to health and well-being. While we also would welcome greater use of experimental studies to enrich our understanding, we do recognize that the prospect of new insights may come up against ethical considerations and where such concerns exist they must take precedence and cannot be justified by reference to any gains established with hindsight. Above all, in exposing the often dire outcomes of workplace aggression for victims, the insights already gained should spur the research community to greater concerted effort to continue disclosing the missing pieces of the jigsaw. Equally, it should encourage employers to utilize existing knowledge to challenge the various forms of aggression in their midst, whether by way of preventative measures, through intervention when problems emerge or rehabilitation where damage to individuals and organizations is already done.

References

Aagestad, C., Tyssen, R., Johannessen, H. A., Gravseth, H. M., Tynes, T., & Sterud, T. (2014). Psychosocial and organizational risk factors for doctor-certified sick leave: A prospective study of female health and social workers in Norway. *BMC Public Health, 14,* 1016. doi:10.1186/1471-2458-14-1016

Abramson, L. Y., Alloy, L. B., & Metalsky, G. I. (1989). Hopelessness depression – a theory-based subtype of depression. *Psychological Review, 96*(2), 358–372. doi:10.1037//0033-295x.96.2.358

Abramson, L. Y., Garber, J., & Seligman, M. E. P. (1980). Learned helplessness in humans: An attributional analysis. In J. Garber & M. E. P. Seligman (Eds.), *Human helplessness. Theory and applications* (pp. 3–34). New York, NY: Academic Press, Inc.

Anderson, C. A., & Bushman, B. J. (2002). Human aggression. *Annual Review of Psychology, 53*(1), 27–51. doi:10.1146/annurev.psych.53.100901.135231

Aquino, K., Douglas, S., & Martinko, M. J. (2004). Overt anger in response to victimization: Attributional style and organizational norms as moderators. *Journal of Occupational Health Psychology, 9*(2), 152–164.

Aquino, K., & Thau, S. (2009). Workplace victimization: Aggression from the target's perspective. *Annual Review of Psychology, 60,* 717–741.

Bakker, A. B., & Demerouti, E. (2006). The job demands-resources model: State of the art. *Journal of Managerial Psychology, 22*(3), 309–328. doi:10.1108/02683940710733115

Balducci, C., Alfano, V., & Fraccaroli, F. (2009). Relationships between mobbing at work and MMPI-2 personality profile, post-traumatic stress symptoms, and suicidal ideation and behavior. *Violence and Victims, 24*(1), 52–67.

Barling, J., Dupré, K. E., & Kelloway, E. K. (2009). Predicting workplace aggression and violence. *Annual Review of Psychology, 60,* 671–692.

Baron, R. A., & Neuman, J. H. (1996). Workplace violence and workplace aggression: Evidence on their relative frequency and potential causes. 1996. *Aggressive Behavior, 22*(3), 161–173. doi:10.1002/(SICI)1098-2337(1996)22:3<161::AID-AB1>3.0.CO;2-Q

Baruch, Y. (2005). Bullying on the net: Adverse behavior on e-mail and its impact. *Information & Management, 42*(2), 361–371.

Beattie, L., & Griffin, B. (2014). Day-level fluctuations in stress and engagement in response to workplace incivility: A diary study. *Work & Stress, 28*(2), 124–142.

Berry, C. M., Ones, D. S., & Sackett, P. R. (2007). Interpersonal deviance, organizational deviance, and their common correlates: A review and meta-analysis. *Journal of Applied Psychology, 92*(2), 410–424.

Berthelsen, M., Skogstad, A., Lau, B., & Einarsen, S. (2011). Do they stay or do they go? A longitudinal study of intentions to leave and exclusion from working life among targets of workplace bullying. *International Journal of Manpower, 32*(2), 178–193. doi:10.1108/01437721111130198

Björkqvist, K., Österman, K., & Hjeltbäck, M. (1994). Aggression among university employees. *Aggressive Behavior, 20*(3), 173–184.

Bond, S. A., Tuckey, M. R., & Dollard, M. (2010). Psychosocial safety climate, workplace bullying, and symptoms of posttraumatic stress. *Organization Development Journal, 28*(1), 28–37.

Bowling, N. A., & Beehr, T. A. (2006). Workplace harassment from the victim's perspective: A theoretical model and meta analysis. *Journal of Applied Psychology, 91*(5), 998–1012.

Bradley, G. L., McColl-Kennedy, J. R., Sparks, B. A., Jimmieson, N. L., & Zapf, D. (2010). Service encounter needs theory: A dyadic, psychosocial approach to understanding service encounters. In W. J. Zerbe, C. E. J. Hartel, & N. M. Ashkanasy (Eds.), *Research on emotions in organizations. Volume 6. Emotions and creativity, learning, change and development* (pp. 231–259). Bingley, UK: Emerald Group Publishers/JAI.

Brodsky, C. M. (1976). *The harassed worker.* Toronto, Canada: Lexington Books.

Burton, J. P., & Hoobler, J. M. (2011). Aggressive reactions to abusive supervision: The role of interactional justice and narcissism. *Scandinavian Journal of Psychology, 52*(4), 389–398. doi:10.1111/j.1467-9450.2011.00886.x

Buss, A. H. (1961). *The psychology of aggression.* New York, NY: John Wiley and Sons, Inc.

Buss, D. M., & Shackelford, T. K. (1997). Human aggression in evolutionary psychological perspective. *Clinical Psychology Review, 17*(6), 605–619. doi:10.1016/S0272-7358(97)00037-8

Carver, C. S., Scheier, M. F., & Weintraub, J. K. (1989). Assessing coping strategies: A theoretically based approach. *Journal of Personality and Social Psychology, 56*(2), 267–283.

Casimir, G., McCormack, D., Djurkovic, N., & Nsubuga-Kyobe, A. (2012). Psychosomatic model of workplace bullying: Australian and Ugandan schoolteachers. *Employee Relations, 34*(4), 411–428. doi:10.1108/01425451211236841

Chen, P. Y., & Spector, P. E. (1992). Relationships of work stressors with aggression, withdrawal, theft and substance use – an exploratory-study. *Journal of Occupational and Organizational Psychology, 65*, 177–184.

Cortina, L. M., Magley, V. J., Williams, J. H., & Langhout, R. D. (2001). Incivility in the workplace: Incidence and impact. *Journal of Occupational Health Psychology, 6*(1), 64–80.

Cropanzano, R., Stein, J. H., & Nadisic, T. (2010). *Social justice and the experience of emotion.* New York, NY: Routledge.

Deery, S., Walsh, J., & Guest, D. (2011). Workplace aggression: The effects of harassment on job burnout and turnover intentions. *Work, Employment and Society, 25*(4), 742–759. doi:10.1177/0950017011419707

de Lange, A. H., Taris, T. W., Kompier, M. A. J., Houtman, I. L. D., & Bongers, P. M. (2005). Different mechanisms to explain the reversed effects of mental health on work characteristics. *Scandinavian Journal of Work Environment & Health, 31*(1), 3–14.

Djurkovic, N., McCormack, D., & Casimir, G. (2004). The physical and psychological effects of workplace bullying and their relationship to intention to leave: A test of the psychosomatic and disability hypotheses. *International Journal of Organization Theory and Behavior, 4*(4), 469–497.

Djurkovic, N., McCormack, D., & Casimir, G. (2006). Neuroticism and the psychosomatic model of workplace bullying. *Journal of Managerial Psychology, 21*(1), 73–88.

Djurkovic, N., McCormack, D., & Casimir, G. (2008). Workplace bullying and intention to leave: The moderating effect of perceived organisational support. *Human Resource Management Journal, 18*(4), 405–422. doi:10.1111/j.1748-8583.2008.00081.x

Dollard, J., Doob, L., Miller, N., Mowrer, O. H., & Sears, R. R. (1939). *Frustration and aggression.* New Haven, CT: Yale University Press.

Duffy, M. K., Ganster, D. C., & Pagon, M. (2002). Social undermining in the workplace. *Academy of Management Journal, 45*(2), 331–351. doi:10.2307/3069350

Einarsen, S. (2000). Harassment and bullying at work: A review of the Scandinavian approach. *Aggression and Violent Behavior, 5*(4), 379–401.

Einarsen, S., Hoel, H., & Notelaers, G. (2009). Measuring exposure to bullying and harassment at work: Validity, factor structure and psychometric properties of the Negative Acts Questionnaire-Revised. *Work and Stress, 23*(1), 24–44.

Einarsen, S., Hoel, H., Zapf, D., & Cooper, C. L. (2011). The concept of bullying and harassment at work: The European tradition. In S. Einarsen, H. Hoel, D. Zapf, & C. L. Cooper (Eds.), *Bullying and harassment in the workplace: Developments in theory, research, and practice* (2nd ed., pp. 3–40). Boca Raton, FL: CRC Press.

Einarsen, S., Matthiesen, S. B., & Skogstad, A. (1998). Bullying, burnout and well-being among assistant nurses. *Journal of Occupational Health and Safety, 14*(6), 563–568.

Einarsen, S., & Nielsen, M. B. (2014). Workplace bullying as an antecedent of mental health problems: A five-year prospective and representative study. *International Archives of Occupational and Environmental Health, 88*(2), 131–142.

Einarsen, S., & Raknes, B. I. (1997). Harassment in the workplace and the victimization of men. *Violence and Victims, 12*(3), 247–263.

Einarsen, S., & Skogstad, A. (1996). Bullying at work: Epidemiological findings in public and private organizations. *European Journal of Work and Organizational Psychology, 5*(2), 185–201.

Eisenberger, N. I., Lieberman, M. D., & Williams, K. D. (2003). Does rejection hurt? An fMRI study of social exclusion. *Science, 302*(5643), 290–292.

Escartin, J., Ceja, L., Navarro, J., & Zapf, D. (2013). Modeling workplace bullying behaviors using catastrophe theory. *Nonlinear Dynamics Psychology and Life Sciences, 17*(4), 493–515.

Escartin, J., Ullrich, J., Zapf, D., Schluter, E., & van Dick, R. (2013). Individual- and group-level effects of social identification on workplace bullying. *European Journal of Work and Organizational Psychology, 22*(2), 182–193.

Eurofound (2012). *Fifth European Working Conditions Survey.* Luxembourg: Publications Office of the European Union.

Felson, R. B. (1992). "Kick 'em when they're down": Explanations of the relationships between stress and interpersonal aggression and violence. *Sociological Quarterly, 33*(1), 1–16.

Finne, L. B., Knardahl, S., & Lau, B. (2011). Workplace bullying and mental distress – a prospective study of Norwegian employees. *Scandinavian Journal of Work, Environment and Health, 37*(4), 276–286.

Frese, M., & Zapf, D. (1994). Action as the core of work psychology: A German approach. *Handbook of industrial and organizational psychology* (vol. 4, 2nd edn., pp. 271–340). Palo Alto, CA: Consulting Psychologists Press, Inc.

Frone, M. R. (1999). Work stress and alcohol use. *Alcohol Research & Health, 23*(4), 284–291.

Geen, R. G. (2001). *Human aggression* (2nd edn.). New York, NY: Taylor & Francis.

Glambek, M., Matthiesen, S. B., Hetland, J., & Einarsen, S. (2014). Workplace bullying as an antecedent to job insecurity and intention to leave: A 6-month prospective study. *Human Resource Management Journal, 24*(3), 255–268.

Glomb, T. M., & Liao, H. (2003). Interpersonal aggression in work groups: Social influence, reciprocal, and individual effects. *Academy of Management Journal, 48*(4), 486–498.

Hansen, A. M., Høgh, A., Garde, A. H., & Persson, R. (2014). Workplace bullying and sleep difficulties: A 2-year follow-up study. *International Archives of Occupational and Environmental Health, 87*(3), 285–294. doi:10.1007/s00420-013-0860-2

Hansen, Å. M., Høgh, A., Persson, A., Karlson, B., Garde, A. H., & Ørbæk, P. (2006). Bullying at work, health outcomes, and physiological stress response. *Journal of Psychosomatic Research, 60*(1), 63–72.

Harvey, P., Stoner, J., Hochwarter, W., & Kacmar, C. (2007). Coping with abusive supervision: The neutralizing effects of ingratiation and positive affect on negative employee outcomes. *Leadership Quarterly, 18*(3), 264–280. doi:10.1016/j.leaqua.2007.03.008

Hauge, L. J., Skogstad, A., & Einarsen, S. (2010). The relative impact of workplace bullying as a social stressor at work. *Scandinavian Journal of Psychology, 51*(5), 426–433.

Hayes, A. F. (2013). *Introduction to mediation, moderation, and conditional process analyses. A regression-based approach.* New York, NY: Guilford Press.

Hershcovis, M. S. (2011). "Incivility, social undermining, bullying ... oh my!": A call to reconcile constructs within workplace aggression research. *Journal of Organizational Behavior, 32*(3), 499–519. doi:10.1002/Job.689

Hershcovis, M. S., & Reich, T. C. (2013). Integrating workplace aggression research: Relational, contextual, and method considerations. *Journal of Organizational Behavior, 34*(S1), S26–S42. doi:10.1002/Job.1886

Hitlan, R. T., Cliffton, R. J., & DeSoto, M. C. (2006). Perceived exclusion in the workplace: The moderating effects of gender on work-related attitudes and psychological health. *North American Journal of Psychology, 8*(2), 217–236.

Hoel, H., Faragher, B., & Cooper, C. L. (2004). Bullying is detrimental to health, but all bullying behaviours are not necessarily equally damaging. *British Journal of Guidance and Counselling, 32*(3), 368–387.

Hofstede, G. H. (2001). *Culture's consequences: Comparing values, behaviors, institutions, and organizations across nations* (2nd edn.). London, UK: Sage.

Hoobler, J. M., & Hu, J. (2013). A model of injustice, abusive supervision, and negative affect. *Leadership Quarterly, 24*(1), 256–269. doi:10.1016/j.leaqua.2012.11.005

Hoobler, J. M., Rospenda, K. M., Lemmon, G., & Rosa, J. A. (2010). A within-subject longitudinal study of the effects of positive job experiences and generalized workplace harassment on well-being. *Journal of Occupational Health Psychology, 15*(4), 434–451. doi:10.1037/A0021000

Høgh, A., Borg, V., & Mikkelsen, K. L. (2003). Work-related violence as a predictor of fatigue: A 5-year follow-up of the Danish Work Environment Cohort Study. *Work & Stress, 17*(2), 182–194.

Høgh, A., Hoel, H., & Carneiro, I. G. (2011). Bullying and employee turnover among healthcare workers: A three-wave prospective study. *Journal of Nursing Management, 19*(6), 742–751.

Jahoda, M. (1981). Work, employment, and unemployment: Values, theories, and approaches in social research. *American Psychologist, 36*(2), 184–191. doi:10.1037/0003-066X.36.2.184

Judge, T. A., Locke, E. A., Durham, C. C., & Kluger, A. N. (1998). Dispositional effects on job and life satisfaction: The role of core evaluations. *Journal of Applied Psychology, 83*(1), 17–34. doi:10.1037//0021-9010.83.1.17

Kääriä, S., Laaksonen, M., Rahkonen, O., Lahelma, E., & Leino-Arjaas, P. (2012). Risk factors of chronic neck pain: A prospective study among middle-aged employees. *Eur J Pain, 16*(6). doi:10.1002/j.1532-2149.2011.00065.x

Kahn, R. L., & Byosiere, P. (1992). Stress in organizations. In M. D. Dunnette & L. M. Hough (Eds.), *Handbook of industrial and organizational psychology* (vol. 3, 2nd edn., pp. 571–650). Palo Alto, CA: Consulting Psychologists Press, Inc.

Keashly, L. (1998). Emotional abuse in the workplace: Conceptual and empirical issues. *Journal of Emotional Abuse, 1*(1), 85–117.

Kivimäki, M., Leino-Arjas, P., Virtanen, M., Elovainio, M., Keltikangas-Järvinen, L., Puttonen, S., . . . Vathera, J. (2004). Work stress and incidence of newly diagnosed fibromyalgia: Prospective cohort study. *Journal of Psychosomatic Research, 57*(5), 417–422.

Lahelma, E., Lallukka, T., Laaksonen, M., Saastamoinen, P., & Rahkonen, O. (2012). Workplace bullying and common mental disorders: A follow-up study. *Journal of Epidemiology and Community Health, 66*(6), e3. doi:10.1136/jech.2010.115212

Law, R., Dollard, M. F., Tuckey, M. R., & Dormann, C. (2011). Psychosocial safety climate as a lead indicator of workplace bullying and harassment, job resources, psychological health and employee engagement. *Accident Analysis and Prevention, 43*(5), 1782–1793. doi:10.1016/j.aap.2011.04.010

Lazarus, R. S., & Folkman, S. (1984). *Stress, appraisal and coping.* New York, NY: Springer.

Lee, R. T., & Brotheridge, C. M. (2006). When prey turns predatory: Workplace bullying as a predictor of counteraggression/bullying, coping, and well-being. *European Journal of Work and Organizational Psychology, 15*(33), 352–377.

Leymann, H. (1990). Mobbing and psychological terror at workplaces. *Violence and Victims, 5*(2), 119–126.

Leymann, H., & Gustafsson, A. (1996). Mobbing at work and the development of post-traumatic stress disorders. *European Journal of Work and Organizational Psychology, 5*(2), 251–275.

Lim, S., Cortina, L. M., & Magley, V. J. (2008). Personal and workgroup incivility: Impact on work and health outcomes. *Journal of Applied Psychology, 93*(1), 95–107. doi:10.1037/0021-9010.93.1.95

Matthiesen, S. B., & Einarsen, S. (2004). Psychiatric distress and symptoms of PTSD among victims of bullying at work. *British Journal of Guidance and Counselling, 32*(3), 335–356.

Mikkelsen, E. G., & Einarsen, S. (2002a). Basic assumptions and symptoms of post-traumatic stress among victims of bullying at work. *European Journal of Work and Organizational Psychology, 11*(1), 87–11.

Mikkelsen, E. G., & Einarsen, S. (2002b). Relationship between exposure to bullying at work and psychological and psychosomatic health complaints: The role of state negative affectivity and generalized self-efficacy. *Scandinavian Journal of Psychology, 43*(5), 397–405.

Miner-Rubino, K., & Reed, W. D. (2010). Testing a moderated mediational model of workgroup incivility: The roles of organizational trust and group regard. *Journal of Applied Social Psychology, 40*(12), 3148–3168. doi:10.1111/j.1559-1816.2010.00695.x

Mitchell, M. S., & Ambrose, M. L. (2007). Abusive supervision and workplace deviance and the moderating effects of negative reciprocity beliefs. *Journal of Applied Psychology, 92*(4), 1159–1168. doi:10.1037/0021-9010.92.4.1159

Moreno-Jiménez, B., Rodríguez-Muñoz, A., Moreno, Y., & Carrosa, E. (2007). The moderating role of assertiveness and social anxiety in workplace bullying: Two empirical studies. *Psychology in Spain, 11*(1), 85–94.

Neall, A. M., & Tuckey, M. R. (2014). A methodological review of research on the antecedents and consequences of workplace harassment. *Journal of Occupational and Organizational Psychology, 87*(2), 225–257.

Neuman, J. H., & Baron, R. M. (2005). Aggression in the workplace: A social-psychological perspective. In S. Fox & P. E. Spector (Eds.), *Counterproductive behavior. Investigations of actors and targets*. Washington, DC: American Psychological Association.

Neuman, J. H., & Baron, R. M. (2011). Social antecedents of bullying: A social interactionist perspective. In S. Einarsen, H. Hoel, D. Zapf, & C. L. Cooper (Eds.), *Bullying and harassment in the workplace. Developments in theory, research, and practice* (2nd edn., pp. 201–225). Boca Raton, FL: CRC Press.

Niedhammer, I., Chastang, J. F., Sultan-Taieb, H., Vermeylen, G., & Parent-Thirion, A. (2013). Psychosocial work factors and sickness absence in 31 countries in Europe. *European Journal of Public Health 23*(4), 622–629. doi:10.1093/eurpub/cks124

Niedhammer, I., David, S., Degioanni, S., Drummond, A., Philip, P., & Phys, O. (2009). Workplace bullying and sleep disturbances: Finding's from a large scale cross-sectional survey in the French working population. *Sleep, 32*(9), 1211–1219.

Nielsen, M. B., & Einarsen, S. (2008). Sampling in research on interpersonal aggression. *Aggressive Behavior, 34*(3), 265–272.

Nielsen, M. B., & Einarsen, S. (2012). Outcomes of workplace bullying: A meta-analytic review. *Work and Stress, 26*(4), 309–332.

Nielsen, M. B., Glasø, L., Matthiesen, S. B., Eid, J., & Einarsen, S. (2013). Bullying and risk-perception as health hazards on oil rigs. *Journal of Managerial Psychology, 28*(4), 367–383.

Nielsen, M. B., Hetland, J., Matthiesen, S. B., & Einarsen, S. (2012). Longitudinal relationships between workplace bullying and psychological distress. *Scandinavian Journal of Work, Environment, and Health, 38*(1), 38–46. doi:10.5271/sjweh.3178

Nielsen, M. B., & Knardahl, S. (2014). Is workplace bullying related to the personality traits of victims? A two year prospective study. *Work & Stress, 29*(2). doi:10.1080/02678373.2015.1032383

Nielsen, M. B., Magerøy, N., Gjerstad, J., & Einarsen, S. (2014). Workplace bullying and subsequent health problems. *Journal for the Norwegian Medical Association, 134*(12/13), 1233–1238. doi:10.4045/tidsskr.13.0880

Nielsen, M. B., Matthiesen, S. B., & Einarsen, S. (2008). Sense of coherence as a protective mechanism among targets of workplace bullying. *Journal of Occupational Health Psychology, 13*(2), 128–136.

Nielsen, M. B., Matthiesen, S. B., & Einarsen, S. (2010). The impact of methodological moderators on prevalence rates of workplace bullying. A meta-analysis. *Journal of Occupational and Organizational Psychology, 83*(4), 955–979. doi:10.1348/096317909x481256

Nielsen, M. B., Tvedt, S. D., & Matthiesen, S. B. (2012). Prevalence and occupational predictors of psychological distress in the offshore petroleum industry: A prospective study. *International Archives of Occupational and Environmental Health, 86*(8), 87–85. doi:10.1007/s00420-012-0825-x

Olweus, D. (1993). *Bullying at schools: What we know and what we can do.* Oxford, UK: Blackwell.

Ortega, A., Christensen, K. B., Høgh, A., Rugulies, R., & Borg, V. (2011). One-year prospective study on the effect of workplace bullying on long-term sickness absence. *Journal of Nursing Management, 19*(6), 752–759. doi:10.1111/j.1365-2834.2010.01179.x

Penney, L. M., & Spector, P. E. (2005). Job stress, incivility, and counterproductive work behavior (CWB): The moderating role of negative affectivity. *Journal of Organizational Behavior, 26*(7), 777–796. doi:10.1002/Job.336

Peterson, C., & Seligman, M. E. P. (1984). Causal explanations as a risk factor for depression: Theory and evidence. *Psychological Review, 91*(3), 347–374.

Quine, L. (1999). Workplace bullying in NHS community trust: Staff questionnaire survey. *BMJ, 318*, 228–232.

Rodríguez-Muñoz, A., Notelaers, G., & Moreno-Jiménez, B. (2011). Workplace bullying and sleep quality: The mediating role of worry and need for recovery. *Behavioral Psychology-Psicologia Conductual, 19*(2), 453–468.

Rugulies, R., Madsen, I. E. H., Hjarsbech, P. U., Høgh, A., Borg, V., Carneiro, I. G., & Aust, B. (2012). Bullying at work and onset of a major depressive episode among Danish female eldercare workers. *Scandinavian Journal of Work Environment & Health, 38*(3), 218–227. doi:10.5271/Sjweh.3278

Salin, D., & Hoel, H. (2011). Organisational causes of workplace bullying. In S. Einarsen, H. Hoel, D. Zapf & C. L. Cooper (Eds.), *Bullying and harassment in the workplace. Developments in theory, research, and practice* (2nd edn., pp. 227–243). Boca Raton, FL: CRC Press.

Schat, A. C. H., & Frone, M. R. (2011). Exposure to psychological aggression at work and job performance: The mediating role of job attitudes and personal health. *Work & Stress, 25*(1), 23–40. doi:10.1080/02678373.2011.563133

Schat, A. C. H., Frone, M. R., & Kelloway, E. K. (2006). Prevalence of workplace aggression in the U.S. workforce: Findings from a national study. In E. K. Kelloway, J. Barling, & J. J. Hurrell (Eds.), *Handbook of workplace violence* (pp. 47–89). Thousand Oaks, CA: Sage.

Schat, A. C. H., & Kelloway, E. K. (2000). Effects of perceived control on the outcomes of workplace aggression and violence. *Journal of Occupational Health Psychology, 5*(3), 386–402. doi:10.1037/1076-8998.5.3.386

Schat, A. C. H., & Kelloway, E. K. (2003). Reducing the adverse consequences of workplace aggression and violence: The buffering effects of organizational support. *Journal of Occupational Health Psychology, 8*(2), 110–122. doi:10.1037/1076-8998.8.2.110

Schat, A. C. H., & Kelloway, E. K. (2005). Workplace aggression. In J. Barling, M. R. Frone, & E. K. Kelloway (Eds.), *Handbook of work stress* (pp. 189–218). Thousand Oaks, CA: Sage.

Schwickerath, J. (2009). *Mobbing am Arbeitsplatz: Stationäre Verhaltenstherapie von Patienten mit Mobbingerfahrungen. [Bullying at the workplace: Inpatient treatment of patients with bullying experiences].* Lengerich, Germany: Pabst Science.

Semmer, N. K., & Beehr, T. A. (2014). Job control and social aspects of work. In M. Peeters, J. de Jonge, & T. Taris (Eds.), *An introduction to contemporary work psychology* (pp. 171–195). Oxford, UK: Wiley-Blackwell.

Semmer, N. K., & Meier, L. L. (2009). Individual differences, work stress, and health. In C. L. Cooper, J. Campbell Quick, & M. J. Schabracq (Eds.), *International handbook of work and health psychology* (3rd edn., pp. 99–121). Chichester, UK: John Wiley and Sons, Ltd.

Spector, P. E., & Fox, S. (2005). The stressor-emotion model of counterproductive work behavior. In S. Fox & P. E. Spector (Eds.), *Counterproductive behavior. Investigations of actors and targets.* Washington, DC: American Psychological Association.

Spector, P. E., & Jex, S. M. (1998). Development of four self-report measures of job stressors and strain: Interpersonal Conflict at Work Scale, Organizational Constraints Scale, Quantitative Workload Inventory and Physical Symptoms Inventory. *Journal of Occupational and Organizational Psychology, 3*(4), 356–367.

Suadicani, P., Olesen, K., Bonde, J. P., & Gyntelberg, F. (2014). Psychosocial work conditions associated with sickness absence among hospital employees. *Occupational Medicine, 64*(7), 503–508. doi:10.1093/occmed/kqu064

Tedeschi, J. T., & Felson, R. B. (1994). *Violence, aggression, and coercive actions.* Washington, DC: American Psychological Association.

Tepper, B. J. (2000). Consequences of abusive supervision. *Academy of Management Journal, 43*(2), 178–190.

Tepper, B. J. (2001). Health consequences of organizational injustice: Tests of main and interactive effects. *Organizational Behavior and Human Decision Processes, 86*(2), 197–215.

Tepper, B. J. (2007). Abusive supervision in work organizations: Review synthesis, and research agenda. *Journal of Management, 33*(3), 261–289.

Tepper, B. J., Duffy, M. K., Henle, C. A., & Lambert, L. S. (2006). Procedural injustice, victim precipitation, and abusive supervision. *Personnel Psychology, 59*(1), 101–123.

Tepper, B. J., Duffy, M. K., & Shaw, J. D. (2001). Personality moderators of the relationship between abusive supervision and subordinates' resistance. *Journal of Applied Psychology, 86*(5), 974–983.

Tepper, B. J., & Henle, C. A. (2011). A case for recognizing distinctions among constructs that capture interpersonal mistreatment in work organizations. *Journal of Organizational Behavior, 32*(3), 487–498. doi:10.1002/Job.688

Tuckey, M. R., & Neall, A. M. (2014). Workplace bullying erodes job and personal resources: Between- and within-person perspectives. *Journal of Occupational Health Psychology, 19*(4), 413–424. doi:10.1037/a0037728

Tynes, T., Johannessen, H. A., & Sterud, T. (2013). Work-related psychosocial and organizational risk factors for headache: A 3-year follow-up study of the general working population in Norway. *Journal of Occupational and Environmental Medicine, 55*(12), 1436–1442. doi:10.1097/JOM.0b013e3182a7e678

van Beest, I., & Williams, K. D. (2006). When inclusion costs and ostracism pays, ostracism still hurts. *Journal of Personality and Social Psychology, 91*(5), 918–928. doi:10.1037/0022-3514.91.5.918

Vie, T. L., Glasø, L., & Einarsen, S. (2010). Does trait anger, trait anxiety or organisational position moderate the relationship between exposure to negative acts and self-labelling as a victim of workplace bullying? *Nordic Psychology, 62*(3), 67–79. doi:10.1027/1901-2276/A000017

Vie, T. L., Glasø, L., & Einarsen, S. (2011). Health outcomes and self-labeling as a victim of workplace bullying. *Journal of Psychosomatic Research, 70*(1), 37–43. doi:10.1016/j.jpsychores.2010.06.007

Vie, T. L., Glasø, L., & Einarsen, S. (2012). How does it feel? Workplace bullying, emotions and musculoskeletal complaints. *Scandinavian Journal of Psychology, 53*(2), 165–173. doi:10.1111/j.1467-9450.2011.00932.x

Wang, W., Mao, J., Wu, W., & Liu, J. (2012). Abusive supervision and workplace deviance: The mediating role of interactional justice and the moderating role of power distance. *Asia Pacific Journal of Human Resources, 50*(1), 43–60.

Wheeler, A. R., Halbesleben, J. R. B., & Whitman, M. V. (2013). The interactive effects of abusive supervision and entitlement on emotional exhaustion and co-worker abuse. *Journal of Occupational and Organizational Psychology, 86*(4), 477–496.

Williams, K. D. (1997). Social ostracism. In R. M. Kowalski (Ed.), *Aversive interpersonal behaviors* (pp. 133–170). New York, NY: Plenum.

Williams, K. D. (2007). Ostracism. *Annual Review of Psychology, 58,* 425–452.

Williams, K. D., & Jarvis, B. (2006). Cyberball: A program for use in research on interpersonal ostracism and acceptance. *Behavior Research Methods, 38*(1), 174–180. doi:10.3758/BF03192765

Williams, K. D., & Sommer, K. L. (1997). Social ostracism by coworkers: Does rejection lead to loafing or compensation? *Personality and Social Psychological Bulletin, 23*(7), 693–706.

Winstanley, S., & Whittington, R. (2002). Anxiety, burnout and coping styles in general hospital staff exposed to workplace aggression: A cyclical model of burnout and vulnerability to aggression. *Work & Stress, 16*(4), 302–315.

Zapf, D., Dormann, C., & Frese, M. (1996). Longitudinal studies in organizational stress research: A review of literature with reference to methodological issues. *Journal of Occupational Health Psychology, 1*(2), 145–169.

Zapf, D., & Einarsen, S. (2005). Mobbing at work: Escalated conflicts in organizations. In S. Fox & P. E. Spector (Eds.), *Counterproductive behavior. Investigations of actors and targets.* Washington, DC: American Psychological Association.

Zapf, D., & Gross, C. (2001). Conflict escalation and coping with workplace bullying: A replication and extension. *European Journal of Work and Organizational Psychology, 10*(4), 497–522.

Zapf, D., Knorz, C., & Kulla, M. (1996). On the relationship between mobbing factors, and job content, social work environment, and health outcomes. *European Journal of Work and Organizational Psychology, 5*(2), 215–238.

11

Proactivity for Mental Health and Well-Being

Francesco Cangiano and Sharon K. Parker

Introduction

Proactive behaviors are self-initiated and future oriented actions that employees take to change and improve themselves or their work environment (Parker, Williams, & Turner, 2006). Being proactive can occur in several domains: for example, by anticipating problems and implementing ideas to prevent them from occurring (Crant, 2000; Frese & Fay, 2001), or by actively seeking feedback from others about one's performance (Ashford, 1986). Recent developments in the context of work have heightened the importance of proactive behavior (Grant, Parker, & Collins, 2009). First, the environment in which organizations operate has become increasingly complex and uncertain. Therefore, employees and managers need to use their own initiative to determine what needs to be done in a given situation (Griffin, Neal, & Parker, 2007). Second, high levels of competition require greater capacity to innovate in order to create competitive advantage (Crant, 2000). Proactivity is an important element of innovation (Unsworth & Parker, 2008). Third, career structures are becoming more unpredictable and flexible, requiring employees to be self-directed and to take charge of their careers (Parker & Collins, 2010). Proactivity is thus a driving force for individual creativity, innovation, adaptability, and flexibility, and hence is crucial for organizations' success.

Because of its importance, research on proactivity at work has primarily focused on the personal and environmental factors that facilitate the onset of proactive behavior. We will briefly review this literature in the current chapter. However, to date there has been little attention given to how engaging in proactivity affects employees' health and well-being, which is our core focus in this chapter. Specifically, we consider how proactivity affects employee well-being and mental health, as well as physical health via stress-related processes. Although proactive behavior might also affect individuals' physical health directly via

The Wiley Blackwell Handbook of the Psychology of Occupational Safety and Workplace Health, First Edition. Edited by Sharon Clarke, Tahira M. Probst, Frank Guldenmund, and Jonathan Passmore. © 2016 John Wiley & Sons Ltd. Published 2020 by John Wiley & Sons Ltd.

influencing occupational safety (Didla, Mearns, & Flin, 2009), our focus here is on well-being and health. For example, questions we consider include: Does being proactive help to fulfill psychological needs, eliciting feelings of competence and autonomy, and thereby promoting well-being? Do the obstacles and resistance faced when engaging in proactivity create feelings of stress? Can proactivity be considered as a resource for employee well-being? Are there factors that mitigate the effect of proactivity on well-being and mental health? Ultimately we propose that proactivity is likely to affect mental health and well-being in multiple ways, and that moderating variables and mediating processes need to be considered.

In the first section of this chapter, we provide a brief overview of research on proactivity, with a particular emphasis on its motivational underpinnings. As we elaborate later, understanding motivation is crucial for exploring the well-being outcomes of proactive behavior. In the second section of the chapter, we introduce our overall model of the effects that proactivity might have on mental health and well-being. In the subsequent sections, we unpack this model. Drawing upon self-determination theory, as well as the broaden-and-build theory of emotions, in the third section we describe how being proactive at work might invigorate employees' well-being and/or prevent stress in the workplace. As part of this discussion, we review previous research that has looked at the interplay between related positive work behaviors (such as contextual performance) and health and well-being (Greguras & Diefendorff, 2010). We also consider how self-directed actions in the workplace have the potential to fuel one's self-confidence at work. However, factors beyond the immediate control of the individual need to be considered when looking at the consequences of proactive behavior.

In the fourth section we introduce the resource-depletion pathway of proactivity, and discuss when and how proactive behavior might be detrimental to employees' mental health and well-being. In section five, we examine the key role of feedback from peers and supervisors in moderating the proactivity/well-being relationship. Specifically, we investigate how receiving negative feedback can thwart needs satisfaction, undermine self-efficacy, and generate negative emotional reactions, thereby reducing the positive consequences of proactivity for well-being and mental health. In section six we discuss how motivations under which proactivity is performed can moderate its effects of well-being. For example, we suggest that controlled forms of proactivity will be more consuming of personal resources and hence might harm individuals' well-being.

In the final section, we suggest practical implications for managers and practitioners of this research, such as how to create a work environment that encourages proactive behavior that is good for mental health, as well as key areas and theoretical issues that need to be addressed in future research.

Proactive Behavior: A Brief Review

Although the term proactivity has been applied to a multitude of organizational behaviors across different topic domains, research has identified two core aspects that define any particular behavior as proactive. First, proactive behavior is anticipatory: it involves thinking ahead about a future situation to prevent future problems or make the most of forthcoming opportunities. The second defining element of proactivity is that it involves taking control of a situation (or an anticipated situation) by initiating change. Thus, anticipating thinking and taking control of the situation are key features of proactivity (Parker et al., 2006). Inherent in both these elements is self-initiation. That is, scholars tend to agree that proactivity is self-starting behavior in which the individual him or herself initiates action, rather than being directed to act. For instance, following instructions to improve a work procedure does not constitute proactivity, whereas self-initiating the implementation of solutions to problems is proactive.

Proactivity has been distinguished from less future-focused and change-oriented behaviors such as core job performance, also referred to as job proficiency, and even adaptivity, which is concerned with adapting to change, rather than initiating it (Griffin et al., 2007). For example, from a performance perspective, employees are considered proficient on a given task based on the extent to which they are able to meet formalized requirements, implying clear standards against which performance can be assessed. Given its self-initiated nature, proactive behavior cannot be easily assessed against standards and indicators (Parker & Collins, 2010). Similarly, proactive career behavior is distinct from other forms of career behavior that are less self-initiated. For example, proactive feedback seeking is distinct from receiving feedback insofar as the former involves actively seeking out feedback rather than waiting for feedback to be given by someone else (Ashford & Cummings, 1985).

Importantly, in contrast to the idea that proactivity is a type of extra-role behavior, the perspective we adopt here is that all kinds of work behavior (e.g., task, extra-role, citizenship, safety) can be carried out more or less proactively (Griffin et al., 2007). For example, an individual can help another individual in a way that is proactive (e.g., anticipating that an individual might need help, and offering this support to them) or that is relatively passive (e.g., an individual might help another when requested). From this perspective, proactivity is a way of behaving, rather than a particular set of behaviors. Taking this perspective further, some scholars (Parker et al., 2012) have argued that proactivity is a process that includes the generation of a proactive goal (envisioning, planning) and then striving for that goal (enacting, reflection).

Distal Antecedents of Proactivity

Unsurprisingly, given the importance of proactive behavior in the workplace, efforts have been made to understand what kind of environment encourages proactivity, and which people are more likely to engage in such behavior (Parker et al., 2006). Among the environmental antecedents of proactivity, previous studies have reported autonomy and coworker trust to be significantly associated with proactivity at work. According to Parker (1998), autonomy stimulates proactivity because it allows people to master new tasks and to take on board greater responsibilities, thereby enhancing employees' self-efficacy, which is an important motivational driver of proactivity (Parker, Bindl, & Strauss, 2010). Job control also facilitates the development of more flexible role orientations in which individuals define their responsibilities broadly, which is a further motivational driver of proactive behavior (Parker, 2000; Parker, Wall, & Jackson, 1997). Research on leadership as an antecedent of proactivity has to date yielded somewhat inconsistent results (Frese & Fay, 2001; Parker & Wu, 2014), suggesting this is a complex relationship. In a recent review, Parker and Wu (2014) proposed multiple pathways through which team-oriented (e.g., transformational leadership) and person-oriented leadership inputs (leader–member exchange) can foster proactivity. For instance, leaders can enhance followers' self-efficacy by supplying them with opportunities to experience feelings of mastery at work (Bandura, 1982, 1986), and leaders can shape the work climate and the work design, which in turn can affect employees' likelihood of behaving proactively (e.g., see Parker et al., 2006).

Regarding personal differences, analyses suggest that some individuals are simply predisposed to be proactive. In this regard, the term proactive personality is generally referred to as the tendency to take action in order to influence one's environment (Bateman & Crant, 1993). Empirical evidence reports that individuals high in proactive personality tend to perform better (Thompson, 2005), have a successful career (Van Dyne & LePine, 1998), and be more creative and innovative (Parker et al., 2006). Thus, it seems that proactive personality, via its effect on proactive behavior, yields several individual and organizational positive outcomes (Zhang, Wang, & Shi, 2012). Other individual differences that predict proactive behavior include learning goal orientation (Sonnentag, 2003), consideration of future consequences (Grant et al., 2009), and need for cognition (Wu, Parker, & de Jong, 2011).

Motivational Underpinnings of Proactive Behavior

Proactivity, with its focus on change, often involves challenging the status quo, so it can be risky to one's image. In addition, proactive behavior can consume a great deal of time, effort, and resources (Bolino, Valcea, & Harvey, 2010). Why then do employees engage in proactive behavior? This is an important question for the current chapter because, as we elaborate shortly, understanding the motivational underpinnings of proactivity will help to unpack its impact on well-being. Parker et al. (2010) proposed a model of proactive motivation in which three key motivational states that prompt and sustain proactivity were identified: can do, reason to, and energized to.

"Can do" motivation

A "*can do*" motivational state includes self-efficacy perceptions (e.g., can I do it?), feasibility appraisals and attributions (e.g., is it attainable?), and the perceived costs associated with the proposed action (e.g., is it risky?). The concept of self-efficacy, originally introduced by Bandura in 1977, is commonly referred to as an individual's confidence about his or her ability to engage in and successfully complete a particular task. Self-efficacy is, therefore, a self-judgment about what one can do, regardless of one's objective skills and abilities (Bandura, 1986).

Self-efficacy perceptions are especially important because proactivity often entails potential psychological risk (Parker et al., 2010) and requires high levels of persistence (Frese & Fay, 2001). Many studies support the importance of self-efficacy perceptions for enhancing proactivity (Frese & Fay, 2001; Parker, 1998; Parker et al., 2006).

"Reason to" motivation

A "reason to" motivation recognizes that people need a motive, or reason, to engage in proactive behavior. Parker et al. (2010) underlined the importance of internalized (or autonomous) motivation as stimulating proactivity, such as feelings of positive affect or engagement, intrinsic motivation/ interest, meaningfulness, flow, and identified motivation. These authors also highlighted the importance of individuals having a personal sense of responsibility. For example, a more flexible role orientation, or feeling ownership for issues and goals beyond one's prescribed tasks (Parker, 2000; Parker et al., 1997), predicts proactive work behavior (Parker et al., 2006).

One important motive for engaging in proactivity is to experience feelings of competence, autonomy, and relatedness. This idea stems from self-determination theory

(Ryan & Deci, 2000). According to self-determination theory, there are three basic and innate psychological needs that are the basis of intrinsically motivated behavior (Ryan & Deci, 2000): the need for competence, autonomy, and relatedness. Deci and Ryan maintain that fulfillment of these needs is essential for human well-being; an assertion that is supported by many studies (2002). Fay and Sonnentag (2012) showed that these basic psychological needs might be a driving force for proactivity. They argued that "proactive behavior is a means to positively influence one's level of experienced competence" (p. 77). This hypothesis was tested in an experience-sampling study with 52 employees. An analysis of within-subject fluctuations in daily proactivity across five working days showed that low self-reports of experienced competence during core tasks predicted a subsequent increase in time spent on proactive behavior. As a result, Fay and Sonnentag's (2012) study seems to corroborate the idea that proactive goals are often challenging, and thus serve to fulfill employees' need to experience competence at work.

"Energized to" motivation

The "*energized to*" motivation is the most affect-related motivational state of proactivity. Parker et al. (2010) proposed that activated positive affect will stimulate proactivity inasmuch as positive affect and vitality help broaden action-thought repertoires (Fredrickson, 2001) and activate approach-action tendencies (Seo, Barrett, & Bartunek, 2004). Bindl, Parker, Totterdell, and Hagger-Johnson (2012) found evidence to support this prediction that positive affect was important in predicting the "envisioning" of proactive goals, as well as their implementation. Additionally, a diary study by Fritz and Sonnentag (2009) showed that positive energized feelings promote taking charge behaviors, and a study by Hahn, Frese, Binnewies, and Schmitt (2012) showed that vigor is an important predictor of personal initiative among business owners.

Related to the "energized to" pathway is the role of engagement in stimulating proactivity. Engagement refers to "a positive, fulfilling, work-related state of mind that is characterized by vigour, dedication and absorption" (Schaufeli, Salanova, González-Romá, & Bakker, 2002, p. 74). Salanova and Schaufeli (2008) showed that workers provided with adequate resources (i.e., job control, feedback, and task variety) were more prone to experience engagement and involvement in their job, which in turn translated into higher levels of proactive behavior (for a review, see Bakker & Demerouti, 2008). In a similar vein, scholars have investigated how positive well-being might promote proactivity. Sonnentag (2003) showed that day-level recovery during off-work time was associated with increased engagement and proactive behavior in the following day. Consistent with Hockey (2000), this suggests that employees are less inclined to invest extra effort when they feel insufficiently recovered. Conversely, when feeling recovered, people are more likely to fully immerse in their job and be more engaged, which in turns increases their likelihood to be proactive at work.

Just as motivation drives proactivity, motivation is also a potential outcome of proactivity, in a dynamic and reciprocal relationship. For example, individuals engage in proactivity when they have self-efficacy, but being proactive might also build self-efficacy. Likewise, while the desire for flow (i.e., a mental state of full immersion, involvement, and enjoyment in the activity) might prompt proactivity, being proactive might then promote flow experiences by yielding a better match between personal skills and task challenges (Csikszentmihalyi, 2000). We discuss these ways in which motivation might be an outcome of proactivity in the next section.

Mental Health and Well-being Outcomes of Proactivity

Many studies have highlighted the positive consequences of proactivity. In a field study, Van Dyne and LePine (1998) reported that employees engaging in voice behavior were rated more favorably in terms of performance by supervisors six months later. In a similar manner, Grant et al. (2009) indicated that individuals displaying high levels of proactive behavior were given better performance ratings by their supervisors, especially when employees had a high prosocial motivation and low negative affect. Thompson (2005) conducted a study on 126 employee-supervisor dyads and suggested that the relationship between proactive personality and job performance might be mediated by proactive behaviors like personal initiative and network building. In a meta-analysis, Fuller and Marler (2009) found positive relationships between proactive personality and supervisor-rated job performance, and added that such an effect on performance "is stronger than that reported for any of the Big Five factors or the Big Five collectively" (p. 329).

However, the benefits of proactive behavior are not confined to superior performance alone. Greenglass and Fiksenbaum (2009) reported that individuals engaging in proactive coping were more likely to have lower absenteeism, and this relationship was mediated by greater levels of positive affect. Research also suggests that proactive individuals are more prone to feel satisfied about their jobs (Wanberg & Kammeyer-Mueller, 2000) and have a more successful career (Blickle, Witzki, & Schneider, 2009). There is thus some evidence of personal benefits from proactivity. Nevertheless, the health and well-being consequences of proactivity need more attention.

It is possible, for example, that an individual might be promoted more rapidly because of their proactivity, but still experience higher levels of psychological strain as a result. Over the past few years different perspectives are arising as to how proactivity may impact on well-being and mental health (Bolino et al., 2010). One crucial issue is whether proactive behavior is beneficial for health and well-being (in a win-win situation), or if its positive effects on organizational performance tend to backfire on employees' well-being. The few articles that have examined this question have held rather different (if not opposite) views on this matter.

We seek to help move this literature forward by proposing a model of the effect of proactivity on mental health and well-being (see Figure 11.1). First, in understanding

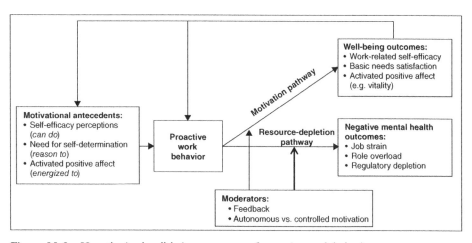

Figure 11.1 Hypothesized well-being outcomes of proactive work behaviour.

the effect of proactivity on well-being and mental health, we suggest it is important to distinguish short-term and more momentary effects from longer-term consequences. While long-term consequences over several years might be hypothesized, our focus in this chapter is to illustrate the shorter term well-being outcomes of proactivity, such as those associated with a particular proactive episode. Second, we propose two potential pathways. The motivation pathway identifies desirable consequences of proactivity and the way in which being proactive at work can boost self-efficacy perceptions, a sense of self-determination, and activated positive affect (e.g., vitality), which in turn can fuel further proactivity. The resource-depletion pathway, in contrast, illustrates how proactive behaviors might in some situations backfire on employee well-being by depleting resources, generating job strain, and role overload (see also Taris & Schaufeli, Chapter 8, this volume). We argue that whether proactivity enhances in a beneficial way, or is detrimental to, well-being is dependent on two key moderators: the type of feedback resulting from proactive behaviors, and one's motivations to be proactive.

Well-being and Mental Health Outcomes of Proactive Behavior: Motivation Pathway

As previously discussed, activated positive affect is a powerful propellant for proactivity (Bindl et al., 2012; Hahn et al., 2012). Scholars have further suggested that such a relationship might be mutual, creating a positive spiral wherein, for example, experiencing vitality and positive affect fuels proactivity, which in turn generates more vitality (Strauss & Parker, 2014a). Successful attempts to be proactive at work are likely to fuel employees' confidence in their ability to carry out work-related tasks (self-efficacy), as well as a broader set of tasks that extends beyond their core duties (Parker, 2000). Hence, this confidence is crucial to determine whether or not an individual will behave proactively again in the near future. Additionally, proactivity can enhance feelings of competence, autonomy and relatedness, which in turn generate activated positive emotions (e.g., vitality) that facilitate the engagement in more proactivity.

A Self-determination Perspective: Satisfaction of Basic Needs as a Mechanism

Drawing on self-determination theory, Strauss and Parker (2014a) argued that proactivity, as a self-initiated and discretionary behavior, can substantially contribute to employees' well-being via the satisfaction of one's basic psychological needs. First, given its self-initiated nature, proactive behavior is less likely to rely on effortful volition, as opposed to more monotonous activities that require self-control, such as repetitive routine tasks. This component of self-initiation has been previously associated with feelings of autonomy and self-direction (Koestner, Ryan, Bernieri, & Holt, 1984). Second, in light of its change-oriented focus, Parker et al. (2010) maintained that being proactive can increase challenging opportunities at work, thus facilitating the experience of competence and mastery (Massimini & Carli, 1988, as cited in Strauss and Parker, 2014a). Finally, in spite of their self-initiated emphasis, engaging in proactive behavior is likely to contribute to meeting the need of relatedness (Strauss & Parker, 2014b). Scholars have emphasized that proactive people are more likely to seek feedback from peers and build social networks, which in turn facilitates their career progression (Belschak & Den Hartog, 2010; Morrison, 2002).

In addition to this, proactivity is potentially a way to actively shape interpersonal relationships and social interactions (Grant & Ashford, 2008), thus raising people's sense of relatedness at work.

In sum, researchers suggest that people engage in proactive behavior motivated by the desire to provide for their basic needs (a "reason to" pathway), and consequently, when they are proactive, individuals are likely to experience greater need fulfillment and, hence, more intrinsic motivation at work. Although a logical prediction, there are no empirical tests yet of the effect of proactivity on need satisfaction and well-being.

Self-efficacy as a Consequence of Proactivity: A Confidence Mechanism

As earlier discussed, self-efficacy perceptions are a crucial antecedent of proactive behaviors in organizational settings (Parker, 2000; Parker et al., 2010). When employees are confident in their ability to successfully complete tasks, they are more likely to engage in proactive behavior. In this section, we propose and discuss why self-efficacy, aside from being a powerful determinant of proactivity, can also represent an important outcome of proactive efforts.

Self-efficacy is a rather malleable trait, subject to considerable intra-individual variations, depending on people's life experiences and emotions. According to Bandura (1982), there are four key experiences that contribute to the development of self-efficacy: enactive mastery (repeated performance accomplishments), modeling (vicarious experiences), verbal persuasion (convincing an individual of his or her ability to complete a task), and emotional arousal (a person's psychological state). The cognitive appraisal and integration of these four cues eventually determines one's self-efficacy. For the purpose of this chapter, we will focus on mastery, since not only it is the most important cue in determining the self-efficacy beliefs, but also the most relevant to our discussion around proactive behaviors.

Mastery is the most important cue in enhancing self-efficacy (Bandura, 1977, 1982). As Gist (1987) states: "mastery is facilitated when gradual accomplishments build the skills, coping abilities, and exposure needed for task performance" (p. 473). This view of mastery as key determinant of self-efficacy is supported by a meta-analysis, in which Sitzmann and Yeo (2013) surveyed 38 studies looking at the self-efficacy/performance relationship and concluded that "past performance enlightens assessments of confidence rather than confidence compelling higher performance" (p. 564). Accordingly, it seems that the impact of past performance on self-efficacy is even more pronounced than vice versa.

These considerations around the experience of mastery are particularly relevant to proactive behavior. Even in favorable circumstances, some individuals may not expose themselves to opportunities for mastery (Gist, 1987). For example, an employee with high job autonomy may perceive that they can control most aspects of their work and follow their initiative, but may hold back from doing so because of fear or incapacity. We speculate that engaging in proactive behavior is to a large extent about mastery, and should therefore enhance perceptions of work-related self-efficacy, above and beyond job characteristics.

Being proactive at work could be particularly beneficial for a specific subset of self-efficacy beliefs: role-breadth self-efficacy (RBSE). Parker (1998) defines RBSE as "the extent to which employees feel confident that they are able to carry out a broader and more proactive role" (p. 835). Again, RBSE has been described as a situation-specific subset of self-efficacy, subject to considerable fluctuations over time (Parker, 1998). Previous research has identified RBSE as a crucial precursor for proactive behavior (Parker, 2000; Parker et al., 2006).

Previous research has indicated that redesigning jobs can be an effective way to build employees' self-efficacy. Indeed, a relationship exists between work characteristics and self-efficacy at work. However, to date this relationship primarily appears to apply to the role of job autonomy. For example, Parker (1998) showed that work redesign practices like job enrichment (involving autonomy) are associated with RBSE, highlighting the potentially pivotal role of job redesign interventions in promoting RBSE. However, this author found that job enlargement (i.e., the breadth of tasks and activities present in a job) was not predictive of RBSE. In a similar vein, a longitudinal study, Axtell and Parker (2003) reported a negative impact of job enlargement on RBSE, and concluded that "expanding the breadth of tasks employees carry out, without simultaneously increasing decision-making influence and involvement (…) is unlikely to enhance RBSE and, indeed, could decrease it." Both sets of authors highlighted the importance of the decision-making responsibility implicit in autonomy for building mastery. Here, we suggest that being proactive is a necessary step in translating greater decisional power and job control and autonomy into heightened feelings of self-confidence. This is because engaging in self-initiated and self-directed actions can provide significant opportunities to experience mastery at work, thus building the belief in one's ability to successfully complete work-related tasks. Indeed Parker and Sprigg (1999) made a similar argument when they showed an interaction between proactive personality, job demands, and job control in predicting job strain. In line with their hypotheses, proactive personality moderated the interaction between job demands, job control, and strain. That is, people need to have some degree of proactivity to make use of their job autonomy and successfully cope with demands at work.

Just as positive mastery experiences can fuel one's self-confidence, negative ones (e.g., failures) can decrease it (Gist, 1987). We discuss the potentially detrimental effect of negative feedback in the link between proactivity and mastery later in this chapter.

A Broaden-and-Build Approach: Affect as a Mechanism

Scholars have further argued that proactivity might have a more dynamic interaction with affect drawing on the Fredrickson's broaden-and-build theory (2001) of positive emotions (Grant & Ashford, 2008; Strauss & Parker, 2014a). This theory seeks to explain how and why positive emotions promote human flourishing. According to Fredrickson, experiencing feelings of positive affect encourages people to broaden their awareness and engage in exploratory actions. As a result, this process helps to create skills and resources, which, in turn, increase one's psychological resilience and the ability to cope with stressors. In a longitudinal study featuring 122 business owners, Hahn et al. (2012) found that entrepreneurs' vigor was positively associated with task and relationship-oriented personal initiative. The researchers argued that business success might explain such a relationship: that is, proactive entrepreneurs are more likely to be successful, which in turn may generate greater psychological well-being (Hahn et al., 2012). Likewise, experiencing positive and activated feelings helps broaden people's thought-action repertoires, thus increasing their likelihood to take personal initiative. However, it should be mentioned that Hahn and colleagues' study is correlational in nature and, therefore, requires cautious interpretation when it comes to causal effects.

On a similar note, Fritz and Sonnentag (2009) maintain that people experiencing positive affective states are more likely to take charge and behave proactively. In turn, being proactive at work can create opportunities to satisfy basic needs and thereby increase vitality in what Strauss and Parker (2014a) call "positive upward spiral of (…) proactivity" (p. 29). Along these lines, Salanova and Schaufeli (2008) have speculated that experiencing feelings of enthusiasm, inspiration, and challenge at work could help broaden habitual ways of thinking and acting, which in turn can facilitate proactive behavior at work.

In sum, scholars have argued that, just as positive emotions can stimulate proactive behavior, proactivity can also result in positive affect, which then has the benefits of broadened thinking and resource building, resulting in more engagement in proactivity. Such a dynamic spiral has not yet been tested.

Empirically, there are very few articles on the potentially positive effects of proactivity on well-being (with the exception of Strauss & Parker, 2014b). However, there is some research on related constructs, such as creativity, innovation and citizenship behaviors, which we briefly consider here.

Creativity refers to the "production of novel and useful ideas in any domain" (Amabile, Conti, Coon, Lazenby, & Herron, 1996, p. 1155); this has some parallels with proactivity (albeit tending to be more focused on generating, rather than implementing, new ideas). The overwhelming majority of research tends to describe workers' creativity as a win-win: not only do organizations that promote individual creativity benefit in terms of effectiveness, but also the very same employees report greater job satisfaction and psychological well-being. This is because creativity creates new challenges for workers, as well as opportunities for personal and professional growth (Amabile et al., 1996). In addition to this, researchers have often associated creativity with the experience of positive energizing emotions such as enthusiasm, optimism, and happiness (Csikszentmihalyi, 2000). According to Belschak and Den Hartog (2010), proactive behavior is also to some extent related to organizational citizenship behavior (OCB). Whilst OCB is distinct from proactivity in that it is not necessarily anticipatory or future-focused, it does share a discretionary emphasis. Meta-analyses have shown a consistent association of OCBs with reduced turnover and job satisfaction (Podsakoff, Whiting, Podsakoff, & Blume, 2009).

The research on creativity, OCBs and well-being suggests largely positive well-being consequences, but there are some major limitations that should be considered. First, it should be noted that, although proactivity shares some common ground with OCBs and creativity, it is distinct. Some of the features of proactivity that make proactivity psychologically risky, and hence potentially threatening to well-being, such as the emphasis of proactivity on self-initiated change, do not apply to creativity or OCBs. Second, research looking at the well-being outcomes of creativity and OCBs is primarily correlational, thus not allowing for causal interpretations. It is quite plausible that more satisfied individuals with greater enthusiasm, for example, will be more likely to engage in these behaviors. Third, little is known about the underlying mechanisms that regulate the effects of innovation and creativity on well-being.

Negative Outcomes of Proactivity: A Resource-Depletion Pathway

One criticism of the literature on proactivity concerns its overwhelming focus on its positive aspects (in terms of organizational effectiveness and career success), with insufficient attention to the potential costs associated with proactivity (Bolino et al., 2010), or the "dark side." In this section, we elaborate on the potentially negative consequences of proactive behavior from a well-being perspective, and discuss the key moderating role of motivation in this process.

Drawing upon conservation of resources theory (COR theory; Hobfoll, 1989), Bolino et al. (2010) identified proactive behaviors as a potential source of employee stress. Previous research has indicated that proactive behavior is likely to necessitate the exertion of energy and resources (Grant & Ashford, 2008). For instance, an employee trying to implement a new administrative procedure, which could result in greater organizational profits, will likely have to undertake extra work to design and test this initiative. The more proactive behaviors require resources, the more they will be stressful. Consequently, some types of voice might be less resource-demanding, and less stressful, compared with behaviors like personal initiative, idea implementation and proactive problem solving.

Empirical evidence for these speculations about the importance of resources has been provided by Parker, Johnson, Collins, and Nguyen (2012) in a quasi-experimental study: in line with COR theory, hospital doctors who did not experience negative affect (suggesting sufficient resources) made use of structural support to engage in greater proactive care and voice. In contrast, doctors who reported high levels of negative affect (suggesting insufficient resources) were more inclined to use the supplied support as a means to protect existing resources, thus resulting in lowered role overload. These findings imply that having a reasonable level of resources is necessary before engaging in proactivity.

Proactivity as a Goal Regulation Process

The above considerations are consistent with the view of proactivity as a goal-regulation process requiring regulatory resources. Bindl et al. (2012) proposed a goal-regulatory model of proactivity at work. Within this framework, the researchers recognized four different core elements of proactive behavior: envisioning, planning, enacting, and reflecting. First, people identify that something can be done to actively change the situation (envisioning); prepare a plan for action (planning); then engage in proactive behavior (enacting); and finally reflect upon the implications of their proactive behavior (reflecting). As a result, proactive behavior is not just about simply acting in a proactive manner, but rather involves a goal-regulation process made of different phases, each of which is vital to yield the positive outcomes of proactive behavior. Conceivably, some of these stages are more resource-demanding than others.

In this regard, an increasing body of research has started to look at self-regulation as a limited resource that, just like a battery, becomes depleted over use. That is, when we exert self-regulation in a task, our performance is likely to be poorer in a subsequent, unrelated task that also requires self-control. The term ego depletion is frequently used to refer to a loss of regulatory resources, which results in subsequent impaired performance in tasks that require the exertion of self-regulation. When people experience this state of depletion, they are more likely to fail to self-regulate afterwards. Accordingly, rather than being solely a matter of trait-like individual differences in personal resources, the ability to regulate one's behaviors, emotions, and impulses largely depends on the regulatory capacity that we can avail of at a certain moment. For example, an experiment by Muraven, Tice, and Baumeister (1998) indicated that controlling emotions impairs subsequent self-regulation. Participants watched an emotionally distressing video clip. Participants who were asked to either show no emotion or exaggerate their emotions performed poorer on a following handgrip exercise compared with participants who spontaneously expressed their natural emotions. This approach, known as the strength model of self-control, has received a considerable amount of empirical support (Hagger, Wood, Stiff, & Chatzisarantis, 2010). Research in this field suggests that this ego depletion effect occurs across various domains; for example, controlling thoughts (Muraven, regulating emotions (Muraven et al., 1998), making decisions (Vohs et al., 2008), help-ing other people (DeWall, Baumeister, Gailliot, & Maner, 2008), and resisting persua-sion (Wheeler, Briñol, & Hermann, 2007). Consistent with COR theory, a considerable amount of research has linked chronic exertion of regulatory depletion (e.g., emotional labor) with outcomes detrimental for well-being and mental health such as burnout and emotional exhaustion (Hülsheger & Schewe, 2011; Schmidt, Neubach, & Heuer, 2007). In fact, burnout is a long-term outcome of stress, resulting from a constant loss of resources without the ability to replenish them successfully (Demerouti, Bakker, Nachreiner, & Schaufeli, 2001).

One question that needs to be asked is whether proactive behavior depletes regula-tory resources and, if so, under what conditions. As a matter of fact, self-control often involves an intra-motivational conflict: we restrain our instincts and impulses in order to maximize our long-term goals. By way of illustration, a person dieting restrains his or her temporary food cravings to achieve the goal of losing weight. In terms of goal-regulation, self-control refers to the ability to guide one's own actions by setting performance stand-ards and monitoring the progression toward these standards (Vohs & Baumeister, 2004). An implication of this is that the amount of goal regulation involved may affect the extent to which proactivity is perceived as demanding by employees. For example, voicing out a concern in a weekly meeting is conceivably a type of proactive behavior that involves less goal regulation compared with longer-sustained activities requiring effortful daily striving, such as implementing a new work procedure. To summarize, when analyzing the potential impact of proactive behavior on well-being, it is important to consider the amount of goal regulation involved in the proactive process.

Although to date, no empirical research has really looked at whether proactivity can deplete resources, the idea that positive organizational behaviors may backfire on employees' well-being has been already been discussed in previous research on similar constructs. For example, Bolino and Turnley (2005) have examined the costs associ-ated with organizational citizenship behaviors (OCBs), showing a positive association between ratings of citizenship behavior at work and role overload, job stress, and work–family conflict. Additionally, individual innovation has been previously considered as an additional demand on employees: innovating may entail challenging the status quo, thus encountering resistance to change from coworkers and supervisors. Along similar lines, taking innovative initiatives has previously been found to be associated with con-flict and frustration at work (Janssen, 2003). A plausible explanation of this relation-ship has been sought in an increased demand of resources: engaging in innovative work often requires complex problem solving, increased workload, and resource investment (Janssen, Van de Vliert, & West, 2004). Fairness in procedures is also a crucial aspect to consider when examining the well-being outcomes of positive organizational behav-iors. In 2004, Janssen carried out a study among first-line managers from six organi-zations which explored the link between innovative behavior on stress and burnout. Consistent with Janssen's predictions, analyses showed that perceptions of distributive fairness moderate the impact of demanding innovative behaviors on stress reactions. Namely, employees perceiving their efforts and investments as "under-appreciated" and "under-rewarded" were more likely to experience high levels of stress, as opposed to innovators perceiving a fair balance between efforts and rewards (Janssen et al., 2004). Bolino and Turnley (2005) examined the costs associated with OCBs, showing a positive association between ratings of citizenship behavior at work and role overload, job stress and work–family conflict.

Although OCBs and personal initiative are different from proactive behavior, there is indeed some theoretical overlap. Research considering the potentially negative effects of

OCBs and personal initiative is mostly correlational and does not allow drawing firm conclusions. However, previous research on the "dark side" of positive organizational behaviors seems to give some support to our model of the effects of proactivity on well-being.

The Moderating Role of Feedback

Feedback is considered a crucial managerial tool that not only provides employees with valuable information about their performance, but can also increase their work motivation (Earley, Northcraft, Lee, & Lituchy, 1990). Feedback is given to notify workers regarding the effectiveness and accuracy of their behaviors at work (Hackman & Oldham, 1976). In relation to motivation, Deci and Ryan (2002) argued that providing positive feedback (i.e., verbal rewards, praise) can support needs satisfaction and infuse a sense of accomplishment in employees that can increase intrinsic motivation at work. In support of these considerations, a meta-analysis of 128 experiments confirmed that while providing extrinsic rewards when achieving goals tends to decrease intrinsic motivation, verbal rewards and praises appear to enhance it (Deci, Koestner, & Ryan, 1999).

Previously we described how being proactive at work can fuel one's self-efficacy perceptions, increase self-determination, and generate positive activate feelings like vigor and vitality. Now, we consider the moderating role of feedback in relation to the motivation and resource-depletion pathways of proactivity. Specifically, we argue that receiving negative feedback can interfere with the development of self-efficacy (or even decrease it), disrupt the self-determination process and needs fulfillment, and potentially elicit negative emotional reactions such as anxiety and depression. Consequently we propose that feedback will moderate the effects of proactivity on self-efficacy, positive affect, need fullfilment, and hence proactivity. In addition to this, we draw upon COR theory to explain why negative feedback can render proactivity more resource-depleting.

How Negative Feedback can Thwart Needs Satisfaction and Undermine Self-Efficacy

Being proactive may expose individuals to criticism, complaints and blaming, which can surely harm the incumbents' well-being. By way of illustration, an employee may suggest a new method for carrying out work that, despite the efforts to be implemented, turns out to be under-appreciated by peers and supervisors. Ironically, even if the outcome of a proactive action was extremely positive for the organization, the way other members or supervisors perceive this type of behavior might be opposite. In fact, the meaning people assign to human behaviors is, to a large extent, socially constructed (Berger & Luckmann, 1966). As a consequence, the way others react and interpret our actions, attitudes, and beliefs is determined by social interactions, and cannot rely on objective evaluations. On this note, Stobbeleir, Ashford, and Luque (2010) maintain that "proactive behaviors are particularly susceptible to social-construction processes" (p. 348). This is indeed due to their discretionary and non-prescribed nature. Along these lines, Grant et al. (2009) found that supervisors' rating of proactive behavior largely depends upon employees' values and level of positive affect.

Although the effects of positive feedback have been widely documented and explored in empirical research, less attention has been devoted to the motivational and well-being effects of negative feedback (Ryan & Deci, 2002). Across three studies, Baron (1988) explored the impact of criticism on task performance and self-efficacy. Consistent with his hypotheses, destructive criticism lowered participants' self-efficacy and hampered their subsequent task performance. From a motivational perspective, Vallerand and Reid (1984) found that providing college students with positive and negative feedback had a differential effect on their intrinsic motivation: as expected, receiving positive feedback increased intrinsic motivation, while negative feedback had a deleterious impact on it. These causal relationships were both mediated by students' perceived competence. Namely, when people receive negative feedback about their performance, this can impair their sense of competence, which in turn decreases intrinsic motivation.

It is important to note that the above mentioned studies on the effects of feedback were mainly focused on task-specific or job performance feedback. In our view, negative feedback is a key moderator in undermining the motivation effects of proactivity and in increasing feelings of resource depletion. We argue that the impact of feedback resulting from proactivity is likely to be more significant than feedback on job proficiency owing to the greater role played by psychological ownership in self-initiated and self-directed behaviors. Adopting self-determination theory as a theoretical framework, Shepherd and Cardon (2009) hypothesized that the intensity of negative emotions triggered by project failure might vary as a function of the previously experienced feelings of self-determination carrying out the project. Namely, dedicating time, effort and energy in pursuit of a project that fuels feelings of autonomy, competence, and relatedness may have intense negative emotional reactions on the individual in case the project failed.

One issue that emerges from this consideration is that feelings of self-determination as a result of proactive actions may actually have a double-edged sword effect on employees' emotional reactions: on one hand, successful attempts of proactive behavior can generate feelings of vitality; on the other hand, when proactivity results in unexpected negative feedback from peers and supervisors, it may generate intense negative emotional reactions, thwart needs satisfaction, and undermine self-efficacy. On the contrary, receiving positive feedback and appreciation from others should elicit positive affect, and provide opportunities to accumulate resources (e.g., work-related self-efficacy). In fact, past research has shown that receiving positive feedback at work can indeed affect motivation and vitality (Mouratidis, Vansteenkiste, Lens, & Sideridis, 2008).

Previously we discussed how being proactive at work can fuel one's confidence at work. However, receiving unfavorable feedback from others after proactivity can interfere with this process. In two experimental studies, Baron (1988) examined how destructive criticism impacts on conflict, self-efficacy perceptions, and task performance. In the first study, in line with his hypotheses, participants who received destructive criticism regarding their task performance reported negative feelings such as tension and anger. In the second experiment, subjects who received destructive criticism indicated lower self-efficacy and were more likely to set lower goals in subsequent tasks, compared with those who received constructive feedback or no feedback at all.

According to Bandura (1977) failures can have a more pronounced impact on self-efficacy beliefs when their causes are attributed to internal factors (e.g., ability), rather than situational factors. Because proactive behavior is by nature self-initiated and self-directed, we speculate that receiving negative feedback as a result of proactive efforts may be perceived more ego threatening than feedback on task performance. As a consequence, an individual's self-efficacy is more likely to be decreased when negative feedback results from self-initiated actions.

Lowering employees' self-efficacy with negative feedback can also undermine future attempts to be proactive. Self-efficacy perceptions are, in fact, a key motivational antecedent of proactivity at work (can do motivation). As an example, if an employee's efforts to be proactive are reciprocated with blaming, reprimands, and destructive criticism, then his or her confidence to be proactive again at a later time is likely to be undermined. Arguably, this effect might be more conspicuous for role-breadth self-efficacy, rather than work-related self-efficacy.

Feedback and Proactivity: A Conservation of Resources Perspective

Being proactive at work often entails going beyond what is technically prescribed for employees. Proactivity, in fact, may well require careful planning, future-oriented thinking, and striving to achieve one's goals. While briefly voicing out a concern during a weekly meeting is still considered proactivity, other behaviors like creating, developing, and implementing a new work procedure may indeed require considerably more time and energy. Such efforts can be an additional burden on employees on top of their core tasks. In other words, proactivity can consume resources. COR theory posits that individuals have an innate drive to create, retain, protect, and foster personal resources (Gorgievski & Hobfoll, 2008; Hobfoll, 1989). Resources can either have an intrinsic value (e.g., support, status, self-esteem, autonomy) or an instrumental value (e.g., money, shelter). According to COR theory, stress ensues when these resources are threatened with loss, lost, or when significant resource investments do not translate into resource gains.

From a conservation of resources perspective, receiving negative feedback or poor appreciation from coworkers and supervisors should trigger a protection of resources mechanism (Hobfoll, 1989). In fact, human beings have an innate desire to retain and protect resources. Within this framework, stress occurs when there is a perceived loss of resources or a lack of substantial gain after resource investments. In light of this, proactive behavior that results in negative feedback from others might be detrimental to their well-being. On the other hand, however, being praised with positive comments and appreciation for one's proactive actions may indeed diminish feelings of depletion and signal the individual that energy and effort have been well invested.

Another crucial aspect to consider is the outcome of proactive behavior. Proactive efforts, in fact, do not always turn out to be successful. For instance, research on individual innovation suggests that experiencing failure may undermine employees' confidence to engage in innovative behavior in the future (Guzzo & Shea, 1992), but also it may cause subsequent reprimands or blaming from peers and supervisors for the unfortunate endeavour. On the other hand, it should be mentioned that successful innovation provides opportunities for recognition and accomplishment at work, which were found to be positively associated with individual well-being (Janssen, Van de Vliert, & West, 2004). Although the research evidence is mainly correlational and necessitates cautious interpretation, it seems plausible that the outcome of one's proactive behavior is likely to determine whether they will do so again in the future.

Autonomous vs. Controlled Proactivity

In the previous section we discussed the moderating role of feedback in relation to the well-being outcomes of proactive behavior. We now turn our attention to another potentially crucial moderator: the motivations under which proactivity is performed. We suggest that the extent to which proactivity drains resources is closely related to the motivations that prompt people to engage in this type of behavior. By definition, proactive behavior is a self-initiated and self-directed action to cause change. Therefore, from a "reason to" perspective, proactivity should be located closer to the autonomous anchor on the autonomous-controlled motivation continuum. That is, proactive actions should be motivated by an innate interest or enjoyment in the task itself (intrinsic motivation) or because the proactivity helps to achieve goals that are extremely important to the self (identified and integrated regulation) (Parker et al., 2010; Ryan & Deci, 2008). For example, an employee constantly seeking feedback from peers and supervisors may not necessarily enjoy the feedback process itself, but would perceive his or her proactive efforts as a means to become more competent at work. It has then been argued that such autonomously motivated proactivity should increase employees' vitality and enhance their well-being at work (Strauss & Parker, 2014a).

However, not all that glitters is gold. Scholars have recognized that organizations sometimes expect proactivity and seek to control it, suggesting this behavior is not always autonomously motivated. Consequently, being consuming of physical and mental energy, proactivity could cause stress, especially when organizations expect individuals to engage in proactive behavior (Bolino et al., 2010) thereby resulting in externally (rather than internally) regulated, or controlled, proactivity (Strauss & Parker, 2014a). For instance, a recently hired employee on probation may engage in proactive behavior with the aim of increasing the likelihood to retain his or her new job. Under this scenario, proactivity is self-initiated, but the goal is to achieve or retain an extrinsic end, which is a more controlled form of proactivity. Such a scenario is arguably becoming increasingly common in organizations, particularly after the economic crisis in 2008 (Heyes, 2011). In a similar manner, restructuring and downsizing may also prompt people to pursue externally motivated actions (Meyer, Becker, & Vandenberghe, 2004). Additionally, proactive behavior may be performed as part of impression management strategies in order to gain promotions and monetary rewards.

According to self-determination theory, controlled behaviors can be extremely motivating. However, there is a differential impact of such motivation on well-being and subjective vitality: the more motivation lays at the intrinsic or autonomous end of the continuum, the greater its ability to generate energy and vitality (Ryan & Deci, 2000, 2008). Consequently, to understand the impact of proactivity on well-being it is necessary to differentiate proactive behavior into two different categories (although not mutually exclusive): controlled proactivity and autonomous proactivity. Autonomously regulated proactive behavior is motivated by intrinsic needs and/or performed for its own sake. Conversely, controlled proactivity is self-serving behavior performed effortfully for extrinsic reasons (e.g., impression management, social influence, job promotions). Under these circumstances, proactivity is more likely to rely on effortful regulation and volition, thus depleting resources and reducing psychological vitality. Even in the case of integrated and identified regulation, proactive behavior may involve self-control and willpower. As Bindl et al. (2012) suggested, some stages of proactivity (e.g., striving) are naturally more effortful and require regulatory mechanisms to achieve the proactive goal. Preliminary evidence for these considerations has been sought by Strauss and Parker (2014b), who investigated how motivation moderates the impact of proactive work behavior on job strain. Specifically, they indicated that, when controlled motivation is high and autonomous motivation is low, proactivity tends to be associated with greater job strain, both in the short (two weeks) and long term (eight months).

Moreover, Fay and Sonnentag (2012) showed that employees engage in proactivity as a means to address their need for competence when their experienced competence in core tasks is low. Arguably, when employees carry out repetitive, tedious and/or boring tasks, they pursue proactive goals to counteract such feelings and experience competence at work. On the other hand, when they feel competent at work, they are less likely to behave proactively. Additionally, Sonnentag (2003) found that day-level recovery was significantly associated with proactive work behavior: rested and refreshed workers are more prone to engage in proactive behavior.

Hence, it appears that a careful consideration of motivational underpinnings is essential to predict whether proactive behavior is bound to have a positive vs. negative effect on an individual's well-being and subjective vitality. Namely, the motivations under which proactive behaviors are performed should moderate the impact of proactivity on well-being and mental health. This is also in line with COR theory, insofar as people perceiving a resource loss (e.g., job stress) have a tendency to preserve existing resources, rather than investing effort in discretionary behavior (Parker et al., 2012).

Practical Implications

The present chapter offers several implications to practitioners. First, our review suggests that there can be many positive effects of proactivity on well-being, and these should be harnessed for positive spirals. Being proactive at work can serve as a powerful means to build one's confidence at work and provide opportunities to feel competent, autonomous, and related to others in the workplace, thus increasing intrinsic motivation. These motivational effects can be particularly important in jobs whose core tasks do not provide many chances to feel self-determined at work (Fay & Sonnentag, 2012). However, taking charge and making things happen at work is a process that requires substantial goal-regulation to be carried out. Past research has indicated that "going the extra mile" and/or using one's personal initiative can often entail further demands on top of core duties (Bolino & Turnley, 2005; Bolino et al., 2010). To prevent role stressors from arising and causing strain, managers should provide structural and emotional support to proactive employees.

It is also essential to acknowledge the potentially pivotal role of feedback in determining the well-being outcomes of proactivity. As we discussed, feedback can interfere considerably with the positive outcomes of proactive behavior. As discussed previously, providing negative feedback to outcomes resulting from proactive behaviors may trigger a conservation of resources mechanism, which may discourage further attempts to be proactive in the future. Feedback, therefore, should be contingent and behavior-oriented, rather than outcome-oriented. Positive reinforcement is also crucially important: employees' proactive actions should be praised by supervisors in order to encourage more proactivity. Given its self-initiated and self-directed nature, supervisors' feedback to proactive behavior should be focused on propelling the subordinates' need for competence, autonomy, and relatedness, as these are key motivators to be proactive in the workplace (Fay & Sonnentag, 2012; Strauss & Parker, 2014a).

Given its goal-regulatory nature, controlled forms of proactive behavior can be detrimental for employees (Strauss & Parker, 2014b). Indeed, organizations should indeed strive to create an environment that facilitates self-directed behaviors and encourages personal initiative. However, it is important to avoid implementing reward systems using incentives that can trigger extrinsic motivations. By way of illustration, formally assessing frequency and valence of proactive behaviors in performance appraisals may give the impression that proactivity is "expected" from employees.

Future Research

The issue regarding the consequences of proactivity on well-being is an intriguing one, which could be usefully explored in future research. The model we proposed in this chapter provides an obvious starting point. From a methodological viewpoint, research looking at the outcomes of proactive behavior from a well-being perspective is scarce and inadequate (mostly correlational). Particularly, we advocate the use of longitudinal studies to unveil the mechanisms through which proactivity may enhance or undermine employees' mental health. Intensive longitudinal methods, such as experience sampling studies (Bolger & Laurenceau, 2013; Larson & Csikszentmihalyi, 1983) are specifically useful to look closely at consequences of proactive work behavior from an episodic type of approach. For instance, scholars should investigate whether, and under what conditions, being proactive at work can increase employees' self-efficacy.

From a theoretical perspective, future research should aim to reveal the role of feedback in relation to well-being and proactivity. As we discussed, feedback is likely to moderate the motivational and resource-depleting effects of proactivity. Understanding how feedback interacts with proactivity can offer particularly useful managerial implications. Research needs to be conducted to establish whether, and under what circumstances, proactivity can deplete regulatory resources. We recommend testing this effect using experimental procedures such as the dual-task paradigm (see Hagger et al., 2010). Although laboratory testing may sound problematic to study self-initiated and self-directed behavior, previous research has attempted to objectively assess proactive behavior in a controlled environment. For instance, Grant and Rothbard (2013) measured proactive behavior in terms of initiatives taken to correct errors in a draft glossary of business terms for high school students. While using experimental procedures may indeed cause external/ecological validity issues, it can be extremely important to investigate the regulatory nature of proactivity. Understanding when and how behaving proactively can cause resource depletion can give useful indications to practitioners as to how they should encourage proactivity at work. In future investigations, it might be also useful to look at the interplay between feedback and motivation. By way of illustration, providing positive feedback and intrinsic rewards on controlled proactivity may ultimately change motivations to be proactive, without generating resource depletion and stress.

Finally, it would be interesting to assess the effects of job insecurity on the motivations to be proactive. In an ever-increasingly globalized world, job insecurity and work intensification are on the rise (Guillén, 2001). Proactive behaviors are crucial for organizations to survive in today's dynamic work contexts. However, a lack of job security may create extrinsic incentives to be proactive at work to impress supervisors, thus increasing the likelihood to retain a job. Feeling compelled to be proactive in order to preserve one's job may well place an additional burden on employees, increasing stressors associated with their role. From a different viewpoint, taking charge and voice behaviors challenging the status quo may threaten one's job security, particularly if the wrong action is taken (Parker et al., 2010).

Conclusions

Taking charge and making things happen at work is an increasingly important behavior for organizations willing to succeed and thrive in complex and dynamic environments. Unsurprisingly, proactivity has generated considerable interest among researchers and practitioners. Yet, over two decades of research on proactive behavior have largely neglected to consider the outcomes of this crucially important behavior from a well-being perspective. In this chapter, we first summarized key research findings on proactivity to identify its distal antecedents and motivational underpinnings. Furthermore, we drew upon key well-being theories and research evidence to suggest pathways through which proactivity can enhance or undermine employees' well-being and mental health.

As we discussed, it is important to distinguish between positive and desirable consequences of proactivity (e.g., self-determination, self-efficacy, and vitality) and potentially negative outcomes (e.g., role overload). We believe it is crucial to understand the variables that determine whether proactive behaviors will energize employees or cause strain. In this chapter, we identified feedback and motivations to be proactive as key moderators in our model. We suggest practitioners design or revise feedback systems and rewards in order to maximise the mental health benefits of proactivity while minimizing its drawbacks. Overall, we recommend that scholars begin to consider the well-being outcomes of proactivity, and advocate the use of longitudinal studies to assess intra-individual change and development in relation to proactive behavior and personal resources.

References

Amabile, T. M., Conti, R., Coon, H., Lazenby, J., & Herron, M. (1996). Assessing the work environment for creativity. *Academy of Management Journal, 39*(5), 1154–1184.

Ashford, S. J. (1986). Feedback-seeking in individual adaptation: A resource perspective. *Academy of Management Journal, 29*(3), 465–487. doi: 10.2307/256219

Ashford, S. J., & Cummings, L. L. (1985). Proactive feedback seeking: The instrumental use of the information environment. *Journal of Occupational Psychology, 58*(1), 67–79. doi:10.1111/j.2044-8325.1985.tb00181.x

Axtell, C. M., & Parker, S. K. (2003). Promoting role breadth self-efficacy through involvement, work redesign and training. *Human Relations, 56*(1), 113–131.

Bakker, A. B., & Demerouti, E. (2008). Towards a model of work engagement. *Career Development International, 13*(3), 209–223.

Bandura, A. (1977). Self-efficacy: Toward a unifying theory of behavioral change. *Psychological Review, 84*(2), 191–215. doi:10.1037/0033-295X.84.2.191

Bandura, A. (1982). Self-efficacy mechanism in human agency. *American Psychologist, 37*(2), 122–147.

Bandura, A. (1986). *Social foundations of thought and action*: Englewood Cliffs, NJ: Prentice Hall.

Baron, R. A. (1988). Negative effects of destructive criticism: Impact on conflict, self-efficacy, and task performance. *Journal of Applied Psychology, 73*(2), 199–207. doi:10.1037/0021-9010.73.2.199

Bateman, T. S., & Crant, J. M. (1993). The proactive component of organizational behavior: A measure and correlates. *Journal of Organizational Behavior, 14*(2), 103–118.

Belschak, F. D., & Den Hartog, D. N. (2010). Pro-self, prosocial, and pro-organizational foci of proactive behaviour: Differential antecedents and consequences. *Journal of Occupational and Organizational Psychology, 83*(2), 475–498. doi: 10.1348/096317909X439208

Berger, P. L., & T. Luckmann (1966), *The social construction of reality: A treatise in the sociology of knowledge*. Garden City, NY: Anchor Books.

Bindl, U. K., Parker, S. K., Totterdell, P., & Hagger-Johnson, G. (2012). Fuel of the self-starter: How mood relates to proactive goal regulation. *Journal of Applied Psychology, 97*(1), 134–150.

Blickle, G., Witzki, A., & Schneider, P. B. (2009). Self-initiated mentoring and career success: A predictive field study. *Journal of Vocational Behavior, 74*(1), 94–101. doi:10.1016/j.jvb.2008.10.008

Bolger, N., & Laurenceau, J. P. (2013). *Intensive longitudinal methods: An introduction to diary and experience sampling research*: New York, NY: Guilford Press.

Bolino, M. C., & Turnley, W. H. (2005). The personal costs of citizenship behavior: The relationship between individual initiative and role overload, job stress, and work–family conflict. *Journal of Applied Psychology, 90*(4), 740–748.

Bolino, M., Valcea, S., & Harvey, J. (2010). Employee, manage thyself: The potentially negative implications of expecting employees to behave proactively. *Journal of Occupational and Organizational Psychology, 83*(2), 325–345. doi: 10.1348/096317910X493134

Crant, J. M. (2000). Proactive behavior in organizations. *Journal of Management, 26*(3), 435–462.

Csikszentmihalyi, M. (2000). *Beyond boredom and anxiety.* San Francisco, CA: Jossey-Bass.

Deci, E. L., Koestner, R., & Ryan, R. M. (1999). A meta-analytic review of experiments examining the effects of extrinsic rewards on intrinsic motivation. *Psychological Bulletin, 125*(6), 627–668.

Deci, E. L., & Ryan, R. M. (2002). *Handbook of self-determination research.* New York, NY: University of Rochester Press.

Demerouti, E., Bakker, A. B., Nachreiner, F., & Schaufeli, W. B. (2001). The Job Demands-Resources model of burnout. *Journal of Applied Psychology, 86*(3), 499–512.

DeWall, C. N., Baumeister, R. F., Gailliot, M. T., & Maner, J. K. (2008). Depletion makes the heart grow less helpful: Helping as a function of self-regulatory energy and genetic relatedness. *Personality and Social Psychology Bulletin, 34*(12), 1653–1662.

Didla, S., Mearns, K., & Flin, R. (2009). Safety citizenship behaviour: A proactive approach to risk management. *Journal of Risk Research, 12*(3–4), 475–483.

Earley, P. C., Northcraft, G. B., Lee, C., & Lituchy, T. R. (1990). Impact of process and outcome feedback on the relation of goal setting to task performance. *Academy of Management Journal, 33*(1), 87–105. doi:10.2307/256353

Fay, D., & Sonnentag, S. (2012). Within-person fluctuations of proactive behavior: How affect and experienced competence regulate work behavior. *Human Performance, 25*(1), 72–93.

Fredrickson, B. L. (2001). The role of positive emotions in positive psychology: The broaden-and-build theory of positive emotions. *American Psychologist, 56*(3), 218–226.

Frese, M., & Fay, D. (2001). Personal initiative: An active performance concept for work in the 21st century. *Research in Organizational Behavior, 23*, 133–187.

Fritz, C., & Sonnentag, S. (2009). Antecedents of day-level proactive behavior: A look at job stressors and positive affect during the workday. *Journal of Management, 35*(1), 94–111.

Fuller Jr, B., & Marler, L. E. (2009). Change driven by nature: A meta-analytic review of the proactive personality literature. *Journal of Vocational Behavior, 75*(3), 329–345. doi:10.1016/j.jvb.2009.05.008

Gist, M. E. (1987). Self-efficacy: Implications for organizational behavior and human resource management. *Academy of Management Review, 12*(3), 472–485. doi:10.2307/258514

Gorgievski, M. J., & Hobfoll, S. E. (2008). Work can burn us out or fire us up: Conservation of resources in burnout and engagement. In J. B. Halbesleben (Ed.), *Handbook of stress and burnout in health care* (pp. 7–22). New York, NY: Nova Science Publishers.

Grant, A., & Ashford, S. (2008). The dynamics of proactivity at work. *Research in Organizational Behavior, 28*, 3–34.

Grant, A. M., Parker, S. K., & Collins, C. G. (2009). Getting credit for proactive behavior: Supervisor reactions depend on what you value and how you feel. *Personnel Psychology, 62*(1), 31–55. doi:10.1111/j.1744-6570.2008.01128.x

Grant, A. M., & Rothbard, N. P. (2013). When in doubt, seize the day? Security values, prosocial values, and proactivity under ambiguity. *Journal of Applied Psychology, 98*(5), 810–819. doi:10.1037/a0032873

Greenglass, E. R., & Fiksenbaum, L. (2009). Proactive coping, positive affect, and well-being. *European Psychologist, 14*(1), 29–39.

Greguras, G. J., & Diefendorff, J. M. (2010). Why does proactive personality predict employee life satisfaction and work behaviors? A field investigation of the mediating role of the self-concordance model. *Personnel Psychology, 63*(3), 539–560. doi:10.1111/j.1744-6570.2010.01180.x

Griffin, M. A., Neal, A., & Parker, S. K. (2007). A new model of work role performance: Positive behavior in uncertain and interdependent contexts. *Academy of Management Journal, 50*(2), 327–347.

Guillén, M. F. (2001). Is globalization civilizing, destructive or feeble? A critique of five key debates in the social science literature. *Annual Review of Sociology, 27*, 235–260.

Guzzo, R. A., & Shea, G. P. (1992). Group performance and intergroup relations in organizations. In M. D. Dunnette & L. M. Hough (Eds.), *Handbook of industrial and organizational psychology* (vol. 3, 2nd edn., pp. 269–313). Paolo Alto, CA: Consulting Psychologists Press.

Hackman, J. R., & Oldham, G. R. (1976). Motivation through the design of work: Test of a theory. *Organizational Behavior and Human Performance, 16*(2), 250–279.

Hagger, M. S., Wood, C., Stiff, C., & Chatzisarantis, N. L. (2010). Ego depletion and the strength model of self-control: a meta-analysis. *Psychological Bulletin, 136*(4), 495–525.

Hahn, V. C., Frese, M., Binnewies, C., & Schmitt, A. (2012). Happy and proactive? The role of hedonic and eudaimonic well-being in business owners' personal initiative. *Entrepreneurship Theory and Practice, 36*(1), 97–114.

Heyes, J. (2011). Flexicurity, employment protection and the jobs crisis. *Work, Employment & Society, 25*(4), 642–657.

Hobfoll, S. E. (1989). Conservation of resources: A new attempt at conceptualizing stress. *American Psychologist, 44*(3), 513–524.

Hockey, G. R. J. (2000). Work environments and performance. In N. Chmiel (Ed.), *Introduction to work and organizational psychology: A European perspective* (pp. 206–230). Oxford, UK: Blackwell.

Hülsheger, U. R., & Schewe, A. F. (2011). On the costs and benefits of emotional labor: A meta-analysis of three decades of research. *Journal of Occupational Health Psychology, 16*(3), 361–389.

Janssen, O. (2003). Innovative behaviour and job involvement at the price of conflict and less satisfactory relations with co-workers. *Journal of Occupational and Organizational Psychology, 76*(3), 347–364.

Janssen, O., Van de Vliert, E., & West, M. (2004). The bright and dark sides of individual and group innovation: A special issue introduction. *Journal of Organizational Behavior, 25*(2), 129–145.

Koestner, R., Ryan, R. M., Bernieri, F., & Holt, K. (1984). Setting limits on children's behavior: The differential effects of controlling vs. informational styles on intrinsic motivation and creativity. *Journal of Personality, 52*(3), 233–248.

Larson, R., & Csikszentmihalyi, M. (1983). The experience sampling method. *New Directions for Methodology of Social & Behavioral Science, 15*, 41–56.

Massimini, F., & Carli, M. (1988). The systematic assessment of flow in daily experience. In M. Csikszentmihalyi & I. S. Csikszentmihalyi (Eds.), *Optimal experience: Psychological studies of flow in consciousness* (pp. 266–287). New York, NY: Cambridge University Press.

Meyer, J. P., Becker, T. E., & Vandenberghe, C. (2004). Employee commitment and motivation: A conceptual analysis and integrative model. *Journal of Applied Psychology, 89*(6), 991–1007.

Morrison, E. W. (2002). Newcomers' relationships: The role of social network ties during socialization. *Academy of Management Journal, 45*(6), 1149–1160.

Mouratidis, A., Vansteenkiste, M., Lens, W., & Sideridis, G. (2008). The motivating role of positive feedback in sport and physical education: Evidence for a motivational model. *Journal of Sport & Exercise Psychology, 30*(2), 240–268.

Muraven, M., Tice, D. M., & Baumeister, R. F. (1998). Self-control as a limited resource: Regulatory depletion patterns. *Journal of Personality and Social Psychology, 74*(3), 774–789.

Parker, S. K. (1998). Enhancing role breadth self-efficacy: The roles of job enrichment and other organizational interventions. *Journal of Applied Psychology, 83*(6), 835–852.

Parker, S. K. (2000). From passive to proactive motivation: The importance of flexible role orientations and role breadth self-efficacy. *Applied Psychology, 49*(3), 447–469.

Parker, S. K., Bindl, U. K., & Strauss, K. (2010). Making things happen: A model of proactive motivation. *Journal of Management, 36*(4), 827–856.

Parker, S. K., & Collins, C. G. (2010). Taking stock: Integrating and differentiating multiple proactive behaviors. *Journal of Management, 36*(3), 633–662.

Parker, S. K., Johnson, A., Collins, C., & Nguyen, H. (2013). Making the most of structural support: Moderating influence of employees' clarity and negative affect. *Academy of Management Journal, 56*(3), 867–892.

Parker, S. K., & Sprigg, C. A. (1999). Minimizing strain and maximizing learning: The role of job demands, job control, and proactive personality. *Journal of Applied Psychology, 84*(6), 925–939.

Parker, S. K., Wall, T. D., & Jackson, P. R. (1997). "That's not my job": Developing flexible employee work orientations. *Academy of Management Journal, 40*(4), 899–929.

Parker, S. K., Williams, H. M., & Turner, N. (2006). Modeling the antecedents of proactive behavior at work. *Journal of Applied Psychology, 91*(3), 636–652.

Parker, S. K., & Wu, C. H. (2014). Leading for proactivity: How leaders cultivate staff who make things happen. In D. V. Day (Ed.), *The Oxford handbook of leadership and organizations* (pp. 380–405). Oxford, UK: Oxford University Press.

Podsakoff, N. P., Whiting, S. W., Podsakoff, P. M., & Blume, B. D. (2009). Individual- and organizational-level consequences of organizational citizenship behaviors: A meta-analysis. *Journal of Applied Psychology, 94*(1), 122–141.

Ryan, R. M., & Deci, E. L. (2000). Self-determination theory and the facilitation of intrinsic motivation, social development, and well-being. *American Psychologist, 55*(1), 68–78.

Ryan, R. M., & Deci, E. L. (2002). Overview of self-determination theory: An organismic-dialectical perspective. In: E. L. Deci & R. M. Ryan (Eds.), *Handbook of self-determination research* (pp. 3–36). New York, NY: University of Rochester Press.

Ryan, R. M., & Deci, E. L. (2008). From ego depletion to vitality: Theory and findings concerning the facilitation of energy available to the self. *Social and Personality Psychology Compass, 2*(2), 702–717.

Salanova, M., & Schaufeli, W. B. (2008). A cross-national study of work engagement as a mediator between job resources and proactive behaviour. *International Journal of Human Resource Management, 19*(1), 116–131.

Schaufeli, W. B., Salanova, M., González-Romá, V., & Bakker, A. B. (2002). The measurement of engagement and burnout: A two sample confirmatory factor analytic approach. *Journal of Happiness Studies, 3*(1), 71–92.

Schmidt, K.-H., Neubach, B., & Heuer, H. (2007). Self-control demands, cognitive control deficits, and burnout. *Work & Stress, 21*(2), 142–154.

Seo, M.-G., Barrett, L. F., & Bartunek, J. M. (2004). The role of affective experience in work motivation. *Academy of Management Review, 29*(3), 423–439.

Shepherd, D. A., & Cardon, M. S. (2009). Negative emotional reactions to project failure and the self-compassion to learn from the experience. *Journal of Management Studies, 46*(6), 923–949.

Sitzmann, T., & Yeo, G. (2013). A meta-analytic investigation of the within-person self-efficacy domain: Is self-efficacy a product of past performance or a driver of future performance? *Personnel Psychology, 66*(3), 531–568.

Sonnentag, S. (2003). Recovery, work engagement, and proactive behavior: A new look at the interface between nonwork and work. *Journal of Applied Psychology, 88*(3), 518–528.

Stobbeleir, K. E., Ashford, S. J., & Luque, M. F. S. (2010). Proactivity with image in mind: How employee and manager characteristics affect evaluations of proactive behaviours. *Journal of Occupational and Organizational Psychology, 83*(2), 347–369.

Strauss, K., & Parker, S. K. (2014a). Effective and sustained proactivity in the workplace: A self-determination theory perspective. In M.Gagne (Ed.), *The Oxford handbook of work engagement, motivation, and self-determination theory* (pp. 50–71). New York, NY: Oxford University Press.

Strauss, K., & Parker, S. K. (2014b). *Proactivity under pressure hurts: Motivation moderates the effects of proactive work behavior on strain.*Manuscript in preparation.

Thompson, J. A. (2005). Proactive personality and job performance: A social capital perspective. *Journal of Applied Psychology, 90*(5), 1011–1017.

Unsworth, K. L., & Parker, S. K. (2008). Proactivity and innovation: Promoting a new workforce for the new workplace. In D. Holman, T. D. Wall, C. W. Clegg, P. Sparrow, & A. Howard (Eds.), *The new workplace: A guide to the human impact of modern working practices,*(pp. 175–196). Chichester, UK: John Wiley & Sons, Ltd.

Vallerand, R. J., & Reid, G. (1984). On the causal effects of perceived competence on intrinsic motivation: A test of cognitive evaluation theory. *Journal of Sport Psychology, 6*(1), 94–102.

Van Dyne, L., & LePine, J. A. (1998). Helping and voice extra-role behaviors: Evidence of construct and predictive validity. *Academy of Management Journal, 41*(1), 108–119.

Vohs, K. D., & Baumeister, R. F. (2004). Ego-depletion, self-control, and choice. In J. Greenberg, S. L. Koole, & T. Pyszczynski (Eds.), *Handbook of experimental existential psychology* (pp. 398–410). New York, NY: Guilford Press.

Vohs, K. D., Baumeister, R. F., Schmeichel, B. J., Twenge, J. M., Nelson, N. M., & Tice, D. M. (2008). Making choices impairs subsequent self-control: A limited-resource account of decision making, self-regulation, and active initiative. *Journal of Personality and Social Psychology, 94*(5), 883–898.

Wanberg, C. R., & Kammeyer-Mueller, J. D. (2000). Predictors and outcomes of proactivity in the socialization process. *Journal of Applied Psychology, 85*(3), 373–385.

Wheeler, S. C., Briñol, P., & Hermann, A. D. (2007). Resistance to persuasion as self-regulation: Ego-depletion and its effects on attitude change processes. *Journal of Experimental Social Psychology, 43*(1), 150–156.

Wu, C. H., Parker, S. K., & de Jong, J. P. J. (2011). Need for cognition as an antecedent of individual innovation behavior. *Journal of Management, 40*(6), 1511–1534. doi:10.1177/0149206311429862

Zhang, Z., Wang, M., & Shi, J. (2012). Leader–follower congruence in proactive personality and work outcomes: The mediating role of leader–member exchange. *Academy of Management Journal, 55*(1), 111–130.

12

Employee Well-Being and Safety Behaviors

Jonathon R. B. Halbesleben and Tom Bellairs

Introduction

In recent years, there has been increasing interest in the impact that reduced employee well-being has on the way employees approach their work (Demerouti, Bakker, & Leiter, 2014). At the same time, a consistent pattern has emerged and suggests that employees who experience lower well-being are more likely to suffer from an occupational illness or injury at work (Ahola, Salminen, Toppinen-Tanner, Koskinen, & Väänänen, 2013; Chung & Wu, 2013; Nahrgang, Morgeson, & Hofmann, 2011). In this chapter, we explore a key mechanism for understanding the employee well-being–safety outcome relationship: safety workarounds (Halbesleben, 2010).

The purpose of this chapter is to outline the psychological mechanisms that would lead one to respond to reduced well-being at work with behaviors that may be unsafe, thus increasing exposure to occupational illness and injury. This conceptualization is outlined in Figure 12.1. To that end, we draw on literature from a variety of occupations and safety settings. In some cases, we may draw upon literature that is not necessarily related to occupational safety, but instead focuses on a different safety context (such as, patient safety; e.g., Debono et al., 2013). However, as many of the psychological processes regarding engaging in safe behavior are consistent across contexts, we believe examination of these other contexts could meaningfully inform the relationships between well-being and occupational safety. Similarly, we take a broad view of lack of well-being, including general constructs such as burnout (Maslach, 1982), as well as more specific stressors such as job insecurity and overload that might lead to more generalized reduced well-being. We also consider research concerning the presence of well-being (e.g., engagement) rather than exclusively focusing on lack of well-being.

The Wiley Blackwell Handbook of the Psychology of Occupational Safety and Workplace Health, First Edition.
Edited by Sharon Clarke, Tahira M. Probst, Frank Guldenmund, and Jonathan Passmore. © 2016 John Wiley & Sons Ltd. Published 2020 by John Wiley & Sons Ltd.

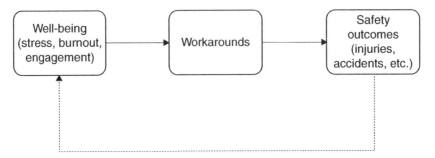

Figure 12.1 Conceptual model linking well-being to safety outcomes through workarounds.

Our chapter integrates several different perspectives in the safety literature and thus helps contribute to our understanding of how employee well-being is linked with safety outcomes. For example, we extend the meta-analysis of Nahrgang et al. (2011) by reviewing the explanatory factors that reside between employee well-being and safety outcomes as opposed to assuming a direct relationship between employee burnout and engagement and safety outcomes. While low employee well-being can indeed have negative physiological effects (Ganster & Rosen, 2013; Melamed, Shirom, Toker, Berliner, & Shapira, 2006; Melamed et al., 1999; Shirom, Westman, Shamai, & Carel, 1997), well-being alone is unlikely to lead to a workplace injury. As a result, we draw upon motivational models of safety (e.g., Christian, Bradley, Wallace, & Burke, 2009; Neal & Griffin, 2006) to bring together the health impairment processes outlined by Nahrgang et al. (2011) with safety outcomes by understanding how employee well-being shapes employees' approaches to work in such a way that increases exposure to injury.

Moreover, though our focus is behavioral in nature, it accounts for extensive literature concerning environmental factors that play a role in safety, such as safety culture/climate and leadership (Clarke, 1999, 2006, 2010, 2013; Clarke & Ward, 2006; et al., 2013; Hofmann & Mark, 2006; Hofmann, Morgeson, & Gerras, 2003; Zohar, 2000, 2003, 2010). As we review below, many of those factors help lead to safety workarounds (Halbesleben & Rathert, 2008) or make them more or less likely in the context of high levels of strain (Leroy et al., 2012). Thus, we are proposing that the notion of safety workarounds offers insight into how several other occupational safety psychology constructs translate to higher levels of exposure to injury, not that safety workarounds replace the long-standing work on these constructs.

In the sections that follow, we first review the literature linking well-being and safety. We then define and review the literature concerning safety workarounds, positioning workarounds as the behavioral mediator between well-being and safety. We review the theories, particularly conservation of resources theory (Hobfoll, 1988, 1989, 1998, 2001), which help clarify the role that workarounds play in occupational health psychology. Finally, we conclude with a description of several future research directions that could help drive the literature in a way that increases our understanding of occupational health psychology theory while, hopefully, reducing injuries in practice.

Well-being and Safety

In this section, we review the literature linking employee well-being with safety, with an emphasis on how reduced well-being can lead to unsafe outcomes. The link between employee well-being and occupational safety has been widely studied (e.g., Halbesleben &

Clark, 2009; Nahrgang et al., 2011). Generally, there is a strong connection between well-being and safety, but the mechanisms are not particularly clear.

Prior to reviewing the literature concerning the links between well-being and safety, it is necessary to establish the criterion space of safety outcomes. This is critical, since, in some cases, safety outcomes have been defined in terms of the behaviors that we argue link well-being to other outcomes (e.g., Burke, Sarpy, Tesluk, & Smith-Crowe, 2002). In other cases, safety outcomes are defined in terms of accidents, injuries, fatalities, and similar events that result in physical harm to the employee (Neal & Griffin, 2006). Since those events are generally low base-rate phenomena, some also explored adverse events such as errors or near misses (e.g., Clarke, Rockett, Sloane, & Aiken, 2002). Still others have combined both approaches under the umbrella of safety outcomes (Nahrgang et al., 2011). No common definition of safety outcomes has been established (Clarke & Robertson, 2005) and any of the above approaches are acceptable if made clear by the authors. For our purposes, we will refer to safety "outcomes" using the latter approach of emphasizing events that result in physical harm to employees. We take this approach to underscore the mediated processes that behaviors have on the links between well-being and safety.

Mirroring arguments of Slovic (2001), who suggested that there should be consideration of both positive and negative outcomes of safety (see also Hollnagel, 2009; Hollnagel, Woods, & Leveson, 2006; Hollnagel, Paries, Woods, & Wreathall, 2011), we can approach the issue of linking well-being with safety from two angles: linking lack of well-being (stress, exhaustion, etc.) to negative safety outcomes (e.g., injuries) or linking the presence of well-being (happiness, health, engagement) to positive safety outcomes. In their meta-analysis linking burnout to safety, Nahrgang et al. (2011) found that burnout was positively related to adverse events (errors, near misses, etc.) and accidents and injuries, but not significantly related to unsafe behavior. It is worth noting that the relationship between burnout and unsafe behavior was tested with only three studies; subsequent studies not included in the meta-analysis found significant relationships between elements of burnout (most notably exhaustion) and unsafe behaviors (e.g., Halbesleben, 2010).

Other broad reviews of relationships between lack of well-being and injuries have also found significant relationships between the two (Johnston, 1995). Research suggests that general work stress has been associated with a variety of injuries, including musculoskeletal strain (Hagen, Magnus, & Vetlesen, 1998; Lindstrom, Leino, Seitsamo, & Torstila, 1997). Chung and Wu (2013) reported positive relationships between burnout and accidents of public transit drivers.

Taking a somewhat different approach by emphasizing specific stressors, Tawatsupa et al. (2013) found a significant relationship between heat stress and occupational injuries among a large sample (>50,000) of Thai workers. In other examinations of specific stressors, scholars found relationships between those stressors and workplace injuries in relatively large samples (e.g., Ahola et al., 2013; Julià, Catalina-Romero, Calvo-Bonacho, & Benavides, 2013; Salminen, Kivimäki, Elovainio, & Vahtera, 2003). In some cases, researchers examined the direct impact that work stressors had on injuries; in others, researchers considered how specific stressors lead to a more negative well-being and the subsequent impact that has on injury (e.g., Turner, Hershcovis, Reich, & Totterdell, 2014).

The evidence linking positive states of well-being and safety outcomes is less clear because there have been fewer studies that have taken this approach. That said, evidence suggests that positive well-being is associated with fewer negative safety outcomes. Nahrgang et al. (2011) reported significant negative relationships between engagement and adverse events in their meta-analyses, but did not find a relationship between engagement and accidents and injuries. They found that satisfaction was negatively related to accidents and injuries as well as adverse events. More recent studies have been establishing a relationship between employee engagement and injuries at work (Baxter, 2013; Halbesleben & Clark, 2009; McCaughey, McGhan, Walsh, Rathert, & Belue, 2014), though several of those studies have not yet been published.

Despite numerous studies linking stressors to negative safety outcomes and the suggestion that positive well-being is linked to positive safety outcomes, the findings are not necessarily consistent or clear (Chau et al., 2011; Palmer, Harris, & Coggon, 2008). It seems unlikely that the stressors alone lead to workplace injuries; burnout by itself should not lead one to experience a traumatic injury, cut, or bruise. Instead, it is likely that the psychological experience of additional stressors leads to behavioral changes that increase exposure to injury, suggesting the need to understand better the behavioral intermediaries between well-being and injury (Ahola et al., 2013). We will focus on one emerging behavior in particular: safety workarounds.

Defining Workarounds

Workarounds occur when an employee experiences a block in workflow and finds a way around that block (Halbesleben, 2010; Halbesleben, Wakefield, & Wakefield, 2008). The block may come from poorly designed processes, difficult coworkers, formal rules, and technology (Friedman et al. 2014; Halbesleben et al., 2008; Koopman & Hoffman, 2003; Koppel, Wetterneck, Telles, & Karsh, 2008). In some cases, the technologies that are worked around are technologies actually intended to improve safety but that create blocks in workflow (Koppel et al., 2010). Workarounds represent a major component of work for many employees. Tucker, Heissler, and Jannisse (2014) estimate that employees in some sectors may spend as much as 10 percent of their work time working around operational failures. Those failures show up, on average, eight times during a typical working shift (Tucker & Spear, 2006), meaning employees frequently encounter situations that deviate from intended work processes. Although much of the workarounds research is in health care settings, workarounds certainly occur in other occupational sectors as well (Schaber et al., 2011).

One of the interesting tensions in the workaround literature is the notion that workarounds can be simultaneously positive and negative (Kahol, Vankipuram, Patel, & Smith, 2011; Wheeler, Halbesleben, & Harris, 2012). On the one hand, workarounds may be necessary to complete tasks, may increase an employee's productivity because the workaround helps bypass perceived workflow blockages, and may result in innovations that improve work processes (Eisenhauer, Hurley, & Dolan, 2007). On the other hand, workarounds typically mean the employee is not completing the task the way it was designed/intended and could create risks to the employee and others (Halbesleben, 2010; Halbesleben, Savage, Wakefield, & Wakefield, 2010). In fact, as Debono et al. (2013) note, several studies refer to workarounds using the term "violations" though the definition of violations in the context of the study is essentially the same as a workaround (e.g., Alper et al., 2012; Fogarty & McKeon, 2006; Taxis & Barber, 2003; see also Chmiel & Hansez, Chapter 7, this volume).

Understanding the positive/negative tension of workarounds in an occupational health setting requires one to consider the timeframe of the workaround consequences. For example, if a home health care worker does not use appropriate lifting equipment to move a patient because the equipment is not readily available (thus, there is a block in the normal workflow), he or she may have the immediate positive result of having moved the patient quickly. If the equipment would not have been available at all (assuming it should have been), one could argue that the workaround was the only way to get the job done. However, negative consequences could occur that are nearly immediate or longer term, such as acute injury to the patient or home health care worker or chronic musculoskeletal pain due to repeatedly engaging in this workaround. Positive outcomes could show up again in the long term if the employee were to come up with an innovative solution to the workaround, either through addressing the block (e.g., suggesting that portable lifting aids be provided to all home health care workers in the organization) or by coming up with a workaround that is just as effective at safely moving the patient as is the intended equipment. In practice, innovative workarounds are rarely communicated in a way that could have a positive impact on work processes? and instead remain idiosyncratic solutions to blocks faced by each employee (Halbesleben et al., 2010; Tucker, Edmondson, & Spear, 2002).

In light of the possibility that workarounds can have both positive and negative valence, one approach is to take a more neutral approach and define workarounds in terms of problem solving (Debono et al., 2013). We do so by defining workarounds as a situation when an employee experiences a block in workflow and figures out a way around that block. Emphasizing the problem solving nature of workarounds helps to underscore the possibility that workarounds resolve workplace issues; however, workarounds may create other future problems. This is consistent with the notion of first-order problem solving, whereby employees address a problem that they face on the job, but do not actually address the underlying causes of the problem (which is second-order problem solving; Tucker & Edmondson, 2002, 2003).

This view is consistent with the role of individuals within socio-technical systems (Besnard & Hollnagel, 2014; Runte, 2010). In situations where safety is an issue, people often have to make adjustments based on a dynamic work environment that may not fit the procedures as they have been presented (Schulman, Roe, Eeten, & Bruijne, 2004). If anything, the mere notion of a near-miss (where a negative safety outcome could have occurred but something was done to avoid it) suggests that safety is more dynamic than simply following safety procedures (Chaplin, 2009; Hodkingson, 2009; Hopkins, 2009; for fascinating case studies, see Haynes, 1991, Wackers, 2006). Consistent with the safety violations literature (e.g., Alper & Karsh, 2009; Besnard & Greathead, 2003), we cannot assume that workarounds are negative and will lead to negative outcomes; the cognitive flexibility of humans suggests that workarounds may be necessary to avoid the negative safety outcomes that are typically the focus of safety research. With that in mind, we turn to a discussion of the psychological and environmental factors that might lead to workarounds.

Antecedents of workarounds

Workarounds result from a variety of factors related to the organization, which include the obstacle preventing task completion and the employee trying to work around the obstacle. Interestingly, though we will consider workarounds as a behavioral response to strain, many of the causes of workarounds are similar to demands that can lead to strains like burnout (Bakker, Demerouti, & Sanz-Vergel, 2014). As such, it is not surprising that employee strain would be associated with greater reliance on workarounds.

With regard to organizational antecedents to workarounds, human resource management issues such as adequate staffing levels and commitment-based human resource management systems tend to be associated with fewer workarounds (Espin, Lingard, Baker, & Regehr, 2006; Fogarty & McKeon, 2006; McKeon, Fogarty, & Hegney, 2006; Wheeler et al., 2012). Staffing levels can be an issue since they impact the amount of workload and the amount of available support when a block appears (e.g., help with lifting an object or person or help clarifying information; Halbesleben et al., 2010; Hutchinson, 1990). Elements of the organization's culture can also impact workarounds, such as perceived psychological safety of the staff to report problems in workflow and continuous quality improvement values (Halbesleben & Rathert, 2008). Interestingly, psychological safety is a double-edged sword because it may lead to the perception that there are more workarounds based on more problems being reported or it may make employees more comfortable engaging in deviations from intended work processes (Tucker & Edmondson, 2002). Chaotic work environments with lots of interruptions can also contribute to workarounds by creating a great number of barriers to workflow (Carayon et al., 2007; O'Neil, Speroni, Dugan, & Daniel, 2010).

Aspects of tasks that make workarounds more or less likely overlap with the organizational antecedents to workarounds. Since much of the workaround literature is focused on health care, and administration of medication in particular, technology has been frequently cited as a block to be worked around (Halbesleben et al., 2010; Koppel et al., 2008; Niazkhani, Pirnejad, van der Sijs, & Aarts, 2011; Van der Sijs, Rootjes, & Aarts, 2010; Vogelsmeier, Halbesleben, & Scott-Cawiezell, 2008). Perhaps again reflecting on the health care focus of the literature, task complexity has been documented as a key factor in workarounds (Fowler, Craig, Fredendall, & Damali, 2008; Kahol et al., 2011; Saleem et al., 2009). Taking a more direct occupational health psychology angle, Halbesleben, Rathert, and Williams (2013) found that nurses' dissatisfaction with the medication administration process increases their likelihood of engaging in workarounds of those processes.

Taking a slightly different angle, Stride et al. (2013) found that experience with or observation of injuries impacts the perceived tension between safety and production in a sample of UK rail employees. Their work suggests that experiencing injuries, either personally or vicariously, might increase the perception that there are barriers to performing work safely and thus lead to a greater reliance on workarounds in the future. It is worth noting, however, that their study was cross-sectional, making it difficult to know for sure if the direction of the causal effect actually suggests observation of the barriers to safety increased the likelihood of injury. However, the idea that the experience of observation of negative safety outcomes would lead one to change behaviors in a way that could actually make the work even less safe is an intriguing notion worthy of further investigation (see also Olson, Grosshuesch, Schmidt, Gray, & Wipfli, 2009).

Many studies link employee factors to workarounds. Most of those studies have focused on employee attitudes toward policies and technologies that they are working around. For example, employees are more likely to work around policies and technology that they do not understand, do not agree with, or thought were not in the best interest of the recipient of their services (Baker, 1997; Furber & Thomson, 2006). Personality and individual belief factors may play a role as well (Dougherty, Sque, & Crouch, 2012; Laumer, Maier, & Eckhardt, 2010. One of the intriguing personality characteristics associated with workarounds is self-efficacy (Halbesleben & Clark, 2009; Tucker et al., 2002). While generally considered advantageous to develop, more self-efficacious employees tend to believe they are good enough at their jobs to solve problems through workarounds and may underestimate safety risks (Krueger & Dickson, 1994).

Dialectical theory and the choice to engage in workarounds

Despite a large number of studies concerning the causes of workarounds, there has been relatively little theory regarding the cognitive processes leading to workarounds (Halbesleben et al., 2010). This is a significant gap because understanding the psychology of workarounds can help (1) determine potential routes of intervention to reduce workarounds, and (2) offer a clearer understanding of the links between workarounds and safety. One way to understand the psychology of workarounds is to position them as a choice between completing work the way it was intended and finishing work quickly (or in some cases, finishing at all) when facing a block in workflow. Such a framing would suggest that employees navigate internal tensions that drive their decision-making.

Dialectics is concerned with inherent contradictions between related constructs and the unique outcomes that result as people seek to manage the natural tension that results from those contradictions (Benson, 1977; Carlo, Lyytinen, & Boland, 2012). Thus, dialectical theories explain how people develop by navigating natural social tensions. Constructs in a dialectic relationship are both interdependent, mutually negating, and fluctuate over time (Bantham, Celuch, & Kasouf, 2003; Baxter, 1990). As an example, one of the most common dialectics examined in the interpersonal relationships literature is the autonomy–connectedness dialectic. In relationships, there is an inherent tension between maintaining one's identity (autonomy) and holding a shared identity (connectedness) with the other person (e.g., as a "couple"). One must comprehend connectedness to truly understand autonomy since autonomy would not be clear unless connection is understood. However, the absence of one pole does not imply presence of the other (no connectedness does not mean one has autonomy). Over time, people navigate the dialectical tension, which creates a need for them to change and grow. For example, if one feels like a relational partner is too "needy" (desires a lot of connectedness), he or she takes steps to move the relationship toward autonomy.

Researchers have extended the relational dialectics perspective to organizational contexts (Benson, 1973, 1977) and suggested that employees manage dialectical tensions in their relationships with organizations (Halbesleben, Whitman, & Crawford, 2014) and coworkers (Bridge & Baxter, 1992). In a safety context, we argue that employees face a tension, when faced with a block in workflow, between following intended procedures and engaging in a workaround; thus, the dialectic exists in the relationship between the employee and his or her work. Like more typical relational dialectics, employees do not constantly experience this tension; it becomes salient when there is a block in the workflow that forces employees to think about their relationship with the task.

The question becomes how the employee addresses the tension and, perhaps even more interesting, how the employee's approach changes over time. Baxter and Montgomery (1996) presented several different approaches that individuals take to address relational dialectics. We will focus on a few that are consistent with past literature concerning workarounds. For example, denying one of the poles of the dialectic is among the most basic ways to address dialectical tensions. For example, the employee may simply stop the work process until the block is removed because he or she does not believe one should engage in workarounds. This approach, however, is typically dysfunctional in relationships because it cannot be sustained (Baxter & Montgomery, 1996); it is difficult to imagine that an employee could continue to leave a task unfinished for an extended period while waiting for the block to be removed. In fact, the whole point of a workaround is to complete the task somehow (Westphal, Lancaster, & Park, 2013).

Another approach, spiraling inversion, occurs when people manage the tension through radical shifts from one pole to the other depending on the context they find themselves in (Baxter & Montgomery, 1996). For example, employees may always follow the proper procedures when supervisors or Occupational Safety and Health Administration (OSHA) inspectors are present, but engage in workarounds when those authorities are not present. Despite its somewhat dramatic name, spiraling inversion is a deliberate employee strategy to manage tension by experiencing both poles but reserving those experiences for the appropriate context.

Over time, employees are likely to address the tension through integration (i.e., the process of bringing the poles together; Baxter, 2011; Bridge & Baxter, 1992). Over time, the employee may perceive the workaround as the most appropriate work process, whereby the tension is resolved by cognitively eliminating it. As we noted, it seems likely that the strategies change over time. Employees attempt to first avoid the workaround pole, then apply it only in specific contexts, and eventually adopt it as a standard operating procedure. However, further research should specifically address the longitudinal responses to the workaround dialectical tension; we will return to this point when we address future research later in the chapter.

Workarounds and Safety Outcomes

Workarounds lead to several consequences; however, the vast majority of studies have emphasized the impact they can have on safety outcomes. This section will review the literature that links workarounds with safety outcomes. This will be a broad review that will address different kinds of safety (e.g., patient/client/customer safety and occupational safety). It will draw heavily on literature from occupational health psychology, but will also include literature from health care (e.g., nursing) and other relevant fields.

With regard to occupational injuries, several studies have found relationships between workarounds or related behaviors (e.g., safety compliance) and injury. In two samples of health care professionals using a cross-lagged panel design with six-month time lags, Halbesleben (2010) reported significant relationships between the number of occupational injuries experienced by the participants and the severity (in terms of missed time from work) of those injuries. In a separate sample of nurses, Halbesleben, Rathert, and Bennett (2013) found that workarounds were positively associated with injury frequency and severity (using the same operationalizations as Halbesleben, 2010). However, they also found that workarounds were negatively associated with reporting those injuries.

Li, Jiang, Yao, and Li (2013) found similar effects in the relationship between safety compliance (Neal & Griffin, 2006) and injuries among crude oil production workers in China. Li et al. (2013) incorporated near misses into their safety outcome measure when conducting their overall structural equation modeling analysis, finding a significant effect. However, the zero-order correlations indicate that safety compliance was significantly associated with near misses ($r = -.09$, p < .05), but not significantly associated with actual injuries ($r = -.07$, *n.s.*). This finding speaks to the advantages of expanding our conceptualization of safety outcomes to include outcomes such as near misses.

Though the focus of this chapter is on occupational health, we would be remiss if we did not acknowledge the large body of research linking workarounds to patient safety from the health care literature (e.g., Halbesleben et al., 2008, 2010; Koppel et al., 2008; Spear & Schmidhofer, 2005). As noted above, there have been frequent suggestions that workarounds can lead to patient safety (see also Bishop, Fleming & Flin, Chapter 20, this volume). However, relatively few studies have actually measured patient safety outcomes to establish that such a relationship exists (Debono et al., 2013).

The basic message of the research linking workarounds and safety outcomes is that workarounds increase exposure to occupational injuries, thereby increasing the likelihood that the employee (or the patient/client) is injured at work. However, few studies have assessed workarounds (or closely related constructs such as safety compliance). More research is needed to establish that relationship and, in particular, boundary conditions that might impact the strength of the relationship (e.g., conditions under which workarounds prevent a likely injury). Further, while there have been some attempts to develop theory-based linkages between strain and injury through workarounds (e.g., Halbesleben, 2010), there are situations still unexplained by current theories that we will attempt to address by extending other theories.

Theoretical Integration

To help address the need for greater theorizing regarding the well-being – workaround – strain relationship, this section will achieve two objectives: (1) to discuss existing theories that have been utilized to understand the proposed relationship, and (2) propose several new theoretical frameworks that might address gaps in the current theorizing. We start with the current theorizing, which has primarily emphasized conservation of resources theory.

Conservation of resources theory

In this section, we will briefly review the relevant tenets of Conservation of Resources (COR) theory (Hobfoll, 1988, 1989, 1998, 2001) and review how the theory has been applied to safety workarounds. We will highlight gaps in the theory that have not been tested and where COR theory – as currently formulated – is unable to guide predictions. We will follow this section by discussing how other theories can fill those gaps.

COR theory proposes that individuals are primarily motivated to retain and acquire resources. Resources are defined as anything that can help an individual to achieve his or her goals (Halbesleben, Neveu, Paustian-Underdahl, & Westman, 2014). COR theory suggests that a loss of or threat to resource loss can decrease employee well-being and increase burnout (Hobfoll & Freedy, 1993). Additionally, strain can result from repeated bad resource investments (Hobfoll, 2001). This could apply in the context of workarounds and further explains the choice to engage in a workaround if the intended work process contributes to lower employee well-being. If, by repeatedly following the specified safety procedures, this leads to outcomes that are perceived as bad investments (e.g., work taking longer or complaints from customers), the strain that results could make a workaround appear more attractive. However, that may not apply in all cases (e.g., cases where the workaround fails or requires higher investment) and the perception is often not that the in-tended work process is problematic as much as the workaround is more efficient or easier.

The value of COR theory is that it helps explain not only what leads employees to experience lower well-being, but also how they respond to the strains that occur as a result of resource losses. As noted above, the theory suggests we are motivated to retain (or protect) our current resources and acquire new resources. Both of these processes, protection and acquisition, have important implications for how people respond to strain. Hobfoll (2001) proposed that when people lose their resources, they engage in defensive strategies to protect their resources. This manifests in the workplace through behaviors such as choosing the easiest path to completing a task or engaging in tasks that may not be as critical to organizational objectives, but may require fewer resources (Halbesleben & Bowler, 2007). Most workarounds, by design, require fewer resources than following the intended work procedure. As a result, we would expect that as individuals have fewer resources, manifesting as strain, they engage in more workarounds (Halbesleben et al., 2008; Rathert, Williams, Lawrence, Halbesleben, 2012).

With regard to resource acquisition, Hobfoll (2001) proposed that those with fewer resources are more likely to make resource investments that lead to further resource losses, creating a loss cycle. In his study of workarounds in occupational safety, Halbesleben (2010) found that employees who engaged in workarounds experienced more injuries and the injuries created further resource declines that further lowered the employees' well-being (see also Lawrence, Halbesleben, & Paustian-Underdahl, 2013). Ironically, despite leading to injuries, workarounds may actually become more likely in those circumstances because resources have been further reduced with fewer available for investment in intended work processes.

While COR theory offers a strong theoretical framework for understanding the relationship between lower well-being and safety outcomes through workarounds, COR theory it has its limitations as well in that context. COR theory is less effective at addressing workarounds that occur when the workaround actually requires more resources than completing the task the appropriate way. As defined, a workaround involves a block in workflow, so there is obviously some difficulty in performing the task as it was intended. However, situations can arise where the workaround is actually more resource-intensive than addressing the block in workflow. COR-based arguments would suggest that when an employee is experiencing strain, he or she should invest the fewest possible resources to finish the task (Hobfoll, 2001).

Another, related and unresolved issue linking strain to workarounds in a COR theory context is sorting out whether workarounds are intentional, thoughtful acts meant to conserve resources in a strategic manner or if the employees experiencing strain simply do not have the cognitive capacity to follow safety procedures as they were designed (Diestel, Cosmar, & Schmidt, 2013; Oosterholt, van der Linden, Maes, Verbraak, & Kompier, 2012; Sandström, Rhodin, Lundberg, Olsson, & Nyberg, 2005). Generally, COR theory emphasizes strategic action on the part of individuals; the corollaries regarding responses to resource loss (defensive investment in particular) suggest as much. However, to the extent that workarounds are a response to strain, they might simply represent the easiest and quickest way to complete tasks.

Finally, although COR theory can explain why individuals chose to engage in workarounds when they suffer from lower well-being, the theory is less clear on how individuals should respond when they have higher well-being (for example, because of higher levels of resources). We have noted that engagement, one indicator of high levels of resources (Gorgievski & Hobfoll, 2008), is associated with lower rates of injury (Baxter, 2013; Halbesleben & Clark, 2009; McCaughey et al., 2014). Normally, engagement is associated with an ability to invest resources in behaviors that require greater resource investments, which could include simply completing tasks as designed (Nahrgang et al., 2011). However, engagement is also associated with behaviors that go beyond expectations (Halbesleben, Harvey, & Bolino, 2009; Rich, Lepine, & Crawford, 2010), including creative activities (Henker, Sonnentag, & Unger, 2015; Park, Song, Yoon, & Kim, 2014). To the extent that one considers engaging in a workaround a creative problem solving endeavor, one might actually expect that those with greater resources to invest are more likely to engage in workarounds.

Other theories

Selection, Optimization, and Compensation (SOC) model   As noted, our application of COR theory to safety workarounds highlights several gaps that cannot be accounted for by COR theory. In this section, we will draw on other theories to help address those gaps and otherwise advance our understanding of the links between well-being and injury through workarounds. One theory that may extend the safety workarounds literature is the SOC model (Baltes, 1997; Baltes & Baltes, 1990). This model suggests that when individuals make resource allocation decisions, they do so by selecting goals, optimizing their current resources to meet those goals, and compensating when something does not allow them to utilize their resources. Well-being may shift the approach individuals take to selection, optimization, and compensation (Zacher & Frese, 2011) and may also impact the relationship between lower well-being and outcomes such as performance (Demerouti et al., 2014). In the context of safety workarounds, individuals prefer to do their work without getting injured. Interesting, however, is consideration of selection in the context of performance and safety. As noted above, safety and task performance can occasionally seem at odds. While the literature typically suggests that individuals focus their attention on task performance when resources are limited (e.g., Hockey, 1997; Holzberger, Philipp & Kunter, 2013), studies of that form of goal selection usually assume that task performance in those contexts can be completed safely. Thus, employees may encounter situations where the goals of task performance and personal safety are at odds. Loss-based selection suggests that individuals might shed goals (safety) in order to focus on task performance goals (Freund & Baltes, 1998; Probst, 2002).

Optimization and compensation are most clearly aligned with the notion of workarounds. The optimization process involves "refinement of resources as a means of reaching higher levels of goal achievement" (Demerouti et al., 2014, p. 98). Presumably, such processes become even more important when resources are threatened or lost. Thus, individuals that engage in high levels of optimization are likely to see a workaround as a way to better configure resources to achieve a goal. The compensation process involves making changes when goal achievement looks unlikely due to inadequate resources. Schmitt, Zacher, and Frese (2012) found that individuals were more likely to rely on others when their workload was higher. In other words, they are compensating for a heavy workload by seeking help from others (see also Halbesleben & Bowler, 2007). Workarounds might be considered a form of compensation when the goal of achieving task completion is blocked.

The SOC model addresses the gap in COR theory regarding situations when the workaround requires more resources than completing the task the prescribed way. The SOC model suggests that aligning selection, optimization, and compensation approaches leads to positive adaptation at work (Baltes & Baltes, 1990). Thus, a workaround can be a means to achieve task performance despite lower levels of resources associated with lower well-being. In this case, the workaround represents loss-based selection whereby the means for achieving the goal must be altered (compensation) due to blocks in workflow. To the extent that the workaround chosen is the best utilization of remaining resources (optimization), the workaround may represent an adaptation that aligns selection, optimization, and compensation strategies.

Broaden-and-build theory Frederickson's (2001; Frederickson & Joiner, 2002) broaden-and-build theory suggests that when individuals experience positive emotions, their repertoire of cognitions and behaviors broadens (Frederickson & Branigan, 2005). This process has several implications for well-being and safety. First, positive emotions can create positive cycles whereby well-being is increased through positive gain spirals similar to what was described in COR theory (Bakker & Demerouti, 2008; Frederickson, 2000; Frederickson & Joiner, 2002) that can negate stressors and downward spirals that can result from repeated blocks in workflow (Garland et al., 2010). The broadening process can also increase psychological resilience and strengthen coping with stressors (Ong, Bergeman, Bisconti, & Wallace, 2006). Thus, positive emotions might make workarounds less likely by improving employee well-being.

To the extent that positive well-being can broaden the employees' base of cognitions and behaviors related to safety, one would expect that those with greater well-being (e.g., those with high levels of work engagement), would be in a better position to evaluate a variety of options for workarounds (Amabile, Barsade, Mueller, & Staw, 2005). While this could increase workarounds, it might also allow employees to account for both the productivity motive and safety motive simultaneously. Thus, the workarounds chosen may be less likely to increase exposure to injury.

In this way, broaden-and-build theory addresses two of the COR gaps discussed above. First, broaden-and-build theory helps us to better understand the processes when employees have more resources. While it suggests some of the same issues with regard to paradoxically increasing workarounds that COR theory does, broaden-and-build theory also helps explain the nature of those workarounds and why they might reduce injuries. Second, it helps address the cognitive capacity issue, effectively suggesting that the processes of lower cognitive capacity and defensive investment work hand-in-hand. As resources increase, individuals increase their cognitive capacity to consider more, and potentially safer, alternatives. Conversely, lower cognitive capacity creates more narrowed thinking and forces individuals to make choices that maximize the outcomes within the resource boundaries they are experiencing.

Certainly, more work is needed to understand where broaden-and-build theory fits within our understanding of well-being and safety. However, research indicates that broaden-and-build theory is an important mechanism in the management of psychological resources in the context of work engagement (Bakker & Demerouti, 2008), so extensions of the theory to fill gaps in COR theory seem like fruitful avenues to explore. To that end, we now turn to a discussion of future research directions linking well-being and injury.

Future Research

Despite a growing body of research, a significant need for more research on the links between well-being and injury and, in particular, the role that workarounds play in that relationship remains. Understanding the underlying psychology of workarounds represents an important priority in the literature. As noted, though there are dozens of studies examining predictors of workarounds, research explaining the cognitive processes leading to those workarounds is needed. We have presented several theoretical directions that require further testing. In this section, we discuss several methodological concerns that must be addressed when testing those theories.

Conceptualization and operationalization of safety workarounds

One of the challenges with studying workarounds is operationalizing them and specifically capturing them as they happen. Several studies have employed very time-intensive observational or interview techniques to learn more about workarounds (e.g., Halbesleben et al., 2010; Tucker & Spear, 2006). While these approaches have helped established the depth of the workaround concept, they are unable to address issues such as prevalence and raise questions about generalizability beyond their limited samples. Thus, measuring workarounds on a larger scale is a significant remaining issue. Halbesleben (2010) presented the first measure of safety workarounds; it was a three-item measure that assessed whether people followed intended safety procedures when it takes longer or is harder to do so. As a basic assessment of safety workarounds, it works well. However, a more comprehensive measure might be useful to address the underlying complexities of workarounds. The measure of Halbesleben, Rathert, and Bennett (2013) offers a starting point because it attempts to measure both the context of workarounds (in other words, the source of the blocks of workflow) and the underlying psychological processes associated with workarounds. They argue that the measure is useful because it allows researchers and managers to focus on the issues most important to their work: either what is causing the workarounds or the underlying processes of those engaging in the workaround. Given the processes they measured were grounded in other empirical work concerning workarounds, adapting their model to safety workarounds (it was written with patient safety in mind) may hold some promise.

Another challenge with measurement is valence of workarounds. Researchers must decide whether workarounds are defined as behaviors independent of their outcome. For example, when discussing broaden-and-build theory, we suggested that positive emotions might actually make workarounds more likely, but that the workarounds would be safer among those with positive emotions because they would have more resources and could consider more workaround options. We have also suggested that sometimes workarounds are a source of good ideas in organizations (Lalley, 2014). Thus, it becomes an issue of whether we measure workarounds independent of whether or not they were effective. Arguments exist for both approaches. Emphasizing the behavior independent of motives or outcomes raises concerns that workarounds are merely safety noncompliance. The line between a workaround and noncompliance is a fine one; the primary difference is that workarounds have the specific motive of working around a block in workflow (Halbesleben et al., 2010). However, incorporating the outcome of the workarounds can only be done in hindsight and may be inappropriate for studies predicting whether someone will engage in a workaround. In the end, a measure that addresses workaround motives, workaround behaviors, and separate outcomes (e.g., safety outcomes) is probably the most appropriate.

Other research design issues

Beyond measurement, several other research design issues exist in the literature. This is evident when we consider several of the alternative theoretical approaches we have proposed. The dialectical perspective suggests that the relationship grows and changes in response to the tensions. Thus, understanding the role of dialectics in workarounds requires longitudinal designs that tap into the dialectical tensions over a period of time. One of the challenges, however, is observing the key points where the tension is triggered since one may experience workflow blocks infrequently. This problem also exists in interpersonal relational dialectics research; researchers in that area have addressed it largely by applying turning points analysis (Becker et al., 2009; Baxter & Bullis, 1986; Bullis & Bach, 1989; Golish, 2000; Surra, 1985, 1987) and have suggested it as an approach to studying relationships in organizations (Halbesleben, 2012). In turning point analysis, the researcher works with the participant to map the trajectory of the relationship over time, identifies times when the relationship has shifted and then explores what occurred during those shifts. Applying this to workarounds, turning points could be identified when workflow was blocked and the employee needed to decide between following intended procedures or working around the block. A turning point requires a shift in the approach. For example, a turning point would occur if the employee had been engaging in workarounds and stopped or had been following procedures and started engaging in workarounds.

Typically, turning point analysis is studied through retrospective recall an emphasis on qualitative methods (cf., Becker et al., 2009); however, one could engage in a prospective

quantitative design whereby data were collected at regular intervals with the hope of capturing the dialectical tension as it was being experienced. Data analysis may be somewhat
challenging given the nonlinear nature of turning points. However, extensions of discontinuous growth modeling might be a possibility whereby the turning points are modeled
as discontinuous moments of change in the data (Singer & Willett, 2003).

The dynamics underlying COR theory and broaden-and-build theory also imply that
more longitudinal research is needed. Given the frequency with which blocks are presented to employees (Tucker & Spear, 2006), designs employing frequent diaries might
be a more useful technique to get at the underlying psychology of workarounds (Ohly,
Sonnentag, Niessen, & Zapf, 2010). While this would require shorter measures of workarounds, complicating several of the issues addressed above with measurement, it could
supplement the current research that is largely cross-sectional and is unable to get at the
moment-to-moment decision to engage in workarounds as blocks are revealed to the
employee.

Conclusion

Several key themes can be drawn from our chapter. First, there is a fairly well established
link between lower well-being and injuries, both in terms of general well-being and
specific stressors. That relationship is consistent across occupations and safety outcomes.
What is less clear, however, is the manner in which lower well-being leads to injuries.
Since it seems unlikely that lower well-being itself causes injury, the focus is increasing on how lower well-being impacts cognitive and behavioral approaches to safety by
employees.

Second, emerging evidence suggests that workarounds might be a key behavioral link
between lower well-being and occupational injuries. Though we all encounter numerous
barriers in our workflow (Tucker & Spear, 2006), those experiencing strain appear more
likely to complete their work using procedures that deviate further from intended safety
practices in ways that jeopardize their personal safety. Because of their limited resources,
strained individuals may be more inclined to navigate the production-safety dialectic by
emphasizing the more immediate production outcomes.

Third, conservation of resources theory offers meaningful explanations to the processes
by which those with strain choose to engage in workarounds and increase their exposure
to occupational injury. However, additional theories can inform situations that are clearly
explained by COR-based processes.

Fourth, much more research is needed on the links between well-being and injury in
general and workarounds in particular. These issues range from conceptual, such as how
researchers separate workarounds from related constructs like deviance and safe violations
(Alper & Karsh, 2009; Besnard & Greathead, 2003) and how researchers measure workarounds (Halbesleben, Rathert, & Bennett, 2013), to interventions designed to improve
well-being and/or reduce workarounds. A key future practical and research concern will be
understanding the ways that workarounds are communicated so that they can be utilized
either as learning opportunities to make the workplace safer or innovative alternatives to
current work processes (Westphal et al., 2013).

Though their incidence is declining, occupational injuries still affect many workers each
year (nearly 3 million in the United States in 2012; BLS, 2013). Understanding the
ties between employee well-being and injuries remains a critical concern for researchers.
Workarounds offer an interesting behavioral mediator that could help improve our understanding of how well-being increases injury incidence.

References

Ahola, K., Salminen, S., Toppinen-Tanner, S., Koskinen, A., & Väänänen, A. (2013). Occupational burnout and severe injuries: An eight-year prospective cohort study among Finnish forest industry workers. *Journal of Occupational Health, 55*(6), 450–457.

Alper, S. J., Holden, R. J., Scanlon, M. C., Patel, N., Kaushal, R., Skibinski, K., Brown, R., & Karsh, B. T. (2012). Self-reported violations during medication administration in two paediatric hospitals. *BMJ Quality & Safety, 21*(5), 408–415.

Alper, S. J., & Karsh, B. T. (2009). A systematic review of safety violations in industry. *Accident Analysis & Prevention, 41*(4), 739–754.

Amabile, T. M., Barsade, S. G., Mueller, J. S., & Staw, B. M. (2005). Affect and creativity at work. *Administrative Science Quarterly, 50*(3), 367–403.

Baker, H. M. (1997). Rules outside the rules for administration of medication: A study in New South Wales, Australia. *Image: The Journal of Nursing Scholarship, 29*(2), 155–158.

Bakker, A. B., & Demerouti, E. (2008). Towards a model of work engagement. *Career Development International, 13*(3), 209–223.

Bakker, A. B., Demerouti, E., & Sanz-Vergel, A. I. (2014). Burnout and work engagement: The JD–R approach. *Annual Review of Organizational Psychology and Organization Behavior, 1,* 389–411.

Baltes, P. B. (1997). On the incomplete architecture of human ontogeny: Selection, optimization, and compensation as foundation of developmental theory. *American Psychologist, 52*(4), 366–380.

Baltes, P. B., & Baltes, M. M. (1990). Psychological perspectives on successful aging: The model of selective optimization with compensation. In P. B. Baltes & M. M. Baltes (Eds.), *Successful aging: Perspectives from the behavioral sciences* (pp. 1–34). New York, NY: Cambridge University Press.

Bantham, J. H., Celuch, K. G., & Kasouf, C. J. (2003). A perspective of partnerships based on interdependence and dialectical theory. *Journal of Business Research, 56*(4), 265–274.

Baxter, L. A. (1990). Dialectical contradictions in relationship development. *Journal of Social and Personal Relationships, 7*(1), 69–88.

Baxter, L. A. (2011). *Voicing relationships: A dialogic perspective.* Thousand Oaks, CA: Sage.

Baxter, L. A., & Bullis, C. (1986). Turning points in developing romantic relationships. *Human Communication Research, 12*(4), 469–493.

Baxter, L. A., & Montgomery, B. M. (1996). *Relating: Dialogues and dialectics.* New York, NY: Guilford Press.

Baxter, L. E. (2013). Supportive leadership, employee engagement and occupational safety: A field study. Unpublished doctoral dissertation. University of Tennessee, Knoxville.

Becker, J. A. H., Johnson, A. J., Craig, E. A., Gilchrist, E. S., Haigh, M. M., & Lane, L. T. (2009). Friendships are flexible, not fragile: Turning points in geographically close and long-distance relationships. *Journal of Social and Personal Relationships, 26*(4), 347–369.

Benson, J. K. (1973). The analysis of bureaucratic-professional conflict: Functional versus dialectical approaches. *Sociological Quarterly, 14*(3), 376–394.

Benson, J. K. (1977). Organizations: A dialectical view. *Administrative Science Quarterly, 22*(1), 1–21.

Besnard, D., & Greathead, D. (2003). A cognitive approach to safe violations. *Cognition, Technology & Work, 5*(4), 272–282.

Besnard, D., & Hollnagel, E. (2014). I want to believe: Some myths about the management of industrial safety. *Cognition, Technology & Work, 16,* 13–23.

Bridge, K., & Baxter, L. A. (1992). Blended relationships: Friends as work associates. *Western Journal of Communication, 56*(3), 200–225.

Bullis, C. A., & Bach, B. W. (1989). Socialization turning points: An examination of change in organizational identification. *Western Journal of Speech Communication, 53*(3), 273–293.

Bureau of Labor Statistics (BLS) (2013). Workplace injury and illness summary. Report USDL-13-2119. http://www.bls.gov/news.release/osh.nr0.htm (accessed 1 June, 2015).

Burke, M. J., Sarpy, S. A., Tesluk, P. E., & Smith-Crowe, K. (2002). General safety performance: A test of a grounded theoretical model. *Personnel Psychology, 55*(2), 429–457.

Carayon, P., Wetterneck, T. B., Hundt, A. S., Ozkaynak, M., DeSilvey, J., Ludwig, B., Ram, P., & Rough, S. S. (2007). Evaluation of nurse interaction with bar code medication administration technology in the work environment. *Journal of Patient Safety, 3*(1), 34–42.

Carlo, L. C., Lyytinen, K., & Boland Jr, R. J. (2012). Dialectics of collective minding: Contradictory appropriations of information technology in a high-risk project. *MIS Quarterly, 36*(4), 1081–1108.

Chaplin, R. (2009). Process safety indicators: Response to Andrew Hopkins. *Safety Science, 47,* 467.

Chau, N., Lemogne, C., Legleye, S., Choquet, M., Falissard, B., & Fossati, P. (2011). Are occupational factors and mental difficulty associated with occupational injury? *Journal of Occupational and Environmental Medicine, 53*(12), 1452–1459.

Christian, M. S., Bradley, J. C., Wallace, J. C., & Burke, M. J. (2009). Workplace safety: A meta-analysis of the roles of person and situation factors. *Journal of Applied Psychology, 94*(5), 1103–1127.

Chung, Y. S., & Wu, H. L. (2013). Effect of burnout on accident involvement in occupational drivers. *Transportation Research Record: Journal of the Transportation Research Board, 2388*(1), 1–9.

Clarke, S. (1999). Perceptions of organizational safety: Implications for the development of safety culture. *Journal of Organizational Behavior, 20*(2), 185–198.

Clarke, S. (2006). The relationship between safety climate and safety performance: A meta-analytic review. *Journal of Occupational Health Psychology, 11*(4), 315–327.

Clarke, S. (2010). An integrative model of safety climate: Linking psychological climate and work attitudes to individual safety outcomes using meta-analysis. *Journal of Occupational and Organizational Psychology, 83*(3), 553–578.

Clarke, S. (2013). Safety leadership: A meta-analytic review of transformational and transactional leadership styles as antecedents of safety behaviours. *Journal of Occupational and Organizational Psychology, 86*(1), 22–49.

Clarke, S., & Robertson, I. (2005). A meta-analytic review of the Big Five personality factors and accident involvement in occupational and non-occupational settings. *Journal of Occupational and Organizational Psychology, 78*(3), 355–376.

Clarke, S. P., Rockett, J. L., Sloane, D. M., & Aiken, L. H. (2002). Organizational climate, staffing, and safety equipment as predictors of needlestick injuries and near-misses in hospital nurses. *American Journal of Infection Control, 30*(4), 207–216.

Clarke, S., & Ward, K. (2006). The role of leader influence tactics and safety climate in engaging employees' safety participation. *Risk Analysis, 26*(5), 1175–1185.

Debono, D. S., Greenfield, D., Travaglia, J. F., Long, J. C., Black, D., Johnson, J., & Braithwaite, J. (2013). Nurses' workarounds in acute healthcare settings: A scoping review. *BMC Health Services Research, 13*(1), 175–189.

Demerouti, E., Bakker, A. B., & Leiter, M. (2014). Burnout and job performance: The moderating role of selection, optimization, and compensation strategies. *Journal of Occupational Health Psychology, 19*(1), 96–107.

Diestel, S., Cosmar, M., & Schmidt, K. H. (2013). Burnout and impaired cognitive functioning: The role of executive control in the performance of cognitive tasks. *Work & Stress, 27*(2), 164–180.

Dougherty, L., Sque, M., & Crouch, R. (2012). Decision-making processes used by nurses during intravenous drug preparation and administration. *Journal of Advanced Nursing, 68*(6), 1302–1311.

Eisenhauer, L. A., Hurley, A. C., & Dolan, N. (2007). Nurses' reported thinking during medication administration. *Journal of Nursing Scholarship, 39*(1), 82–87.

Espin, S., Lingard, L., Baker, G. R., & Regehr, G. (2006). Persistence of unsafe practice in everyday work: An exploration of organizational and psychological factors constraining safety in the operating room. *Quality and Safety in Health Care, 15*(3), 165–170.

Fogarty, G. J., & McKeon, C. M. (2006). Patient safety during medication administration: The influence of organizational and individual variables on unsafe work practices and medication errors. *Ergonomics, 49*(5–6), 444–456.

Fowler, P. H., Craig, J., Fredendall, L. D., & Damali, U. (2008). Perioperative workflow: Barriers to efficiency, risks, and satisfaction. *AORN Journal, 87*(1), 187–208.

Fredrickson, B. L. (2000). Cultivating positive emotions to optimize health and well-being. *Prevention & Treatment, 3*(1), 1a.

Fredrickson, B. L. (2001). The role of positive emotions in positive psychology: The broaden-and-build theory of positive emotions. *American Psychologist, 56*(3), 219–226.

Fredrickson, B. L., & Branigan, C. (2005). Positive emotions broaden the scope of attention and thought-action repertoires. *Cognition & Emotion, 19*(3), 313–332.

Fredrickson, B. L., & Joiner, T. (2002). Positive emotions trigger upward spirals toward emotional well-being. *Psychological Science, 13*(2), 172–175.

Freund, A. M., & Baltes, P. B. (1998). Selection, optimization, and compensation as strategies of life management: Correlations with subjective indicators of successful aging. *Psychology and Aging, 13*(4), 531–543.

Friedman, A., Crosson, J. C., Howard, J., Clark, E. C., Pellerano, M., Karsh, B. T., Crabtree, B., Jaén, C. R., & Cohen, D. J. (2014). A typology of electronic health record workarounds in small-to-medium size primary care practices. *Journal of the American Medical Informatics Association, 21*(e1), e78–e83.

Furber, C. M., & Thomson, A. M. (2006). "Breaking the rules" in baby-feeding practice in the UK: Deviance and good practice? *Midwifery, 22*(4), 365–376.

Ganster, D. C., & Rosen, C. C. (2013). Work stress and employee health: A multidisciplinary review. *Journal of Management, 39*(5), 1085–1122.

Garland, E. L., Fredrickson, B., Kring, A. M., Johnson, D. P., Meyer, P. S., & Penn, D. L. (2010). Upward spirals of positive emotions counter downward spirals of negativity: Insights from the broaden-and-build theory and affective neuroscience on the treatment of emotion dysfunctions and deficits in psychopathology. *Clinical Psychology Review, 30*(7), 849–864.

Golish, T. D. (2000). Changes in closeness between adult children and their parents: A turning point analysis. *Communication Reports, 13*(2), 79–97.

Gorgievski, M. J., & Hobfoll, S. E. (2008). Work can burn us out or fire us up: Conservation of resources in burnout and engagement. In J. R. B. Halbesleben (Ed.), *Handbook of stress and burnout in health care* (pp. 7–22). Hauppauge, NY: Nova Science.

Hagen, K., Magnus, P., & Vetlesen, K. (1998). Neck/shoulder and low-back disorders in the forestry industry: Relationship to work tasks and perceived psychosocial job stress. *Ergonomics, 41*(10), 1510–1518.

Halbesleben, J. R. B. (2010). The role of exhaustion and workarounds in predicting occupational injuries: A cross-lagged panel study of health care professionals. *Journal of Occupational Health Psychology, 15*(1), 1–16.

Halbesleben, J. R. B. (2012). Positive coworker interactions. In L. Eby and T. Allen (Eds.), *Personal relationships: The effect of supervisory, co-worker, team, customer and non-work exchanges on employee attitudes, behavior, and well-being* (pp. 107–130). Hoboken, NJ: John Wiley & Sons, Inc.

Halbesleben, J. R., & Bowler, W. M. (2007). Emotional exhaustion and job performance: the mediating role of motivation. *Journal of Applied Psychology, 92*(1), 93–106.

Halbesleben, J. R. B., & Clark, S. K. (2009). Work engagement and occupational injuries: Investing resources in safety. Paper presented at APA/NIOSH Work, Stress, and Health 2009: Global Concerns and Approaches Conference, San Juan, Puerto Rico.

Halbesleben, J. R. B., Harvey, J., & Bolino, M. C. (2009). Too engaged? A conservation of resources view of the relationship between work engagement and work interference with family. *Journal of Applied Psychology, 94*(6), 1452–1465.

Halbesleben, J. R. B., Leroy, H., Dierynch, B., Simons, T., Savage, G., McCaughey, D., & Leon, M. R. (2013). Living up to safety values in healthcare: Effects of a leaders' behavioral integrity on occupational safety. *Journal of Occupational Health Psychology, 18*(4), 395–405.

Halbesleben, J. R., Neveu, J. P., Paustian-Underdahl, S. C., & Westman, M. (2014). Getting to the "COR": Understanding the role of resources in conservation of resources theory. *Journal of Management, 40,* 1334–1364.

Halbesleben, J. R. B., & Rathert, C. (2008). The role of continuous quality improvement and psychological safety in predicting workarounds. *Health Care Management Review, 33*(2), 134–144.

Halbesleben, J. R. B., Rathert, C., & Bennett, S. F. (2013). Measuring nursing workarounds: Tests of the reliability and validity of a tool. *Journal of Nursing Administration, 43*(1), 50–55.

Halbesleben, J. R. B., Rathert, C., & Williams, E. S. (2013). Emotional exhaustion and medication administration workarounds: The moderating role of nurse satisfaction with medication administration. *Health Care Management Review, 38,* 95–104.

Halbesleben, J. R. B., Savage, G. T., Wakefield, D. S., & Wakefield, B. J. (2010). Rework and workarounds in nurse medication administration processes. *Health Care Management Review, 35*(2), 124–133.

Halbesleben, J. R. B., Wakefield, D. S., & Wakefield, B. J. (2008). Work-arounds in health care settings: Literature review and research agenda. *Health Care Management Review, 33*(1), 2–12.

Halbesleben, J. R. B., Whitman, M. V., & Crawford, W. S. (2014). A dialectical theory of the decision to attend work: Bringing together absenteeism and presenteeism. *Human Resource Management Review, 24*(2), 177–192.

Haynes, A. (1991). Transcript of the presentation given at the NASA Ames Research Center, May 24, 1991. http://www.panix.com/~jac/aviation/haynes.html (accessed June 1, 2015).

Henker, N., Sonnentag, S., & Unger, D. (2015). Transformational leadership and employee creativity: The mediating role of promotion focus and creative process engagement. *Journal of Business and Psychology, 30*(2), 235–247.

Hobfoll, S. E. (1988). *The ecology of stress.* New York, NY: Hemisphere.

Hobfoll, S. E. (1989). Conservation of resources: A new attempt at conceptualizing stress. *American Psychologist, 44*(3), 513–524.

Hobfoll, S. E. (1998). *Stress, culture, and community.* New York, NY: Plenum.

Hobfoll, S. E. (2001). The influence of culture, community, and the nested self in the stress process: Advancing conservation of resources theory. *Applied Psychology: An International Review, 50*(3), 337–370.

Hobfoll, S. E., & Freedy, J. (1993). Conservation of resources: A general stress theory applied to burnout. In W. B. Schaufeli, C. Maslach, & T. Marek (Eds.), *Professional burnout: Recent developments in theory and research* (pp. 115–129). Washington, DC: Taylor & Francis.

Hockey, G. R. (1997). Compensatory control in the regulation of human performance under stress and high workload: A cognitive-energetical framework. *Biological Psychology, 45*(1), 73–93.

Hodkinson, M. (2009). Process safety indicators: Response to Andrew Hopkins. *Safety Science, 47,* 469.

Hofmann, D. A., & Mark, B. (2006). An investigation of the relationship between safety climate and medication errors as well as other nurse and patient outcomes. *Personnel Psychology, 59*(4), 847–869.

Hofmann, D. A., Morgeson, F. P., & Gerras, S. J. (2003). Climate as a moderator of the relationship between LMX and content-specific citizenship behavior: Safety climate as an exemplar. *Journal of Applied Psychology, 88*(1), 170–178.

Hollnagel, E. (2009). Extending the scope of the human factor. In E. Hollnagel (Ed.), *Safer complex industrial environments* (pp. 37–61). Boca Raton, FL: Taylor & Francis.

Hollnagel, E., Paries, J., Woods, D. D., & Wreathall, J. (Eds.) (2011). *Resilience engineering in practice: A guidebook.* Farnham, UK: Ashgate.

Hollnagel, E., Woods, D. D., & Leveson, N. G. (2006). *Resilience engineering: Concepts and precepts.* Aldershot, UK: Ashgate.

Holzberger, D., Philipp, A., & Kunter, M. (2013). How teachers' self-efficacy is related to instructional quality: A longitudinal analysis. *Journal of Educational Psychology, 105*(3), 774.

Hopkins, A. (2009). Thinking about process safety indicators. *Safety Science, 47,* 460–465.

Hutchinson, S. A. (1990). Responsible subversion: A study of rule-bending among nurses. *Research and Theory for Nursing Practice, 4*(1), 3–17.

Johnston, J. J. (1995). Occupational injury and stress. *Journal of Occupational and Environmental Medicine, 37*(10), 1199–1203.

Julià, M., Catalina-Romero, C., Calvo-Bonacho, E., & Benavides, F. G. (2013). The impact of job stress due to the lack of organisational support on occupational injury. *Occupational and Environmental Medicine, 70*(9), 623–629.

Kahol, K., Vankipuram, M., Patel, V. L., & Smith, M. L. (2011). Deviations from protocol in a complex trauma environment: Errors or innovations? *Journal of Biomedical Informatics, 44*(3), 425–431.

Koopman, P., & Hoffman, R. R. (2003). Work-arounds, make-work, and kludges. *IEEE Intelligent Systems, 18*(6), 70–75.

Koppel, R., Wetterneck, T., Telles, J. L., & Karsh, B. (2008). Workarounds to barcode medication administration systems: Their occurrences, causes and threats to patient safety. *Journal of the American Medical Informatics Association, 15*(4), 408–423.

Krueger, N., & Dickson, P. R. (1994). How believing in ourselves increases risk taking: Perceived self-efficacy and opportunity recognition. *Decision Sciences, 25*(3), 385–400.

Lalley, C. (2014). Workarounds and obstacles: Unexpected source of innovation. *Nursing Administration Quarterly, 38*(1), 69–77.

Laumer, S., Maier, C., & Eckhardt, A. (2010). Why do they resist? An empirical analysis of an individual's personality trait resistance regarding the adoption of new information systems. ECIS Proceedings, Paper 31. http://aisel.aisnet.org/ecis2010/31 (accessed June 1, 2015)

Lawrence, E., Halbesleben, J. R. B., & Paustian-Underdahl, S. (2013). The impact of financial and job security on work–family reactions to occupational injuries. *Journal of Occupational Health Psychology, 18*(4), 371–383.

Leroy, H., Dierynch, B., Anseel, F., Simons, T., Halbesleben, J. R. B., McCaughey, D., Savage, G., & Sels, L. (2012). Behavioral integrity for safety, priority of safety, psychological safety, and patient safety: A team level study. *Journal of Applied Psychology, 97*(6), 1273–1281.

Li, F., Jiang, L., Yao, X., & Li, Y. (2013). Job demands, job resources and safety outcomes: The roles of emotional exhaustion and safety compliance. *Accident Analysis & Prevention, 51,* 243–251.

Lindstrom, K., Leino, T., Seitsamo, J., & Torstila, I. (1997). A longitudinal study of work characteristics and health complaints among insurance employees in VDT work. *International Journal of Human–Computer Interaction, 9*(4), 343–368.

Maslach, C. (1982). *Burnout: The cost of caring.* Englewood Cliffs, NJ: Prentice Hall.

McCaughey, D., McGhan, G., Walsh, E. M., Rathert, C., & Belue, R. (2014). The relationship of positive work environments and workplace injury: Evidence from the National Nursing Assistant Survey. *Health Care Management Review, 39*(1), 75–88.

McKeon, C. M., Fogarty, G. J., & Hegney, D. G. (2006). Organizational factors: Impact on administration violations in rural nursing. *Journal of Advanced Nursing, 55*(1), 115–123.

Melamed, S., Shirom, A., Toker, S., Berliner, S., & Shapira, I. (2006). Burnout and risk of cardiovascular disease: Evidence, possible causal paths, and promising research directions. *Psychological Bulletin, 132*(3), 327–353.

Melamed, S., Ugarten, U., Shirom, A., Kahana, L. Lerman, Y., & Froom, P. (1999). Chronic burnout, somatic arousal and elevated cortisol levels. *Journal of Psychosomatic Research, 46*(6), 591–598.

Nahrgang, J. D., Morgeson, F. P., & Hofmann, D. A. (2011). Safety at work: A meta-analytic investigation of the link between job demands, job resources, burnout, engagement, and safety outcomes. *Journal of Applied Psychology, 96*(1), 71–94.

Neal, A., & Griffin, M. A. (2006). A study of the lagged relationships among safety climate, safety motivation, safety behavior, and accidents at the individual and group levels. *Journal of Applied Psychology, 91*(4), 946–953.

Niazkhani, Z., Pirnejad, H., van der Sijs, H., & Aarts, J. (2011). Evaluating the medication process in the context of CPOE use: The significance of working around the system. *International Journal of Medical Informatics, 80*(7), 490–506.

Ohly, S., Sonnentag, S., Niessen, C., & Zapf, D. (2010). Diary studies in organizational research. *Journal of Personnel Psychology, 9*(2), 79–93.

Olson, R., Grosshuesch, A., Schmidt, S., Gray, M., & Wipfli, B. (2009). Observational learning and workplace safety: The effects of viewing the collective behavior of multiple social models on the use of personal protective equipment. *Journal of Safety Research, 40*(5), 383–387.

O'Neil, S., Speroni, K. G., Dugan, L., & Daniel, M. G. (2010). A 2-tier study of direct care providers assessing the effectiveness of the red rule education project and precipitating factors surrounding red rule violations. *Quality Management in Healthcare, 19*(3), 259–264.

Ong, A. D., Bergeman, C. S., Bisconti, T. L., & Wallace, K. A. (2006). Psychological resilience, positive emotions, and successful adaptation to stress in later life. *Journal of Personality and Social Psychology, 91*(4), 730–749.

Oosterholt, B. G., van der Linden, D., Maes, J. H., Verbraak, M. J. P. M., & Kompier, M. A. (2012). Burned out cognition – Cognitive functioning of burnout patients before and after a period with psychological treatment. *Scandinavian Journal of Work, Environment & Health, 38*(4), 358–369.

Palmer, K. T., Harris, E. C., & Coggon, D. (2008). Chronic health problems and risk of accidental injury in the workplace: A systematic literature review. *Occupational and Environmental Medicine, 65*(11), 757–764.

Park, Y. K., Song, J. H., Yoon, S. W., & Kim, J. (2014). Learning organization and innovative behavior: The mediating effect of work engagement. *European Journal of Training and Development, 38*(1/2), 75–94.

Probst, T. M. (2002). Layoffs and tradeoffs: Production, quality, and safety demands under the threat of job loss. *Journal of Occupational Health Psychology, 7*(3), 211–220.

Rathert, C., Williams, E. S., Lawrence, E. R., & Halbesleben, J. R. (2012). Emotional exhaustion and workarounds in acute care: Cross sectional tests of a theoretical framework. *International Journal of Nursing Studies, 49*(8), 969–977.

Rich, B. L., Lepine, J. A., & Crawford, E. R. (2010). Job engagement: Antecedents and effects on job performance. *Academy of Management Journal, 53*(3), 617–635.

Runte, E. (2010). Productivity and safety: Adjustments at work in socio-technical systems. Doctoral dissertation, Mines-ParisTech, France.

Saleem, J. J., Russ, A. L., Justice, C. F., Hagg, H., Ebright, P. R., Woodbridge, P. A., & Doebbeling, B. N. (2009). Exploring the persistence of paper with the electronic health record. *International Journal of Medical Informatics, 78*(9), 618–628.

Salminen, S., Kivimäki, M., Elovainio, M., & Vahtera, J. (2003). Stress factors predicting injuries of hospital personnel. *American Journal of Industrial Medicine, 44*(1), 32–36.

Sandström, A., Rhodin, I. N., Lundberg, M., Olsson, T., & Nyberg, L. (2005). Impaired cognitive performance in patients with chronic burnout syndrome. *Biological Psychology, 69*(3), 271–279.

Schaber, S. D., Gerogiorgis, D. I., Ramachandran, R., Evans, J. M., Barton, P. I., & Trout, B. L. (2011). Economic analysis of integrated continuous and batch pharmaceutical manufacturing: A case study. *Industrial & Engineering Chemistry Research, 50*(17), 10083–10092.

Schmitt, A., Zacher, H., & Frese, M. (2012). The buffering effect of selection, optimization, and compensation strategy use on the relationship between problem solving demands and occupational well-being: A daily diary study. *Journal of Occupational Health Psychology, 17*(2), 139–149.

Schulman, P., Roe, E., Eeten, M. V., & Bruijne, M. D. (2004). High reliability and the management of critical infrastructures. *Journal of Contingencies and Crisis Management, 12*(1), 14–28.

Shirom, A., Westman, M., Shamai, O., & Carel, R. S. (1997). Effects of work overload and burnout on cholesterol and triglycerides levels: The moderating effects of emotional reactivity among male and female employees. *Journal of Occupational Health Psychology, 2*(4), 275–288.

Singer, J. D., & Willett, J. B. (2003). *Applied longitudinal data analysis: Modeling change and event occurrence.* New York, NY: Oxford University Press.

Slovic, P. (2001). The risk game. *Journal of Hazardous Materials, 86*(1–3), 17–24.

Spear, S. J., & Schmidhofer, M. (2005). Ambiguity and workarounds as contributors to medical error. *Annals of Internal Medicine, 142*(8), 627–630.

Stride, C. B., Turner, N., Hershcovis, S. M., Reich, T. C., Clegg, C. W., & Murphy, P. (2013). Negative safety events as correlates of work–safety tension. *Safety Science, 53*, 45–50.

Surra, C. A. (1985). Courtship types: Variations in interdependence between partners and social networks. *Journal of Personality and Social Psychology, 49*(2), 357–375.

Surra, C. A. (1987). Reasons for changes in commitment: Variations by courtship type. *Journal of Social and Personal Relationships, 4*(1), 17–33.

Tawatsupa, B., Yiengprugsawan, V., Kjellstrom, T., Berecki-Gisolf, J., Seubsman, S. A., & Sleigh, A. (2013). Association between heat stress and occupational injury among Thai workers: Findings of the Thai Cohort Study. *Industrial Health, 51*(1), 34–46.

Taxis, K., & Barber, N. (2003). Causes of intravenous medication errors: An ethnographic study. *Quality and Safety in Health Care, 12*(5), 343–347.

Tucker, A. L., & Edmondson, A. C. (2002). Managing routine exceptions: A model of nurse problem solving behavior. In L. H. Friedman, J. Goes, & G. T. Savage (Eds.), *Advances in health care management* (vol. 3, pp. 87–113). Bingley, UK: Emerald Group Publishing Ltd.

Tucker, A. L., & Edmondson, A. C. (2003). Why hospitals don't learn from failures. *California Management Review, 45*(2), 55–72.

Tucker, A. L., Edmondson, A. C., & Spear, S. (2002). When problem solving prevents organizational learning. *Journal of Organizational Change Management, 15*(2), 122–137.

Tucker, A. C., Heisler, W. S., & Janisse, L. D. (2014). Designed for workarounds: A qualitative study of the causes of operational failures in hospitals. *Permanente Journal, 18*(3), 33–41.

Tucker, A. L., & Spear, S. J. (2006). Operational failures and interruptions in hospital nursing. *Health Services Research, 41*(3), 643–662.

Turner, N., Hershcovis, M. S., Reich, T. C., & Totterdell, P. (2014). Work–family interference, psychological distress, and workplace injuries. *Journal of Occupational and Organizational Psychology, 87*(4), 715–732.

Van der Sijs, H., Rootjes, I., & Aarts, J. (2010). The shift in workarounds upon implementation of computerized physician order entry. *Studies in Health Technology and Informatics, 169*, 290–294.

Vogelsmeier, A. A., Halbesleben, J. R. B., & Scott-Cawiezell, J. R. (2008). Technology implementation and workarounds in the nursing home. *Journal of the American Medical Informatics Association, 15*(1), 114–119.

Wackers, G. (2006). Vulnerability and robustness in a complex technological system: Loss of control and recovery in the 2004 Snorre A gas blow-out. Research report 42/2006, University of Maastricht, the Netherlands.

Westphal, J., Lancaster, R., & Park, D. (2013). Work-arounds observed by fourth-year nursing students. *Western Journal of Nursing Research, 36*(8), 1002–1018.

Wheeler, A. R., Halbesleben, J. R., & Harris, K. J. (2012). How job-level HRM effectiveness influences employee intent to turnover and workarounds in hospitals. *Journal of Business Research, 65*(4), 547–554.

Zacher, H., & Frese, M. (2011). Maintaining a focus on opportunities at work: The interplay between age, job complexity, and the use of selection, optimization, and compensation strategies. *Journal of Organizational Behavior, 32*(2), 291–318.

Zohar, D. (2000). A group-level model of safety climate: Testing the effect of group climate on micro-accidents in manufacturing jobs. *Journal of Applied Psychology, 85*(4), 587–596.

Zohar, D. (2003). The influence of leadership and climate on occupational health and safety. In D. A. Hofmann, & L. E. Tetrick (Eds.), *Health and safety in organizations: A multilevel perspective* (pp. 201–230). San Francisco, CA: Jossey-Bass.

Zohar, D. (2010). Thirty years of safety climate research: Reflections and future directions. *Accident Analysis and Prevention, 42*(5), 1517–1522.

13

Organizational Climate

Sara Guediri and Mark A. Griffin

Introduction

Historically, research on workplace health and safety has focused less on organizational factors and instead approached employee health from an individual or job perspective and workplace safety from a technical-engineering perspective. However, a growing body of evidence has drawn attention to the organizational context as a key contributing factor in promoting health and safety at work. Addressing organizational factors has the potential for a more wide-reaching impact on improving health and safety than efforts aimed at certain job or individual characteristics (e.g., Carr, Schmidt, Ford, & DeShon, 2003; Dextras-Gauthier, Merchand, & Haines, 2012). As part of this interest for organizational factors in health and safety research, the concept of organizational climate has gained prominence. Organizational climate describes "the shared perceptions of and the meaning attached to policies, practices and procedures employees experience and the behaviors they observe getting rewarded and that are supported and expected" (Schneider, Ehrhart, & Macey, 2013, p. 362). Thus, organizational climate is a summary profile of the formal and informal policies, practices, and procedures and has sometimes been described as the "atmosphere" within an organization (Schulte, Ostroff, & Kinicki, 2006).

Organizational climate has been examined as an individual-level as well as a unit-level property (Schneider et al., 2013; Schulte et al., 2006). At the individual level, climate refers to employees' individual experience of organizational practices, policies, procedures, and norms. At the group or organizational level, organizational climate refers to shared perceptions or perceptual consensus about organizational practices, policies, procedures, and norms. There has been a considerable amount of debate on the issue of level of climate (Glick, 1985; Jones & James, 1979; Schneider et al., 2013; Zohar & Luria, 2005). The term *psychological climate* is used to refer to climate at the individual level whereas the term *organizational climate* is used when referring to shared perceptions (James & Jones, 1974; Schneider et al., 2013; Schulte et al., 2006). In addition, literature on organizational climate recognizes that practices, policies, and procedures vary for different domains within

The Wiley Blackwell Handbook of the Psychology of Occupational Safety and Workplace Health, First Edition.
Edited by Sharon Clarke, Tahira M. Probst, Frank Guldenmund, and Jonathan Passmore. © 2016 John Wiley & Sons Ltd. Published 2020 by John Wiley & Sons Ltd.

an organization (Ostroff, Kinicki, & Tamkins, 2003; Schneider, 1975; Schneider et al., 2013). Thus, organizations can have several sub-climates that refer to specific domains. For example, the wider organizational literature has explored domain-specific climates such as climate for service (e.g., Liao & Chuang, 2007) or climate for innovation (e.g., Mathisen, Torsheim, & Einarsen, 2006). The term *molar* organizational climate has been used to describe overarching organizational climate and the term *strategic* climate refers to domain-specific climates (e.g., Carr et al., 2003). Research in the area of health and safety has advanced the understanding of molar organizational climate as well as of various strategic climates for enhancing health and safety at work. One of the most prominent strategic climates that has stimulated a large volume of conceptual and empirical work is safety climate. Safety climate refers to perceptions about organizational practices, policies, and procedures specifically related to safety matters and has been identified as a key indicator of workplace safety (Clarke, 2006; Neal & Griffin, 2006; Zohar, 1980, 2000, 2010). Luria in Chapter 16 of this volume discusses safety climate as a group-level concept.

Although in practice, organizations tend to approach health and safety as one common objective, research has usually focused on health or safety. Thus, this chapter begins by reviewing literature on organizational climate and workplace health and well-being and then addresses research on organizational factors and workplace safety with a particular focus on the concepts of safety culture and safety climate. The final section of the chapter discusses emerging research that explores the dependencies between employee health, well-being, and safety and the role of organizational factors within these interconnections.

Organizational Climate, Health, and Well-being

Research on predictors of workplace health and well-being has often focused on individual-level variables, such as personal coping and individual differences, or job-level variables such as job demands and job-level resources (e.g., see Häusser, Mojzisch, Niesel, & Schulz-Hardt, 2010; van der Doef & Maes, 1999). Several chapters in this volume provide reviews of individual- and job-level perspectives and their relevance for understanding workplace health and safety: Chapter 11 by Cangiano and Parker on individual differences in proactivity, Chapter 7 by Chmiel and Hansez on work design and job demands, as well as Chapter 8 by Taris and Schaufeli on the job demands-resource model. These strands of research have made valuable advances in understanding the more immediate factors that impact on employee health and well-being. However, there is a growing body of research that points to the wider organizational context as an important impact factor for health and well-being in the workplace (Dextras-Gauthier et al., 2012; Jex, Sliter, & Britton, 2014; Morgeson, Dierdorff, & Hmurovic, 2010; Wilson, DeJoy, Vandenberg, Richardson, & McGrath, 2004; Zwetsloot & Leka, 2010). In particular, organizational climate, which subsumes multiple organizational factors, has been considered as a potent concept to explain workplace health and well-being.

This organizational approach to health and well-being can be related to context theory, which focuses on the importance of contextual determinants of organizational behavior (Bamberger, 2008; Johns, 2006; Rousseau & Fried, 2001). Bamberger (2008) discusses that closing the micro–macro gap in management research requires conjoining individual micro-level research (e.g., on individuals' health and well-being) with contextual concepts. Consistent with this perspective, a number of studies have addressed social support as an organizational factor that can enhance employee health and well-being (e.g., Kumari & Sharma, 1990; Rhoades & Eisenberger, 2002). However, it has been argued that research should move beyond social support and explore perceptions about the wider work environment as a determinant of health and well-being (Terry, Callan, & Sartori, 1996). Most conceptualizations of organizational climate include social support but in addition encompass a range of other organizational elements related to processes of the wider work environment, role, job, and leader, although there is no agreed framework on the structure of organizational climate (Martin, Jones, & Callan, 2005; Patterson et al., 2005).

DeJoy and Southern (1993) called for a more integrative perspective on how to promote employee health and well-being. They proposed a model with three layers referring to (1) the wider societal and economical situation, (2) physical and social aspects of the work environment (e.g., organizational climate), and (3) individual employee characteristics and job demands. They suggest that each level can directly or indirectly, through one of the other levels, influence employee health and well-being. Similarly, Cooper and Cartwright (1994; Cartwright, Cooper, Murphy, 1995) argue that achieving a "healthy organization" requires interventions that are targeted at more macro-level factors. They develop a research framework that outlines organizational-level climate as an antecedent of employee stress at the individual level, which in turn impacts on organizational-level consequences such as absenteeism and turnover rates. Others have also adopted theoretical frameworks, which extend the approach to workplace health by including organizational climate as a central element that shapes employees' experience at work (e.g., Dextras-Gauthier et al., 2012; Hart & Cooper, 2001; Michela, Lukaszewski, & Allegrante, 1995). Thus, underlying the relationship of organizational climate to employee health and well-being is the assumption that aspects of the overarching organizational functioning can influence lower-level job conditions and consequently affect individuals' health and well-being (Cummings & DeCotiis, 1973; Hart & Cooper, 2001; Wilson et al., 2004).

Since these earlier theorizations a number of empirical studies have explored the relationship of organizational climate to health and well-being outcomes. This body of literature has assessed specific psychological or physical health symptoms, but has also used broader measures, which reflect the more encompassing construct of employee well-being (Danna & Griffin, 1999). While there is no clear-cut definition, it is generally agreed that well-being goes beyond the sheer absence of ill-health and instead includes overall positive life experience (Danna & Griffin, 1999; Warr, 1990). Within organizational research this can include measures such as job engagement or job satisfaction. Thus, the discussion below focuses on the role of organizational climate for health and well-being.

It has been argued that research on the relationship of climate to health and well-being is somewhat dispersed due to the different dimensions of organizational climate, inconsistencies in labeling of dimensions, as well as different types of domain-specific climates of organizational climate (Carr et al., 2003). One broad categorization of studies is whether they investigated overall organizational climate (i.e., molar climate) or a domain-specific climate (i.e., strategic climate). Thus, the following parts of the chapter will first discuss research that has linked overall organizational climate with health and well-being and will then review research on specific facets of organizational climate and their link to workplace health and well-being.

In a meta-analysis Carr et al. (2003) summarized research on the relationship of organizational climate with work-relevant outcomes including psychological well-being. Based on an earlier taxonomy by Ostroff (1993), they distinguish organizational climate in terms of three components: affective (referring to social relations and interpersonal involvement), cognitive (referring to cognitive involvement such as job autonomy), and instrumental (referring to involvement in tasks and impact within the organization). The findings from their meta-analysis showed that all three organizational climate components were significantly, positively related to psychological well-being, but with effects of moderate to small magnitude. The affective organizational climate component showed the strongest relationship with psychological well-being (r = .17 based on 13 studies), whereas correlations between the instrumental (r = .11 based on nine studies) and cognitive (r = .07 based on nine studies) components with well-being were lower. These results suggest that aspects of organizational climate related to interpersonal and social involvement might be more important for influencing employee well-being than instrumental or cognitive involvement. Moreover, their study showed that the link between organizational climate components and psychological well-being was mediated by job satisfaction, suggesting a key pathway through which organizational climate impacts on psychological well-being.

Parker et al. (2003) also conducted a meta-analysis on climate and a range of work-related criterion measures including psychological well-being. A difference to Carr et al.'s (2003) meta-analysis is that they assessed psychological climate with reference to individual-level perceptions about organizational practices rather than climate perceptions aggregated to a higher unit. Based on a framework by James and James (1989) they differentiate five dimensions of psychological climate: (1) job-related (e.g., autonomy), (2) role-related (e.g., ambiguity), (3) leader-related (e.g., leader support), (4) work group-related (e.g., cooperation), and (5) organization-related (e.g., information sharing). Results showed that all five psychological climate dimensions were positively related to psychological well-being. Leader-related (r = .44 based on three studies) and role-related dimensions (r = .35 based on 11 studies) of psychological climate were most strongly correlated with psychological well-being, indicating that certain aspects of climate are more relevant for influencing employee well-being.

While both meta-analyses make an important contribution by summarizing the research findings on the link between climate and well-being, they also illustrate why synthesis of research in this area can be difficult. The two meta-analyses have relied on different frameworks to distinguish between different dimensions of climate. The findings of both studies converge by indicating that certain dimensions are more strongly related to well-being. Carr and her colleagues find that "affective climate" is most strongly related to well-being and Parker and colleagues find that the leader-related and job-related dimensions are most strongly correlated with psychological well-being. However, the different underlying frameworks make it difficult to draw overall conclusions about the aspects of organizational climate that are most critical for enhancing employee health and well-being.

Since the publication of the above two meta-analyses further research attention has been given to the influence of organizational climate on health and well-being, although empirical investigations are relatively limited. For example, Arnetz, Lucas, and Arnetz (2011) investigated the relationship between four aspects of organizational climate (i.e., social climate, participation, goal clarity, and performance feedback) to occupational stress and employee mental health. Based on a sample of 5316 Swedish hospital employees, the results showed that the link between the four organizational climate dimensions with stress and health was partially mediated by organizational efficiency. That is, organizational climate was linked to organizational efficiency, which in turn was negatively related to occupational stress, which ultimately had an influence on employee mental health. In a longitudinal study, Ylipaavalniemi et al. (2005) linked climate to employee depression. Their measure of climate included aspects such as support for innovation, support for participation, and commitment to excellence, which they combined into a total climate measure and aggregated to the team level. Based on a sample of 4815 Finnish hospital employees, results showed that team climate was related to doctor-diagnosed depression two years later, while controlling for baseline psychological distress. In addition, they investigated factors such as procedural justice and relational justice, which although not conceptualized as formal elements of organizational climate, describe practices from the wider working environment. The results revealed that high levels of procedural justice and relational justice were negatively related to future depression in employees.

There is also evidence that climate can be an effective strategy in promoting employee health and well-being during particularly stressful times such as organizational change. Martin et al. (2005) investigated psychological climate as a determinant of employee stress during an organizational change period. They showed that positive perceptions of psychological climate dimensions were linked to higher levels of psychological well-being with some of the effects being mediated through reduced change-related stress and increased change self-efficacy. Other studies have further broadened the range of health and well-being outcomes and linked organizational climate to criteria such as return from work after illness (Holmgren, Ekbladh, Hensing, & Dellve, 2013) and somatic health symptoms (Kawano, 2008).

Thus, empirical research lends support for organizational climate as an origin of employee health and well-being. This suggests that the scope of health and well-being interventions should include organizational factors. It has been shown that organizational climate encompasses a range of different aspects of the work environment and therefore is a broad spanned source that is applicable to a variety of job roles within an organization (Burke, Borucki, & Kaufman, 2002; Hall, Dollard, Winefield, Dormann, & Bakker, 2013; Martin et al., 2005). Thus, interventions aimed at climate perceptions might offer the potential for a more wider-reaching impact for improving health and well-being compared with narrower interventions focused on specific worker or job characteristics (Burke et al., 2002; Hall et al., 2013). This makes organizational climate perceptions an attractive prospect for efficient, cost-effective interventions. A potential peril of such a broad span approach is that it might lose relevance to the stressors and strains that employees experience at work (Hemingway & Smith, 1999). Thus, it remains critical that efforts to enhance health and well-being through organizational climate ensure that these match the stressors in the specific work environment (e.g., de Jonge & Dormann, 2006; Hemingway & Smith, 1999).

As noted above, while some studies have examined the role of molar organizational climate, other research has focused on domain-specific climates and their relationship with employee health and well-being (for a review see Jex et al., 2014). Among this body of research, psychosocial safety climate is a domain-specific climate that is rapidly gaining increasing research attention as a function to enhance workplace health and well-being (Bond, Tuckey, & Dollard, 2010; Dollard & Bakker, 2010; Garrick et al., 2014; Hall et al., 2013; Idris & Dollard, 2011; Law, Dollard, Tuckey, & Dormann, 2011). Studies investigating psychosocial safety climate have found support for it as a precursor to job demands experienced by employees (e.g., Idris, Dollard, & Yulita, 2014) as well as a resource that moderates the strain–health relationship (e.g., Garrick et al., 2014; Hall et al., 2013). Zadow and Dollard (Chapter 18 in this volume) provide a detailed discussion of the psychological safety climate construct and review evidence on its relationship with workplace health and well-being.

In addition to psychosocial safety climate, research has linked other domain-specific climates to employee health and well-being. In a review, Jex et al. (2014) identified studies that have related health and well-being outcomes with service climate (e.g., Drach-Zahavy, 2010; Grandey, Foo, Groth, & Goodwin, 2012; Kao, Cheng, Kuo, & Huang, 2014; Liao & Searcy, 2012;), organizational justice climate (e.g., Moliner, Martínez-Tur, Peiró, Ramos, & Cropanzano, 2005; Spell & Arnold, 2007), interpersonal relations climate such as incivility climate (e.g., Griffin, 2010; Leiter, Laschinger, Day, & Oore, 2011; Lim, Cortina, & Magley, 2008; Miner-Rubino & Cortina, 2004), climate for competitiveness (e.g., Arnold, Flaherty, Voss, & Mowen, 2009) as well as collective perceptions about efficacy (e.g., Jex & Bliese, 1999) and organizational control and support (e.g., Bachrach & Bamberger, 2007). They also identified safety climate as a strategic climate linked to workplace health. A separate detailed discussion of safety climate follows in the second part of this chapter.

Overall, studies of strategic domain-specific climates show the potential for these climates to influence employee health and well-being. Some argue that strategic climates can provide a more precise understanding when organizations are aiming to improve specific areas of employee health and well-being (Patterson et al., 2005). An interesting development within this literature is that research has begun to explore climates that have potential detrimental effects on health and well-being. So far, most research has addressed desirable strategic climates that organizations should foster to reduce ill-health and increase well-being (e.g., psychosocial safety climate, organizational justice climate, climate for support). Research on climates concerned with organizational processes such as incivility suggests that companies might want to discourage the development of these climates to prevent negative effects on health and well-being.

Multiple strategic climates create the potential for conflict between competing organizational goals. For example, perceptions about competitiveness might benefit overall performance but carry the risk of decreasing health and well-being among employees. Schneider et al. (2013) suggest that future research should pay attention to interactions between different strategic climates. Future research could investigate whether fostering a positive psychosocial safety climate as well as organizational justice climate brings incremental benefits for the promotion of health and well-being. Moreover, Schneider et al. (2013) discuss the role of molar organizational climate in developing specific strategic climates and suggests that molar climate sets the foundation for creating specific strategic climates. While research has theorized on the connection between organizational climate and domain-specific strategic climates, empirical investigations of this relationship are rare with a few exceptions (Clarke, 2010; Neal, Griffin, & Hart, 2000; Wallace, Popp, & Mondore, 2006). Thus, a further avenue for future research is to examine how overarching organizational climate and strategic climates can work in tandem to promote workplace health and well-being.

Overall, research indicates that organizational climate and domain-specific climates play a role in shaping workplace health and safety. An interesting pattern within this emerging literature is that studies report, for organizational climate as well as domain-specific climates, positive relationships to desirable outcomes (such as work engagement) and negative associations with poor well-being and ill-health. High levels of well-being go beyond the sheer absence of stress or ill-health and refer to an active positive life experience (Hall et al., 2013). Thus, research evidence on organizational climate is promising as it suggests that climate-focused interventions can be an effective strategy for reducing ill-health as well as proactively promoting health and well-being.

Organizational Climate and Workplace Safety

Research has traditionally explored safety as an engineering and ergonomic problem (Cox & Cheyne, 2000; Zohar, 2002). Organizations, governments, and regulators have made significant progress in accident reduction through implementation of strategies aimed at the control of physical hazards, technological advances in machinery and equipment, and safety management systems. However, major accident events such as the sinking of the Herald of Free Enterprise (Sheen, 1987) and Piper Alpha (Cullen, 1990) have highlighted organizational aspects as key factors that contributed to the incidents. This recognition initiated a shift toward organizational and social factors within safety research. However, while research on organizational approaches to safety has made substantial progress, investigations of recent major accident events such as Deepwater Horizon (President's Commission, 2011), continue to identify organizational factors as underlying causes. Thus, organizational conditions that were identified as contributory to accidents that happened over two decades ago still emerge as underlying causes in disasters. This continuity highlights that although academics, practitioners and industry leaders generally recognize organizational factors as an important aspect of workplace safety, research is still needed to advance the understanding of organizational factors for safety and how changes can be implemented in practice.

Within the organizational approach to safety, the two concepts of safety culture and safety climate have attracted much attention. This chapter will introduce safety culture and safety climate and will then focus on the construct of safety climate, discussing how safety climate can be differentiated from safety culture, the dimensionality of safety climate, and empirical developments on safety climate as an indicator of safety outcomes. Guldenmund in Chapter 19 of this volume reviews the safety culture literature and discusses the development of safety culture.

Safety culture

The International Atomic Energy Agency (IAEA, 1991) introduced the term *safety culture* following the nuclear reactor accident in Chernobyl in April 1986. Following the Chernobyl disaster, organizational deficiencies were identified as a cause in other large-scale accidents and the concept of safety culture rapidly gained interest across different industries. Since then there has been a considerable amount of scientific research on safety culture (Blazsin & Guldenmund, 2014; Choudry, Fang, & Mohamed, 2007; Clarke, 1999, 2003; Edwards, Davey, & Armstrong, 2013; Grote, 2008; Hale, 2000; Pidgeon & O'Leary, 2000; Reason, 1997, 1998; Wu, Liu, & Lu, 2007). The safety culture approach recognizes that it is too restrictive to view accident reduction from a purely technical-engineering or human factors perspective and acknowledges organizational conditions and social factors as underlying causes of accidents (Choudry et al., 2007; Clarke, 1999, 2000; Flin, 2007; Parker, Lawrie, & Hudson, 2006; Vredenburgh, 2002). Pidgeon (1991) defines safety culture "as the constructed system of meanings through which a given people or group understand the hazards of the world. Such a constructed meaning system specifies what is important and legitimate to them, and explains their relationship to matters of life and death, work and danger" (p. 135).

Safety culture is based on the concept of organizational culture, which is often described as "the way we do things around here" and refers to shared values, beliefs, and norms (Guldenmund, 2000). Several comprehensive reviews have been published on organizational culture (e.g., Brinkmann, 2007; Ehrhart, Schneider, & Macey, 2014; Schein, 2010; Schneider et al., 2013). The concept of general organizational culture does not consider that behavioral norms, values, and beliefs might vary with regard to different organizational dimensions such as technology, financial decision-making, or service quality. Thus, it has been argued that culture requires a facet-specific perspective (Guldenmund, 2000; Richter & Koch, 2004; Zohar, 1980). Safety culture describes a "facet" (Cooper, 2000) or "subset" (Clarke, 1999; O'Toole, 2002) of the overarching organizational culture specifically focused on health and safety matters.

Safety climate

As part of the shift of attention from individual-level factors toward organizational contributions to accidents, safety climate has become a prevalent concept within safety research

(Clarke, 2006; Flin, Mearns, O'Connor, & Bryden, 2000; Neal & Griffin, 2006; Mearns, Whitaker, & Flin, 2003; Zohar, 1980, 2000, 2010). Within the safety literature, safety climate is a key variable for understanding the role of organizational factors and could be referred to as the central tenet in a socio-organizational approach to safety. Safety climate subsumes a range of organizational characteristics and processes. It is described as "the workforce's perceptions of the organizational atmosphere" (Flin et al., 2000, p. 178) with regard to safety. Safety climate is defined as shared perceptions of policies, procedures, and practices relating to safety in the workplace (Griffin & Neal, 2000; Neal & Griffin, 2006). There is considerable evidence that safety climate is associated with a range of safety outcomes such as safety behaviors (Clarke, 2006; Neal & Griffin, 2006; Neal et al., 2000) and injury and safety incident rates (Barling, Loughlin, & Kelloway, 2002; Christian, Bradley, Wallace, & Burke, 2009; Clarke, 2006, 2013; Dedobbeleer & Béland, 1991; Hofmann & Stetzer, 1996; Mearns et al., 2003; Zohar, 1980, 2000).

Drawing on social learning theory (Bandura, 1977), it is theorized that employees make sense of their work environment and infer the behaviors that are desired, valued, and rewarded from interactions with managers, supervisors, coworkers, and other stakeholders. These repeated interactions communicate the value of safety within the workplace and hence shape employees' perceptions of safety climate (Zohar, 1980; Zohar & Tenne-Gazit, 2008). Therefore, safety climate provides employees with information about the status of safety and functions as "a frame of reference for guiding appropriate and adaptive task behavior" (Zohar, 1980, p. 96).

An important conceptual and measurement attribute of safety climate is that it captures the *relative* priority of safety. Safety often stands in direct competition with other organizational goals or demands such as cost or productivity. The status of safety might differ in a project that is within budget and on time compared with a project that is running behind schedule or under tight cost constraints. Thus, safety climate perceptions are based on *true* priorities, describing the value of safety relative to other demands (Shannon & Norman, 2009; Zohar, 2008, 2010; Zohar & Tenne-Gazit, 2008). Zohar (2010) refers to "espoused and enacted" values, with safety climate perceptions being derived from the enacted priority of safety. He emphasizes that it is important to reflect this relative value of safety in conceptualizations as well as operationalizations of safety climate.

Mirroring the conceptual link between safety culture and organizational culture, safety climate is a specific facet of universal organizational climate (James & James, 1989; Schneider et al., 2013; Zohar, 2010). As outlined in the introduction to this chapter, organizations' policies and practices are prioritized to differing degrees with regard to specific domains, so that an organization might have different "climates" referring to different organizational facets (Schneider, 1975; Schneider, Wheeler, & Cox, 1992). Therefore safety climate refers to prioritization of safety. However, as noted above this does not mean that safety climate is unrelated to the wider organizational context. Neal et al. (2000) demonstrated in a sample of Australian hospital employees that perceptions about a workplace's general organizational climate influence safety climate perceptions, which in turn are related to safety outcomes. They conclude that initiatives to enhance safety climate should therefore be embedded within the wider organizational climate. In line with this, Smith-Crowe, Burke, and Landis (2003) showed in a sample from the nuclear waste industry that transfer of a safety training initiative had stronger effects on employees' safety knowledge and safety performance under conditions of an overall supportive organizational climate.

Safety Climate Versus Culture

Safety climate is closely related to the concept of safety culture and there has been a substantial amount of debate about how these two constructs are distinguished from each other (Clarke, 2000; Cox & Flin, 1998; Denison, 1996; Guldenmund, 2000; Mearns & Flin, 1999; Mearns, Flin, Gordon, & Fleming, 1998). Clarke (2000) discusses that one difference lies in the theoretical origins of safety culture and safety climate. The term safety culture developed out of accident investigations and was only after its emergence conceptually linked to organizational culture. The concept of safety climate is directly based on the organizational climate literature, which provides it with a constitutive conceptual ground. For some time there has been inconsistency in how the two terms were used causing some confusion and controversy. A key distinction between the two constructs is that safety climate presents a "snapshot" picture of an organization's more enduring safety culture (Flin et al., 2000). Similarly, Shannon and Norman (2009) explain that safety culture describes "the way we do things around here, while safety climate captures perceptions about what is actually done" (p. 327). Through common attitudes and behaviors safety climate is the "manifestation" of a more deeply ingrained safety culture (Cox & Flin, 1998). There is consensus among most researchers within the field of organizational safety on this main distinction and it could be proclaimed that the debate on the conceptual relationship between safety climate and safety culture has reached settlement. Describing safety climate as a momentary representation of safety culture has implications for the two constructs' measurement and potential for change. It suggests that safety climate as a surface-level portrayal of shared attributes and behaviors can be readily measured (e.g., through a questionnaire) and is open to change, while an organization's deep-rooted safety culture is more difficult to access (Glendon & Stanton, 2000; Guldenmund, 2000; Shannon & Norman, 2009). This is reflected in the focus of empirical safety research on safety climate with a volume of studies investigating safety climate, but relatively few empirical works on safety culture, although some investigations often through qualitative case research exist (e.g., Atak & Kingma, 2011; Blazsin & Guldenmund, 2014; Brooks, 2005, 2008).

Structure of Safety Climate

A substantial amount of empirical research has investigated the construct of safety climate. Most studies operationalize safety climate through a questionnaire measure and numerous safety climate surveys have been developed (e.g., Cox & Cheyne, 2000; Kines et al., 2011; Silva, Lima, & Baptista, 2004; Zohar, 2000; Zohar & Luria, 2005). From a practical perspective, development of safety climate scales offers overcoming limitations of traditional safety indicators such as accident records, which are retrospective and only provide limited information about risk exposure and wider safety issues (Glendon & Litherland, 2001; Seo, Torabi, Blair, & Ellis, 2004). Safety climate is usually viewed as multidimensional and there has been much debate about the "dimensions," "facets," or "scales" that compose overall safety climate (for reviews see Flin et al., 2000; Gadd & Collins, 2002; Guldenmund, 2000, 2007).

Zohar (1980) developed one of the first safety climate scales in a sample of Israeli production workers from different factories. Using principal components analysis, he identified eight factors:

1. perceived importance of safety training programs;
2. perceived management attitudes toward safety;
3. perceived effects of safe conduct on promotion;
4. perceived level of risk at workplace;
5. perceived effects of required work pace on safety;
6. perceived status of safety officer;
7. perceived effects of safe conduct on social status; and
8. perceived status of safety committee.

Results showed that the first two factors, importance of safety training and management attitudes, explained 60 percent of variance. Brown and Holmes (1986) used the same safety climate questionnaire in a sample of US production workers, but could not replicate Zohar's (1980) factor structure. Instead they found support for a three-factor solution. Dedobbeleer and Béland (1991) tested a modified version of Brown and Holmes' (1986) safety climate questionnaire in a sample of US construction workers. Contrary to Brown and Holme's (1986) three factors, they found the most appropriate fit for a two-factor solution. The two factors were interpreted as management commitment and worker involvement in safety. These early investigations on the dimensionality of safety climate show a lack of consensus on a common factor structure of safety climate.

Subsequent studies continued to report inconsistencies in safety climate dimensions, which added to concerns whether a stable set of safety climate factors can be established (e.g., Cheyne, Cox, Oliver, & Tomás, 1998; Cox & Cheyne, 2000; Cox & Cox, 1991; Coyle, Sleeman, & Adams, 1995; Diaz & Cabrera, 1997; Mearns et al., 1998, 2003; Niskanen, 1994; Varonen & Mattila, 2000). Coyle et al. (1995) developed a safety climate questionnaire that combined some of Zohar's (1980) original items with additional new items. They distributed the questionnaire in two Australian health care and social services organizations. Results from principal components analysis showed that the factor sets differed for the two organizations, identifying a seven-factor solution in one organization and a three-factor solution in the second organization. Niskanen (1994) assessed the dimensionality of a safety climate survey in the Finnish road maintenance and road construction sector. His sample consisted of frontline workers and their supervisors. Separate factor analyses for these two participant groups identified a four-factor structure for both the worker and supervisor sample. However, the items making up the four factors differed between the worker and supervisor sample. Niskanen's (1994) as well as Coyle et al.'s (1995) study have been criticized for lacking methodological rigor, as they did not test for reliability or validity of the safety climate dimensions (Seo et al., 2004). Cox and Cheyne (2000) tested the Safety Climate Assessment Toolkit in the offshore industry. They proposed nine dimensions and found support for a nine-factor structure using confirmatory analysis. Mearns et al. (2003) used a different safety climate survey in the offshore industry, the Offshore Safety Questionnaire, and reported 11 factors and 10 factors for two slightly different versions of the questionnaire. However, the authors did not discuss details on the factor analysis, as this was not the central objective of their study. Fullarton and Stokes (2007), using a sample of 1238 employees from nine Australian companies, failed to find support for a nine-factor structure that had previously been reported for the safety climate scale that was used in their study. The authors question whether safety climate is best represented through a single higher-order factor. Others have also tested safety climate as one higher-order factor (e.g., Hofmann & Stetzer, 1996), although the additional detail that multiple first-order factors provide is generally recognized (Griffin & Neal, 2000).

Thus, measurement scales of safety climate vary in their number and labels of safety climate dimensions. The emergence of different safety climate measures throughout the 1990s and early 2000s without a unifying factor structure, led to safety climate research being criticized for proliferation of dimensions (Coyle et al., 1995; Flin et al., 2000; Glendon & Litherland, 2001; Guldenmund, 2000, 2007). Guldenmund (2000, 2007) conducted two reviews of safety climate measures. In his earlier review based on 15 studies, he considers a number of methodological issues that have contributed to the lack of coherence in safety climate factor structures. This discussion includes the appropriateness of factor analysis and principal component analysis for data that is not strictly interval scaled and the common use of orthogonal factor rotations, which constrains factors to be uncorrelated. A further reason for the disparity in safety climate dimensions might be inconsistent labeling of factors, which obscures similarities between the factors identified by different studies (Gadd & Collins, 2002; Guldenmund, 2000). However, labeling does not explain the differences in the number of safety climate factors identified. In his 2007 review, Guldenmund adds the multilevel nature of safety climate as a further issue in determining the generic dimensions of safety climate. It has also been reasoned that safety climate instruments might be specific to the industry for which they were initially developed, resulting in discrepancies in factor structures between studies using the same instrument in different contexts (Cox & Flin, 1998). However, Shannon and Norman (2009) point out that many safety climate questionnaires use generic item wordings that are applicable to various settings.

Another reason for the difficulties in establishing a common structure of safety climate might be differences in the conceptualizations underlying the various safety climate measures. In a review of the safety climate literature, Clarke (2006) distinguished three different theoretical approaches: (1) a perceptual approach, (2) an attitudinal approach, (3) a mixed approach combining attitudes and perceptions. Williamson, Feyer, Cairns, and Biancotti (1997) compared attitudinal and perceptual items as part of the development of a safety climate scale in a sample of 660 manufacturing workers from different organizations. They found that attitudinal items were more likely to be skewed than perceptual items, with a large proportion of participants giving favorable responses if items assessed safety attitudes. The authors suggest that attitudes and perceptions provide two distinct viewpoints of safety climate and discuss that perceptions are a description of actual safety processes in the workplace, whereas safety attitudes represent someone's stereotypical stance on safety. However, Guldenmund (2007) argues that perceptions and attitudes are not separate from each other, but that perceptions about safety are a reflection of someone's attitudes toward safety.

With the objective to synthesize the array of safety climate dimensions, Flin et al. (2000) reviewed 18 different safety climate surveys and categorized the scales' dimensions into common themes. They identified three themes that were included in two-thirds of the reviewed studies, related to: (1) management attitudes and behaviors, (2) safety system (e.g., safety committees, safety policies, safety auditing procedures, safety equipment), and (3) risk (e.g., perceptions about risk and hazard exposure, risk-taking behavior, and attitudes toward risk). Flin et al. (2000) reported "work pressure" and "competence" as two further themes that appeared in one-third of the included studies. A sixth, less frequent theme that was only included in three of the 18 studies referred to "procedures and rules." Thus, their thematic review identified management, safety systems, and risk as the most common dimensions of safety climate measures. While individual questionnaire measures of safety climate continue to differ in content and factorial structure, Flin et al.'s (2000) research has made a strong contribution toward a common taxonomy of the core safety climate features. Since then, some studies have reported empirical support for successful replications of safety climate dimensions. Seo et al. (2004) discuss that existing safety climate measures are rarely reused and reassessed by other researchers, contributing to the lack of consensus on safety climate dimensions. They developed a safety climate questionnaire based on a literature review of existing scales and showed a consistent five-factor structure in a calibration sample and validation sample. Glendon and Litherland (2001) assessed the dimensions of the Safety Climate Questionnaire (SCQ) and were able to confirm a factor structure that resembled the results of previous research using the same questionnaire. Pousette, Larsson, and Törner (2008) cross-validated a safety climate questionnaire that was first developed by Cheyne et al. (1998). In their initial study, Cheyne et al. (1998) used the safety climate questionnaire in a sample from the manufacturing sector and reported five factors. Pousette et al. (2008) distributed a modified version of the questionnaire to Swedish construction workers and were able to replicate Cheyne et al.'s (1998) five-factor solution, although they relabeled the dimensions. They also discuss that the five dimensions thematically fit with the core features of safety climate as identified by Flin et al. (2000) and Seo et al. (2004). Moreover, Pousette et al. (2008) collected data at three successive time points and found that the factor structure for the safety climate scale was invariant across time. Kines et al. (2011) developed the Nordic Safety Climate Questionnaire (NOSACQ-50) and initially tested the measure in a sample of construction employees from five Nordic countries. Exploratory and confirmatory factor analysis identified seven dimensions, referring to:

1. management safety priority, commitment, and competence;
2. management safety empowerment;
3. management safety justice;
4. workers' safety commitment;
5. workers' safety priority and risk non-acceptance;
6. safety communication, learning, and trust in coworkers' safety competence; and
7. workers' trust in the efficacy of safety systems.

The researchers were able to replicate these factors fairly well in three subsequent studies, which included different occupational groups from different Nordic nations. Kines et al. (2011) stress the importance of replicable safety climate measures to allow for comparative studies, such as cross-cultural investigations, in safety climate research.

Other studies have indicated that the structure of safety climate is stable over time (Tharaldsen, Olsen, & Rundmo, 2008), across different job groups (Cheyne, Tomás, Cox, & Oliver, 2003), and industries (Hahn & Murphy, 2008; Olsen, 2010 – but see Cheyne, Tomás, Cox, & Oliver, 1999 for differences in safety structure across sectors). These studies indicate that there is stronger agreement on the core features that underlie safety climate and which can be replicated across different contexts. Bahari and Clarke (2013) investigated whether the structure of a safety climate measure that was developed in Western culture could be replicated in a Malaysian sample. Their results showed that a safety climate model that was validated in Western countries could not be transferred to the Malaysian sample without alterations. The authors point to other studies that also had difficulty in replicating safety climate structures between nations or cultures (e.g., Pfeiffer & Manser, 2010; Smits, Christiaans-Dingelhoff, Wagner, van der Wal, & Groenewegen, 2008). This raises the issue of cross-cultural transferability of safety climate models as a next challenge for research.

As discussed in the introduction to this chapter, climate can be investigated as an individual-level or higher unit-level property. Safety climate has also been conceptualized and empirically tested at different levels (Zohar, 2000, 2010). The value placed on safety can vary considerably between work groups, sites, or plants so that solely assessing safety climate at the organizational level is likely to be too crude (Hofmann & Stetzer, 1996, 1998; Zohar, 2000). However, assessing individuals' perceptions of safety climate without taking into consideration within-group agreement does not properly represent the *shared* aspect of safety climate. Thus, safety climate can be examined at the individual level, group level, and organizational level. At the individual-level safety climate is referred to as "psychological safety climate" representing individuals' perceptions, while at higher levels safety climate refers to the shared perceptions of the unit (Clarke, 2010; Zohar & Luria, 2004, 2005). Luria in Chapter 16 of this volume discusses safety climate as a group-level construct.

A further conceptual refinement of safety climate involves distinguishing between climate *valence* and *strength* (González-Romá, Peiró, Tordera, 2002; Zohar & Luria, 2004, 2005). Within the safety climate literature reference has often been made to a "good" or "poor" safety climate. While a safety climate can be of positive or negative valence, the degree to which perceptions about the value of safety are shared or the *strength* of consensus among a group provides another important element of information (Luria, 2008; Zohar & Luria, 2004, 2005).

Safety Climate as a Leading and Lagging Indicator

The concept of safety climate has stimulated a large amount of empirical research investigating its relationship with a range of safety-related outcomes across different industries and work settings. This body of research has highlighted safety climate as an important "leading indicator" of safety as it represents a proactive measure giving insight into the state of workplace safety before failure occurs (Mearns & Flin, 1999; Neal & Griffin, 2006; Payne, Bergman, Beus, Rodriguez, & Hennig, 2009; Yule, Flin, & Murdy, 2007; Zohar, 1980, 2002, 2010).

Based on the proposition that safety climate acts as a guide for individuals' decisions and behavior with regard to safety, numerous studies have explored the link between safety climate and employees' safety performance. Griffin and Neal (2000) demonstrated in two separate studies with samples from the mining and manufacturing sector, that a positive safety climate was associated with higher levels of employee safety performance. They divide safety performance into two components: safety compliance and safety participation. The former refers to core safety behaviors such as employees' adherence to safety rules, regulations, and procedures. The latter describes employees' voluntary engagement or extra effort for safety that goes beyond formal role prescriptions such as participating in a safety committee, helping others with safety matters or attending a voluntary safety meeting. This differentiation is based on the organizational model of task performance and contextual performance as sub-components of job performance (Borman & Motowildo, 1993). Many subsequent studies on safety performance have adopted Griffin and Neal's (2000) two-dimension model. In their study, Griffin and Neal (2000) find support that favorable safety climate perceptions are linked to higher levels of safety compliance as well as safety participation. Moreover, the results of their study indicate that the relationship between safety climate and safety performance is partially mediated by employees' safety knowledge as well as motivation (although to a lesser extent). This finding provides insight into the mechanisms through which safety climate affects individuals' safety behavior. Other studies have also reported that safety climate influences safety behaviors by enhancing safety knowledge and safety motivation (e.g., Christian et al., 2009; Neal et al., 2000).

The relationship between safety climate and safety performance has been explored across a range of different industries such as manufacturing (e.g., Zohar & Luria, 2005) offshore oil and gas (Dahl & Olsen, 2013; Mearns et al., 2003), construction (Gillen, Baltz, Gassel, Kirsch, & Vaccaro, 2002; Pousette et al., 2008; Siu, Phillips, & Leung, 2004) and health care (Flin, 2007; Katz-Navon, Naveh, & Stern, 2005). Zacharatos, Barling, and Iverson (2005) showed in a combined sample from a petrochemical plant and telecommunications company that positive safety climate perceptions were linked with stronger personal-safety orientation (i.e., a global variable that constitutes safety knowledge, safety motivation, safety compliance, and initiative for safety). Bosak, Co-etsee, and Cullinane (2013) found in a sample of 623 South African workers from a chemical manufacturing company that safety climate was related to employees' risk-taking behavior. They also investigated the interaction between different safety climate sub-dimensions (i.e., management commitment to safety, priority of safety, and pressure for production). The authors reported that if production pressures within an organiza-tion were low, but priority for safety was high, the effect of management commitment to safety on risk behaviors was nullified. However, if production pressures were high, management commitment and priority given to safety were significant in reducing risk-taking behaviors. Katz-Navon et al. (2005) in a sample of Israeli hospital employees found similar interactions between sub-dimensions of safety climate (i.e., safety priority, safety procedures, safety information, managerial safety practices). They conclude that interventions for enhancing safety climate need to attune the effects of individual di-mensions to ensure maximum benefits for safety. Interestingly their study also reported a curvilinear relationship between safety procedures (which they tested as a safety cli-mate dimension) and treatment errors. Insufficient procedures as well as overly detailed procedures were related to higher rates of treatment errors. Associations between safety climate and safety performance have also been reported in samples from industry sectors where risks and hazards might be somewhat less salient, but where ensuring safe working is nevertheless of importance. Barling et al. (2002) linked safety climate to safety compli-ance and participation in the service industry. DeJoy, Schaffer, Wilson, Vandenberg, and Butts (2004) linked safety climate to perceptions of hazard exposure in a large sample of participants from a retail chain.

In addition to safety performance behaviors as an outcome criterion, numerous stud-ies have established links between safety climate and accident, incident or injury rates (e.g., Barling et al., 2002; Christian et al. 2009; Clarke, 2006, 2013; Dedobbeleer & Béland, 1991; Hofmann & Stetzer, 1996; Mearns et al., 2003; Silva et al., 2004; Singer, Lin, Falwell, Gaba, & Baker, 2009; Siu et al., 2004; Vinodkumar & Bhasi, 2009; Zohar, 1980, 2000). Within this body of research, several studies have employed a prospective study design, which relates safety climate to future safety performance, accident and in-jury rates (e.g., Cooper & Phillips, 2004; Johnson, 2007; Neal & Griffin, 2006; Nielsen, Rasmussen, Glasscock, & Spangenberg, 2008; Pousette et al., 2008; Zohar, Huang, Lee, & Robertson, 2014). Pousette et al. (2008) found in a sample of Swedish construction workers that safety climate predicted employee safety behavior seven months later. Zohar et al. (2014) investigated the safety climate–behavior link in a sample of truck drivers and reported that safety climate perceptions predicted driving safety six months later. Their study makes a contribution by showing that safety climate is influential for safety in lone-working occupations. Neal and Griffin (2006) tested the relationship between group-level safety climate and safety outcomes over a five-year period. They found that safety climate forecasts future safety participation and safety motivation. Safety climate did not signifi-cantly predict accident rates three and five years later, but the results were in the expected direction with positive group-level safety climate perceptions being associated with lower accident rates. Together these studies offer support for the predictive validity of safety climate and underline the concept as a "leading indicator" of safety.

In addition to safety performance and accident rates, a more favorable safety climate has been associated with a range of other safety outcomes such as accident under-reporting (Probst & Estrada, 2010), safety control (Huang, Ho, Smith, & Chen, 2006), and attribution of the causes of workplace accidents (Hofmann & Stetzer, 1998). Most studies have theorized safety climate as a direct or indirect (mediated through other variables) predictor and empirically tested safety climate as a main effect on employees' safety behaviors and accident and injury rates. Alternatively, safety climate can be viewed as a contextual factor that impacts on the influence of other variables on workplace safety. In line with this, some studies have empirically explored safety climate as a moderator that augments or mitigates the relationship between other variables with safety-related outcomes. Hofmann, Morgeson, and Gerras (2003) demonstrated that safety climate augmented the positive relationship between high-quality leadership and safety citizenship behavior. Jiang, Yu, Li, and Li (2010) reported that safety climate moderated the relationship of coworkers' safety knowledge and safety behavior to employee safety compliance and participation. Probst (2004) found that a positive safety climate buffered against the negative effects of job insecurity on safety outcomes. Thus, several studies support safety climate as a contextual condition that can enhance or mitigate the effects of other factors on safety.

Three main meta-analyses have integrated research in the relationship of safety climate to safety performance and ultimately accidents and injury rates (Beus, Payne, Bergman, & Arthur, 2010; Christian et al., 2009; Clarke, 2006) and will be reviewed below. Clarke (2006) meta-analytically tested the link of safety climate to safety compliance, safety participation, and accident involvement. Results showed corrected correlation coefficients between safety climate and safety compliance of $r = .43$ (based on 12 studies), safety participation of $r = .50$ (based on eight studies) and accident involvement of $r = .22$ (based on 28 studies). In addition, the meta-analysis tested study design (prospective vs. retrospective) as a moderator of the relationship between safety climate and accident involvement. The results showed that safety climate was more strongly related to future accidents (corrected $r = .35$) than to accidents that were retrospectively measured (corrected $r = .22$). This lends further support for safety climate as a proactive measure of safety, although the finding was based on a small number of longitudinal studies. Christian et al. (2009) conducted a meta-analysis of the relationship of safety climate to safety performance and accidents. Mean-corrected correlations showed a significant, moderate relationship between safety climate and safety performance, with a stronger association between safety climate and safety participation (for individual-level climate $r = .59$; for group-level climate $r = .59$) than with safety compliance (for individual-level climate $r = .48$; for group-level climate $r = .40$). Relationships between safety climate and accident/injury rates were less strong for group-level safety climate ($r = -.39$) and of even lower magnitude for individual-level safety climate ($r = -.14$). These estimates are generally higher than those reported by Clarke (2006), which might be attributed to a larger number of primary studies (Christian et al., 2009). The results also showed that criterion source (i.e., self-reported accidents/safety performance vs. objective accident records/supervisor-rated performance) acted as a moderator in the above relations. In addition, Christian et al. (2009) found support for a path model whereby safety climate influenced safety knowledge and motivation, which affects safety performance, which in turn impacts on accident and injury rates. In a further meta-analysis, Beus et al. (2010) examined the link between safety climate and injuries with a particular focus on whether safety climate functions as a leading as well as a lagging indicator. That is, they tested whether safety climate influences injury rates, but also whether past injuries predict subsequent safety climate perceptions.

Results from the meta-analysis show support for a safety climate → injury link as well as for an injury → safety climate link. Moreover, for safety climate at the organizational-level, injuries were a stronger predictor of safety climate (corrected p = −.29) than safety climate of injuries (corrected p = −.24).

Two further meta-analyses have been conducted, which provided additional evidence for the association between safety climate and safety outcomes (Clarke, 2010; Nahrgang, Morgeson, & Hoffmann, 2011). These are discussed further below as investigations that have integrated safety climate into the wider health and well-being literature by including non-safety specific variables into their models.

Overall, meta-analytical evidence supports safety climate as an important antecedent of safety behavior and safety incidents, although several meta-analyses have shown that moderators such as study design and source of the criterion are important to take into consideration. There is also a trend amongst meta-analyses that safety climate as a group-level phenomenon shows a stronger relationship with safety outcomes compared with individual-level safety climate perceptions.

Evidence for safety climate as an important leading indicator has sparked interest in factors that foster or create a strong, positive safety climate. A substantial number of studies have focused on leadership as a key antecedent of safety climate (e.g., Barling et al., 2002; Clarke, 2010, 2013; Kelloway, Mullen, & Francis, 2006; Martínez-Córcoles, Gracia, Tomás, & Peiró, 2011; O'Dea & Flin, 2001; Zohar & Polachek, 2014). The relationship between safety climate and leadership has been explained as a social learning process whereby subordinates interpret the relative value of safety (i.e., safety climate) from their observations and interactions with their leader (Dragoni, 2005; Zohar, 2000). In particular, transformational leadership has received considerable attention as a leadership style that is positively related to subordinates' safety climate perceptions (e.g., Barling et al., 2002; Christian et al., 2009; Clarke, 2013; Hoffmeister et al., 2014; Mullen & Kelloway, 2009). There is also evidence that leaders who adopt a passive leadership style have a detrimental impact on safety climate (Kelloway et al., 2006; Zohar, 2002). The relationship between leadership and workplace safety is comprehensively discussed by Wong, Kelloway, and Makhan in Chapter 5 in this volume.

Research on determinants of safety climate other than leadership is now emerging, but is less structured. Some studies have explored how aspects of the wider organizational climate affect safety climate (e.g., Colley, Lincolne, & Neal, 2013; DeJoy et al., 2004; Hsu, Lee, Wu, & Takano, 2008; Wallace et al., 2006; Zacharatos et al., 2005). Zacharatos et al. (2005) showed that high-performance work systems, which they treated as a global variable consisting of different organizational practices such as selective hiring, employment security, information sharing, and extensive training, are positively related with safety climate. DeJoy et al. (2004) showed that organizational support, organizational communication, coworker support, and environmental conditions (e.g., excessive noise, poor lighting) were related to safety climate perceptions. Similarly, Wallace et al. (2006) linked organizational support and positive manager–employee relations to a more positive safety climate, which in turn was related to lower occupational injury rates. Other variables that have been linked to safety climate are job demands (Phipps, Malley, & Ashcroft, 2012) and mean work site tenure (Beus, Bergman, & Payne, 2010). These findings place emphasis on the wider social work environment to foster a positive, strong safety climate and prevent workplace accidents. This is an important growing body of research as it has been argued that the focus within organizational safety research is too much on safety climate with little exploration of other organizational factors that might be critical for accident reduction (Mullen, 2004). The above studies indicate safety climate as an important influence variable for safety, which itself is influenced by other (non-safety specific) organizational aspects.

Linking Health and Safety

As noted in our introduction, although practitioners and academics alike tend to view health and safety as a single domain, research has often investigated the relationship of climate to either health or safety. Thus, the above sections have discussed evidence on the influence of climate on health and safety respectively. As part of a progression toward a more holistic approach to "health and safety", studies have begun to explore how organizational factors link to well-being as well as safety outcomes in combined models (Clarke, Guediri, & O'Connor, 2013). For example, Tholén, Pousette, and Törner (2013) argue that there is a need to embed safety climate within the broader organizational context. In a four-wave longitudinal study with employees from 44 work units, they found some support for safety climate as a mediator of the influence of psychosocial conditions (this included information sharing, sense of community, possibilities for development, social support, and quality of leadership) on safety behaviors. The results also showed some indication that psychosocial conditions and safety climate might share common determinants. The authors provide an example, discussing that the project site where data was collected experienced changes in staffing during the study period, which might have influenced perceptions of psychosocial conditions as well as of safety climate.

Clarke (2010) developed an integrative model that combines the processes of generic psychological climate as well as safety climate on work attitudes (i.e., organizational commitment, job satisfaction), safety behaviors and health and well-being. More specifically, Clarke's (2010) model proposes that generic psychological climate influences safety climate which in turn impacts directly on well-being and safety behaviors, which finally affects occupational accident rates. In addition, the model includes work attitudes as an indirect pathway through which safety climate affects safety behaviors. Through meta-analysis Clarke (2010) found support for the model. The study makes important contributions by empirically supporting a knock-on effect of generic psychological climate on safety climate and demonstrating evidence for interconnections between health outcomes, safety outcomes, and wider work attitudes. Nahrgang et al. (2011) also conducted a meta-analysis that synthesized research on non-domain specific organizational factors, safety climate, and health-related as well as safety-specific outcomes. They used the job demands-resource model as a framework for their meta-analysis and tested the effect of job demands (i.e., risks and hazards, physical demands, job complexity) and job resources (i.e., safety knowledge, autonomy, social support, leadership, safety climate) on burnout, engagement, and safety outcomes (unsafe behavior, accidents and injuries, adverse events). Results showed that safety-specific job demands (e.g., risks and hazards) and safety-specific resources (e.g. safety climate) were significantly related to non-safety-specific well-being outcomes (e.g., burnout and satisfaction). This demonstrates a crossover of safety-related demands and resources with health and well-being outcomes. Moreover, a final path model suggested that safety climate influences adverse safety events through safety compliance as well as through burnout. Overall, the study shows that safety-related demands such as exposure to high levels of risk, do not only impact on employees' safety behavior but also have consequences for employee health and well-being.

Future Research

The above review identified some practical and theoretical issues that deserve more systematic attention. Next, we identify some opportunities for further research that will benefit safety and health outcomes. Cross-cultural issues in health and safety are particularly important for future research. Organizations increasingly operate across national boundaries and global economic factors influence the nature of operations in industries. For example, many mining companies operate across multiple countries and the safety systems appropriate in one context might be ineffective in another. Better understanding of the way national cultures interact with organizational culture to influence effective practices is needed to support positive health and safety outcomes. Developing countries in particular face many barriers to better health and safety that might be supported by understanding the way health and safety systems operate in different cultural contexts. Measures, constructs, and interventions might operate differently across cultural domains and there is little systematic information about the macro-level factors that might moderate the effective translation of knowledge and practice from one context to another (Bahari & Clarke, 2013).

Methodological issues and debates have played a major role in the development of organizational culture and climate concepts. A positive outcome of this process is a rich set of concepts and tools to tackle new problems. Some of the areas where further methodological development will support new insights is the way multiple types and forms of climate interact with each other (Kuenzi & Schminke, 2009). We noted that interaction among specific types of climate might be important for health and safety outcomes. For example, a competitive climate might interact with a participative safety climate to reduce its effectiveness. The growing attention to both positive and negative climate attributes also raises the possibility that there might be interactions among these dimensions of climate. The measurement and evaluation of these types of interaction create complexities that might be addressed by future research that examines more complex climate profiles (Colley et al., 2013).

Complexity also increases when the different forms of climate are considered. For example, the distribution of perceptions within a particular climate is now recognized as an important attribute that should be considered in its own right, somewhat independently from the overall level of a particular attribute. For example, there is evidence that the dispersion of climate perceptions conveys information that goes beyond the mean level of a perception (Beus, Bergman, & Payne, 2010). To date, most attention has been given to dispersion in terms of the width of simple distributions. Future research might extend this work by examining multi-modal distributions where sub-groups have distinct perceptions of the climate. In these situations, the mean and standard deviation can mask important attributes of the organizational factors that influence health and safety.

Another methodological opportunity arises through changes in technology that allow for rapid collection and dissemination of climate and culture data. Traditional data collection procedures typically require an organization-wide process involving surveys and interviews. The nature of this procedure limits the frequency of measurement while economies of scale usually encourage whole organization measurement. The wide availability of smartphones and other devices mean a more continuous process of measurement where individuals and business units provide less data per occasion but provide data on multiple occasions. New methods of analyzing this kind of intensive longitudinal data are becoming more widely available (Tan, Shiyko, Li, Li, & Dierker, 2012) and create new opportunities for understanding how climate changes over time. They also create the opportunity for more accurate and detailed insight about the internal perceptions and behavior of groups.

Technology change also enables better integration of data systems such as safety incidents, health records, with perceptual measures of climate and culture. Advances in areas such as customer service analytics and business diagnostics are only beginning to be applied to the study of organizational climate and culture (Guzzo, Nalbantian, & Parra, 2014).

There is great potential to integrate this kind of data with other information about human resource and organization development systems. Research using this type of integrated data can provide much more diagnostic information about business units. The integration of multiple data sources creates the possibility to develop a more complete and flexible model of the causes of health and safety that can guide strategic planning and organizational change.

Conclusion

Our review identified research linking multiple dimensions of organizational climate and culture to broad areas of health and safety. This research indicates that the organizational context exerts substantial influence on individual perceptions and behaviors. Organizational climate has a pervasive impact on a wide range of health and safety outcomes ranging from work injuries to chronic health outcomes. Until recently, these outcomes have been considered somewhat separately. However, there is now progress toward a more holistic and integrated view of the way organizational climate shapes health, well-being, and safety.

Organizational climate represents an important point of intervention for health and safety interventions. Although climate shows a degree of stability over time, there is also evidence that interventions designed to improve organizational climate result in changes that contribute to better health, well-being, and safety for employees. In contrast to individual-focused interventions that have a more local impact, the design and implementation of organizational change strategies have great potential for improving outcomes across broad groups and organizational units.

References

Arnetz, B. B., Lucas, T., & Arnetz, J. E. (2011). Organizational climate, occupational stress, and employee mental health: Mediating effects of organizational efficiency. *Journal of Occupational and Environmental Medicine, 53*, 34–42.

Arnold, T., Flaherty, K. E., Voss, K. E., & Mowen, J. C. (2009). Role stressors and retail performance: The role of perceived competitive climate. *Journal of Retailing, 85*, 194–205.

Atak, A., & Kingma, S. (2011). Safety culture in an aircraft maintenance organisation: A view from the inside. *Safety Science, 49*, 268–278.

Bachrach, S. B., & Bamberger, P. A. (2007). 9/11 and New York City firefighters' post hoc unit support and control climates: A context theory of the consequences of involvement in traumatic work-related events. *Academy of Management Journal, 50*, 849–868.

Bahari, S. F., & Clarke, S. (2013). Cross-validation of an employee safety climate model in Malaysia. *Journal of Safety Research, 45*, 1–6.

Bamberger, P. (2008). From the editors beyond contextualization: Using context theories to narrow the micro-macro gap in management research. *Academy of Management Journal, 51*, 839–846.

Bandura, A. (1977). Self-efficacy: Toward a unifying theory of behavioral change. *Psychological Review, 84*, 191–215.

Barling, J., Loughlin, C., & Kelloway, E. K. (2002). Development and test of a model linking safety-specific transformational leadership and occupational safety. *Journal of Applied Psychology, 87*, 488–496.

Beus, J. M., Bergman, M. E., & Payne, S. C. (2010). The influence of organizational tenure on safety climate strength: A first look. *Accident Analysis & Prevention, 42*, 1431–1437.

Beus, J. M., Payne, S. C., Bergman, M. E., & Arthur W. Jr, (2010). Safety climate and injuries: An examination of theoretical and empirical relationships. *Journal of Applied Psychology, 95*, 713–727.

Blazsin, H., & Guldenmund, F. (2014). The social construction of safety: Comparing three realities. *Safety Science, 71*, 16–27.

Bond, S. A., Tuckey, M. R., Dollard, M. F. (2010). Psychosocial safety climate, workplace bullying, and symptoms of posttraumatic stress. *Organization Development Journal, 28*, 37–56.

Borman, W. C., & Motowidlo, S. M. (1993). Expanding the criterion domain to include elements of contextual performance. In N. Schmitt and W. C. Borman (Eds.), *Personnel selection in organizations* (pp. 71–98). San Francisco, CA: Jossey-Bass.

Bosak, J., Coetsee, W. J., & Cullinane, S. J. (2013). Safety climate dimensions as predictors for risk behavior. *Accident Analysis & Prevention, 55*, 256–264.

Brinkmann, S., (2007). Culture as practices: A pragmatist conception. *Journal of Theoretical and Philosophical Psychology, 27*, 192–212.

Brooks, B. (2005). Not drowning, waving! Safety management and occupational culture in an Australian commercial fishing port. *Safety Science, 43*, 795–814.

Brooks, B. (2008). The natural selection of organizational and safety culture within a small to medium sized enterprise (SME). *Journal of Safety Research, 39*, 73–85.

Brown, R. L., & Holmes, H. (1986). The use of a factor-analytic procedure for assessing the validity of an employee safety climate model. *Accident Analysis & Prevention, 18*, 455–470.

Burke, M. J., Borucki, C. C., & Kaufman, J. D. (2002). Contemporary perspectives on the study of psychological climate: A commentary. *European Journal of Work and Organizational Psychology, 11*, 325–340.

Carr, J. Z., Schmidt, A. M., Ford, J. K., & DeShon, R. P. (2003). Climate perceptions matter: A meta-analytic path analysis relating molar climate, cognitive and affective states, and individual level work outcomes. *Journal of Applied Psychology, 88*, 605–619.

Cartwright, S., Cooper, C. L., & Murphy, L. R. (1995). Diagnosing a healthy organization: A proactive approach to stress in the workplace. In L. R. Murphy, J. J. Hurrell, Jr, S. L. Sauter, & G. P. Keita (Eds.), *Job stress interventions* (pp. 217–233). Washington, DC: American Psychological Association.

Cheyne, A., Cox, S., Oliver, A., & Tomás, J. M. (1998). Modelling safety climate in the prediction of levels of safety activity. *Work & Stress, 12*, 255–271.

Cheyne, A., Tomás, J. M., Cox, S., & Oliver, A. (1999). Modelling employee attitudes to safety. *European Psychologist, 4*, 1–10.

Cheyne, A., Tomás, J. M., Cox, S., & Oliver, A. (2003). Perceptions of safety climate at different employment levels. *Work & Stress, 17*, 21–37.

Choudhry, R. M., Fang, D., & Mohamed, S. (2007). The nature of safety culture: A survey of the state-of-the-art. *Safety Science, 45*, 993–1012.

Christian, M. S., Bradley, J. C., Wallace, J. C., & Burke, M. J. (2009). Workplace safety: A meta-analysis of the roles of person and situation factors. *Journal of Applied Psychology, 94*, 1103–1127.

Clarke, S. (1999). Perceptions of organizational safety: Implications for the development of safety culture. *Journal of Organizational Behavior, 20*, 185–198.

Clarke, S. (2000). Safety culture: Under-specified and overrated? *International Journal of Management Reviews, 2*, 65–90.

Clarke, S. (2003). The contemporary workforce: Implications for organisational safety culture. *Personnel Review, 32*, 40–57.

Clarke, S. (2006). The relationship between safety climate and safety performance: A meta-analytic review. *Journal of Occupational Health Psychology, 11*, 315–327.

Clarke, S. (2010). An integrative model of safety climate: Linking psychological climate and work attitudes to individual safety outcomes using meta-analysis. *Journal of Occupational and Organizational Psychology, 83*, 553–578.

Clarke, S. (2013). Safety leadership: A meta-analytic review of transformational and transactional leadership styles as antecedents of safety behaviours. *Journal of Occupational and Organizational Psychology, 86*, 22–49.

Clarke, S., Guediri, S., & O'Connor, E. (2013). Creating a safe and healthy work environment: The latest thinking and research evidence. In R. J. Burke & C. L. Cooper (Eds.), *The fulfilling workplace: The organization's role in achieving individual and organizational health* (pp. 265–285). Burlington, VT: Gower.

Colley, S. K., Lincolne, J., & Neal, A. (2013). An examination of the relationship amongst profiles of perceived organizational values, safety climate and safety outcomes. *Safety Science, 51*, 69–76.

Cooper, C. L., & Cartwright, S. (1994). Healthy mind, healthy organization – A proactive approach to occupational stress. *Human Relations, 47*, 455–471.

Cooper, M. D. (2000). Towards a model of safety culture. *Safety Science, 36*, 111–136.

Cooper, M. D., & Phillips, R. A. (2004). Exploratory analysis of the safety climate and safety behavior relationship. *Journal of Safety Research, 35*, 497–512.

Cox, S. J., & Cheyne, A. J. T. (2000). Assessing safety culture in offshore environments. *Safety Science, 34*, 111–129.

Cox, S., & Cox, T. (1991). The structure of employee attitudes to safety: A European example. *Work & Stress, 5*, 93–106.

Cox, S., & Flin, R. (1998). Safety culture: Philosopher's stone or man of straw? *Work & Stress, 12*, 189–201.

Coyle, I. R., Sleeman, S. D., & Adams, N. (1995). Safety climate. *Journal of Safety Research, 26*, 247–254.

Cullen, W. (1990). *Report of the official inquiry into the Piper Alpha disaster*. London, UK: HMSO.

Cummings, L. L., & DeCotiis, T. A. (1973). Organizational correlates of perceived stress in a professional organization. *Public Personnel Management, 2*, 275–282.

Dahl, Ø., & Olsen, E. (2013). Safety compliance on offshore platforms: A multi-sample survey on the role of perceived leadership involvement and work climate. *Safety Science, 54*, 17–26.

Danna, K., & Griffin, R. W. (1999). Health and well-being in the workplace: A review and synthesis of the literature. *Journal of Management, 25*, 357–384.

Dedobbeleer, N., & Béland, F. (1991). A safety climate measure for construction sites. *Journal of Safety Research, 22*, 97–103.

de Jonge, J., & Dormann, C. (2006). Stressors, resources, and strain at work: A longitudinal test of the triple-match principle. *Journal of Applied Psychology, 91*, 1359–1374.

DeJoy, D. M., Schaffer, B. S., Wilson, M. G., Vandenberg, R. J., & Butts, M. M. (2004). Creating safer workplaces: Assessing the determinants and role of safety climate. *Journal of Safety Research, 35*, 81–90.

DeJoy, D. M., & Southern, D. J. (1993). An integrative perspective on work-site health promotion. *Journal of Occupational and Environmental Medicine, 35*, 1221–1230.

Denison, D. R. (1996). What is the difference between organizational culture and organizational climate? A native's point of view on a decade of paradigm wars. *Academy of Management Review, 21*, 619–654.

Dextras-Gauthier, J., Marchand, A., & Haines V. III, (2012). Organizational culture, work organization conditions, and mental health: A proposed integration. *International Journal of Stress Management, 19*, 81–104.

Díaz, R. I., & Cabrera, D. D. (1997). Safety climate and attitude as evaluation measures of organizational safety. *Accident Analysis & Prevention, 29*, 643–650.

Dollard, M. F., & Bakker, A. B. (2010). Psychosocial safety climate as a precursor to conducive work environments, psychological health problems, and employee engagement. *Journal of Occupational and Organizational Psychology, 83*, 579–599.

Drach-Zahavy, A. (2010). How does service workers' behavior affect their health? Service climate as a moderator in the service behavior–health relationships. *Journal of Occupational Health Psychology, 15*, 105–119.

Dragoni, L. (2005). Understanding the emergence of state goal orientation in organizational work groups: The role of leadership and multilevel climate perceptions. *Journal of Applied Psychology, 90*, 1084–1095.

Edwards, J. R., Davey, J., & Armstrong, K. (2013). Returning to the roots of culture: A review and re-conceptualisation of safety culture. *Safety Science, 55*, 70–80.

Ehrhart, M.G., Schneider, B., & Macey, W.H. (2014). *Organizational climate and culture: An introduction to theory, research and practice*. New York, NY: Routledge.

Flin, R. (2007). Measuring safety culture in healthcare: A case for accurate diagnosis. *Safety Science, 45*, 653–667.

Flin, R., Mearns, K., O'Connor, P., & Bryden, R. (2000). Measuring safety climate: Identifying the common features. *Safety Science, 34,* 177–192.

Fullarton, C., & Stokes, M. (2007). The utility of a workplace injury instrument in prediction of workplace injury. *Accident Analysis & Prevention, 39,* 28–37.

Gadd, S., & Collins, A. M. (2002). *Safety culture: A review of the literature* [HSL/2002/25]. Sheffield, UK: Health and Safety Laboratory.

Garrick, A., Mak, A. S., Cathcart, S., Winwood, P. C., Bakker, A. B., & Lushington, K. (2014). Psychosocial safety climate moderating the effects of daily job demands and recovery on fatigue and work engagement. *Journal of Occupational and Organizational Psychology, 87,* 694–714.

Gillen, M., Baltz, D., Gassel, M., Kirsch, L., & Vaccaro, D. (2002). Perceived safety climate, job demands, and coworker support among union and non-union injured construction workers. *Journal of Safety Research, 33,* 33–51.

Glendon, A. I., & Litherland, D. K. (2001). Safety climate factors, group differences and safety behaviour in road construction. *Safety Science, 39,* 157–188.

Glendon, A. I., & Stanton, N. A. (2000). Perspectives on safety culture. *Safety Science, 34,* 193–214.

Glick, W. H. (1985). Conceptualizing and measuring organizational and psychological climate: Pitfalls in multilevel research. *Academy of Management Review, 10,* 601–616.

González-Romá, V., Peiró, J. M., & Tordera, N. (2002). An examination of the antecedents and moderator influences of climate strength. *Journal of Applied Psychology, 87,* 465–473.

Grandey, A., Foo, S. C., Groth, M., & Goodwin, R. E. (2012). Free to be you and me: A climate of authenticity alleviates burnout from emotional labor. *Journal of Occupational Health Psychology, 17,* 1–14.

Griffin, B. (2010). Multilevel relationships between organizational-level incivility, justice and intention to stay. *Work & Stress, 24,* 309–323.

Griffin, M. A., & Neal, A. (2000). Perceptions of safety at work: A framework for linking safety climate to safety performance, knowledge, and motivation. *Journal of Occupational Health Psychology, 5,* 347–358.

Grote, G. (2008). Diagnosis of safety culture: A replication and extension towards assessing "safe" organizational change processes. *Safety Science, 46,* 450–460.

Guldenmund, F. W. (2000). The nature of safety culture: A review of theory and research. *Safety Science, 34,* 215–257.

Guldenmund, F. W. (2007). The use of questionnaires in safety culture research – an evaluation. *Safety Science, 45,* 723–743.

Guzzo, R. A., Nalbantian, H. R., & Parra, L. F. (2014). A big data, say-do approach to climate and culture: A consulting perspective. In B. Schneider & K. M. Barbera (Eds.), *The Oxford handbook of organizational climate and culture* (pp. 197–211). New York, NY: Oxford University Press.

Hahn, S. E., & Murphy, L. R. (2008). A short scale for measuring safety climate. *Safety Science, 46,* 1047–1066.

Hall, G. B., Dollard, M. F., Winefield, A. H., Dormann, C., & Bakker, A. B. (2013). Psychosocial safety climate buffers effects of job demands on depression and positive organizational behaviors. *Anxiety, Stress & Coping, 26,* 355–377.

Hart, P. M., & Cooper, C. L. (2001). Occupational stress: Toward a more integrated framework. In N. Anderson, D. S. Ones, H. K. Sinangil, & C. Viswesvaran (Eds.), *Handbook of industrial, work, and organizational psychology* (vol. 2, pp. 93–114). Thousand Oaks, CA: Sage.

Hale, A. R. (2000). Culture's confusion. *Safety Science, 34,* 1–14.

Häusser, J. A., Mojzisch, A., Niesel, M., & Schulz-Hardt, S. (2010). Ten years on: A review of recent research on the job demand-control (-support) model and psychological well-being. *Work & Stress, 24,* 1–35.

Hemingway, M. A., & Smith, C. S. (1999). Organizational climate and occupational stressors as predictors of withdrawal behaviours and injuries in nurses. *Journal of Occupational and Organizational Psychology, 72,* 285–299.

Hoffmeister, K., Gibbons, A. M., Johnson, S. K., Cigularov, K. P., Chen, P. Y., & Rosecrance, J. C. (2014). The differential effects of transformational leadership facets on employee safety. *Safety Science, 62,* 68–78.

Hofmann, D. A., Morgeson, F. P., & Gerras, S. J. (2003). Climate as a moderator of the relationship between leader-member exchange and content specific citizenship: Safety climate as an exemplar. *Journal of Applied Psychology, 88*, 170–178.

Hofmann, D. A., & Stetzer, A. (1996). A cross-level investigation of factors influencing unsafe behaviors and accidents. *Personnel Psychology, 49*, 307–339.

Hofmann, D. A., & Stetzer, A. (1998). The role of safety climate and communication in accident interpretation: Implications for learning from negative events. *Academy of Management Journal, 41*, 644–657.

Holmgren, K., Ekbladh, E., Hensing, G., & Dellve, L. (2013). The combination of work organizational climate and individual work commitment predicts return to work in women but not in men. *Journal of Occupational and Environmental Medicine, 55*, 121–127.

Hsu, S. H., Lee, C. C., Wu, M. C., & Takano, K. (2008). A cross-cultural study of organizational factors on safety: Japanese vs. Taiwanese oil refinery plants. *Accident Analysis & Prevention, 40*, 24–34.

Huang, Y. H., Ho, M., Smith, G. S., & Chen, P. Y. (2006). Safety climate and self-reported injury: Assessing the mediating role of employee safety control. *Accident Analysis & Prevention, 38*, 425–433.

IAEA (1991). *Safety culture* (Safety Series 75-INSAG-4). Vienna, Austria: International Atomic Energy Agency.

Idris, M. A., & Dollard, M. F. (2011). Psychosocial safety climate, work conditions, and emotions in the workplace: A Malaysian population-based work stress study. *International Journal of Stress Management, 18*, 324–347.

Idris, M. A., & Dollard, M. F., Yulita (2014). Psychosocial safety climate, emotional demands, burnout, and depression: A longitudinal multilevel study in the Malaysian private sector. *Journal of Occupational Health Psychology, 19*, 291–302.

James, L. A., & James, L. R. (1989). Integrating work environment perceptions: Explorations into the measurement of meaning. *Journal of Applied Psychology, 74*, 739–751.

James, L. R., & Jones, A. P. (1974). Organizational climate: A review of theory and research. *Psychological Bulletin, 81*, 1096–1112.

Jex, S. M., & Bliese, P. D. (1999). Efficacy beliefs as a moderator of the impact of work-related stressors: A multilevel study. *Journal of Applied Psychology, 84*, 349–361.

Jex, S. M., Sliter, M. T., & Britton, A. (2014). Employee stress and well-being. In B. Schneider & K. M. Barbera (Eds.), *The Oxford handbook of organizational climate and culture* (pp. 177–196). New York, NY: Oxford University Press.

Jiang, L., Yu, G., Li, Y., & Li, F. (2010). Perceived colleagues' safety knowledge/behavior and safety performance: Safety climate as a moderator in a multilevel study. *Accident Analysis & Prevention, 42*, 1468–1476.

Johns, G. (2006). The essential impact of context on organizational behavior. *Academy of Management Review, 31*, 386–408.

Johnson, S. E. (2007). The predictive validity of safety climate. *Journal of Safety Research, 38*, 511–521.

Jones, A. P., & James, L. R. (1979). Psychological climate: Dimensions and relationships of individual and aggregated work environment perceptions. *Organizational Behavior and Human Performance, 23*, 201–250.

Kao, F. H., Cheng, B. S., Kuo, C. C., & Huang, M. P. (2014). Stressors, withdrawal, and sabotage in frontline employees: The moderating effects of caring and service climates. *Journal of Occupational and Organizational Psychology, 87*, 755–780.

Katz-Navon, T. A. L., Naveh, E., & Stern, Z. (2005). Safety climate in health care organizations: A multidimensional approach. *Academy of Management Journal, 48*, 1075–1089.

Kawano, Y. (2008). Association of job-related stress factors with psychological and somatic symptoms among Japanese hospital nurses: Effect of departmental environment in acute care hospitals. *Journal of Occupational Health, 50*, 79–85.

Kelloway, E. K., Mullen, J., & Francis, L. (2006). Divergent effects of transformational and passive leadership on employee safety. *Journal of Occupational Health Psychology, 11*, 76–86.

Kines, P., Lappalainen, J., Mikkelsen, K. L., Olsen, E., Pousette, A., Tharaldsen, J., Tómasson, K., & Törner, M. (2011). Nordic Safety Climate Questionnaire (NOSACQ-50): A new tool for diagnosing occupational safety climate. *International Journal of Industrial Ergonomics, 41,* 634–646.

Kuenzi, M., & Schminke, M. (2009). Assembling fragments into a lens: A review, critique, and proposed research agenda for the organizational work climate literature. *Journal of Management, 35,* 634–717.

Kumari, K., & Sharma, S. (1990). Social support, organizational role stress and well-being: A study of medicos. *Psychological Studies, 35,* 163–169.

Law, R., Dollard, M. F., Tuckey, M. R., & Dormann, C. (2011). Psychosocial safety climate as a lead indicator of workplace bullying and harassment, job resources, psychological health and employee engagement. *Accident Analysis & Prevention, 43,* 1782–1793.

Leiter, M. P., Laschinger, H. K. S., Day, A., & Oore, D. G. (2011). The impact of civility interventions on employee social behavior, distress, and attitudes. *Journal of Applied Psychology, 96,* 1258–1274.

Liao, H., & Chuang, A. (2007). Transforming service employees and climate: A multilevel, multisource examination of transformational leadership in building long-term service relationships. *Journal of Applied Psychology, 92,* 1006.

Liao, H., & Searcy, D. W. (2012). Positive exchange relationships with customers. In L. T. Eby, & T. D. Allen (Eds.), *Personal relationships: The effect on employee attitudes, behavior, and well-being* (pp. 235–260). New York, NY: Taylor & Francis.

Lim, S., Cortina, L. M., & Magley, V. J. (2008). Personal and workgroup incivility: Impact on work and health outcomes. *Journal of Applied Psychology, 93,* 95–107.

Luria, G. (2008). Climate strength – How leaders form consensus. *Leadership Quarterly, 19,* 42–53.

Martin, A. J., Jones, E. S., & Callan, V. J. (2005). The role of psychological climate in facilitating employee adjustment during organizational change. *European Journal of Work and Organizational Psychology, 14,* 263–289.

Martínez-Córcoles, M., Gracia, F., Tomás, I., & Peiró, J. M. (2011). Leadership and employees' perceived safety behaviours in a nuclear power plant: A structural equation model. *Safety Science, 49,* 1118–1129.

Mathisen, G. E., Torsheim, T., & Einarsen, S. (2006). The team-level model of climate for innovation: A two-level confirmatory factor analysis. *Journal of Occupational and Organizational Psychology, 79,* 23–35.

Mearns, K. J., & Flin, R. (1999). Assessing the state of organizational safety – culture or climate? *Current Psychology, 18,* 5–17.

Mearns, K., Flin, R., Gordon, R., & Fleming, M. (1998). Measuring safety climate on offshore installations. *Work & Stress, 12,* 238–254.

Mearns, K., Whitaker, S. M., & Flin, R. (2003). Safety climate, safety management practice and safety performance in offshore environments. *Safety Science, 41,* 641–680.

Michela, J. L., Lukaszewski, M. P., & Allegrante, J. P. (1995). Organizational climate and work stress: A general framework applied to inner-city schoolteachers. In S. L. Sauter & L. R. Murphy (Eds.), *Organizational risk factors for job stress* (pp. 61–80). Washington, DC: American Psychological Association.

Miner-Rubino, K., & Cortina, L. M. (2004). Working in a context of hostility toward women: Implications for employees' well-being. *Journal of Occupational Health Psychology, 9,* 107–122.

Moliner, C., Martínez-Tur, V., Peiró, J. M., Ramos, J., & Cropanzano, R. (2005). Relationships between organizational justice and burnout at the work-unit level. *International Journal of Stress Management, 12,* 99–116.

Morgeson, F. P., Dierdorff, E. C., & Hmurovic, J. L. (2010). Work design in situ: Understanding the role of occupational and organizational context. *Journal of Organizational Behavior, 31,* 351–360.

Mullen, J. (2004). Investigating factors that influence individual safety behavior at work. *Journal of Safety Research, 35,* 275–285.

Mullen, J. E., & Kelloway, E. K. (2009). Safety leadership: A longitudinal study of the effects of transformational leadership on safety outcomes. *Journal of Occupational and Organizational Psychology*, 82, 253–272.

Nahrgang, J. D., Morgeson, F. P., & Hofmann, D. A. (2011). Safety at work: A meta-analytic investigation of the link between job demands, job resources, burnout, engagement, and safety outcomes. *Journal of Applied Psychology*, 96, 71–94.

Neal, A., & Griffin, M. A. (2006). A study of the lagged relationships among safety climate, safety motivation, safety behavior, and accidents at the individual and group levels. *Journal of Applied Psychology*, 91, 946–953.

Neal, A., Griffin, M. A., & Hart, P. M. (2000). The impact of organizational climate on safety climate and individual behavior. *Safety Science*, 34, 99–109.

Nielsen, K. J., Rasmussen, K., Glasscock, D., & Spangenberg, S. (2008). Changes in safety climate and accidents at two identical manufacturing plants. *Safety Science*, 46, 440–449.

Niskanen, T. (1994). Safety climate in the road administration. *Safety Science*, 17, 237–255.

O'Dea, A., & Flin, R. (2001). Site managers and safety leadership in the offshore oil and gas industry. *Safety Science*, 37, 39–57.

Olsen, E. (2010). Exploring the possibility of a common structural model measuring associations between safety climate factors and safety behaviour in health care and the petroleum sectors. *Accident Analysis & Prevention*, 42, 1507–1516.

Ostroff, C. (1993). The effects of climate and personal influences on individual behavior and attitudes in organizations. *Organizational Behavior and Human Decision Processes*, 56, 56–90.

Ostroff, C., Kinicki, A. J., & Tamkins, M. M. (2003). Organizational culture and climate. In W. C. Borman, D. R. Ilgen, & R. J. Kinicki (Eds.), *Handbook of psychology – industrial and organisational psychology* (vol. 12, pp. 565–594). Hoboken, NJ: John Wiley & Sons, Inc.

O'Toole, M. (2002). The relationship between employees' perceptions of safety and organizational culture. *Journal of Safety Research*, 33, 231–243.

Parker, C. P., Baltes, B. B., Young, S. A., Huff, J. W., Altmann, R. A., Lacost, H. A., & Roberts, J. E. (2003). Relationships between psychological climate perceptions and work outcomes: A meta-analytic review. *Journal of Organizational Behavior*, 24, 389–416.

Parker, D., Lawrie, M., & Hudson, P. (2006). A framework for understanding the development of organisational safety culture. *Safety Science*, 44, 551–562.

Patterson, M. G., West, M. A., Shackleton, V. J., Dawson, J. F., Lawthom, R., Maitlis, S., Robinson, D. L., & Wallace, A. M. (2005). Validating the organizational climate measure: Links to managerial practices, productivity and innovation. *Journal of Organizational Behavior*, 26, 379–408.

Payne, S. C., Bergman, M. E., Beus, J. M., Rodríguez, J. M., & Henning, J. B. (2009). Safety climate: Leading or lagging indicator of safety outcomes? *Journal of Loss Prevention in the Process Industries*, 22, 735–739.

Pfeiffer, Y., & Manser, T. (2010). Development of the German version of the Hospital Survey on Patient Safety Culture: Dimensionality and psychometric properties. *Safety Science*, 48, 1452–1462.

Phipps, D. L., Malley, C., & Ashcroft, D. M. (2012). Job characteristics and safety climate: The role of effort-reward and demand-control-support models. *Journal of Occupational Health Psychology*, 17, 279–289.

Pidgeon, N., & O'Leary, M. (2000). Man-made disasters: Why technology and organizations (sometimes) fail. *Safety Science*, 34, 15–30.

Pidgeon, N. F. (1991). Safety culture and risk management in organizations. *Journal of Cross-Cultural Psychology*, 22, 129–140.

Pousette, A., Larsson, S., & Törner, M. (2008). Safety climate cross-validation, strength and prediction of safety behaviour. *Safety Science*, 46, 398–404.

President's Commission (2011). *Deep water: The Gulf Oil disaster and the future of offshore drilling.* Report to the President National Commission on the BP Deepwater Horizon Oil Spill and Offshore Drilling. US Government, January 2011.

Probst, T. M. (2004). Safety and insecurity: Exploring the moderating effect of organizational safety climate. *Journal of Occupational Health Psychology*, 9, 3–10.

Probst, T. M., & Estrada, A. X. (2010). Accident under-reporting among employees: Testing the moderating influence of psychological safety climate and supervisor enforcement of safety practices. *Accident Analysis & Prevention, 42*, 1438–1444.

Reason, J. (1997). *Managing the risks of organizational accidents.* Aldershot, UK: Ashgate.

Reason, J. (1998). Achieving a safe culture: Theory and practice. *Work & Stress, 12*, 293–306.

Rhoades, L., & Eisenberger, R. (2002). Perceived organizational support: A review of the literature. *Journal of Applied Psychology, 87*, 698–714.

Richter, A., & Koch, C. (2004). Integration, differentiation and ambiguity in safety cultures. *Safety Science, 42*, 703–722.

Rousseau, D. M., & Fried, Y. (2001). Location, location, location: Contextualizing organizational research. *Journal of Organizational Behavior, 22*, 1–13.

Schein, E. H. (2010). *Organizational culture and leadership* (4th edn.). San Francisco, CA: Jossey-Bass.

Schneider, B. (1975). Organizational climates: An essay. *Personnel Psychology, 28*, 447–479.

Schneider, B., Ehrhart, M. G., & Macey, W. H. (2013). Organizational climate and culture. *Annual Review of Psychology, 64*, 361–388.

Schneider, B., Wheeler, J. K., & Cox, J. F. (1992). A passion for service: Using content analysis to explicate service climate themes. *Journal of Applied Psychology, 77*, 705–716.

Schulte, M., Ostroff, C., & Kinicki, A. J. (2006). Organizational climate systems and psychological climate perceptions: A cross-level study of climate-satisfaction relationships. *Journal of Occupational and Organizational Psychology, 79*, 645–671.

Seo, D. C., Torabi, M. R., Blair, E. H., & Ellis, N. T. (2004). A cross-validation of safety climate scale using confirmatory factor analytic approach. *Journal of Safety Research, 35*, 427–445.

Shannon, H. S., & Norman, G. R. (2009). Deriving the factor structure of safety climate scales. *Safety Science, 47*, 327–329.

Sheen, J. (1987). *M.V. Herald of Free Enterprise* (Report of Court No. 8074). London, UK: HMSO Department of Energy.

Silva, S., Lima, M. L., & Baptista, C. (2004). OSCI: An organisational and safety climate inventory. *Safety Science, 42*, 205–220.

Singer, S., Lin, S., Falwell, A., Gaba, D., & Baker, L. (2009). Relationship of safety climate and safety performance in hospitals. *Health Services Research, 44*, 399–421.

Siu, O. L., Phillips, D. R., & Leung, T. W. (2004). Safety climate and safety performance among construction workers in Hong Kong: The role of psychological strains as mediators. *Accident Analysis & Prevention, 36*, 359–366.

Smith-Crowe, K., Burke, M. J., & Landis, R. S. (2003). Organizational climate as a moderator of safety knowledge-safety performance relationships. *Journal of Organizational Behavior, 24*, 861–876.

Smits, M., Christiaans-Dingelhoff, I., Wagner, C., van der Wal, G., & Groenewegen, P. P. (2008). The psychometric properties of the "Hospital Survey on Patient Safety Culture" in Dutch hospitals. *BMC Health Services Research, 8*, 230–239.

Spell, C. S., & Arnold, T. J. (2007). A multi-level analysis of organizational justice climate, structure, and employee mental health. *Journal of Management, 33*, 724–751.

Tan, X., Shiyko, M. P., Li, R., Li, Y., & Dierker, L. (2012). A time-varying effect model for intensive longitudinal data. *Psychological Methods, 17*(1), 61–77.

Terry, D. D. J., Callan, V. J., & Sartori, G. (1996). Employee adjustment to an organizational merger: Stress, coping and intergroup differences. *Stress Medicine, 12*, 105–122.

Tharaldsen, J. E., Olsen, E., & Rundmo, T. (2008). A longitudinal study of safety climate on the Norwegian continental shelf. *Safety Science, 46*, 427–439.

Tholén, S. L., Pousette, A., & Törner, M. (2013). Causal relations between psychosocial conditions, safety climate and safety behaviour: A multi-level investigation. *Safety Science, 55*, 62–69.

Van der Doef, M., & Maes, S. (1999). The job demand-control (-support) model and psychological well-being: A review of 20 years of empirical research. *Work & Stress, 13*, 87–114.

Varonen, U., & Mattila, M. (2000). The safety climate and its relationship to safety practices, safety of the work environment and occupational accidents in eight wood-processing companies. *Accident Analysis & Prevention, 32*, 761–769.

Vinodkumar, M. N., & Bhasi, M. (2009). Safety climate factors and its relationship with accidents and personal attributes in the chemical industry. *Safety Science, 47,* 659–667.

Vredenburgh, A. G. (2002). Organizational safety: which management practices are most effective in reducing employee injury rates? *Journal of Safety Research, 33,* 259–276.

Wallace, J. C., Popp, E., & Mondore, S. (2006). Safety climate as a mediator between foundation climates and occupational accidents: A group-level investigation. *Journal of Applied Psychology, 91,* 681–688.

Warr, P. (1990). The measurement of well-being and other aspects of mental health. *Journal of Occupational Psychology, 63,* 193–210.

Williamson, A. M., Feyer, A. M., Cairns, D., & Biancotti, D. (1997). The development of a measure of safety climate: The role of safety perceptions and attitudes. *Safety Science, 25,* 15–27.

Wilson, M. G., DeJoy, D. M., Vandenberg, R. J., Richardson, H. A., & McGrath, A. L. (2004). Work characteristics and employee health and well-being: Test of a model of healthy work organization. *Journal of Occupational and Organizational Psychology, 77,* 565–588.

Wu, T., Liu, C., & Lu, M. (2007). Safety climate in university and college laboratories: Impact of organizational and individual factors. *Journal of Safety Research, 38,* 91–102.

Ylipaavalniemi, J., Kivimäki, M., Elovainio, M., Virtanen, M., Keltikangas-Järvinen, L., & Vahtera, J. (2005). Psychosocial work characteristics and incidence of newly diagnosed depression: A prospective cohort study of three different models. *Social Science & Medicine, 61,* 111–122.

Yule, S., Flin, R., & Murdy, A. (2007). The role of management and safety climate in preventing risk-taking at work. *International Journal of Risk Assessment and Management, 7,* 137–151.

Zacharatos, A., Barling, J., & Iverson, R. D. (2005). High-performance work systems and occupational safety. *Journal of Applied Psychology, 90,* 77–93.

Zohar, D. (1980). Safety climate in industrial organizations: Theoretical and applied implications. *Journal of Applied Psychology, 65,* 96–102.

Zohar, D. (2000). A group-level model of safety climate: Testing the effect of group climate on microaccidents in manufacturing jobs. *Journal of Applied Psychology, 85,* 587–596.

Zohar, D. (2002). The effects of leadership dimensions, safety climate, and assigned priorities on minor injuries in work groups. *Journal of Organizational Behavior, 23,* 75–92.

Zohar, D. (2010). Thirty years of safety climate research: Reflections and future directions. *Accident Analysis & Prevention, 42,* 1517–1522.

Zohar, D., Huang, Y. H., Lee, J., & Robertson, M. (2014). A mediation model linking dispatcher leadership and work ownership with safety climate as predictors of truck driver safety performance. *Accident Analysis & Prevention, 62,* 17–25.

Zohar, D., & Luria, G. (2004). Climate as a social-cognitive construction of supervisory safety practices: Scripts as proxy of behavior patterns. *Journal of Applied Psychology, 89,* 322–333.

Zohar, D., & Luria, G. (2005). A multilevel model of safety climate: Cross-level relationships between organization and group-level climates. *Journal of Applied Psychology, 90,* 616–628.

Zohar, D., & Polachek, T. (2014). Discourse-based intervention for modifying supervisory communication as leverage for safety climate and performance improvement: A randomized field study. *Journal of Applied Psychology, 99,* 113–124.

Zohar, D., & Tenne-Gazit, O. (2008). Transformational leadership and group interaction as climate antecedents: A social network analysis. *Journal of Applied Psychology, 93,* 744–757.

Zwetsloot, G., & Leka, S. (2010). Corporate culture, health, and well-being. In S. Leka & J. Houdmont (Eds.), *Occupational health psychology* (pp. 250–268). Oxford, UK: Wiley-Blackwell.

Part III

Improving Occupational Safety and Workplace Health in Organizations

14
Behavior-Based Approaches to Occupational Safety

E. Scott Geller and Zechariah J. Robinson

Introduction

For more than three decades, behavior-based safety (BBS) has been flourishing in industrial settings across the USA, and more recently throughout the world. Several books detail the principles and procedures of BBS (e.g., Geller, 1996a, 1998a, 1996b, 2001d; Geller & Williams, 2001; Krause, 1995; Krause, Hidley, & Hodson, 1996; McSween, 1995; Petersen, 1989; Sulzer-Azaroff, 1998; Williams, 2010). Moreover, a number of systematic reviews of the literature provide solid evidence for the success of this approach to injury prevention (e.g., Al-Hemoud & Al-Asfoor, 2006; Chen & Tian, 2012; Choudhry, 2014; Foster, Parand, & Bennett, 2008; Grindle, Dickinson, & Boettcher, 2000; Ismail et al., 2012; Lingard & Rowlinson,1997; McAfee & Winn, 1989; Parand & Foster, 2006; Petersen, 1989; Sulzer-Azaroff & Austin, 2000).

Safety professionals readily relate to the term "behavior," because they realize human behavior is involved to some extent in almost every environmental hazard, personal injury, and fatality. So improving safety-related behavior is key to preventing injuries. In other words, safety leaders and consultants recognize that unsafe or at-risk behavior contributes to most minor and major injuries, and fatalities in the workplace; and therefore substituting safe behavior for at-risk behavior is critical for an upstream proactive approach to industrial health and safety. Unfortunately, there has been much distortion and confusion among safety professionals and consultants regarding BBS. There is much more to BBS than believing behavior change is critical for injury prevention. This chapter details the theoretical and empirical foundation of BBS, as well as practical applications and directions for future research.

The Wiley Blackwell Handbook of the Psychology of Occupational Safety and Workplace Health, First Edition. Edited by Sharon Clarke, Tahira M. Probst, Frank Guldenmund, and Jonathan Passmore. © 2016 John Wiley & Sons Ltd. Published 2020 by John Wiley & Sons Ltd.

Principles of Applied Behavioral Science

Ideally, BBS adheres to the seven key Applied Behavioral Science (ABS) principles described below. These should serve as criteria to consider when evaluating whether a particular safety-management practice reflects BBS appropriately, as well as guidelines to follow when developing a behavior-based method or tool for proactive safety management. Each principle is broad enough to encompass a wide range of practical operations, but narrow enough to guide the development of cost-effective procedures for managing the human dynamics of safety and health.

Focus intervention on observable behavior

The BBS approach is founded on behavioral science as conceptualized and researched by B. F. Skinner (1938, 1953, 1974). Experimental behavior analysis, and later applied behavior analysis, emerged from Skinner's research and teaching, and laid the groundwork for numerous therapies and interventions to improve the quality of life of individuals, groups, and entire communities (Goldstein & Krasner, 1987; Greene, Winett, Van Houten, Geller, & Iwata, 1987). Whether working one-on-one in a clinical setting or with work teams throughout an organization, the intervention procedures always target specific behaviors relevant to producing constructive change. In other words, BBS focuses on what people do, analyzes why they do it, and then applies a research-supported intervention strategy to improve what people do.

The focus is on *acting people into thinking differently* rather than targeting internal awareness or attitudes in order to *think people into acting differently*. This latter approach is used successfully by many clinical psychologists in professional therapy sessions, but it is not cost effective in a group or organizational setting. To be effective, attitude-focused intervention requires extensive one-on-one interaction between a client and a specially trained intervention specialist. Even if time and facilities were available to intervene on internal and unobservable person states, few safety professionals or consultants possess the educational background, training, skills, and experience to implement such an approach. Thus, whatever the intervention approach, the focus is on behavior. It is behavior-based training, behavior-based commitment, behavior-based goal-setting, behavior-based feedback, behavior-based recognition, behavior-based incentives and rewards, and so on.

Look for external factors to understand and improve behavior

Skinner did not deny the existence of internal determinants of behavior (such as personality characteristics, perceptions, attitudes, and values); rather, he rejected such unobservable inferred constructs for *scientific study* as causes or outcomes of behavior. We obviously do what we do because of factors in both our external and internal worlds. However, given the difficulty in objectively defining internal states or traits, it is more cost effective to identify environmental conditions that influence behavior and then to change those factors when behavior change is desired.

When BBS became a "hot" topic at company safety meetings and professional development conferences in the 1990s, Hans (1996) reported this quote from the Director of the National Safety Council's consulting division: "The all-consuming focus on employee behaviors can mask management inadequacies that otherwise might come to light" (pp. 45–46).

In fact, the opposite is true. A systematic behavior analysis of risky work practices can pinpoint many determinants of such behavior, including inadequate management systems

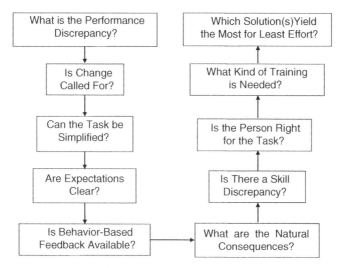

Figure 14.1   The sequential questions for a behavioral safety analysis.

or supervisor behaviors that promote or inadvertently encourage at-risk work. Without the upstream and objective problem solving perspective fostered by the BBS principles, these inadequacies may never be identified (or they might be revealed only after a "close call" or injury).

Examining external factors to explain and improve behavior is a primary focus of organizational behavior management (e.g., Austin, 2000; Austin, Carr, & Agnew, 1999; Bailey & Austin, 1996; Gilbert, 1978). In occupational safety this approach has been termed behavioral safety analysis (Geller, 2000, 2001a). It involves a search for answers to the following questions in the order given here and summarized in Figure 14.1.

Can the task be simplified?   Before designing an intervention to improve behavior, it is critical to implement all possible engineering "fixes." In other words, the first step is to consider how the environment could be changed to reduce physical effort, reach, and repetition. That is, procedures to make the job more user-friendly are entertained before deciding what behaviors are needed to prevent injury. This is, of course, the rationale behind ergonomics and the search for engineering solutions to occupational safety and health (Kroemer, 1991).

Sometimes environmental facilitators can be added, such as: (a) control designs with different shapes so they can be discriminated by touch as well as sight, (b) clear instructions placed at the point of application, (c) color codes to aid memory and task differentiation (Norman, 1988), or (d) convenient machine lifts or conveyor rollers to help with physical jobs. In addition, complex assignments might be redesigned to involve fewer steps or more people; or to reduce boredom or repetition, simple tasks might allow for job swapping. Thus, BBS professionals ask the following questions at the start of a behavioral safety analysis:

- Can an engineering intervention make the job more user-friendly?
- Can the task be redesigned to reduce physical demands?
- Can a behavior facilitator be added to improve response differentiation, reduce memory load, or increase reliability?

- Can the challenges of a complex task be shared?
- Can boring, repetitive jobs be cross-trained and swapped?

Is a quick fix available? From their more than 60 combined years of analyzing and solving human performance problems, Mager and Pipe (1997) concluded that many discrepancies between real and ideal behavior can be eliminated with relatively little effort. More specifically, behavior might be more at-risk than desired because expectations are unclear, resources are inadequate, or feedback is unavailable. In these cases, behavior-based instruction or demonstration can overcome ill-informed expectations, and behavior-based feedback can enable continuous improvement. A work team could decide what resources are needed to make a safe behavior more convenient, comfortable, or efficient. When conducting this aspect of a behavioral safety analysis, BBS professionals ask these questions:

- Does the individual know what safety precautions are expected?
- Are there obvious barriers to safe work practices?
- Is the equipment as safe as possible under the circumstances?
- Is personal protective equipment (PPE) readily available and as comfortable as possible?
- Do employees receive frequent behavior-based feedback related to their personal safety?

Is safe behavior punished? In some work cultures, the interpersonal consequences for reporting an environmental hazard or minor injury are more negative than positive. After all, those situations imply that someone was irresponsible or careless. Sometimes workers are teased or ridiculed for wearing protective gear or using an equipment guard. In some work cultures, it might even be considered "cool" or "macho" to work unprotected and take risky short cuts. The hidden agenda might be that "only a 'chicken' would wear fall protection." Mager and Pipe (1997) refer to these situations as "upside-down consequences," and suggest they contribute to many of the undesirable behaviors occurring in the workplace. The BBS facilitator asks these questions during a behavioral safety analysis:

- What are the consequences for safety-related behavior?
- Are there more negative than positive consequences for safe behavior?
- What negative consequences for safe behavior can be reduced or removed?

Is at-risk behavior rewarded? At-risk behavior is often followed by natural positive consequences, including comfort, convenience, and efficiency. Short-cuts are usually taken to save time and can lead to a faster rate of output. Therefore, taking an at-risk short-cut may be considered "efficient" behavior. Most people perform the way they do because they expect to achieve soon, certain, and positive consequences, or they expect to avoid soon, certain, and negative consequences. People take calculated risks because they expect to gain something positive and/or avoid something negative. The BBS professional asks these questions:

- What are the soon, certain, and positive consequences for at-risk behavior?
- Do workers receive more attention, prestige, or status from coworkers for their at-risk than safe behavior?
- What rewarding consequences for at-risk behavior can be reduced or removed?

Are extra consequences applied effectively? Since the natural consequences of comfort, convenience, and efficiency usually support at-risk over safe behavior, it is often necessary to add extra consequences. These usually take the form of incentive/reward or disincentive/

penalty contingencies. Unfortunately, many of these programs do more harm than good because they are implemented ineffectively (Geller, 1996b, 2001a). Disincentives are often ineffective because they are used inconsistently and motivate avoidance behavior rather than achievement. In addition, safety incentives based on outcomes can stifle employee participation in the development and administration of an effective BBS incentive/reward program (Geller, 2002). Therefore, BBS professionals ask the following questions when analyzing the impact of using extra consequences to motivate improved safety performance:

- Can contingent negative consequences be implemented consistently and fairly?
- Can the safety incentive stifle the reporting of injuries, close calls, and injuries?
- Do the safety incentives motivate the achievement of safety-process goals?
- Do monetary rewards foster participation for only a financial payoff and thus conceal the real benefit of performing safety-related behavior – injury prevention?
- Are workers recognized individually *and* in teams for completing process activities related to safety improvement?

Is there a skill discrepancy? What about those times when the individual does not know how to perform the prescribed safe behavior? The person is "unknowingly at-risk." This situation might call for training, which is a relatively expensive approach to corrective action. Mager and Pipe (1997) claim that undesirable work behavior is usually not caused by lack of knowledge or skill. People can usually perform the recommended safe behavior if the conditions and the consequences are right. So training should be used relatively infrequently for corrective action. The BBS professional asks the following questions to determine whether the behavioral discrepancy is caused by a lack of knowledge or skill:

- Could the person perform the task safely if his or her life depended on it?
- Are the person's current skills adequate for the task?
- Did the employee ever know how to perform the job safely?
- Has the worker forgotten the safest way to perform the task?

What kind of training is needed? Answers to the last two questions can help pinpoint the kind of intervention needed to eliminate a skill discrepancy. More specifically, a "yes" answer to these questions implies the need for a skill-maintenance program. Skill maintenance might be needed to help a person stay skilled, as when police officers practice regularly on a pistol range to stay ready to use their guns effectively in the rare situation when they need it. This is the rationale behind periodic emergency training.

People need to practice the behaviors that could prevent injury or save a life during an emergency. Fortunately, emergencies don't happen very often; but since they don't, people need to go through the motions just to "stay in practice." Then if the infrequent event does occur, they will be ready to do the right thing.

A very different situation also calls for skill-maintenance training. This is when certain behaviors occur regularly, but discrepancies still exist. Contrary to circumstances requiring emergency training, this problem is not due to lack of practice; rather, the person gets plenty of practice doing the behavior ineffectively or unsafely. In this case, practice does not make perfect but rather serves to entrench a bad (or at-risk) habit.

Vehicle driving is perhaps the most common and relevant example of this second kind of situation in need of behavior-based skill-maintenance training. Most drivers know how to drive a vehicle safely, and at one time performed most of their driving behaviors safely, as prescribed in their driver-training classes. For many drivers, however, the frequency of safe-driving practices decreases considerably over time, with some behaviors dropping out of a driving repertoire completely.

Practice with appropriate behavior-based feedback is critical for solving both types of skill discrepancies. However, if the skill is already used frequently but has deteriorated (as in the driving example), it is often necessary to add an extra feedback intervention to overpower the natural consequences that caused the behavior to drift from the ideal. (This critical component of BBS is explained later in this chapter.) Competent BBS professionals ask the following questions to determine whether the cause of the apparent skill discrepancy is due to lack of practice or lack of behavioral feedback:

- How often is the desired skill performed?
- Does the performer receive regular behavioral feedback relevant to skill maintenance?
- How does the performer find out how well he or she is doing?

Is the person right for the job?   A skill discrepancy can be handled in one of two ways – change the job or change the behavior. The first approach is exemplified by simplifying the task, while the latter approach is reflected in practice and behavior-based feedback. But what if a person's interests, skills, or prior experiences are incompatible with the job?

Before investing in skill training for a particular individual, it is a good idea to assess whether the person is right for the task. If the person does not have the motivation or the physical and mental capabilities for a particular assignment, the cost-effective solution is to replace the performer. Not doing this sub-optimizes work output and increases the risk for personal injury. The following questions address whether an individual has the potential to handle the job safely and effectively:

- Does the person have the physical capability to perform the task as desired?
- Does the person have the mental capability to handle the complexities of the task?
- Is the worker over-qualified for the job and thus prone to boredom or dissatisfaction?
- Can the person learn how to do the job as desired?

Before deciding on an intervention approach, BBS professionals conduct a careful analysis of the situation, the target behavior(s), and the individual(s) involved in any observed discrepancy between desired and actual (observed) behavior(s). They do not impulsively assume corrective action to improve behavior requires training or "discipline"; rather, as summarized here, a behavioral safety analysis will likely give priority to a number of alternative intervention approaches.

Direct with activators and motivate with consequences

This principle enables an understanding of why behavior occurs, and guides the design of interventions to improve behavior. It can run counter to common sense or "pop psychology." When people are asked why they did something, they offer statements like, "Because I wanted to do it," "Because I needed to do it," or "Because I was told to do it." These answers imply the cause of behavior precedes it, and is supported by a multitude of "pop psychology" self-help books that claim we motivate our behavior with self-affirmations, positive thinking, optimistic intentions, or hopeful expectations. The fact is, however, we do what we do because of the consequences we expect to get for doing it. As Dale Carnegie (1936) put it, "Every act you have ever performed since the day you were born was performed because you wanted something" (p. 62). Indeed, Carnegie (1936) cited the research and scholarship of B. F. Skinner as the foundation of this motivation principle.

The important point here is that activators (or signals preceding behavior) are only as powerful as the consequences supporting them. In other words, activators tell us what to do in order to receive a consequence, from the ringing of a telephone or doorbell to the instructions from a training seminar or one-on-one coaching session. We follow through with the particular behavior activated to the extent doing so will provide a pleasant consequence or enable avoidance of an unpleasant consequence.

This principle is typically referred to as the ABC model or three-term contingency, with A for activator, B for behavior, and C for consequence. Proponents of the BBS approach use this ABC principle to design interventions for improving behavior at individual, group, and organizational levels. More than 50 years of behavioral science research has demonstrated the efficacy of this general approach to directing and motivating behavior change. The next principle provides more specific direction for designing an intervention to improve behavior.

Focus on positive consequences to motivate behavior

B. F. Skinner's concern for people's feelings and attitudes is reflected in his antipathy toward the use of punishment (or negative consequences) to motivate behavior: "The problem is to free men, not from control, but from certain kinds of control" (Skinner, 1971, p. 41). He goes on to explain why control by negative consequences must be reduced in order to increase perceptions of personal freedom.

To be sure, the same situation can be viewed as control by negative consequences for undesired behavior or control by positive consequences for desired behavior. For example, some students are motivated to avoid failure (e.g., a poor grade), whereas other students are motivated to achieve success (e.g., a good grade or even increased knowledge). Which of these groups of students feel more in control of their course grade and thus have a better attitude toward the class? You know the answer to this question because you can reflect on your own feelings or attitude in similar situations where you perceived your behavior was influenced by positive versus negative consequences.

More than 50 years ago, Atkinson and his associates (e.g., Atkinson, 1957, 1964; Atkinson & Litwin, 1960) compared the decision-making of individuals with a high need to avoid failure versus those with a high need to achieve success, and found dramatic differences. While those motivated to achieve positive consequences set challenging but attainable goals, those participants with a high need to avoid failure were apt to set goals that were either overly easy or overly difficult.

An easy goal assures avoidance of failure, whereas an unrealistic goal provides a readily available excuse for failure – termed self-handicapping by later researchers (e.g., Berglas & Jones, 1978; Rhodewalt, 1994; Rhodewalt & Fairfield, 1991). Thus, a substantial amount of behavioral research and motivational theory justifies advocating the use of positive consequences rather than negative contingencies, whether contrived to improve someone else's behavior or imagined to motivate personal rule-governed behavior (Malott, 1992; Sidman, 1989).

Of course, disincentive/penalty contingencies are relatively easy to implement on a large scale. That's why governments select this approach to behavior management. Just pass a law and enforce it. And when monetary fines (i.e., penalties) are paid for transgressions, the controlling agency obtains financial support for continuing its enforcement efforts.

In many domains of large-scale behavior management, especially transportation management, control by negative consequences is seemingly the only feasible approach. As a result, the side effects of aggressive driving and road rage are common and observed by anyone who drives. Furthermore, most drivers have experienced the unpleasant emotional reaction of seeing the flashing blue light of a police vehicle in their rear-view mirror. And the temporary behavioral impact of this enforcement threat is readily experienced or observed. However, classic research in behavioral science taught us to expect only temporary suppression of a punished behavior (Azrin & Holz, 1966), and to predict that some drivers in their "Skinner box on wheels" will actually drive faster to compensate for the time they lost when slowing down in an "enforcement zone" (Estes & Skinner, 1941).

Practical ways to apply positive-consequence contingencies for influencing driving-related behaviors are available (e.g., Geller, Kalsher, Rudd, & Lehman, 1989; Kalsher, Geller, Clarke, & Lehman, 1989; Hagenzieker, 1991; Rudd & Geller, 1985), but much more long-term research is needed in this domain. Specifically, various incentive/reward contingencies need to be evaluated with regard to their success at offsetting the negative side effects of the existing disincentive/penalty contingencies.

Regarding industrial safety, it is often possible to increase people's perceptions that they are working to achieve success rather than working to avoid failure. Even verbal behavior directed toward another person, perhaps as a statement of genuine approval or appreciation for a task well done (Geller, 2014a), can influence motivation in ways that increase perceptions of personal freedom and empowerment. Of course, we can't be sure our intervention will have the effect we intended. Therefore, it is important to measure objectively the impact of an intervention process, as reflected by the next basic principle of BBS.

Apply the scientific method to improve intervention

Some safety professionals have suggested that dealing with the human dynamics of safety requires only "good common sense" (cf. Eckenfelder, 1996). It is hoped readers of this book realize the absurdity of such a premise. Common sense is based on people's selective attention, listening, and interpretation, and is usually founded on what sounds good to the particular individual, not necessarily on what works (cf. Daniels, 2001). In contrast, systematic objective observation enables the kind of feedback needed to know what works and what doesn't work to improve a particular target behavior.

The occurrence of specific behaviors can be objectively observed and measured before and after the implementation of an intervention process. This application of the scientific method provides feedback that enables improvement. As depicted in Figure 14.2, the acronym "DO IT" illustrates this process, and is useful for teaching this principle of BBS to employees who are empowered to intervene on behalf of their coworkers' safety and want to continuously improve their intervention skills. This process puts people in control of improving safety-related behaviors and preventing injuries.

"D" for define   The process begins by defining specific behaviors to target. These are safe behaviors that need to occur more often or at-risk behaviors that need to occur less often. Avoiding at-risk behaviors often requires certain safe behaviors, and therefore safe targets might be behaviors to substitute for particular at-risk behaviors. On the other hand, a safe target behavior can be defined independently of an associated at-risk behavior. The definition of a safe target might be as basic as using certain personal protective equipment (PPE) or "walking within pedestrian walkways." Or, the safe target could be a process requiring a particular sequence of safe behaviors, as when lifting a heavy load or locking out an energy source.

Deriving a precise definition of a DO IT target is facilitated with the development of a critical behavioral checklist (CBC) that can be used to evaluate whether a certain target behavior or process is being performed safely. Developing such behavioral definitions for

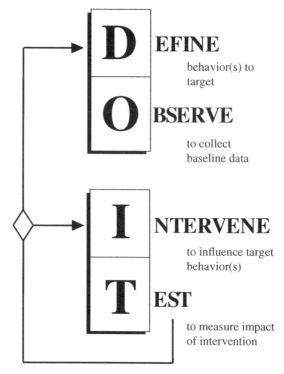

Figure 14.2 The "DO IT" process for applied behavioral science (ABS).

a CBC provides a valuable learning experience. When people get involved in deriving a CBC, they own a training process that can improve human dynamics on both the outside (behaviors) and the inside (feelings and attitudes) of people. A worksheet for developing a CBC is depicted in Figure 14.3.

From the relevant operating procedures, work teams define the specific behaviors on their job that are safe and at-risk. They derive their own customized CBC, with the critical behaviors listed and a column to check for safe observations and at-risk observation, as well as a column to record factors that may influence the behavior(s) observed. This column is depicted on the sample CBC shown in Figure 14.4.

"O" for observe   When people observe each other for certain safe and at-risk behaviors, they realize everyone performs at-risk behavior, sometimes without even realizing it. The observation stage is not a fault-finding procedure, but is a fact-finding learning process to facilitate the discovery of behaviors and conditions that need to be changed or continued in order to prevent injuries. Thus, no behavioral observation is made without awareness and explicit permission from the person being observed. The observer should be open to learning as much (if not more) from the post-observation feedback conversation as she or he expects to teach from completing the CBC.

When designing a CBC and an observation-and-feedback process, teams of workers should answer the following questions:

- What is the operational definition of each behavior on the CBC?
- Who will conduct the behavioral observations and complete the CBC?

Operating procedures	Safe observation	At-risk observation
BODY POSITIONING/PROTECTING Positioning/protecting body parts (e.g., avoiding line of fire, using PPE, equipment guards, barricades, etc.).		
VISUAL FOCUSING Eyes and attention devoted to ongoing task(s).		
COMMUNICATING Verbal or nonverbal interaction that affects safety.		
PACING OF WORK Rate of ongoing work (e.g., spacing breaks appropriately, rushing, etc.).		
MOVING OBJECTS Body mechanics while lifting, pushing/pulling.		
COMPLYING WITH LOCKOUT/TAGOUT Following procedures for lockout/tagout.		
COMPLYING WITH PERMITS Obtaining, then complying with permit(s) (e.g., confined space entry, hot work, excavation, open line, hot tap, etc.).		

Figure 14.3 A worksheet for developing a critical behavior checklist (CBC) (adapted from Geller, 2001d).

- How often will the observations be conducted?
- How will data from the CBC be summarized and interpreted?
- How will workers be informed of the results from an observation process?

Critical Behavior Checklist			
Area: _____ Immediate follow-up needed: YES NO			
Date: _____ Observer: _____			
	Safe	At-Risk	Comments
1 PPE			
A. Eye/Face			
B. Hearing			
C. Head			
D. Breathing			
E. Body			
2 Body positioning			
A. Cramped			
B. Ergonomics			
C. Extended			
D. Lifting			
E. Line of fire			
F. Pinch points			
3 Tools and equipment:			
A. Use			
B. Condition			

Figure 14.4 A sample critical behavior checklist (CBC).

One generic observation procedure is not possible for every situation, and the observation/feedback process for a particular setting should be continuously refined, depending on changing circumstances and the results of prior CBC results. It is often beneficial to begin with a limited number of behaviors and a relatively simple CBC. This reduces the possibility that some employees will feel overwhelmed at the start. Beginning small also enables the broadest range of voluntary participation, and provides numerous opportunities to successively improve the process by expanding its coverage of both behaviors and work areas. Details on how to design and use a CBC for constructive observation and feedback are given elsewhere (Geller, 1998b, 2001d; Geller & Williams, 2001; Krause et al., 1996; McSween, 1995; Roberts, 2014; Williams, 2010).

"I" for intervene   During this stage, interventions are designed and implemented in an attempt to increase the occurrence of safe behavior and/or decrease the frequency of at-risk behavior. A BBS intervention implies changing external conditions of the system in order to make safe behavior more likely than at-risk behavior. When designing interventions, it is important to realize the most motivating consequences are soon, certain, and sizable; and positive consequences are preferable to negative consequences.

The process of observing and recording the frequency of safe and at-risk behavior on a CBC provides an opportunity to give individuals and groups valuable behavior-based feedback. When the results of a behavioral observation are shown to individuals or groups, they receive the kind of information that enables practice to improve performance.

Considerable research has shown that providing workers with feedback regarding their ongoing behavior is a very cost-effective intervention approach (see, for example, the seminal analysis of the Hawthorne Effect by Parsons, 1974; comprehensive reviews by Alvero, Bucklin, & Austin, 2001, and Balcazar, Hopkins, & Suarez, 1986, as well as a historical review and meta-analysis of feedback interventions by Kluger & DeNisi, 1996).

Furthermore, occupational safety has significantly improved following the feedback display of workers' percentages of safe versus at-risk behavior (e.g., Austin, Kessler, Riccobono, & Bailey, 1996; Sulzer-Azaroff & de Santamaria, 1980; Williams & Geller, 2000; Zohar, Cohen, & Azar, 1980).

In addition to behavioral feedback, researchers have found a number of other intervention strategies to be effective at increasing safe work practices. These include worker-designed safety slogans, "close-call" and corrective-action reporting, individual and group goal setting, BBS coaching, as well as behavior-focused incentive/reward programs for individuals or groups (Geller, 1996a, 1998b, 2001d, 2014b; McSween, 1995; Petersen, 1989; Williams, 2010). In addition, Geller (2001, 2014b) explains the social validity and impact of safe behavior promise cards and actively-caring thank-you cards.

"T" for test   The test phase of DO IT provides work teams with the information they need to refine or replace a behavior-change intervention, and thereby improve the process. If observations indicate significant improvement in the target behavior has not occurred, the work team analyzes and discusses the situation. The workers might refine the intervention or choose another intervention approach. On the other hand, if the target behavior(s) reach the desired frequency level, the participants turn their attention to one or more other behaviors. They might add new critical behaviors to their CBC, thus expanding the domain of their behavioral observations. Alternatively, they might design a new intervention procedure to focus only on new behaviors.

Every time the participants evaluate an intervention approach, they learn more about how to improve safety-related behavior. They have essentially become behavioral scientists, using the DO IT process to: (a) diagnose a behavior-based issue, (b) monitor the behavioral impact of a behavior-change intervention, and (c) refine an intervention for continuous improvement. The results from such testing provide motivating consequences to support this learning process and keep the participants involved. The systematic evaluation of a number of DO IT processes can lead to a body of knowledge worthy of integration into a theory. This is reflected in the next principle.

Use theory to integrate information, not to limit possibilities

While much, if not most, research is theory driven, Skinner (1950) was critical of designing research projects to test theory. The theory-driven deductive approach can narrow the perspective of the investigator and limit the extent of findings from the scientific method. In other words, applying the DO IT process to merely test a theory can be like putting blinders on a horse. It can limit the amount of information gained from systematic observation.

Many important findings in behavioral science have resulted from exploratory investigation. That is, systematic observations of behavior occurred before and after an intervention or treatment procedure to simply answer the question, "I wonder what will happen if…?," rather than "Is my theory correct?" With this inductive approach to theory development, the investigators were not expecting a particular result, but were open to finding anything relevant to the target domain. Subsequently, they modified their research design or observation process according to their behavioral observations, not a particular theory. In other words, their innovative research was data driven rather than theory driven.

This is an important perspective for safety professionals, especially when applying the DO IT process. It is often better to be open to many possibilities for improving safety performance than to be motivated to support a certain process. Numerous intervention procedures are consistent with a BBS approach, and an intervention process that is effective in one situation will not necessarily be successful in another setting. Thus, BBS safety leaders are advised to make an educated guess about what intervention procedures to use at the start of a BBS process, but be open to results from a DO IT process and refine their procedures accordingly. Of course, the first four BBS principles introduced here should be used as a guide when designing an intervention process for behavior change.

After many systematic applications of the DO IT process, distinct consistencies will likely be found. Certain procedures will work better in some situations than others, with some individuals than others, and with some behaviors than others. Summarizing relationships between intervention impact and specific situational or interpersonal characteristics can lead to the development of a research-based theory of what type of intervention is most effective under particular circumstances. This implies the use of theory to integrate information gained from systematic behavioral observation. Skinner (1950) approved of this inductive use of theory, but cautioned that premature theory development can lead to premature theory testing and limited profound knowledge.

Design interventions with consideration of internal feelings and attitudes

As discussed above, B. F. Skinner was concerned about unobservable attitudes and feeling states. This is evidenced by his criticism of behavioral control with negative consequences because of its impact on people's feelings or perceptions. This perspective also reflects a realization that intervention procedures influence person-states, and these can be pleasant or unpleasant, desirable or undesirable. In other words, internal feelings or attitudes are influenced indirectly by the type of behavior-focused intervention procedure implemented, including the delivery method; and such relationships require careful consideration by the developers and managers of a BBS process.

The rationale for using more positive than negative consequences to motivate behavior is based on the differential feeling states provoked by positive versus negative consequences. Similarly, the way an intervention process is implemented can increase or decrease feelings of empowerment, build or destroy trust, or cultivate or inhibit a sense of teamwork or belonging (Geller, 2001d, 2002, 2014a). Therefore, it is important to assess feeling states or perceptions that occur concomitantly with an intervention process. This can be accomplished informally through one-on-one interviews and group discussions, or formally with a perception survey (O'Brien, 2000; Petersen, 2001).

Decisions regarding which intervention to implement and how to refine existing intervention procedures should be based on both objective behavioral observations and subjective evaluations of person-states. Often, however, it is possible to evaluate the indirect internal impact of an intervention by merely imagining oneself going through a particular set of intervention procedures and asking, "How would I feel?" Perhaps in this case, one's common sense is as good as any evidence one could gather from subjective evaluations of another person's feeling states.

From Principles to Applications

The first author used the term BBS in the late 1970s when researching applications of behavioral science to increase the use of vehicle safety belts throughout Blacksburg, VA, the home of Virginia Tech (VT). Research students took to the streets with pens and clipboards, and obtained empirical records of drivers' use of safety belts before, during, and after the implementation of a community-based intervention. In contrast to the current ubiquitous disincentive/penalty approach of "Click it or Ticket," the community-based interventions were all positive. For example, "if-then" incentive/reward contingencies were set up throughout the town. Banks and fast-food restaurants gave customers lottery coupons or bingo numbers at the drive-by windows if they were buckled up. Local merchants donated various prizes for winners of lotteries and "BELTS Bingo." When directing traffic on campus, police officers used pocket-size tape recorders to document the license-plate numbers of drivers who were buckled-up. Later these numbers were translated into lottery coupons for weekly "Get Caught Buckled Up" drawings. Each week, the VT President drew winners whose names were published in the local newspapers, along with the prizes and the businesses that donated them.

This approach offered positive consequences for all. Banks and fast-food restaurants got more patrons using their drive-by windows; local businesses were recognized in local media for their contributions; and most importantly, drivers significantly increased their use of safety belts. These win-win interventions, along with positive media attention, more than doubled the use of safety belts throughout the Blacksburg community and on the VT campus (Geller et al., 1989; Geller & Rudd, 1985).

Word spread beyond Blacksburg, and the US Department of Transportation and the National Highway Traffic Safety Administration (NHTSA) funded several follow-up studies of this positive approach to improving road safety. In 1982, the Corporate Safety Director for Ford Motor Company requested this application of BBS principles to increase the use of vehicle safety belts among Ford employees at approximately 110 faculties. This led to the development of training materials to teach change agents how to *Define* a target behavior (in this case, vehicle safety-belt use), *Observe* and record its frequency of occurrence, *Intervene* with positive prompts, incentives, and rewards to increase the frequency of safety-belt use, and then to *Test* the impact of the intervention by comparing frequencies of belt use during Baseline, Intervention, and Withdrawal phases (Geller, 1982; Geller, Lehman, Kalsher, 1987). This was called the "DO IT" process, as discussed above.

Safety-belt use among all Ford employees increased from 9 percent to 54 percent in 1984, saving at least 20 lives, reducing injuries to more than 800 other vehicle occupants, and saving an estimated $22 million (Gray, 1984). Following the success of this corporate-wide BBS program, the Corporate Safety Director asked the first author to expand the BBS principles and procedures to address the human side of occupational safety within Ford plants. This led to the first author delivering BBS workshops at the facilities of several automobile-manufacturing companies, including Ford, General Motors, and Chrysler. Then the safety professionals of particular plants represented at these workshops implemented BBS interventions to increase the frequency of safe behavior and decrease occurrences of at-risk (or unsafe) behavior.

Every intervention process included some form of behavioral observation and feedback, but the operations varied significantly. Plus, some BBS programs included an incentive/reward intervention whereby various types of rewards (e.g., baseball caps and shirts with a safety logo, lottery coupons, and gift cards) were offered for specific safety-related behaviors (e.g., completing a specific number of observation/feedback sessions, reporting an analysis of a "near miss" or the correction of an environmental hazard, or achieving a certain group percent-safe goal from the CBC). Unfortunately, the methods and results of these BBS programs were not documented for formal dissemination, but success stories were communicated at safety conferences and contributed to making the BBS approach extremely popular.

The popularity of BBS

In the 1990s, and subsequently throughout the world, BBS became increasingly popular in industrial settings across the USA. Our sampling of the research literature identified reports of successful BBS interventions well beyond the USA to the UK (Foster, Parand,

& Bennett, 2008; Parand & Foster, 2006), Kuwait (Al-Hemoud & Al-Asfoor, 2006), Malaysia (Ismail et al., 2012), China (Chen & Tian, 2012), and Hong Kong (Choudhry, 2014; Lingard & Rowlinson, 1997).

The general BBS procedures followed by these authors were consistent with the behavioral observation-and-feedback principles discussed above (i.e., the DO IT process) and included: (1) defining safe and unsafe target behaviors and developing a behavioral checklist (a CBC) to use during an observation session, (2) applying this checklist when observing and recording relevant safe and unsafe (or at-risk) behaviors of individual workers, (3) following the observation session (which varied from 1 to 15 minutes, depending on the number of behaviors observed), with a discussion of the results between the observer and the employee observed. Often a "percent-safe" score is calculated after the observation session by dividing the number of safe behaviors by the total number of observations and multiplying by 100 (Geller, 1996a, 2001d, 2014b; Williams, 2010).

The nature of the interpersonal feedback conversations cannot be determined from most of the research publications, but most BBS professionals recommend a nondirective approach whereby the checklist results are shown to the individual observed for his or her comments (Geller, 1996b; Geller, Perdue, & French, 2004; Roberts, 2014). The observer does not give directions but offers behavioral feedback from a fact-finding and actively caring stance (Geller & Veazie, 2014). For example, instead of telling a worker certain behaviors observed were unsafe, the observer might ask, "Is there a safer way to do that task?"

Consistent with a behavioral safety analysis explained earlier in this chapter, a critical aspect of each post-observation discussion is the identification of contextual and management-system factors that could have influenced the occurrence of at-risk behavior, as well as those factors serving as potential barriers or inhibitors of safe behavior. While observing the employee, the observer notes these potential determinants of safe vs. at-risk behavior in the "comments" column of the CBC, as described above. Specifying these factors during the post-observation feedback session facilitates the identification of hazards, conditions, or contingencies that would improve workplace safety if changed.

Most often the results of each observation session are entered into a computer program capable of comparing percent-safe scores across work areas and/or teams. Sometimes the observer's statements in the "comments" column are entered into a computer program for a subsequent content analysis and identifications of common facilitators of at-risk behavior and barriers to safe behavior. The aim is not to find fault with any individual or work team, but to discover behavior and conditions that need follow-up attention and intervention.

Deviations from the principles

The popularity of analyzing and summarizing the CBC data with computer-assisted technology is noteworthy, because it often leads to excessive focus on the data-sheet checkmarks in lieu of constructive peer-to-peer feedback conversations about the observed behaviors and conditions that put people at risk for personal injury. Geller and Veazie (2014) note this deviation from an optimal application of the CBC. They claim the primary purpose of formal observation-and-feedback sessions is not to obtain behavioral data for a computer program, but rather to give employees practice at talking to each other about their safe vs. at-risk behavior under specific circumstances. It is hoped such formal BBS observation-and-feedback communication will lead to daily informal coaching for workplace safety, eventually resulting in a brother/sister keeper's culture in which employees continually look out for the safety of themselves and others with an interdependent mindset.

The evolution to a culture in which workers "have each other's back" is impossible if supervisors conduct the behavioral observations. However, this is often the case because it is efficient at getting data for a computer program, and does not require costly education and training of line workers. Too often, even the work supervisors do not receive the necessary *education* to understand the research-based principles underlying a behavioral observation-and-feedback process, nor do they receive proper *training* on how to complete a CBC and deliver behavioral feedback so it is accepted and appreciated by the individual observed.

Most published reports of a BBS process indicate that employer "training" was a component of the intervention, but the nature of the training is rarely specified. Was the format a lecture or an interactive discussion? Was there sufficient role playing and behavioral feedback to justify the label "training session"? Was the "education" sufficient to teach the rationale of the BBS process and thereby convince participants of its meaningfulness?

Indeed, it is likely many of the BBS consultants from around the world are not even aware of the behavioral-science foundation of BBS, as reviewed in this chapter. As a result, they present incomplete and narrow perspectives of BBS. Too often they offer a quick-fix, step-by-step behavior-change *program* rather than the behavioral science philosophy and principles from which a behavior-improvement *process* can be customized for a particular concern, circumstance, context, and culture.

One example of the unfortunate and ill-informed teaching and misinterpretation of BBS that persists to this day is that many BBS consultants "sell" their BBS program on the premise that "95% or more of workplace accidents are caused by behavior." To make their point, some of these safety consultants show videos of workers engaged in extremely risky behaviors and/or experience a workplace "accident," seemingly resulting from unsafe behavior.

When these BBS sales pitches became popular in the 1990s, leaders of labor unions objected vehemently and justifiably (Hans, 1996; Howe, 1998; Lessin, 1997; Smith 1995) because claiming behaviors cause workplace injuries and property damage places blame on the employee and dismisses management's responsibility. "Don't blame people for problems caused by the system," warned W. Edwards Deming (1991).

As this chapter explains, this blame-the-worker perspective is not consistent with the behavioral science principles of BBS. It is wrong to presume behavior is a "cause" of an injury or property damage. Behavior is one of several contributing factors to an injury, along with environmental and engineering factors, management factors, cultural factors, and even person-states. Indeed, behavior should be considered an outcome of a system of interactive external and internal variables, and identifying these factors inform the design and implementation of an effective behavior-change intervention.

It is ironic the United Auto Workers (UAW) were most vociferous in their objection to BBS because the BBS methodology taught at workshops for Ford Motor Company in 1982 was appreciated by the UAW (Geller, 1982; Geller, Lehman, & Kalsher, 1987). Later, BBS became ill-defined by some consultants who marketed and taught their own interpretations of BBS procedures which often lacked the profound knowledge of behavioral science as conceptualized and researched by B. F. Skinner (1938, 1953, 1974), and reviewed earlier in this chapter.

The Challenge of Sustaining Behavior Change

The protocol of the BBS interventions reported in the research literature varies dramatically, and we found limited demonstration or discussion of long-term behavior change. For example, no research report documented a transition from formal to informal behavioral observations and feedback, as advocated by Geller and Veazie (2014). Although the senior author is aware of several companies that have continued a successful BBS process for several years, the long-term effectiveness of BBS is not reported in the research literature (but can be accessed on a website: www.safetyperformance.com).

At the 2014 annual safety conference sponsored by Safety Performance Solutions, the six facilitators of BBS for the 1500 employees of an oil-drilling company in southern California reported annual results of their observation-and-feedback process that was initiated in 1997 (E. Williams et al., 2014). Specifically, these individuals showed graphs of "man hours," reported injuries, and total recordable injury rates (TRIR)[1] per year for 19 consecutive years. As depicted in Table 14.1, annual man hours did not vary significantly over this time period, but the number of reported injuries and the TRIR decreased rather successively and dramatically after a peer-to-peer BBS coaching process was initiated in 1997; and the BBS process was sustained thereafter with continuous refinements per observations reported on CBCs.

Often researchers remove a BBS process after several months in order to demonstrate functional control. In other words, the clear impact of an observation-and-feedback process is demonstrated with a significant improvement in the target behavior(s) over baseline and then by a return to prior baseline levels after the BBS intervention is removed. While this ABA reversal design offers convincing evidence the BBS intervention influenced behavior, evidence of long-term behavior change is not provided.

Table 14.1 Annual outcome results from a company that has sustained peer-to-peer BBS observation and feedback since 1997.

Year	Number of man hours	Number of injuries	TRIR
1995	2,750,000	82	6.26
1996	2,900,000	80	5.47
1997	3,100,000	71	4.41
1998	3,000,000	50	3.35
1999	2,500,000	53	3.86
2000	3,000,000	60	3.99
2001	2,950,000	39	2.64
2002	2,500,000	28	2.22
2003	2,500,000	24	1.94
2004	2,600,000	21	1.62
2005	2,750,000	30	2.21
2006	2,850,000	23	1.06
2007	2,900,000	21	1.43
2008	3,200,000	19	1.16
2009	2,300,000	8	0.68
2010	2,800,000	11	0.78
2011	3,200,000	13	0.79
2012	3,900,000	10	0.52
2013	4,400,000	13	0.59

Some behavioral scientists consider long-term behavior change to be primarily a challenge of institutionalizing the ABC contingencies of the intervention process (Malott, 2001; McSween & Matthews, 2001). In other words, the external and extrinsic activators and consequences need to be transferred from the intervention agent to the indigenous personnel of the organizational setting in which the target behavior occurs. Thus, the intervention is not actually removed; rather those who deliver the intervention contingencies are changed.

Other behavioral scientists talk about this maintenance challenge in terms of the behavior continuing in the absence of the external and extrinsic intervention (Baer, 2001; Boyce & Geller, 2001; Geller, 2001b; Stokes & Baer, 1977). Some presume the objectives of the intervention are internalized, and people act themselves into thought processes consistent with the new behavior (Geller, 2001a). As such, personal change is viewed as a continuous spiral of behavior causing thinking, thinking inducing more behavior, and then this additional behavior influencing more thinking consistent with the behavior, and so on. However, programmatic research indicates that some interventions do not facilitate an attendant change in thinking. This is reflected profoundly in Bem's (1972) classic theory of self-perception.

Behavioral self-perception

Bem (1972) prefaced his behavioral presentation of self-perception theory with " individuals come to 'know' their own attitudes, emotions, and other internal states by inferring them from observations of their own overt behavior and/or the circumstances in which this behavior occurs" (p. 2). In other words, we write mental scripts or make internal attributions about ourselves from our observations and interpretations of the various ABC contingencies that enter our life space, and "if external contingencies seem sufficient to account for the behavior, then the individual will not be led into using the behavior as a source of evidence for his self-attributions" (p. 19).

Thus, children who had the excuse of a severe threat for not playing with a "forbidden toy" did not internalize a rule, and therefore played with the forbidden toy when the threat contingency was removed (Lepper & Green, 1978). Similarly, college students paid $20 for telling other students a boring task was fun did not develop a personal view that the task was enjoyable (Festinger & Carlsmith, 1959). The incentive/reward contingency made their behavior implausible as a reflection of their personal belief or self-perception.

In contrast, participants who received a mild threat or low compensation (only $1) to encourage their behavior developed a self-perception consistent with their behavior. The children avoided playing with the forbidden toy in a subsequent situation with no threat, and the college students who lied for low compensation decided they must have liked the boring task. In theory, these participants viewed their behavior as a valid guide for inferring their private views, since their behavior was not under strong contingency control.

The more outside control, the less self-persuasion

Much additional research supports the notion that self-persuasion is more likely when the extrinsic control of the ABC contingency is less obvious or perhaps indirect. In other words, when there are sufficient external consequences to justify the amount of effort required for a particular behavior, the performer does not develop an internal justification for the behavior. There is no self-persuasion (Aronson, 1999) and performing the behavior does not alter self-perception (Bem, 1972). Under these circumstances the maintenance of the behavior is unlikely, unless it is possible to keep a sufficient accountability system (e.g., incentives or disincentives) in place over the long term, as was in fact the case for a 13-year incentive/reward process that successfully reduced injuries in an open-pit mine (Fox, Hopkins, & Anger, 1987).

Intervening to improve behavior over the long term is more complex than applying the ABC contingency. Not only is it necessary to consider whether the performer needs instruction, motivation, or only support to improve or maintain behavior (Geller, 2001a), it seems internal cognitive factors are important whenever external contingencies cannot remain in place to hold people accountable. This implicates self-persuasion and self-directed behavior, topics not typically considered in BBS. These concepts imply that indirect influence is more likely to lead to sustained behavior change than direct persuasion, thus the focus on nondirective presentations of feedback from a CBC, as discussed earlier.

Direct persuasion   Advertisers use direct persuasion. They show us people enjoying positive consequences or avoiding negative consequences by using their products. As such, they apply the three-term contingency or ABC model to sell their goods and services. The activator (or "A" of the ABC contingency) announces the availability of a reinforcing consequence (the "C" of the ABC contingency) if the purchasing behavior is performed (the "B" of the ABC contingency). Note, however, the purpose of an advertisement is to persuade a consumer to select a certain brand of merchandise they already use. This boils down to merely choosing one commodity over another at the retail store. This is hardly a burdensome change in lifestyle.

Safety-related behavior is usually more inconvenient and requires more effort than switching brands at a supermarket. In other words, long-term participation in a safety-related work process is far more cumbersome and lifestyle-changing than the consumer behavior targeted by advertisers. In fact, direct attempts to persuade people to make inconvenient changes in their lifestyle have often yielded disappointing results. For example, communication strategies have generally been unsuccessful at persuading smokers to quit smoking (Elder, Geller, Hovell, & Mayer, 1994), drivers to stop speeding (Geller, 1998a), homeowners to conserve water (Geller, Erikson, & Buttram, 1983) or insulate their water heaters (Geller, 1981), bigoted individuals to cease prejudicial behavior, or sexually active people to use condoms (Aronson, 1999). Similarly, the "Just Say No to Drugs" campaigns have not influenced much behavior change.

The direct approach can give the impression the target behavior is accomplished for someone else's benefit. This can cause a disconnection between the behavior and self-perception. There is no self-persuasion – a mindset needed for lasting change in the absence of incentives/rewards, disincentives/penalties, or another type of extrinsic accountability system.

The indirect approach   Self-persuasion is more likely to occur when the motivational strategy is less obvious. For example, compliments regarding a person's performance are often more powerful when they are more indirect than direct (Allen, 1990; Geller, 1997, 2014a). Personal experience probably verifies this. Suppose you overhear a person tell someone else about your superb achievement on a particular assignment. Or, what if a friend gives you secondhand recognition by sharing what another person said about your special talents. Both of these situations reflect indirect commendation, and would likely have more influence on your self-perception than a direct interpersonal statement of praise. Why, because the direct approach is tainted by the possibility the flattery is given for an ulterior motive.

Indirect persuasion deviates significantly from the standard "command and control" method of promoting compliance with safety regulations. Both approaches might be equally effective at motivating behavior change, but an indirect (or nondirective) approach will be far more successful at enhancing the kind of internal dialogue needed to maintain behavior in the absence of an external motivator or accountability system.

Defining intervention conditions that can make this happen is not easy, but start by asking "Does the situation promote individual choice, ownership, and personal accountability?" "Does the context in which safety participation is desired contribute to connecting or disconnecting the link between what people do and what they think of themselves?" "Are the safety-related activities only behaviors or do they stimulate supportive cognitive activity or self-persuasion?" These questions reflect the role of psychological states, or expectancies in facilitating safety-related behavior.

Indeed, if certain feelings or beliefs affect people's participation in safety-related activities, then enhancing these states could be a powerful indirect way to improve safety-related behaviors over the long term. We mention these here to introduce a need for future research: to identify what factors need to be added or subtracted from applications of BBS to enhance its long-term beneficial impact on safety-related behavior.

Future Research

The previous section on the challenges of sustaining behavior change implicates research literature beyond the traditional domain of ABS, including theories of self-perception (Bem, 1972) and self-motivation (e.g., Deci, 1975; Ryan & Deci, 2000). This extension, as well as inaccurate presentations and distortions of BBS, led the first author to introduce a new label for applying psychological science to occupational safety – people-based safety (PBS). The term "psychological science" rather than behavioral science is used here, because PBS draws from areas of psychology beyond ABS, including cognitive science, social science, as well as research on perception, emotion, and personality.

The PBS approach was not introduced as an alternative to BBS, but rather an evolution (Geller, 2005, 2008). The overall approach is represented with the acronym ACTS: *Acting, Coaching, Thinking*, and *Seeing*. The *Acting* and *Coaching* components implicate BBS, except self-coaching and self-management techniques are incorporated (cf. Geller & Clarke, 1999). These added processes are supported through self-talk, which involve the *Thinking* component of PBS. The *Seeing* dimension of PBS takes into account the divergent perceptions of safety-related issues held by employers, supervisors, and managers, which are assessed with a perception survey prior to designing an intervention process for a particular work culture.

Entertaining these additional components of PBS is beyond the scope of this chapter, but these domains of occupational safety and health are addressed in other chapters in this Handbook. They are mentioned here as determinants of PBS intervention in order to set the stage for a primary empirical question and a critical direction for future research: namely, what aspects of the PBS evolution from BBS are functional, especially with regard to sustaining long-term improvements in safety-related behavior.

Consider, for example, the data in Table 14.1 as presented by six of the PBS coaches who were among those educated and trained in 1997 to lead the PBS approach for the 1500 employees of an oil-drilling company in southwestern California. They referred to their safety program as PBS because their intervention program was derived from PBS textbooks (Geller, 2005, 2008), but the essence of their program was peer-to-peer behavior-based observation and feedback. Thus, it cannot be determined whether any psychological science concepts beyond ABS were instrumental in facilitating the impressive long-term benefits of their PBS approach to addressing the human dynamics of injury prevention.

Factors other than the PBS coaching process could have been key determinants of the impressive outcome data in Table 14.1. These data will never appear in the research literature, as is the case for many other reports of impressive results from application of BBS and PBS documented by safety professionals, consultants, and hourly employees and presented at regional and national safety conferences. This defines a basic research need: long-term systematic evaluations of BBS and PBS programs that are sufficiently rigorous for publication in a refereed research journal.

The PBS facilitators who reported the impressive long-term outcome data in Table 14.1 indicated the following as key to their remarkable success: (a) maintaining open relationships with the field workers, and keeping them in mind at every level of our efforts; (b) promoting interpersonal trust and the theme that PBS is for the benefit of all employees; and (c) validating employee ownership of the PBS coaching process by making it visible that workers' peers are involved in every aspect of PBS implementation, from training new employees, upgrading and refining materials and procedures to analyzing and interpreting the results from the CBCs.

We hope this discussion suggests obvious directions for future research. Consider for example, the following empirical questions relevant to finding ways to increase the long-term beneficial impact of BBS or PBS interventions:

1   Beyond an observation-and-behavioral-feedback process, what additional intervention components of BBS enhance the sustainability of safe work practices?
2   To what extent are BBS principles other than behavior-based observation and feedback (i.e., coaching) practiced effectively (e.g., a behavioral safety analysis as outlined in Figure 14.1, a behavior-based incentive/reward program, applications of a DO IT process to continuously improve behavior-focused interventions, and periodic assessment of employee attitudes related to a BBS or PBS program)?
3   What factors can facilitate a transition from a formal observation-and-feedback process with a CBC to an informal "brother/sister keeper's" culture, whereby workers give each other supportive and corrective behavioral feedback periodically without a structured accountability system?
4   What intervention factors increase workers' perceptions of choice, competence, and community, and thereby enhance their engagement in a BBS or PBS process without extrinsic accountability contingencies?
5   To what extent does the active involvement of management (e.g., first-line supervisors) enhance or diminish the beneficial impact of a BBS or PBS program?

Conclusion

Seven fundamental principles of ABS were detailed as they have been applied successfully in numerous industries worldwide to prevent workplace injuries by increasing the frequency of safe behaviors and decreasing the frequency of at-risk behaviors. A key process is behavior-based observation and feedback, whereby employees use a CBC to observe and record occurrences of safe and at-risk behaviors of their coworkers and then offer them supportive and corrective behavioral feedback. The popular label for this widely practiced approach to empowering workers to intervene on behalf of the safety of their peers is termed behavior-based safety (BBS), although an evolution to people-based safety (PBS) incorporates factors beyond ABS to enhance self-motivated involvement of the wage workers.

The effectiveness of the behavior-based approach to injury prevention has been shown internationally and documented in a variety of research journals. However, most of these demonstrations are relatively short term, and questions remain with regard to those process components (or ABS principles) necessary for long-term success. Indeed, a majority of the research reports of successful BBS or PBS interventions omit details about employee education and training, accountability systems, relative management involvement, the development, application, and refinement of a CBC, and the process of presenting behavioral feedback to individuals and groups. Thus, substantial follow-up research is needed to identify those components of a BBS process that are necessary and sufficient for long-term success.

It is likely the components of an effective BBS or PBS process will vary as a function of the work culture. Then the challenge becomes: How should a culture be assessed in order to define ways to make a BBS or PBS intervention most successful? While academics ponder these and other intriguing research questions, consultants will continue to attract more clients who want to progress beyond top-down enforcement of safety rules and regulations. They will continue to help organizations empower their employees to adopt the available BBS/PBS tools, and thereby enable the bottom-up employee engagement necessary to achieve an injury-free workplace. By exploring answers to the research questions posed in this chapter, applied behavioral scientists will improve this process by providing evidence-based ways to benefit current BBS/PBS techniques and procedures, and by adding intervention tools to make BBS/PBS more cost effective and durable.

Note

1   TRIR is a measure of the rate of recordable workplace injuries, normalized per 100 workers per year, and is derived by multiplying the number of recordable injuries in a calendar year by 200,000 (100 employees working 2000 hours per year) and dividing this value by the total man-hours actually worked in the year.

References

Al-Hemoud, A. M., & Al-Asfoor, M. M. (2006). A behavior based safety approach at a Kuwait research institution. *Journal of Safety Research, 37*(2), 201–206.

Allen, J. (1990). *I saw what you did and I know who you are: Bloopers, blunders and success stories in giving and receiving recognition.* Tucker, GA: Performance Management Publications.

Alvero, A. M., Bucklin, B. R., & Austin, J. (2001). An objective review of the effectiveness and characteristics of performance feedback in organizational settings (1985–1998). *Journal of Organizational Behavior Management, 21*(1), 3–29.

Aronson, E. (1999). The power of self-persuasion. *American Psychologist, 54*(11), 875–884.

Atkinson, J. W. (1957). Motivational determinants of risk-taking behavior. *Psychological Review, 64*(6), 359–372.

Atkinson, J. W. (1964). *An introduction to motivation.* Princeton, NJ: Van Nostrand.

Atkinson, J. W., & Litwin, G. F. (1960). Achievement motive and test anxiety conceived as motive to approach success and motive to avoid failure. *Journal of Abnormal and Social Psychology, 60*, 52–63.

Austin, J. (2000). Performance analysis and performance diagnostics. In J. Austin & J. E. Carr (Eds.), *Handbook of applied behavior analysis* (pp. 321–349). Reno, NV: Context Press.

Austin, J., Carr, J. E., & Agnew, J. (1999). The need for assessing maintaining variables in OBM. *Journal of Organizational Behavior Management, 19*(2), 59–87.

Austin, J., Kessler, M. L., Riccobono, J. E., & Bailey, J. S. (1996). Using feedback and reinforcement to improve the performance and safety of a roofing crew. *Journal of Organizational Behavior Management, 16*(2), 49–75.

Azrin, N. H., & Holz, W. C. (1966). Punishment. In W. K. Honig (Ed.), *Operant behavior: Areas of research and application.* New York, NY: Appleton-Century-Crofts.

Baer, D. M. (2001). Since safety maintains our lives, we need to maintain maintaining. *Journal of Organizational Behavior Management, 21*(1), 61–64.

Bailey, J. S., & Austin, J. (1996). Evaluating and improving productivity in the workplace. In B. Thyer & M. Mattaini (Eds.), *Behavior analysis and social work* (pp. 179–200). Washington, DC: American Psychological Association.

Balcazar, F., Hopkins, B. L., & Suarez, I. (1986). A critical, objective review of performance feedback. *Journal of Organizational Behavior Management, 7*(3–4), 65–89.

Bem, D. J. (1972). Self-perception theory. In L. Berkowitz (Ed.), *Advances in experimental social psychology* (vol. 6, pp. 1–60). New York, NY: Academic Press.

Berglas, S., & Jones, E. E. (1978). Drug choice as a self-handicapping strategy in response to noncontingent success. *Journal of Personality and Social Psychology, 36*(4), 405–417.

Boyce, T. E., & Geller, E. S. (2001). Applied behavior analysis and occupational safety: The challenge of response maintenance. *Journal of Organizational Behavior Management, 21*(1), 31–60.

Carnegie, D. (1936). *How to win friends and influence people.* New York: Simon and Schuster.

Chen, D., & Tian, H. (2012). Behavior based safety for accidents prevention and positive study in china construction project. *Procedia Engineering, 43,* 528–534.

Choudhry, R. M. (2014). Behavior-based safety on construction sites: A case study. *Accident Analysis & Prevention, 70,* 14–23.

Daniels, A. C. (2000). *Bringing out the best in people: How to apply the astonishing power of positive reinforcement* (2nd edn.). New York, NY: McGraw-Hill.

Daniels, A. C. (2001). *Other people's habits: How to use positive reinforcement to bring out the best in people around you.* New York, NY: McGraw-Hill.

Deci, E. L. (1975). *Intrinsic motivation.* New York, NY: Plenum

Deming, W. E. (1991). *Quality, productivity, and competitive position.* Four-day workshop presented in Cincinnati, OH by Quality Enhancement Seminars, Inc.

Eckenfelder, D. J. (1996). *Values-driven safety.* Rockville, MD: Government Institutes, Inc.

Elder, J. P., Geller, E. S., Hovell, M. F., & Mayer, J. A. (1994). *Motivating health behavior.* New York, NY: Delmar Publishers.

Estes, W. K., & Skinner, B. F. (1941). Some quantitative properties of anxiety. *Journal of Experimental Psychology, 29*(5), 390–400.

Festinger, L., & Carlsmith, J. M. (1959). Cognitive consequences of forced compliance. *Journal of Abnormal and Social Psychology, 58,* 203–210.

Foster, P. J, Parand, A., & Bennett, J. (2008). Improving the safety performance of the UK quarrying industry through a behavioural-based safety intervention. *Journal of the Southern African Institute of Mining and Metallurgy – Surface Mining, 108*(11), 683–690.

Fox, D. K., Hopkins, B. L., & Anger, W. K. (1987). The long-term effects of a token economy on safety performance in open-pit mining. *Journal of Applied Behavior Analysis, 20*(3), 215–224.

Geller, E. S. (1981). Evaluating energy conservation programs: Is verbal report enough? *Journal of Consumer Behavior, 8*(3), 331–334.

Geller, E. S. (1982). *Corporate incentives for promoting safety-belt use.* Washington, DC: US Department of Transportation.

Geller, E. S. (1996a). *The psychology of safety: How to improve behaviors and attitudes on the job.* Radnor, PA: Chilton Book Company.

Geller, E. S. (1996b). The truth about safety incentives. *Professional Safety, 41*(10), 34–39.

Geller, E. S. (1997). Key processes for continuous safety improvement: Behavior-based recognition and celebration. *Professional Safety, 42*(10), 40–44.

Geller, E. S. (1998a). *Applications of behavior analysis to prevent injury from vehicle crashes* (2nd edn.). Cambridge, MA: Cambridge Center for Behavioral Studies.

Geller, E. S. (1998b). *Understanding behavior-based safety: Step-by-step methods to improve your workplace* (2nd edn.). Neenah, WI: J. J. Keller & Associates, Inc.

Geller, E. S. (2000). Behavioral safety analysis: Precursor to corrective action. *Professional Safety, 45*(3), 29–32.

Geller, E. S. (2001a). Behavior-based safety in industry: Realizing the large-scale potential of psychology to promote human welfare. *Applied & Preventive Psychology, 10*(2), 87–105.

Geller, E. S. (2001b). *Beyond safety accountability.* Rockville, MD: Government Institutes.

Geller, E. S. (2001c). Dream – Operationalize – Intervene – Test: If you want to make a difference – Just DO IT. *Journal of Organizational Behavior Management, 21*(1), 109–121.

Geller, E. S. (2001d). *The psychology of safety handbook.* Boca Raton, FL: CRC Press.

Geller, E. S. (2002). *The participation factor: How to get more people involved in occupational safety.* Des Plaines, IL: American Society of Safety Engineers.

Geller, E. S. (2005). *People-based safety: The source.* Virginia Beach, VA: Coastal Training and Technologies Corporation.

Geller, E. S. (2008). *Leading people-based safety: Enriching your culture.* Virginia Beach, VA: Coastal Training and Technologies Corporation.

Geller, E. S. (2014a). Leading with AC4P communication. In E. S. Geller (Ed.), *Actively caring for people: Cultivating a culture of compassion* (4th edn., pp. 151–174). Newport, VA: Make-A-Difference, LLC.

Geller, E. S. (2014b). The psychology of AC4P. In E. S. Geller (Ed.) *Actively caring for people: Cultivating a culture of compassion* (4th edn., pp. 35–62). Newport, VA: Make-A-Difference, LLC.

Geller, E. S., & Clarke, S. W. (1999). Safety self-management: A key behavior-based process for injury prevention. *Professional Safety, 44*(7), 29–33.

Geller, E. S., Erickson, J. B., & Buttram, B. A. (1983). Attempts to promote residential water conservation with educational, behavioral, and engineering strategies. *Population and Environment, 6*(2), 96–112.

Geller, E. S., Kalsher, M. J., Rudd, J. R., & Lehman, G. (1989). Promoting safety-belt use on a university campus: An integration of commitment and incentive strategies. *Journal of Applied Social Psychology, 19*(1), 3–19.

Geller, E. S., Lehman, G. R., & Kalsher, M. J. (1987). *Behavior analysis training for occupational safety.* Detroit, MI: Ford Motor Company.

Geller, E. S., Perdue, S., & French, A. (2004). Behavior-based safety coaching: Ten guidelines for successful application. *Professional Safety, 49* (7), 42–49.

Geller, E. S., & Rudd, J. R. (1985). University-wide incentives for encouraging safety-belt use: A comprehensive evaluation. *Proceedings of the Fourth Symposium on Traffic Safety Effectiveness (Impact) Evaluation Projects.* National Safety Council, Chicago, IL.

Geller, E. S., & Veazie, R. A. (2014). Behavior-based safety versus actively caring: From other-directed compliance to self-directed commitment. *Professional Safety, 59*(10), 44–50.

Geller, E. S., & Williams, J. (Eds.) (2001). *Keys to behavior-based safety from Safety Performance Solutions.* Rockville, MD: Government Institutes.

Gilbert, T. F. (1978). *Human competence: Engineering worthy performance.* New York, NY: McGraw-Hill.

Goldstein, A. P., & Krasner, L. (1987). *Modern applied psychology.* New York, NY: Pergamon Press

Gray, D. (1984). Personal communication to E. S. Geller, February 7, 1984.

Greene, B. F., Winett, R. A., VanHouten, R., Geller, E. S., & Iwata, B. A. (Eds.) (1987). *Behavior analysis in the community: Readings from the Journal of Applied Behavior Analysis.* University of Kansas, Lawrence.

Grindle, A. C., Dickinson, A. M., & Boettcher, W. (2000). Behavioral safety research in manufacturing settings: A review of the literature. *Journal of Organizational Behavior Management, 20*(1), 29–68.

Hagenzieker, M. P. (1991). Enforcement or incentive? Promoting safety-belt use among military personnel in the Netherlands. *Journal of Applied Behavior Analysis, 24*(1), 23–30.

Hans, M. (1996). Does behavior-based safety work? *Safety and Health,* National Safety Council, June, 44–49.

Howe, J. (1998, January). *A union critique of behavioral safety.* Paper presented at the ASSE Behavioral Safety Symposium, Orlando, FL.

Ismail, F., Hashim, A. E., Zuriea, W., Ismail, W., Kamarudin, H., & Baharom, Z. A. (2012). Behaviour-based approach for quality and safety environment improvement: Malaysian experience in the oil and gas industry. *Procedia – Social and Behavioral Sciences 35,* 586–594.

Kalsher, M. J., Geller, E. S., Clarke, S. W., & Lehman, G. R. (1989). Safety-belt promotion on a naval base: A comparison of incentives vs. disincentives. *Journal of Safety Research, 20*(3), 103–113.

Kluger, A. N., & DeNisi, A. (1996). The effects of feedback interventions on performance: A historical review, a meta-analysis, and a preliminary feedback intervention theory. *Psychological Bulletin, 119*(2), 254.

Krause, T. R. (1995). *Employee-driven systems for safe behavior: Integrating behavioral and statistical methodologies*. New York, NY: Van Nostrand Reinhold.

Krause, T. R., Hidley, J. H., & Hodson, S. J. (1996). *The behavior-based safety process: Managing improvement for an injury-free culture* (2nd edn.). New York, NY: Van Nostrand Reinhold.

Kroemer, K. H. (1991). Ergonomics. *Encyclopedia of Human Biology* (vol. 3, pp. 473–480). New York, NY: Academic Press.

Lepper, M., & Green, D. (1978). *The hidden cost of reward*. Hillsdale, NJ: Erlbaum.

Lessin, N. (1997). Workers need real rights. *Industrial Safety & Hygiene News, 31*(10), 42.

Lingard, H., & Rowlinson, S. (1997). Behavior-based in Hong-Kong's safety management construction industry. *Journal of Safety Research, 2*(4), 243–256.

Mager, R. F., & Pipe, P. (1997). *Analyzing performance problems or you really oughta wanna* (3rd edn.). Atlanta, GA: Center for Effective Performance, Inc.

Malott, R. W. (1992). A theory of rule-governed behavior and organizational behavior management. *Journal of Organizational Behavior Management, 12*(2), 45–65.

Malott, R. W. (2001). Occupational safety and response maintenance: An alternative view. *Journal of Organizational Behavior Management, 21*(1), 85–102.

McAfee, R. B., & Winn, A. R. (1989). The use of incentives/feedback to enhance workplace safety: A critique of the literature. *Journal of Safety Research, 20*(1), 7–19.

McSween, T. E. (1995). *The values-based safety process: Improving your safety culture with a behavioral approach*. New York, NY: Van Nostrand Reinhold.

McSween, T., & Matthews, G. A. (2001). Maintenance in organizational safety management. *Journal of Organizational Behavior Management, 21*(1), 75–83.

Norman, D. A. (1988). *The psychology of everyday things*. New York, NY: Basic Books.

O'Brien, D. P. (2000). *Business measurements for safety performance*. New York, NY: Lewis Publishers.

Parand, A., & Foster, P. J. (2006) *Behavioural-based safety in the minerals industry: A research based methodology carried out in the UK quarrying sector*. Queensland Resources Council Mining Health & Safety Conference, Townsville, Queensland.

Parsons, H. M. (1974). What happened at Hawthorne? *Science, 183*, 922–932.

Petersen, D. (1989). *Safe behavior reinforcement*. Goshen, NY: Aloray, Inc.

Petersen, D. (2001). *Authentic involvement*. Itasca, IL: National Safety Council.

Rhodewalt, F. (1994). Conceptions of ability achievement goals, and individual differences in self-handicapping behavior: On the application of implicit theories. *Journal of Personality, 62*(1), 67–85.

Rhodewalt, F., & Fairfield, M. (1991). Claimed self-handicaps and the self-handicapper: The relations of reduction in intended effort to performance. *Journal of Research in Personality, 25*(4), 402–417.

Roberts, D. S. (2014). Actively caring for occupational safety: Preventing injuries with people-based safety. In E. S. Geller (Ed.). *Actively caring for people: Cultivating a culture of compassion* (4th edn., pp. 181–197). Newport, VA: Make-A-Difference, LLC.

Rudd, J. R., & Geller, E. S. (1985). A university-based incentive program to increase safety-belt use: Toward cost-effective institutionalization. *Journal of Applied Behavior Analysis, 18*(3), 215–226.

Ryan, R. M., & Deci, E. L. (2000). Self-determination theory and the foundation of intrinsic motivation, social development, and well-being. *American Psychologist, 55*, 68–75.

Sidman, M. (1989). *Coercion and its fallout*. Boston, MA: Authors Cooperative, Inc., Publishers.

Skinner, B. F. (1938). *The behavior of organisms: An experimental analysis*. Acton, MA: Copley Publishing Group.

Skinner, B. F. (1950). Are theories of learning necessary? *Psychological Review, 57*(4), 193–216.

Skinner, B. F. (1953). *Science and human behavior*. New York, NY: Macmillan.

Skinner, B. F. (1971). *Beyond freedom and dignity*. New York, NY: Alfred A. Knopf.

Skinner, B. F. (1974). *About behaviorism*. New York, NY: Alfred A. Knopf.

Smith, T. A. (1995). Viewpoint: Rebutting behaviorism. *Industrial Safety & Hygiene News, 40*(3), 40.

Stokes, T. F., & Baer, D. M. (1977). An implicit technology of generalization. *Journal of Applied Behavior Analysis, 10*(2), 349–367.

Sulzer-Azaroff, B. (1998). *Who killed my daddy? A behavioral safety fable.* Cambridge, MA: Cambridge Center for Behavioral Studies.

Sulzer-Azaroff, B., & Austin, J. (2000). Does BBS work? Behavior-based safety and injury reduction: A survey of the evidence. *Professional Safety, 45*(7), 19–24.

Sulzer-Azaroff, B., & de Santamaria, M. C. (1980). Industrial safety hazard reduction through performance feedback. *Journal of Applied Behavior Analysis, 13*(2), 287–295.

Williams, E., Eusquiano, M., Holland, W., Cabs, D., Escobar, J., & Gibbons, G. (2014, August). *Maintaining momentum: Increasing employee participation, strengthening leadership and supervisor support: Utilizing behavior-based safety processes since 1997.* Break-out session at the 18th Annual Safety Performance Solutions Conference, Roanoke, VA.

Williams, J. H. (2010). *Keeping people safe: The human dynamics of injury prevention.* Lanham, MD: Scarecrow Press, Inc.

Williams, J. H., & Geller, E. S. (2000). Behavior-based intervention for occupational safety: Critical impact of social comparison feedback. *Journal of Safety Research, 31*(3), 135–142.

Zohar, D., Cohen, A., & Azar, N. (1980). Promoting increased use of ear protectors in noise through information feedback. *Human Factors, 22*(1), 69–79.

15

Safety Training

Michael J. Burke and Caitlin E. Smith Sockbeson

Introduction

The focus of this chapter is on how modifying individual and team characteristics through safety training affects the exhibition of safe work behaviors and the reduction of negative outcomes such as accidents, illnesses, and injuries. Safety training and the transfer of safety training take place within work systems. Here, we review the extant safety training literature in order to assess our current state of knowledge with respect to a *worker characteristic–work criteria–work context* framework and identify where, with respect to estimating relationships in such a framework or work system, future research might be directed. In doing so, we concentrate our discussion on safety training research involving working adults.

Our chapter unfolds as follows. Initially, we present a general framework for studying relations between worker characteristics affected by safety training programs, safety-relevant criteria for evaluating the effectiveness of such interventions, and work-context factors that may promote or inhibit the transfer of safety training to the job. In the second section, we discuss the nature of safety training interventions with respect to the targets, content, and modes for the delivery of safety training. The third section focuses on what we know about relationships between safety training and safety-relevant criteria, and how such relationships are moderated by work context factors. The fourth section is concerned with the limits of our current knowledge and practice in regard to worker safety training and the types of research needed to expand those limits.

A General Framework for Studying Safety Training Interventions

In discussing a general framework for organizing the safety training literature, we begin with broad dependent variable categories in Figure 15.1 that are posited to be either directly or indirectly affected by safety training interventions. In large part, safety performance,

The Wiley Blackwell Handbook of the Psychology of Occupational Safety and Workplace Health, First Edition. Edited by Sharon Clarke, Tahira M. Probst, Frank Guldenmund, and Jonathan Passmore. © 2016 John Wiley & Sons Ltd. Published 2020 by John Wiley & Sons Ltd.

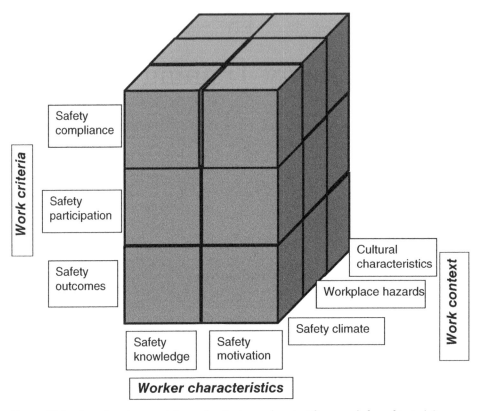

Figure 15.1 A *worker characteristic–work criteria–work context* framework for safety training.

or the safety-related actions that workers engage in, can be viewed with respect to two broad content categories, often labeled *safety compliance* and *safety participation*, respectively. *Safety compliance* refers to mandated or expected safety behaviors, whereas *safety participation* includes actions that are more discretionary in nature (see Neal, Griffin, & Hart, 2000). Although a fair amount of research on behavioral aspects of safety treats these broad content categories as unitary constructs (e.g., see Hofmann, Morgeson, & Gerras, 2003; Neal et al., 2000), qualitative research and factor analytic work on measures of safety performance indicate otherwise (see Burke, Sarpy, Tesluk, & Smith-Crowe, 2002a; Cagno, Micheli, Jacinto, & Masi, 2014; Marchand, Simard, Carpentier-Roy, & Ouellet, 1998). Both Burke et al. and Marchand et al. found that a two-factor model of safety performance (with factors relating to safety compliance and safety initiative) did not provide a good fit to the data. For instance, Burke et al. confirmed, across 23 jobs, a grounded theoretical model of general safety performance with four factors. Several of their confirmed factors (e.g., using personal protective equipment and engaging in work practices to reduce risk) would fall within the domain of safety compliance, whereas other confirmed factors (e.g., exercising employee rights and responsibilities) are closer to the notion of safety participation. Notably, these factors related to both individual and group work.

Together, conceptual and empirical research on the factor structure of behavioral safety performance would suggest that safety training researchers, across disciplinary boundaries, may benefit from attending to potentially useful construct distinctions when behavioral measures are used as criteria for evaluating the effectiveness of safety training. This point may be particularly relevant to the consideration of criteria for evaluating team safety training where process-oriented constructs and measures such as coordination and adaptive capacity might be taken into account. That said, the notions of safety compliance and safety participation are useful content distinctions for organizing discussions of the relative effectiveness of safety training interventions insofar as such programs focus on modifying individual and team characteristics to influence expected or discretionary behaviors, respectively.

Along with safety performance, we include a general category in Figure 15.1 pertaining to safety outcomes. *Safety outcomes* refer to accidents, near misses, illness/disease, and injury that are viewed within most models of workplace safety as consequent to unsafe work behavior (see Christian, Bradley, Wallace, & Burke, 2009; Paul & Maiti, 2007). Although safety training is largely aimed at improving workers' knowledge for engaging in actions that will preclude such negative outcomes, safety training interventions are occasionally evaluated with respect to actual reductions in negative outcomes. For instance, in the case of occupational contact dermatitis, Held, Mygind, Wolff, Gyntelberg, and Anger (2002) evaluated the effectiveness of safety training with respect to the reduction of symptoms themselves as determined via clinical examinations.

In regard to worker characteristics that safety training interventions are aimed at modifying, we organize our discussions around two broad categories: safety knowledge and safety motivation. For the purposes of our discussion, the term *safety knowledge* refers to both the factual or declarative knowledge that training focuses on and the procedural skills or know-how related to conducting safety-related work. We use the broader term safety knowledge due to the fact that many safety training programs concurrently emphasize the acquisition of facts and skills. For instance, the literature is full of such examples, which can be further broken down into four more specific areas: fundamental knowledge and skills (e.g., related to using personal protective equipment, Sadler & Montgomery, 1982), recognition and awareness knowledge and skills (e.g., collecting information about workplace hazards, Caparaz, Rice, Graumlich, Radike, & Morawetz, 1990), problem solving and decision-making skills (e.g., related to using union and management resources, Lapping & Parsons, 1980), and empowerment skills (e.g., empowering workers to take collective action, Luskin, Somers, Wooding, & Levenstein, 1992).

Safety training programs can also be directed at modifying workers' *safety motivation*, workers' regulatory behavior in regard to exerting effort when on the job to engage in safe work behavior (Ford & Tetrick, 2008). For instance, some safety training programs emphasize the development of self-efficacy or confidence for dealing with particular situations, while others focus on establishing goals for engaging in safe work behavior with accompanying feedback on the job. Although self-efficacy can be influenced by multi-session training involving practice and feedback, Wallace and colleagues (Wallace & Chen, 2006; Wallace, Little, & Shull, 2008) have also noted the potential importance for workers of adopting a particular regulatory focus. That is, they stress the importance of workers adopting a prevention focus (i.e., a focus on performing tasks accurately and in accordance with one's duties) versus a promotion focus (i.e., a focus on accomplishing more tasks, more quickly) in regard to promoting workplace safety.

In terms of situational characteristics that might moderate effects associated with safety training programs, we focus on safety climate, workplace hazards, and cultural characteristics in Figure 15.1. For the purposes of our discussion, *safety climate* refers to work environment characteristics such as safety policies, practices, and procedures that affect members of the workgroup or organization (see Guediri & Griffin, Chapter 13, this volume). At the individual level of analysis, a number of studies have examined the factor structure of workers' safety climate perceptions (see Flin, Mearns, O'Connor, & Bryden,

2000; Zohar, 2011 for reviews). A general conclusion is that a somewhat common set of dimensions, albeit with different factor labels, underlie individual perceptions or psychological climate in regard to workplace safety (i.e., management commitment, management support, safety systems, human resource management practices, risk, group processes, and work pressure; Neal & Griffin, 2004). Many of these factors are important or relevant at the workgroup level as well (Zohar, 2011).

Further, consistent with conceptual arguments in the general domain of work climate (see James et al., 2008 for a review), we view safety climate as having a hierarchical structure at both the individual (psychological) and group levels of analysis. At the higher-order factor level, safety climate can be conceptualized with respect to employees' perceptions of how the work environment affects their personal well-being as well as the well-being of other, relevant stakeholders (e.g., the public in relation to hazardous waste work). That is, at the higher order factor level, we view first-order climate factors (e.g., supervisory support, risk, work pressure) as driven by an employee's emotional evaluation of the degree to which the work environment is perceived as personally beneficial or detrimental to oneself and to relevant others (e.g., organizational safety orientation in relation to the public). Burke, Borucki, and Kaufman (2002b) and Burke and Signal (2010) offer more detailed discussions of the first-order factors that would comprise higher-order safety climate factors relative to employees and other stakeholders.

While other researchers have posited a single, higher-order safety climate factor in relation to employees' personal well-being (see Christian et al., 2009; Griffin & Neal, 2000; Neal & Griffin, 2004), we view such a perspective as potentially construct-deficient with respect to capturing an organization's safety climate in terms of how it affects all organizational constituencies. We will return to a discussion of this point below. However, given that the extant literature has largely focused on safety climate dimensions that more directly relate to worker well-being, we provisionally begin with a general safety climate category in Figure 15.1. Although this factor has been variously labeled in the literature as Safety Climate General (SCg) (Neal & Griffin, 2004), Concern for Employees (Burke et al., 2002b), and overall Safety Climate (Christian et al., 2009), we adopt the more straightforward label of "safety climate" for this higher-order factor. Viewing safety climate as a higher-order factor is also consistent with how the literature on safety climate has been meta-analytically integrated (i.e., with respect to overall measures of safety climate, see Clarke, 2006). Importantly, at the organization or workgroup level, an important indicator of safety climate is workers' shared perceptions of work environment characteristics as they pertain to safety matters that affect group members (e.g., Neal & Griffin, 2004; Zohar & Luria, 2005; see also Luria, Chapter 16, this volume).

Turning to workplace hazards as situational characteristics, we view the category *workplace hazards* (e.g., biological, chemical, radiological, and noise) along a continuum, going from being less severe (e.g., slips, overexertion, repetitive motion) to being more severe (e.g., the contraction of hepatitis or HIV resulting from needle sticks, exposure to harmful substances and environments). In doing so, we begin with a general workplace hazards category. Viewing workplace hazards along a continuum is consistent with the Bureau of Labor Statistics' Occupational Injury and Illness Classification System (OIICS) (see Biddle, 1998), which hierarchically arranges workplace hazards to reflect the increasing potential for severe illness, injury, or death due to hazardous event or exposure. Although considerable discussion exists in the workplace safety literature for researchers to focus on perceived as opposed to objective risk factors (e.g., see Morrow & Crum, 1998; Pidgeon, 1991), as discussed below, we believe there are conceptual and empirical bases for safety training researchers to reconsider the role of workplace hazards themselves as moderators of safety training–safety criterion relationships.

Finally, the category of *cultural characteristics* in Figure 15.1 refers to cultural dimensions (see Hofstede, 2001; Schwartz, 1999) such as uncertainty avoidance, power distance, and masculinity–femininity that would be expected to underlie aspects of the political economy of nations and states that, in turn, would be expected to influence safety training itself and its transfer to the job. Here, we refer to political economy as the political, economic, and legal systems of countries and states. As discussed in detail within Burke and Signal (2010), cultural values would be expected to drive the social justice orientation, fiscal capacity of nations and states, and the capacity for labor to organize. For instance, Burke and Signal discuss how nations and states characterized by higher levels of power distance and masculinity have fewer regulatory bodies to focus on workplace safety, less fiscal capacity for enforcement of safety-related laws and regulations, and an emphasis on industry over labor with the result being that workers in these nations and states face greater potential exposure to workplace hazards. Several studies have documented associations between cultural dimensions and the nature of safety training (Burke, Chan-Serafin, Salvador, Smith, & Sarpy, 2008); safety outcomes, including the responsibility for accident occurrence (Gyekye & Salminen, 2005; Infortunio, 2006); and organizational safety climate (Håvold, 2007).

Safety Training Interventions

Organizations may institute health and safety interventions to comply with national or local laws and regulations (e.g., Occupational Safety and Health Administration regulations in the United States), in response to specific incidents or accidents in the workplace, or in an effort to proactively promote the safety and health of workers as individuals, groups, teams, or work units, and other organizational stakeholders. These interventions may focus on different types of knowledge and skill (e.g., using protective equipment, recognizing and reporting hazards) and may take different forms (e.g., lectures, computer-based training, and role playing). In this section, we discuss the varying targets, content, and modes for the delivery of safety training.

Prior to discussing how safety training interventions differ with respect to targets, content, and method of delivery, we note that safety training often has safety and health implications for not only workers, but also for other stakeholders (e.g., patients, suppliers, customers, and community members). For example, hospital workers may be trained to protect themselves from injuries (e.g., due to improper lifting techniques or incorrect needle use), which may have important implications for patient safety and health (e.g., Benning et al., 2011; Evanoff, Bohr, & Wolf, 1999; Lee, Allen, & Daly, 2012; Yao et al., 2013; see also Bishop, Fleming, & Flin, Chapter 20, this volume). Employees who work with food often need training in the correct use of knives and proper personal hygiene for their safety and health as well as consumers' health (e.g., Fenton, LaBorde, Radhakrishna, Brown, & Cutter, 2006; Mancini, Murray, Chapman, & Powell, 2012; McIntyre, Vallaster, Wilcott, Henderson, & Kosatsky, 2013; Park, Kwak, & Chang, 2010). Similarly, training for pilots (e.g., Kearns, 2011; Salas, Fowlkes, Stout, Milanovich, & Prince, 1999) is not merely aimed at protecting those employees, but also the safety of passengers and others who could be affected by flight operations.

Training to promote worker safety and the well-being of other stakeholders varies widely in regard to the specific purposes of training. For instance, fishermen may be trained in emergency response to prevent drowning (e.g., Dzugan, 2010), farm workers may be trained in work practices to avoid pesticide poisoning to themselves and food-borne illness to consumers (e.g., Levesque, Arif, & Shen, 2012; Nieto-Montenegro,

Brown, & LaBorde, 2008; Zhang et al., 2011), and construction workers may be trained in fall protection to prevent minor as well as severe injury or death (e.g., Bena, Berchialla Coffano, Debernardi, & Icardi, 2009; Fullen, 2010; Kaskutas, Dale, Lipscomb, & Evanoff, 2013). On the other hand, workers in a number of occupations may be trained in sun safety to prevent the onset of skin cancer (e.g., Girgis, Sanson-Fisher, & Watson, 1994; Madgwick, Houdmont, & Randall, 2011; Mayer et al., 2009) or proper posture and movement to avoid the development of musculoskeletal disorders (Gagnon, 2003; Videman et al., 1989). Notably, these examples indicate that safety training across occupations and industries can be conducted with respect to workplace hazards that vary in the likelihood of severe injury/illness potential due to an event or exposure, or where the onset of injury or illness is due to chronic exposure.

While the specific aims of training and nature of workplace hazards differ across occupations and industries, the content and objectives of safety training can nevertheless be grouped into categories or types of training programs that apply more generally. These categories relate to the acquisition of fundamental knowledge and skills (e.g., using personal protective equipment; Foster 1996), recognition knowledge and skills (e.g., collecting and communicating information about workplace hazards; Robins, Hugentobler, Kaminski, & Klitzman, 1990), problem solving and decision-making skills (e.g., controlling a hazard or handling an emergency; Lapping & Parsons, 1980), and empowerment skills (e.g., taking collective action or exercising one's rights and responsibilities; Wallerstein & Wenger 1992). To illustrate this point, take, for example, the category of fundamental knowledge and skill and the use of personal protective equipment as a learning objective. Here, we could consider training targeted at the use of basic protective equipment such as eyewear, which could include items such as goggles, face shields, and safety glasses and relate to workers in many occupations and industries such as manufacturing, construction, service, and retail (Forst et al., 2006; Lipscomb, 2000; Lombardi, Verma, Brennan, & Perry, 2009; Reif, Fraser, & Liffers, 2013).

In addition to the type of training, safety training interventions can be considered with respect to the method used to deliver the training. At a more passive level, warnings and information may be provided on posted signs or labels in the workplace (McGrath, 2011), with training provided to recognize what the warning symbols mean (e.g., Chan & Ng, 2010). Greater learner involvement is required for programs like hazard mapping, wherein employees are taught to locate and identify hazards, communicate information on such hazards to management, and thus target hazards for elimination from the workplace (e.g., Anderson, Collins, Devlin, & Renner, 2012). This movement from passive to more activity-based means of learning may be reflected in a variety of activities and methods: attending lectures or reading materials and manuals (e.g., Gettle, 2009); viewing videos (e.g., Cherrett, Wills, Price, Maynard, & Dror, 2009; Nielsen, Sigurdsson, & Austin, 2009); participating in computer- or web-based learning (e.g., Mancini, Cazzell, Kardong-Edgren, & Cason, 2009; Cerecero & Charlton, 2012; Ho & Dzeng, 2010; Kearns, 2011), simulations (e.g., Orr, Mallet, & Margolis, 2009; West, Slatin, Sanborn, & Volicer, 2009), tactical decision games (e.g., Crichton, 2009); role-playing (Calabro, Weltge, Parnell, Kouzekanani, & Ramirez, 1998); staging of a hazardous event including the recreation of an historical event with an after-action review (Becker & Burke, 2012); and hands-on learning (Jensen & Friche, 2007).

Of course, safety training methods are not necessarily mutually exclusive, as computer-based training could include videos or lecture-based classroom instruction could include role-playing, to name just a few combinations. Noting this point, and relying on arguments from dialogical and experiential theories of learning, Burke and colleagues, in a series of publications (see Burke et al., 2006; Burke et al., 2011; Burke, Scheuer, &

Meredith, 2007), have discussed how the method or means of safety training delivery can be considered along an engagement continuum. Here, engagement refers to characteristics of the training method and, more specifically, the degree to which training incorporates or promotes action (such as role-playing or practice), dialogue (i.e., intra- and interpersonal dialogue, and with respect to actions taken or considered) and reflection (i.e., thinking about contradictions, dilemmas, and possibilities). The implication of a dialogical-based experiential approach for the acquisition of safety-related knowledge and skills and the notion of an engagement continuum is that learning methods that are more engaging (in the sense of incorporating elements of action, dialogue, and reflection) will enhance knowledge acquisition relative to lesser engaging means of knowledge development. Arguably, more engaging methods of learning force trainees to infer causal and conditional relations between actions and events. In this regard, more engaging safety training methods can alter trainees' ways of thinking and acting, particularly in unique or unforeseen situations. In effect, more engaging forms of learning are expected to not only improve knowledge acquisition and its transfer to the job, but also to the development of anticipatory thinking for avoiding accidents and unwanted exposures in all types of safety work.

While traditional methods of safety training such as lecture or some forms of computer-based training may be categorized as lower in engagements, this discussion indicates that they need not necessarily be low in engagement characteristics. That is, trainers can consider how different forms of action, dialogue, and reflection can be incorporated into all means of safety training to improve the level of engagement of the training method. Future research on the role of dialogue and reflection, especially within traditionally lesser engaging training methods, has considerable potential for advancing our understanding of how to optimally develop safety knowledge and safety motivation. As pointed out within the broader educational literature, the form, structure, and instructional activities would likely be somewhat specific to the nature of the safety training intervention, the level of skill being acquired, and the size of the training group (Frederiksen, 1999; Gorsky, Caspi, & Trumper, 2006).

Finally, we note that safety training can be targeted at an individual, group, work unit, or team. The methods discussed above may be employed for group training, alone or in conjunction, such as classroom training that includes videos and role-plays (e.g., Rabol et al., 2012). When deciding whether to train individuals or groups, one needs to consider the nature of the work and the organizational role of the trainee. Training can be administered in groups (particularly with classroom training) even if the employees themselves do not work together as a team (i.e., no common goal or interdependence). For example, Lee et al. (2012) implemented a program to increase safety through better communication, where training was given to groups of hospital workers across departments and functions.

Alternatively, when safety training is targeted at a work unit (e.g., a department or business unit), the aim is to improve the safe working behavior of all unit members or to improve overall health and safety within the work unit. While all workers in the unit can participate in the intervention (e.g., see Komaki, Collins, & Penn, 1982), in many cases the work unit manager or operator takes part in the training, and is then expected to disseminate the information or lead by example. The effectiveness of the training is evaluated relative to overall safety and health improvements in the work unit, not just in changes in the leader's knowledge or behavior. For instance, farm operators have participated in agricultural safety interventions with the aim of improving the overall safety of farm operations and health of farm workers (e.g., Landsittel, Murphy, Kiernan, Hard, & Kassab, 2001). As several other examples, Cotterchio, Gunn, Coffill, Tormey, and Barry (1998) evaluated a restaurant manager training program on the overall safety and health of restaurant operations; Bush et al. (2009) conducted workshops for restaurant and food service owners/managers to teach them to provide health and safety training to their employees; Smith, Anger, and Uslan (1978) studied the efficacy of a first-line shipyard supervisor safety training intervention on the accident rates of shipfitter crews that they supervised; Kaskutas et al. (2013) trained construction foremen in the hope that falls and fall hazards would decrease at worksites; and Pedersen et al. (2010) tested an intervention to encourage safety feedback to construction managers in the hope of improving overall safety.

At times, it may be beneficial to train a team as a whole. If intact teams are to be trained, then several issues need to be considered. As Kozlowski, Brown, Weissbein, Cannon-Bowers, and Salas (2000) discuss, when compilation processes are involved (that is, when higher-level variables like performance are a result of related but different lower-level processes rather than being isomorphic across levels) training team members together is necessary for the best outcomes. In short, when competencies such as cooperation, coordination, communication, and possibly adaptation are important for the workers to accomplish their work, then team training may be necessary (Gregory, Feitosa, Driskell, Salas, & Vessey, 2013). Training can help teams develop mental models and build tacit knowledge so that team members can work more effectively and more safely. In addition, team adaptive training has been shown to be beneficial in general, perhaps especially under instances of high stress (Entin & Serfaty, 1999). This may be helpful for safety training as well, particularly under high hazard or crisis conditions (and thus, high stress).

Team safety training has been implemented in a variety of settings. For example, in the oil and gas industry, action teams have been trained in team tactical decision games to aid in team decision-making and communication to help improve safety (Crichton, 2009). Air traffic controllers have also been trained in dyadic teams to improve coordination, communication, and error management (Malakis & Kontogiannis, 2012). Crew resource management (CRM) training has been used for decades in the aviation industry to reduce error and accidents and seems to be effective, but most evaluations of this type of training have been done using simulations, so transfer to real settings needs more research (Salas, Burke, Bowers, & Wilson, 2001; Salas & Cannon-Bowers, 2001). Group and team training has also been used to improve competencies in numerous other types of safety-related work such as healthcare (Lee et al., 2012; Rabol et al., 2012), military operations (Entin & Serfaty, 1999), and manufacturing (Lazovich et al., 2002). Finally, we note that a fair amount of highly engaging training involves individual instruction that is coupled with some form of workgroup or dyadic/team training activity.

Relationships between Safety Training Interventions and Safety-relevant Criteria

Over the last 30 years, a considerable body of literature has developed on experimental and quasi-experimental effects associated with safety training interventions. These studies have been reported with respect to a wide variety of occupational samples (e.g., coal miners, drivers, firefighters, and nurses) and industries (e.g., health care, agriculture, manufacturing and construction industries), and within various fields of inquiry (e.g., occupational medicine, industrial hygiene, management, and applied psychology). Across occupations and industries, the type of knowledge being acquired is often associated with the training method. That is, as one moves from training programs aimed at workers' acquisition of fundamental knowledge to more advanced skills such as problem solving and decision-making skills, the method of safety training tends to become more engaging. Furthermore, irrespective of occupation or industry, these evaluation studies have focused on workers' knowledge acquisition and exhibition of safe work behavior as dependent variables, and to a lesser extent on reductions in more distal outcomes such as accidents and injuries. Given these points, the following discussion will emphasize training method-training outcome relationships for lesser engaging training methods versus more highly engaging training methods and with respect to broad dependent variable categories of safety knowledge, safety performance, and safety and health outcomes.

We note that dependent variable measures vary within our broad dependent variable categories. For instance, safety knowledge acquisition is typically measured via a self-rating or test of knowledge; safety performance is measured with respect to self, supervisory, coworker, or observer ratings of a worker or workgroup's safety behavior; and safety and health outcomes are often based on different types of information relative to accidents, near misses, injuries, and illnesses. Although the measures and their reliability differ within dependent variable categories, study effects (in many cases) have been converted to standardized effects (i.e., d-statistics) within various meta-analyses and systematic reviews. As a result, our discussion below takes this cumulative literature into account and discusses findings relative to standardized effects and broad dependent variable categories. Also, since Burke et al.'s (2006) meta-analysis of safety training found minimal differences in results for within-subjects vs. between-subjects designs, we do not emphasize this study design distinction for the purposes of our review below.

Safety knowledge as the dependent variable

A relatively large number of safety training evaluation studies would be characterized as having employed a lesser engaging means of training and examined knowledge as a dependent variable. A common form of instruction is a lecture and discussion that may include some takeaway such as a booklet, brochure, or pamphlet (Finch & Daniel, 2005; Girgis et al., 1994; Harrington & Walker, 2002; Kowalski-Trakofler & Barrett, 2003; Martyny, Buchan, Keefe, & Blehm, 1988; Peterson, McGlothlin, & Blue, 2004; Porru et al., 1993; Seto, Ching, Chu, & Fielding, 1990; Symes, Graveling, & Campbell, 1992). Another common type of lesser engaging training is a lecture and discussion accompanied with some form of video presentation (e.g., Arcury, Quandt, Austin, Preisser, & Cabrera, 1999; Barnett et al., 1984; Bosco & Wagner, 1988; Brnich, Derick, Mallett, & Vaught, 2002; Ewigman, Kivlahan, Hosokawa, & Horman, 1990; Lynch et al., 1990; Uwakwe, 2000; Yarrall, 1986). Notably, the vast majority of evaluation studies aimed at workers' knowledge acquisition via lesser engaging training methods are concerned with workers' potential exposure to harmful substances or environments.

In regard to highly engaging means of training directed at workers' knowledge acquisition, a common method is to conduct a lecture and discussion followed by role-playing/behavioral modeling and feedback, simulation training, practice or some form of hands-on experience (Albers et al., 1997; Carlton, 1987; Cohen & Jensen, 1984; Curwick, Reeb-Whitaker, & Connon, 2003; Daltroy et al., 1993; Eckerman et al., 2004; Huang et al., 2002; Lueveswanij, Nittayananta, & Robison, 2000; Luskin et al., 1992; Lynch & Freund, 2000; Rundio, 1994). The latter training frequently concerns hazards related to bodily reaction and exertion or exposure to harmful substances and environments, and to a lesser extent dealing with assaults and violent acts (e.g., Coutts, Graham, Braun, & Wells, 2000; Hurlebaus & Link, 1997) or operating machinery and equipment to avoid accidents (e.g., Cohen & Jensen, 1984).

While there is meaningful variation in standardized effects across training evaluation studies, highly engaging forms of training are often considerably more effective than lesser engaging methods of training with respect to knowledge acquisition (Burke et al., 2011). On average, the effects associated with highly engaging training are approximately

70 percent greater than the effects for lesser engaging methods. This percentage difference is based on respective average standardized effects for lesser and highly engaging training methods (for safety knowledge as the dependent variable) of approximately .35 and .60 reported within Burke et al. (2011), respectively. These findings are consistent with results from meta-analyses in other domains where the relative effectiveness of less versus more active forms of learning on knowledge acquisition have been examined (e.g., Taylor, Russ-Eft, & Chan, 2005).

Safety performance as the dependent variable

Likewise, when safety performance is the dependent variable, the majority of safety training evaluation studies have involved lesser engaging training methods. Lecture and discussion is a common training method in such evaluation studies (Azizi et al., 2000; Dortch & Trombly, 1990; Froom, Kristal-Boneh, Melamed, Shalom, & Ribak, 1998; Inman & Blanciforti, 2002; Kerrigan et al., 2006; Leslie & Adams, 1973; Ma et al., 2002; Mayer et al., 2007; Parkinson et al., 1989; Rasmussen et al., 2003; Sadler & Montgomery, 1982). In addition, many of these interventions have concerned applications of reinforcement or feedback theories aimed at modifying the exhibition of safe work behavior (Alavosius & Sulzer-Azaroff, 1986; Al-Hemoud & Al-Asfoor, 2006; Askari & Mehring, 1992; Chan & Ng, 2010; Chhokar & Wallin, 1984; Fox & Sulzer-Azaroff, 1987; Greene, DeJoy, & Olejnik, 2005; Johnsson, Carlosson, & Lagerstrom, 2002; Komaki, Heinzmann, & Lawson, 1980; Ludwig & Geller, 1997; Marsh & Kendrick, 1998; Mattila, 1990; Mattila & Hyodynmaa, 1988; Patros, 2001; Perry & Layde, 2003; Ray, Bishop, & Wang, 1997; Reber, Wallin, & Chhokar, 1984; Saari & Nasanen, 1989; Stephens & Ludwig, 2005; Whitby, Stead, & Najman, 1991; Williams & Geller, 2000; Wong et al., 1991; Yarrall, 1986). Together, the lesser engaging training methods aimed at modifying safe work behavior have concerned the full range of potentially hazardous events and exposures that workers may encounter.

Highly engaging training methods directed at modifying workers' safety performance are often similar to those focused on knowledge acquisition with heavy emphasis on behavioral modeling, simulation training, practice, or some form of hands-on experience. A fair amount of this training evaluation work has involved workers in a variety of occupations such as floor layers (Jensen & Friche, 2007), groundskeepers and custodians (Hultman, Nordin, & Ortengren, 1984; McCauley, 1990), health professionals (Yassi et al., 2001), and office workers (Nieuwenhuijsen, 2004), whose work may lead to injury associated with bodily reaction and exertion. In addition, highly engaging training methods are commonly employed for training workers who face potential exposure to harmful substances or environments such as direct care workers for clients with mental disabilities (Baker, 1998), coal miners (Cole et al., 1988), community health workers (Forst et al., 2004), wetwork employees (Held et al., 2002), agricultural workers (Knobloch & Broste, 1998), and professional and technical employees (Vaught, Brinch, & Kellner, 1988).

Highly engaging forms of safety training are, on average, more effective than lesser engaging methods of training with respect to improving safety performance (Burke et al., 2011). More specifically, the average standardized effects for lesser and highly engaging training methods (for safety performance as the dependent variable) were reported in Burke et al. (2011) as approximately .20 and .40, respectively. This pattern of effects is also evident in studies where training is delivered to the work unit as a whole or the owner/manager of the business unit. The majority of the work unit training has been more engaging, often involving some form of practice, and produced moderate effect size changes in the safe work behavior of employees within restaurants (Bush et al., 2009; Cotterchio et al., 1998), construction workers within residential building companies (Kaskutas et al., 2013), employees within food processing departments (Komaki et al., 1982), and healthcare workers within hospital units (Lee et al., 2012).

Recent primary studies have yielded moderate to large effects for more engaging simulation-based training methods or training conducted over multiple sessions (e.g., Taylor & Alvero, 2012; Yao et al., 2013). While the overall, average effects for more engaging training have been meaningful, there has been notable variation in training effects suggesting the presence of moderators. We will return to a discussion of possible moderator variables below. Nevertheless, the overall findings are consistent with results from primary and meta-analytic studies in other domains where the relative effectiveness of less versus more active forms of learning on performance have been examined (e.g., Bell & Kozlowski, 2008; Taylor et al., 2005).

In addition to meta-analytic research examining safety training–safety performance relationships, several systematic reviews of safety interventions have been conducted over the last 20 years (Cohen & Colligan, 1998; Robson et al., 2010, 2012; Tompa, Dolinschi, Oliverira, & Irvin, 2009). While the Tompa et al. (2009) review focused on ergonomic equipment and control interventions where safety training was a component of the overall intervention (e.g., see Collins, Wolf, Bell, & Evanoff, 2004; Rempel et al., 2006), the Robson et al. (2010) qualitative review directly evaluated the impact of safety training engagement on safety performance. Notably, Robson et al.'s systematic review culled only 14 studies for their final analyses (Banco, Lapidus, Monopoli, & Zavoski, 1997; Brisson, Montreuil, & Punnett, 1999; Eklöf & Hagberg, 2006; Greene et al., 2005; Harrington & Walker, 2004; Held et al., 2002; Hickman & Geller, 2003; Hong, Ronis, Lusk, & Kee, 2006; Loffler, Bruckner, Diepen, & Effendy, 2006; Perry & Layde, 2003; Rasmussen et al., 2003; Wang, Fennie, He, Burgess, & Williams, 2003; Wright, Turner, & Daffin, 1997). These studies represented experimental studies that were judged by the authors to have adequate controls for making causal inferences. As with the Burke et al. (2006) meta-analysis, Robson et al. (2010) found minimal differences between lesser and highly engaging training methods in terms of their impact on safety-related behaviors. As such, Robson et al. (2010) concluded that there was insufficient evidence with respect to observed effects (i.e., effects that were uncorrected for dependent variable reliability) of single-session high engagement training as having a greater effect on safety-related behaviors compared with low/medium engagement training for a single session.

The difference between the Burke et al. (2011) meta-analysis, which found a meaningful overall effect of training method engagement on safety performance as discussed above, and the other reviews is likely due to several reasons. First, in contrast to Burke et al. (2006), the Burke et al. (2011) study had a markedly higher number of studies and effects included in their analyses (i.e., 91 versus 67 effects), which led to more robust findings. On the other hand, the differences between Robson et al.'s qualitative findings and the meta-analytic results reported in Burke et al.'s (2011) are likely due to Robson et al.'s (2010) selective study inclusion criteria (e.g., safety training studies published subsequent to Cohen and Colligan's 1998 review) and several somewhat arbitrary primary study exclusion criteria (e.g., excluding studies with nonrandom assignment due to time constraints on the review team). These criteria led to a very small sample of studies to integrate. In short, and in contrast to the more comprehensive review by Burke et al. (2011), the Burke et al. (2006) and Robson et al. (2010) reviews were subject to greater second-order sampling of studies and lower statistical power for detecting experimental effects.

Safety and health outcomes as dependent variables

Relative to other types of dependent variables, comparably fewer studies have evaluated safety training with respect to health and safety outcomes (e.g., Daltroy et al., 1993; Evanoff et al.,1999; Feldstein, Valanis, Vollmer, Stevens, & Overton, 1993; Haiduven, DeMaio, & Stevens, 1992; Infantino & Musingo, 1985; Maples, Jacoby, Johnson, Ter Haar, & Buckingham, 1982; Melhorn, 1996; Parenmark, Engvall, & Malmkvist, 1988; Reddell, Congleton, Huchingson, & Montgomery, 1992; Rhoton, 1980; Saarela, Saari, & Alltonen, 1989; Schwartz, 1989; Sulzer-Azaroff & de Santamaria, 1980; van Poppel, Koes, van der Ploeg, Smid, & Bouter, 1998; Wang et al., 2003). These and other studies were cumulatively integrated by Burke et al. (2006) in regard to least, moderate, and highly engaging training methods. Whereas other meta-analyses and systematic reviews have categorized computer-based instruction and feedback techniques within a lesser engaging training methods category, the Burke et al. (2006) meta-analysis considered these methods within a separate (i.e., moderately engaging) category. For their meta-analysis, effects associated with highly engaging training methods were, on average, greater than the moderately engaging training methods in regard to reducing negative health and safety outcomes.

A closer examination of the Burke et al. (2006) findings indicates that moderate and highly engaging training methods had somewhat comparable effects when studies were broken down by between-subjects and within-subjects designs, and when a moderately engaging training study with a very large sample size was taken into account. For instance, studies with within-subjects designs had respective standardized effects for moderate and highly engaging training methods of –.32 and –.34. The standardized effects were lower for between-subjects designs. Notably, very few safety training evaluation studies have employed a lesser engaging training method with just lecture and discussion when evaluating training relative to health and safety outcomes (e.g., Carrabba, Field, Tormoehlen, & Talbert, 2000).

More recent studies provide similar evidence for the relative effectiveness of safety training methods with respect to the reduction of negative health and safety outcomes. For instance, Mujuru, Helmkamp, Mutambuzdi, Hu, and Bell (2009) found small decrements, over an eight-year period, in logging workers' injury claims, which were emphasized in a low engagement video-based safety training intervention. On the other hand, more engaging, multi-session educational interventions have produced moderate to large effects with respect to the reduction of a variety of occupational injuries for construction workers (Bena et al., 2009) and needlestick injuries for nursing students (Yao et al., 2013). This pattern in findings for training engagement in relation to safety and health outcomes is also evident in studies where training is delivered to the work unit as a whole or the owner/manager of the business unit (e.g., Lansittel et al., 2001; Lazovich et al., 2002). Consistent with meta-analytic findings, variation in primary study effects is evident with respect to training engagement. For example, Gettle (2009) found a moderate effect associated with a relatively low engagement, one-hour training session for manufacturing workers; whereas Yu et al. (2013) found a very small effect for a more engaging, participatory training program aimed at reducing musculoskeletal disorders.

Finally, although not addressing safety and health outcomes per se, a meta-analysis by Salas et al. (2008) found that team training can have a positive effect on team cognitive and performance outcomes. Training intact teams seems to have particular impact on performance outcomes, and large teams may also benefit the most from training in terms of performance outcomes, though affective, process, and cognitive outcomes may be more improved in teams of small or medium size.

Safety motivation as a dependent variable

Safety motivation is a theoretically important variable, being posited and studied as a direct antecedent to safety performance (Christian et al., 2009; Griffin & Neal, 2000) and a mediator of the relationship between safety training and safety performance (Vinodkumar & Bhasi, 2010). Several studies (Burke et al., 2011; Weinstein, 2000) indicate that how training stresses the severity and likelihood of dangerous events or hazard exposures may affect subsequent motivation to engage in safe work behavior. In addition, a number of motivational theories would lead to the conclusion that feedback during and subsequent to training may have an important impact on the safety motivation and the maintenance of safe work behavior. As discussed above (also see Sulzer-Azaroff & Austin, 2000), a number of studies have found feedback interventions to be moderately effective with respect to improving the exhibition of safe work behavior.

As a training outcome itself, safety motivation is infrequently studied. In many cases, changes in attitudes and behavioral intentions are evaluated (e.g., Harrington & Walker, 2002, 2004; Mayer et al., 2013), with the implication that such assessments reflect the motivation to engage in safety work behavior. While these studies indicate that safety training can have relatively large effects on changes in attitudes and behavioral intentions, the measurement of attitudes as dependent variables arguably does not provide information on changes in motivation associated with safety training. A notable exception is Greene et al.'s (2005) evaluation of a computer-based ergonomics training program where changes in employees' self-efficacy beliefs and outcome expectations were assessed within a randomized control study. Greene et al. found sizeable increases in self-efficacy beliefs for engaging in particular work practices to reduce musculoskeletal disorders.

Greene et al.'s (2005) training study and other non-training studies (e.g., Neal et al., 2000; Vindokumar & Bhasi, 2010) demonstrate how safety motivation can be measured quantitatively. In addition, other efforts provide sound examples for how safety motivation can be measured qualitatively such as through conducting and coding interviews (Lingard, 2002). Recently, Pedersen and Kines (2011) developed brief scales to measure different components of safety motivation, and found that normative safety motivation (i.e., what is expected) has the largest relationship with safety compliance in comparison to social and calculative aspects of safety motivation. This measurement development effort could be improved upon in regard to the expansion of item pools to produce longer scales with adequate psychometric properties. Progress in this area would be helpful for future research studying the direct effect of safety training on safety motivation or the role of safety motivation within causal models of workplace safety.

Moderators of relationships between safety training, safety performance, and safety-related outcomes

A longstanding argument in the applied psychology literature is that organizational or workgroup environments that are more restrictive in nature (e.g., more centralized and less supportive of employees) are likely to attenuate relationships between individual difference variables (e.g., see James, Demaree, Mulaik, & Ladd, 1992). The primary reason for this occurrence is that more restrictive or less positive work environments are expected to substantively restrict variability in individual differences possibly by inhibiting the display of acquired knowledge and skill, resulting in lower relationships between individual difference variables in more vs. less restrictive environments.

In the realm of workplace safety, Smith-Crowe, Burke, and Landis (2003) adopted this general argument as a basis for suggesting why business-unit safety climate would be expected to moderate the relationship between safety knowledge (acquired via training) and safety performance. Smith-Crowe et al. found evidence for a stronger relationship between safety training and safety performance in a less restrictive, more positive safety climate. In a related manner, Brahm and Singer (2013) found that, for panel data from 2,787 Chilean firms, an organization's occupational safety and health capabilities and commitment may attenuate or lower the relative effectiveness of more (in comparison to lesser) engaging safety training methods.

Other studies have provided similar support for the expected moderating role of safety climate on safety training–outcome relationships. For instance, Jiang, Yu, Li, and Li (2010), in a study of 23 work units within two petroleum and chemical companies, found that work unit safety climate moderated the relationship between workers' self-reports of safety skills and safety performance, with stronger relationships in more positive safety climates. Likewise, Burke et al. (2008), using data from 68 organizations, found that organizational safety climate moderated not only the relationship between safety training and safety performance, but it also moderated the relationship between safety training and safety outcomes. For the latter relationship, more positive safety climates were associated with a stronger relationship between training and the reduction of accidents and injuries.

DeJoy (1996) suggested that safety climate might interact with structural characteristics of work environments to affect health and safety outcomes. In particular, DeJoy argued that a more positive safety climate serves to augment the effect of workplace factors that are conducive to safe work behavior. In a test of this expectation with 280 nursing units in 143 hospitals, Mark et al. (2007) found that safety climate moderated the relationship between an aggregated (to the nursing unit level) measure that focused on workgroup expertise (labeled work engagement) and needlestick injuries. At higher levels of safety climate, higher levels of work engagement were associated with fewer needlestick injuries. Together, research demonstrating the moderating role of safety climate on relationships between safety training and safety criteria are consistent with a substantial body of literature supporting the importance of safety climate as a key situational moderator of individual difference relationships as well as relationships between organizational-level variables (e.g., Katz-Navon, Naveh, & Stern, 2005; Probst, 2004; Probst & Estrada, 2010; Sinclair, Martin, & Sears, 2010).

Another set of potential moderator variables concerns culture. For example, Burke et al. (2008) found that the cultural dimension of uncertainty avoidance, the extent to which members of a culture attempt to avoid uncertain or ambiguous situations (Hofstede, 1991), moderated the relationship between safety training and the reduction in accidents and injuries. More specifically, their results indicated that as uncertainty avoidance, or the tendency to ensure predictability, increases, the relationship between safety training and the reduction of negative safety outcomes decreases. The authors suggested that this finding may be due to the tendency of organizations in high uncertainty avoidant cultures training workers with respect to standardized, less engaging training methods, which could lessen workers' ability to adaptively respond to critical safety situations.

Uncertainty avoidance is not the only important cultural dimension when it comes to safety training. Qualitative research by Carruth et al. (2010) indicated that Vietnamese culture affected shrimp fishermen's preferred types of safety training, including that captains should be trained first, a certificate of completion was important, training should be hands-on, and training should be conducted in the primary language of the trainees. Research has also indicated that indigenous (American) workers may have different preferences for information dissemination than Latino immigrant workers and that immigrant workers may not benefit from the same training that helps native workers, due to language, educational, and cultural differences (Arcury, Estrada, & Quandt, 2010; Samples et al., 2009).

Finally, we note that the potential severity of a hazardous event/exposure may interact with the nature of safety training to affect worker motivation and, thus, the relative effectiveness of different types of safety training (Burke et al., 2011). When event/exposure severity is high (e.g., needlestick injuries resulting in infections such as HIV), higher levels of training engagement are associated with improved safety work behavior; but when severity is low (e.g., repetitive-motion injuries), training that is more or less engaging was equally effective with respect to safety performance. Clearly, more primary research is needed to directly evaluate the expected interaction of training engagement and workplace hazard severity on safe work behavior where multiple hazards are being considered within a study. Nevertheless, the overall meta-analytic finding concerning the interaction of training engagement and hazard severity has important implications for organizations implementing training interventions, as highly engaging programs may be more costly than less engaging ones, and whether that cost is justified may depend on the nature of the hazards employees will be exposed to.

Future Research

Our above review summarized the state of knowledge concerning the relative effectiveness of safety training interventions and identified areas of needed research. In this section, we highlight additional questions concerning the role of demographic and cultural variables in the conduct and transfer of safety training, questions regarding the role of technology and web-based safety training, research directions for enhancing our understanding of the economic implications of safety training, and questions concerning the decay in safety training effects.

Questions concerning the role of racial/ethnic and language variables in the conduct of safety training

In both developing and developed economies, different racial/ethnic groups or socioeconomic groups are at times disproportionately exposed to potentially hazardous work events and environments. Within the USA, higher cancer rates for African-American men relative to White-American men have been, in part, attributed to differential exposures to hazardous occupational conditions (Briggs et al., 2003). In addition, in comparison to other racial groups, Hispanic workers in particular regions within the USA experience high occupational injury rates and lost work days due to illness and injury (Forst et al., 2013; Richardson, Loomis, Bena, & Bailer, 2009; Strong & Zimmerman, 2005). These figures signal a need to develop safety training programs and training evaluation studies that take into account the background of workers along with information on workplace hazards to enhance workers' motivation to learn how to avoid hazardous events and exposures, especially with respect to hazards that may appear to be benign to the untrained worker (e.g., toxic black mold or sawdust).

Language barriers are also an important issue. Failure to speak fluently can affect the transfer of safety training as workers may not understand the material and may not be able to properly ask questions to gain clarification. In instances where workers speak different languages and need to address a common safety issue, translated training materials may need to be developed. For example, during the Deepwater Horizon/Gulf Oil Spill clean-up effort, training booklets were translated into English, Spanish, and Vietnamese (National Institute of Environmental Health Sciences, 2010). Obviously such translation requires an additional expense and duplication of materials, but such efforts may be necessary if the workers cannot understand the primary language. In some cases, workers' literacy skills may be deficient, calling for both alternative means to communicate health and safety information to such workers and to evaluate the efficacy of safety training (e.g., see Leprevost, Storm, Blanchard, Asuaje, & Cope, 2013).

Questions regarding the use of technology and online safety training

In recent years, computer-based and online safety training has become more prevalent as technology has improved and such methods have become more affordable. While these forms of safety training can be helpful in training relatively large numbers of individuals in a self-paced manner and with respect to multiple languages (e.g., Calandra & Harmon, 2012), questions remain as to how to design such programs to enhance trainees' cognitive and affective engagement (Cherrett et al., 2009; Ho & Dzeng, 2010). In addition, issues related to workers' background characteristics such as the degree of formal education, computer experience, and learning styles are salient, with relatively little research on such individual differences in the domain of worker safety training (Anger et al., 2006; Arcury et al., 2010). Finally, we would note that while computer-based and web-based safety training may not necessarily be more effective in comparison to more traditional in-class forms of instruction, considerable labor cost benefits may be realized from such training and more assessments of this nature would be helpful (e.g., Cerecero & Charlton, 2012).

Also, virtual reality training has been successfully used in safety-related work, particularly within military and pilot operations, and is gaining traction in terms of training workers to deal with workplace hazards and hazardous circumstances (Orr et al., 2009; Zhao & Lucas, 2014). Research focused on promoting trainee engagement is needed in this domain as are studies that directly compare virtual reality training with more traditional instructional methods. We raise these points as virtual reality technology is continuously improving, with advancements like the Oculus Rift, a small, immersive headset that was developed for gaming but has implications for training as well (e.g., Reiners et al., 2014). In addition, while in situ simulations have been successfully employed for team training within medical settings (see Kobayashi et al., 2012), we know little about the applicability and efficacy of such training for workgroups and teams in the broader domain of workplace safety. This point would also hold for other means of in situ training such as staff rides, which have been proposed as a means for recreating critical incidents for workers to learn about and how to handle in extremis, life-threatening events (Becker & Burke, 2014).

Questions pertaining to the economic implications of safety training

While Tompa et al.'s (2009) systematic review, as noted above, provided useful information concerning the financial implications of safety interventions within several industry sectors (e.g., healthcare, manufacturing, and warehousing), their review identified a number of deficiencies in the evaluation studies. First, safety training evaluations or effectiveness assessments were often disconnected from the economic analyses in that factors such as the study design and unit of analysis differed between the two. In addition, studies commonly failed to consider the time value of money, adjust monetary values from different time periods for inflation, or assess the robustness of results to the assumptions that were made such as through a sensitivity analysis.

Notably, decision theoretic utility analysis procedures developed within the applied psychology and management fields can assist in addressing most of the deficiencies noted within Tompa et al.'s (2009) review. In particular, decision-theoretic utility analysis procedures (see Cascio, 2000, for a review) provide a straightforward means for integrating the evaluation of safety training with the estimate of economic utility, and at the same time they allow for adjusting utility estimates to reflect the time value of money. For instance, Morrow, Jarrett, and Rupinski (1997) illustrate how decision-theoretic utility analysis procedures can be used to estimate the economic implications of safety training. Importantly, decision-theoretic utility analysis procedures can be effectively applied to situations where the work group or unit is the focus of the safety training intervention, where organizationally relevant metrics other than dollars are of interest (e.g., injuries, lives saved), and where one is interested in estimating the net incremental benefit as opposed to just the cost savings associated with safety training. Future studies directed at the application of decision-theoretic utility analysis procedures to safety training and particularly at the workgroup, team, and work unit levels of analysis to estimate the net incremental benefits of safety training would be informative.

Questions related to the decay in safety training effects

A main question in the safety training literature that remains to be answered is how long the benefits of training interventions can be expected to last. There have been some longitudinal studies in this domain, but questions pertaining to whether the type of training impedes decay, how often "refresher" training needs to be implemented, and whether the severity or frequency of the hazards faced plays a role in retention remain unanswered. For instance, a review of safety training of commercial fishermen indicated that such training appears to be efficacious in preventing deaths, but that there is significant training decay after only a month and that skills deteriorated even further after a few years (Dzugan, 2010). This review also revealed that even trained fishermen were unlikely to run safety drills that might help them better retain their training.

Studies that do measure the impact of training interventions over time often have employed somewhat short, 30–60 day, post-intervention follow-up periods (e.g., Lynch & Freund, 2000), leaving questions about long-term efficacy of safety training. We would like to encourage more studies with methods similar to Porru et al. (1993), who studied the effects of safety and health training on lead-exposed workers after four months and again after one year. The authors measured actual lead levels in the blood, not just safety knowledge, and found that a one-hour lecture-based training program (with a booklet of illustrations) was still having a positive effect (that is, decreased lead levels in the blood were maintained) after one year.

Turning to refresher training, in a study of medical flight crews, Wynn and Black (1998) found that a refresher course greatly improved (32 percent increase) safety knowledge from a baseline (1–1.5 years after prior training), but six months later, mean knowledge levels had dropped to just 5 percent above pre-refresher-training levels. Nevertheless, research in education indicates that refresher training may be integral in aiding retention; an issue in Wynn and Black's (1998) study may have been that the refresher training occurred too long after the initial training period. Pashler, Rohrer, and Cepeda (2006) recommend that the optimal spacing be 10–20 percent of the retention interval, though benefits seemed to increase with longer spacing between training sessions. This finding still leaves open some questions about what spacing should be like when the desired retention period is the length of a person's career in an occupation, not just a year or two, and the authors did note that the spacing does not work within all learning domains (e.g., visuospatial skills).

Together, the above studies and findings indicate that much still remains to be learned about the maintenance/decay of knowledge subsequent to safety training and the means for how to enhance knowledge retention. Clearly, more in the way of longitudinal studies with multiple criterion measures and adequate control groups would add to our understanding of the long-term effects of safety training.

Conclusion

In this chapter, we critically reviewed research on workplace safety training from a variety of disciplines and fields within business, engineering, psychology, public health, and medicine. Our discussion highlighted what is known about safety training with respect to a *worker characteristic–work criteria–work context* framework and where future safety training research might be directed to advance our understanding of relationships within such a framework. Importantly, our discussion emphasized the role of training engagement, in regard to the extent that a training method promotes dialogue, action, and reflection, as a key driver of the relative effectiveness of safety training with respect to knowledge acquisition, demonstration of safe work behavior, and the reduction in negative safety and health outcomes. Furthermore, our review stressed the importance of safety climate, cultural values and variables, and workplace hazards as key situational moderators of safety training effects, and the types of research that are needed to expand our understanding of the role of work context factors in the transfer to-the-job of safety training. While our review points to the fact that safety training can have meaningful behavioral, health, and economic impacts, our discussion also signals that much work can be done to improve our conceptualization and measurement of constructs within a *worker characteristic–work criteria–work context* framework to study safety training at individual, workgroup, and business unit levels of analysis.

References

Alavosius, M. P., & Sulzer-Azaroff, B. (1986). The effects of performance feedback on the safety of client lifting and transfer. *Journal of Applied Behavior Analysis, 19*, 261–267. doi:10.1901/jaba.1986.19-261

Albers, J. T., Li, Y., Lemasters, G., Sprague, S., Stinson, R., & Bhattacharya, A. (1997). An ergonomic education and evaluation program for apprentice carpenters. *American Journal of Industrial Medicine, 32*, 641–647. doi:10.1002/(SICI)1097-0274(199712)32:6<641::AID-AJIM10>3.0.CO;2-1

Al-Hemoud, A. M., & Al-Asfoor, M. M. (2006). A behavior based safety approach at a Kuwait research institution. *Journal of Safety Research, 37*, 201–206. doi:10.1016/j.jsr.2005.11.006

Anger, K. W., Stupfel, J., Ammerman, T., Tamulinas, A., Bodner, T., & Rohlman, D. (2006). The suitability of computer-based training for workers with limited formal education: A case study from the U.S. agricultural sector. *International Journal of Training and Development, 10*, 269–284. doi:10.1111/j.1468-2419.2006.00260.x

Anderson, J., Collins, M., Devlin, J., & Renner, P. (2012). Using hazard maps to identify and eliminate workplace hazards: A union-led health and safety training program. *New Solutions: A Journal of Environmental and Occupational Health Policy, 22*(3), 325–342.

Arcury, T. A., Estrada, J. M., & Quandt, S. A. (2010). Overcoming language and literacy barriers in safety and health training of agricultural workers. *Journal of Agromedicine, 15*(3), 236–248.

Arcury, T. A., Quandt, S. A., Austin, C. K., Preisser, J., & Cabrera, L. F. (1999). Implementation of EPA's Worker Protection Standard training for agricultural laborers: An evaluation using North Carolina data. *Public Health Reports, 114*, 459–468. doi:10.1093/phr/114.5.459

Askari, E., & Mehring, J. (1992). Human immunodeficiency virus/acquired immunodeficiency syndrome training from a union perspective. *American Journal of Industrial Medicine, 22,* 711–720. doi:10.1002/ajim.4700220509

Azizi, E., Flint, P., Sadetzki, S., Solomon, A., Lerman, Y., Harari, G., & Rosenberg, L. (2000). A graded work site intervention program to improve sun protection and skin cancer awareness in outdoor workers in Israel. *Cancer Causes and Control, 11,* 513–521. doi:10.1023/A:1008970224998

Baker, D. J. (1998). Effects of video-based staff training with manager led exercises in residential support. *Mental Retardation, 36,* 198–204. doi:10.1352/0047-6765(1998)036<0198:EOVSTW>2.0.CO;2

Banco, L., Lapidus, G., Monopoli, J., & Zavoski, R. (1997). The safe teen work project: A study to reduce cutting injuries among young and inexperienced workers. *American Journal of Industrial Medicine, 31*(5), 619–622.

Barnett, P. G., Midtling, J. E., Velasco, A. R., Romero, P., O'Malley, M., Clements, C., & Barbaccia, J. C. (1984). Educational intervention to prevent pesticide-induced illness of field workers. *Journal of Family Practice, 19*(1), 123–125.

Becker, W. S., & Burke, M. J. (2012). The staff ride: An approach to qualitative data generation and analysis. *Organizational Research Methods, 15,* 316–335.

Becker, W., & Burke, M. J. (2014). Instructional staff rides for management learning and education. *Academy of Management Learning & Education, 13*(4), 510–524.

Bell, B. S., & Kozlowski, S. W. J. (2008). Active learning: Effects of core training design elements on self-regulatory processes, learning, and adaptability. *Journal of Applied Psychology, 93,* 296–316. doi:10.1037/0021-9010.93.2.296

Bena, A., Berchialla, P., Coffano, M. E., Debernardi, M. L., & Icardi, L. G. (2009). Effectiveness of the training program for workers at construction sites of the high-speed railway line between Torino and Novara: Impact on injury rates. *American Journal of Industrial Medicine, 52*(12), 965–972.

Benning, A., Dixon-Woods, M., Nwulu, U., Ghaleb, M., Dawson, J., Barber, N., ..., & Lilford, R. (2011). Multiple component patient safety intervention in English hospitals: Controlled evaluation of second phase. *British Medical Journal, 342,* 1–16: d199. doi:10.1136/bmj.d199

Biddle, E. (1998). Development and application of an occupational injury and illness classification system. In J. Stellman (Ed.), *Encyclopaedia of occupational safety and health, vol. 1: The body, health care, management and policy, tools and approaches* (4th edn., pp. 32.12–32.18). Geneva, Switzerland: International Labour Office.

Bosco, J., & Wagner, J. (1988). A comparison of the effectiveness of interactive laser disc and classroom video tape for safety instruction of General Motors workers. *Educational Technology, 28*(6), 15–22.

Brahm, F., & Singer, M. (2013). Is more engaging safety training always better in reducing accidents? Evidence of self-selection from Chilean panel data. *Journal of Safety Research, 47,* 85–92.

Briggs, N. C., Levine, R. S., Hall, H. I., Cosby, O., Brann, E. A., & Hennekens, C. H. (2003). Occupational risk factors for selected cancers among African American and White men in the United States. *American Journal of Public Health, 93*(10), 1748–1752.

Brisson, C., Montreuil, S., & Punnett, L. (1999). Effects of an ergonomic training program on workers with video display units. *Scandinavian Journal of Work, Environment and Health, 25*(3), 255–263.

Brnich, M. J., Derick, R. L., Mallett, L., & Vaught, C. (2002). Innovative alternatives to traditional classroom health and safety training. In R. H. Peters (Ed.), *Strategies for improving miners' training* (pp. 19–25). Washington, DC: US Department of Health and Human Services.

Burke, M. J., Borucki, C. C., & Kaufman, J. D. (2002b). Contemporary perspectives on the study of psychological climate: A commentary. *European Journal of Work and Organizational Psychology, 11*(3), 325–340.

Burke, M. J., Chan-Serafin, S., Salvador, R., Smith, A., & Sarpy, S. A. (2008). The role of national culture and organizational climate in safety training effectiveness. *European Journal of Work and Organizational Psychology, 17*(1), 133–152.

Burke, M. J., Salvador, R. O., Smith-Crowe, K., Chan-Serafin, S., Smith, A., & Sonesh, S. (2011). The dread factor: How hazards and safety training influence learning and performance. *Journal of Applied Psychology, 96*(1), 46–70. doi:10.1037/a0021838

Burke, M. J., Sarpy, S., Smith-Crowe, K., Chan-Serafin, S., Salvador, R. O., & Islam, G. (2006). Relative effectiveness of worker safety and health training methods. *American Journal of Public Health, 96*, 315–324. doi:10.2105/AJPH.2004.059840

Burke, M. J., Sarpy, S. A., Tesluk, P. E., & Smith-Crowe, K. (2002a). General safety performance: A test of a grounded theoretical model. *Personnel Psychology, 55*(2), 429–457.

Burke, M. J., Scheuer, M., & Meredith, R. (2007). A dialogical approach to skill development: The case of safety skills. *Human Resource Management Review, 17*(2), 235–250.

Burke, M. J., & Signal, S. M. (2010). Workplace safety: A multilevel, interdisciplinary perspective. In H. Liao, J. J. Martocchio, & A. Joshi (Eds.), *Research in Personnel and Human Resources Management* (vol. 29, pp. 1–47). Bingley, UK: Emerald Group Publishing Ltd.

Bush, D., Paleo, L., Baker, R., Dewey, R., Toktogonova, N., & Cornelio, D. (2009). Restaurant supervisor safety training: Evaluating a small business training intervention. *Public Health Reports, 124*(Suppl 1), 152.

Cagno, E., Micheli, G. J. L., Jacinto, C., & Masi, D. (2014). An interpretive model of occupational safety performance for samll- and medium-sized enterprises. *International Journal of Industrial Ergonomics, 44*(1), 60–74.

Calabro, K., Weltge, A., Parnell, S., Kouzekanani, K., & Ramirez, E. (1998). Intervention for medical students: Effective infection control. *American Journal of Infection Control, 26*(4), 431–436.

Calandra, B., & Harmon, S. W. (2012). A unique design for high-impact safety and awareness training. *Educational Media International, 49*(2), 97–108.

Caparaz, A., Rice, C., Graumlich, S., Radike, M., & Morawetz, J. (1990). Development and pilot evaluation of a health and safety training program for foundry workers. *Applied Occupational Environmental Hygiene, 5*(9), 595–603.

Carlton, R. S. (1987). The effects of body mechanics instruction on work performance. *American Journal of Occupational Therapy, 41*(1), 16–20.

Carrabba, J. J., Field, W. E., Tormoehlen, R. L., & Talbert, B. A. (2000). Effectiveness of the Indiana 4–H Tractor Program at instilling safe tractor operating behaviors and attitudes in youth. *Journal of Agricultural Safety and Health, 6*(3), 179–189.

Carruth, A. K., Levin, J. L., Gilmore, K., Bui, T., Gallardo, G., Evert, W., & Sealey, L. (2010). Cultural influences on safety and health education among Vietnamese fishermen. *Journal of Agromedicine, 15*(4), 375–385.

Cascio, W. F. (2000). *Costing human resources: The financial impact of behavior in organizations.* Cincinnati, OH: Southwestern Publishing.

Cerecero, J. A., & Charlton, M. A. (2012). Designing, implementing, and conducting a web-based radiation safety training program to meet Texas Standards for Radiation Protection. *Health Physics, 103*(5S), S188–S193.

Chan, A. H. S., & Ng, A. W. Y. (2010). Effects of sign characteristics and training methods on safety sign training effectiveness. *Ergonomics, 53*, 1325–1346. doi:10.1080/00140139.2010.524251

Cherrett, T., Wills, G., Price, J., Maynard, S., & Dror, I. E. (2009). Making training more cognitively effective: Making videos interactive. *British Journal of Educational Technology, 40*, 1124–1134. doi:10.1111/j.1467-8535.2009.00985.x

Chhokar, J. S., & Wallin, J. A. (1984). A field study of the effect of feedback frequency on performance. *Journal of Applied Psychology, 69*, 524–530. doi:10.1037/0021-9010.69.3.524

Christian, M. S., Bradley, J. C., Wallace, J. C., & Burke, M. J. (2009). Workplace safety: A meta-analysis of the roles of person and situation factors. *Journal of Applied Psychology, 94*(5), 1103–1127.

Clarke, S. (2006). The relationship between safety climate and safety performance: A meta-analytic review. *Journal of Occupational Health Psychology, 11*(4), 315–327.

Cohen, A., & Colligan, M. J. (1998). *Assessing occupational safety and health training.* Cincinnati, OH: National Institute for Occupational Safety and Health. NIOSH Publication 98–145.

Cohen, H. H., & Jensen, R. C. (1984). Measuring the effectiveness of an industrial lift truck safety training program. *Journal of Safety Research, 15*, 125–135. doi:10.1016/0022-4375(84)90023-9

Cole, B. L., Mallet, L. G., Haley, J. V., Berger, P. K., Lacefield, W. E., Wasielewski, R. D., & Wala, A. M. (1988). *Research and evaluation methods for measuring nonroutine mine health and safety skills* (vol. 1). Pittsburgh, PA: US Bureau of Mines.

Collins, J. W., Wolf, L., Bell, J., & Evanoff, B. A. (2004). An evaluation of a "best practices" musculoskeletal injury prevention program in nursing homes. *Injury Prevention, 10*(4), 206–211.

Cotterchio, M., Gunn, J., Coffill, T., Tormey, P., & Barry, M. A. (1998). Effect of a manager training program on sanitary conditions in restaurants. *Public Health Reports, 113*(4), 353–359.

Coutts, M. C., Graham, K., Braun, K., & Wells, S. (2000). Results of a pilot program for training bar staff in preventing aggression. *Journal of Drug Education, 30*, 171–191. doi:10.2190/HFDB-3XDG-59D1-GG8P

Crichton, M. T. (2009). Improving team effectiveness using tactical decision games. *Safety Science, 47*(3), 330–336.

Curwick, C. C., Reeb-Whitaker, C. K., & Connon, C. L. (2003). Reaching managers at an industry association conference: Evaluation of ergonomics training. *AAOHN Journal, 51*(11), 464–469.

Daltroy, L. H., Iversen, M. D., Larson, M. G., Ryan, J., Zwerling, Z., Fossel, A. H., & Liang, M. H. (1993). Teaching and social support: Effects on knowledge, attitudes, and behaviors to prevent low back injuries in industry. *Health Education Quarterly, 20*(1), 43–62.

DeJoy, D. M. (1996). Theoretical models of health behavior and workplace self-protective behavior. *Journal of Safety Research, 27*(2), 61–72.

Dortch, H. L., & Trombly, C. A. (1990). The effects of education on hand use with industrial workers in repetitive jobs. *American Journal of Occupational Therapy, 44*(9), 777–782.

Dzugan, J. (2010). The development and efficacy of safety training for commercial fishermen. *Journal of Agromedicine, 15*(4), 351–356.

Eckerman, D. A., Abrahamson, K., Ammerman, T., Fercho, H., Rohlman, D., & Anger, K. (2004). Computer-based training for food services workers at a hospital. *Journal of Safety Research, 35*, 317–327. doi:10.1016/j.jsr.2003.11.008

Eklöf, M., & Hagberg, M. (2006). Are simple feedback interventions involving workplace data associated with better working environment and health? A cluster randomized controlled study among Swedish VDU workers. *Applied Ergonomics, 37*(2), 201–210.

Entin, E. E., & Serfaty, D. (1999). Adaptive team coordination. *Human Factors: The Journal of the Human Factors and Ergonomics Society, 41*(2), 312–325.

Evanoff, B. A., Bohr, P. C., & Wolf, L. D. (1999). Effects of a participatory ergonomics team among hospital orderlies. *American Journal of Industrial Medicine, 35*(4), 358–365.

Ewigman, B. G., Kivlahan, C. H., Hosokawa, M. C., & Horman, D. (1990). Efficacy of an intervention to promote use of hearing protective devices by firefighters. *Public Health Reports, 105*(1), 53–59.

Feldstein, A., Valanis, B., Vollmer, W., Stevens, N., & Overton, C. (1993). The back injury prevention project pilot study. *Journal of Occupational and Environmental Medicine, 35*(2), 114–120.

Fenton, G. D., LaBorde, L. F., Radhakrishna, R. B., Brown, J. L., & Cutter, C. N. (2006). Comparison of knowledge and attitudes using computer-based and face-to-face personal hygiene training methods in food processing facilities. *Journal of Food Science, 5*(3), 45–50.

Finch, C., & Daniel, E. (2005). Food safety knowledge and behavior of emergency food relief organization workers: Effects of food safety training intervention. *Journal of Environmental Health, 67*(9), 30–34.

Flin, R., Mearns, K., O'Connor, P., & Bryden, R. (2000). Measuring safety climate: Identifying the common features. *Safety Science, 34*(1), 177–192.

Ford, M. T., & Tetrick, L. E. (2008). Safety motivation and human resource management in North America. *International Journal of Human Resource Management, 19*(8), 1472–1485.

Forst, L., Ahonen, E., Zanoni, J., Holloway-Beth, A., Oschner, M., Kimmel, L., …, & Sokas, R. (2013). More than training: Community-based participatory research to reduce injuries among Hispanic construction workers. *American Journal of Industrial Medicine, 56*(8), 827–837.

Forst, L., Lacey, S., Chen, H. Y., Jimenez, R., Bauer, S., Skinner, S., & Conroy, L. (2004). Effectiveness of community health workers for promoting use of safety eyewear by Latino farm workers. *American Journal of Industrial Medicine, 46*, 607–613. doi:10.1002/ajim.20103

Forst, L., Noth, I. M., Lacey, S., Bauer, S., Skinner, S., Petrea, R., & Zanoni, J. (2006). Barriers and benefits of protective eyewear use by Latino farm workers. *Journal of Agromedicine, 11*(2), 11–17.

Foster, L. (1996). Manual handling training and changes in work practices. *Occupational Health, 48*(11), 402–406.

Fox, C. J., & Sulzer-Azaroff, B. (1987). Increasing completion of accident reports. *Journal of Safety Research, 18*, 65–71. doi:10.1016/0022-4375(87)90086-7

Frederiksen, C. H. (1999). Learning to reason through discourse in a problem-based learning group. *Discourse Processes, 27*(2), 135–160.

Froom, P., Kristal-Boneh, E., Melamed, S., Shalom, A., & Ribak, J. (1998). Prevention of needlestick injury by the scooping-resheathing method. *American Journal of Industrial Medicine, 34*, 15–19. doi:10.1002/(SICI)1097-0274(199807)34:1<15::AID-AJIM3>3.0.CO;2-P

Fullen, M. D. (2010). The development, diffusion and evaluation of a fall hazard safety training program for residential construction workers utilizing instructor led and new media delivery. *Dissertation Abstracts International*, Section A, 70.

Gagnon, M. (2003). The efficacy of training for three manual handling strategies based on the observation of expert and novice workers. *Clinical Biomechanics, 18*, 601–611. doi:10.1016/S0268-0033(03)00076-7

Gettle, M. K. (2009). *Examining the relationship between safety training and incidence of occupational injury* (Order No. 3359012). Available from ProQuest Dissertations & Theses Global (305164069). http://search.proquest.com/docview/305164069 (accessed June 14, 2015).

Girgis, A., Sanson-Fisher, R. W., & Watson, A. (1994). A workplace intervention for increasing outdoor workers' use of solar protection. *American Journal of Public Health, 84*, 77–81. doi:10.2105/AJPH.84.1.77

Gorsky, P., Caspi, A., & Trumper, R. (2006). Campus-based university students' use of dialogue. *Studies in Higher Education, 31*(1), 71–87.

Greene, B. L., DeJoy, D. M., & Olejnik, S. (2005). Effects of an active ergonomics training program on risk exposure, worker beliefs, and symptoms in computer users. *Work, 24*(1), 41–52.

Gregory, M. A., Feitosa, J., Driskell, T., Salas, E., & Vessey, W. B. (2013). Designing, delivering, and evaluating team training in organizations: Principles that work. In E. Salas, S. I. Tannenbaum, D. Cohen, & G. Latham (Eds.), *Developing and enhancing teamwork in organizations* (pp. 441–487). San Francisco, CA: Jossey-Bass.

Griffin, M. A., & Neal, A. (2000). Perceptions of safety at work: A framework for linking safety climate to safety performance, knowledge, and motivation. *Journal of Occupational Health Psychology, 5*(3), 347–358.

Gyekye, S. A., & Salminen, S. (2005). Responsibility assignment at the workplace: A Finnish and Ghanaian perspective. *Scandinavian Journal of Psychology, 46*(1), 43–48.

Haiduven, D. J., DeMaio, T. M., Stevens, D. A. (1992). A five-year study of needlestick injuries: Significant reduction associated with communication, education, and convenient placement of sharps containers. *Inject Control Hasp Epidemiology, 13*(5), 265–271.

Harrington, S. S., & Walker, B. L. (2002). A comparison of computer-based and instructor-led training for long-term care staff. *Journal of Continuing Education in Nursing, 33*(1), 39–45.

Harrington, S. S., & Walker, B. L. (2004). The effects of ergonomics training on the knowledge, attitudes, and practices of teleworkers. *Journal of Safety Research, 35*(1), 13–22.

Håvold, J. I. (2007). National cultures and safety orientation: A study of seafarers working for Norwegian shipping companies. *Work & Stress, 21*(2), 173–195.

Held, E., Mygind, K., Wolff, C., Gyntelberg, F., & Anger, T. (2002). Prevention of work related skin problems: An intervention study in wet work employees. *Occupational and Environmental Medicine, 59*(8), 556–561.

Hickman, J. S., & Geller, E. (2003). A safety self-management intervention for mining operations. *Journal of Safety Research, 34*, 299–308. doi:10.1016/S0022-4375(03)00032-X

Ho, C., & Dzeng, R. (2010). Construction safety training via e-Learning: Learning effectiveness and user satisfaction. *Computers & Education, 55*, 858–867. doi:10.1016/j.compedu.2010.03.017

Hofmann, D. A., Morgeson, F. P., & Gerras, S. J. (2003). Climate as a moderator of the relationship between leader–member exchange and content specific citizenship: Safety climate as an exemplar. *Journal of Applied Psychology, 88*(1), 170–178.

Hofstede, G. H. (1991). *Cultures and organizations: Software of the mind*. London, UK; and New York, NY: McGraw-Hill.

Hofstede, G. H. (2001). *Culture's consequences: Comparing values, behaviors, institutions and organizations across nations*. Thousand Oaks, CA: Sage.

Hong, O., Ronis, D. L., Lusk, S. L., & Kee, G. S. (2006). Efficacy of a computer-based hearing test and tailored hearing protection intervention. *International Journal of Behavioral Medicine, 13*, 304–314. doi:10.1207/s15327558ijbm1304_5

Huang, J., Jiang, D., Wang, X., Liu, Y., Fennie, K., Burgess, J., & Williams, A. (2002). Changing knowledge, behavior and practice related to universal precautions among hospital nurses in China. *Journal of Continuing Education in Nursing, 33*(5), 217–224.

Hultman, G., Nordin, M., & Ortengren, R. (1984). The influence of a preventive educational programme on trunk flexion in janitors. *Applied Ergonomics, 15*, 127–133. doi:10.1016/0003-6870(84)90288-6

Hurlebaus, A. E., & Link, S. (1997). The effects of an aggressive behavior management program on nurses' levels of knowledge, confidence, and safety. *Journal of Nursing Staff Development, 13*(5), 260–265.

Infantino, A., & Musingo, S. Y. (1985). Assaults and injuries among staff with and without training in aggression control techniques. *Hospital and Community Psychology, 36*(12), 1312–1314.

Infortunio, F. A. (2006). An exploration of the correlations between fatal accident rates across nations and the cultural dimensions of power distance, uncertainty avoidance, individuality, and masculinity. *Dissertation Abstracts International, 67*, 1809.

Inman, C., & Blanciforti, L. (2002). *Observed versus reported behaviors and a theoretically-based eye injury intervention for carpenters: Injury insights*. Itasca, IL: National Safety Council Research and Statistical Services.

James, L. R., Choi, C. C., Ko, C.-H. E., McNeil, P. K., Minton, M. K., Wright, M. A., & Kim, K. (2008). Organizational and psychological climate: A review of theory and research. *European Journal of Work and Organizational Psychology, 17*(1), 5–32.

James, L. R., Demaree, R. G., Mulaik, S. A., & Ladd, R. T. (1992). Validity generalization in the context of situational models. *Journal of Applied Psychology, 77*, 3–14.

Jensen, L. K., & Friche, C. (2007). Effects of training to implement new tools and working methods to reduce knee load in floor layers. *Applied Ergonomics, 38*, 655–665. doi:10.1016/j.apergo.2006.03.008

Jiang, L., Yu, G., Li, Y., & Li, F. (2010). Perceived colleagues' safety knowledge/behavior and safety performance: Safety climate as a moderator in a multilevel study. *Accident Analysis & Prevention, 42*(5), 1468–1476.

Johnsson, C., Carlosson, R., & Lagerstrom, M. (2002). Evaluation of training in patient handling and moving skills among hospital and home care personnel. *Ergonomics, 45*(12), 850–865.

Kaskutas, V., Dale, A., Lipscomb, H., & Evanoff, B. (2013). Fall prevention and safety communication training for foremen: Report of a pilot project designed to improve residential construction safety. *Journal of Safety Research, 44*, 111–118. doi:10.1016/j.jsr.2012.08.020

Katz-Navon, T. A. L., Naveh, E., & Stern, Z. (2005). Safety climate in health care organizations: a multidimensional approach. *Academy of Management Journal, 48*(6), 1075–1089.

Kearns, S. (2011). Online single-pilot resource management: Assessing the feasibility of computer-based safety training. *International Journal of Aviation Psychology, 21*(2), 175–190. doi:10.1080/10508414.2011.556499

Kerrigan, D., Moreno, L., Rosario, S., Gomez, B., Jerez, H., Barrington, C., … , & Sweat, M. (2006). Environmental–structural interventions to reduce HIV/STI risk among female sex workers in the Dominican Republic. *American Journal of Public Health, 96*, 120–125. doi: 10.2105/AJPH.2004.042200

Knobloch, M. J., & Broste, S. K. (1998). A hearing conservation program for Wisconsin youth working in agriculture. *Journal of School Health, 68*, 313–318. doi:10.1111/j.1746–1561.1998. tb00591.x

Kobayashi, L., Dunbar-Vivieros, Devine, J., Jones, M. S., Overly, F. L., Gosbee, J. W., & Jay, G. D. (2012). Pilot-phase findings from high-fidelity in situ medical simulation investigation of emergency deparment procedural sedation. *Simulation in Healthcare, 7*(2), 81–94.

Komaki, J. L., Collins, R. L., & Penn, P. (1982). The role of performance antecedents and consequences in work motivation. *Journal of Applied Psychology, 67*(3), 334–340.

Komaki, J., Heinzmann, A. T., & Lawson, L. (1980). Effect of training and a component analysis of a behavioral safety program. *Journal of Applied Psychology, 65*, 261–270. doi:10.1037/0021-9010.65.3.261

Kowalski-Trakofler, K. M., & Barrett, E. (2003). The concept of degraded images applied to hazard recognition training in mining for reduction of lost time injuries. *Journal of Safety Research, 34*, 515–525. doi:10.1016/j.jsr.2003.05.004

Kozlowski, S. W. J., Brown, K. G., Weissbein, D. A., Cannon-Bowers, J. A., & Salas, E. (2000). A multilevel approach to training effectiveness: Enhancing horizontal and vertical transfer. In K. J. Klein & S. W. J. Kozlowski (Eds.), *Multilevel theory, research, and methods in organizations: Foundations, extensions, and new directions* (pp. 157–210). San Francisco, CA: Jossey-Bass.

Landsittel, D. P., Murphy, D. J., Kiernan, N. E., Hard, D. L., & Kassab, C. (2001). Evaluation of the effectiveness of educational interventions in the Pennsylvania central region farm safety pilot project. *American Journal of Industrial Medicine, 40*(2), 145–152.

Lapping, J. E., & Parsons, M. A. (1980). The impact of training in the construction industry. *Professional Safety, 25*, 13–18.

Lazovich, D. Parker, D. L., Brosseau, L. M., Miton, F. T., Dugan, S. K., Pan, W., & Hock, L. (2002). Effectiveness of a worksite intervention to reduce an occupational exposure: The Minnesota wood dust study. *American Journal of Public Health, 92*(9), 1498–1505.

Lee, P., Allen, K., & Daly, M. (2012). A "communication and patient safety" training programme for all healthcare staff: Can it make a difference? *BMJ Quality & Safety, 21*(1), 84–88.

Leprevost, C. E., Storm, J. F., Blanchard, M. R., Asuaje, R., & Cope, W. G. (2013). Engaging Latino farmworkers in the development of symbols to improve pesticide safety and health education and risk communication. *Journal of Immigrant and Minority Health, 15*(5), 975–981.

Leslie, J. H., & Adams, S. K. (1973). Programmed safety through programmed learning. *Human Factors, 15*(3), 223–236.

Levesque, D. L., Arif, A. A., & Shen, J. (2012). Effectiveness of pesticide safety training and knowledge about pesticide exposure among hispanic farmworkers. *Journal of Occupational and Environmental Medicine, 54*(12), 1550–1556. doi:10.1097/JOM.0b013e3182677d96

Lingard, H. (2002). The effect of first aid training on Australian construction workers' occupational health and safety motivation and risk control behavior. *Journal of Safety Research, 33*(2), 209–230.

Lipscomb, H. J. (2000). Effectiveness of interventions to prevent work-related eye injuries. *American Journal of Preventive Medicine, 18*(4S), 27–33

Löffler, H., Bruckner, T., Diepgen, T., & Effendy, I. (2006). Primary prevention in health care employees: A prospective intervention study with a 3-year training period. *Contact Dermatitis, 54*(4), 202–209.

Lombardi, D. A., Verma, S. K., Brennan, M. J., & Perry, M. J. (2009). Factors influencing worker use of personal protective eyewear. *Accident Analysis & Prevention, 41*, 755–762. doi:10.1016/j. aap.2009.03.017

Ludwig, T. D., & Geller, E. S. (1997). Assigned versus participative goal setting and response generalization: Managing injury control among professional pizza deliverers. *Journal of Applied Psychology, 82*, 253–261. doi:10.1037/0021-9010.82.2.253

Lueveswanij, S., Nittayananta, W., & Robison, V. A. (2000). Changing knowledge, attitudes, and practices of Thai oral health personnel with regard to AIDS: An evaluation of an educational intervention. *Community Dental Health, 17*(3), 165–171.

Luskin, J., Somers, C., Wooding, J., & Levenstein, C. (1992). Teaching health and safety: Problems and possibilities for learner-centered training. *American Journal of Industrial Medicine, 22,* 665–676. doi:10.1002/ajim.4700220505

Lynch, P., Cummings, M. J., Roberts, P. L., Herriott, M. J., Yates, B., & Stamm, W. E. (1990). Implementing and evaluating a system of generic infection precautions: Body substance isolation. *American Journal of Infection Control, 18,* 1–12. doi:10.1016/0196-6553(90)90204-6

Lynch, R. M., & Freund, A. (2000). Short-term efficacy of back injury intervention project for patient care providers at one hospital. *American Industrial Hygiene Association Journal, 61,* 290–294. doi:10.1202/0002-8894(2000)0612.0.CO;2

Ma, S., Dukers, N. H., van den Hoek, A., Yuliang, F., Zhiheng, C., Jiangting, F., & Xiusing, Z. (2002). Decreasing STD incidence and increasing condom use among Chinese sex workers following a short term intervention: A prospective cohort study. *Sexually Transmitted Infections, 78,* 110–114. doi:10.1136/sti.78.2.110

Madgwick, P., Houdmont, J., & Randall, R. (2011). Sun safety measures among construction workers in Britain. *Occupational Medicine, 61,* 430–433. doi:10.1093/occmed/kqr054

Malakis, S., & Kontogiannis, T. (2012). Refresher training for air traffic controllers: Is it adequate to meet the challenges of emergencies and abnormal situations? *International Journal of Aviation Psychology, 22,* 59–77. doi:10.1080/10508414.2012.635127

Mancini, R., Murray, L., Chapman, B. J., & Powell, D. A. (2012). Investigating the potential benefits of on-site food safety training for Folklorama, a temporary food service event. *Journal of Food Protection, 75*(10), 1829–1834.

Mancini, M. E., Cazzell, M., Kardong-Edgren, S., & Cason, C. L. (2009). Improving workplace safety training using a self-directed CPR-AED learning program. *AAOHN Journal, 57*(4), 159–169.

Maples, T. W., Jacoby, J. A., Johnson, D. E., Ter Haar, G., & Buckingham, F. M. (1982). Effectiveness of employee training and motivation programs in reducing exposure to inorganic lead and lead alkyls. *American Industrial Hygiene Association Journal, 43*(9), 692–694.

Marchand, A., Simard, M., Carpentier-Roy, M. C., & Ouellet, F. (1998). From a unidimensional to a bidimensional concept and measurement of workers' safety behavior. *Scandinavian Journal of Work, Environment & Health, 24*(4), 293–299.

Mark, B. A., Hughes, L. C., Belyea, M., Chang, Y., Hofmann, D., Jones, C. B., & Bacon, C. T. (2007). Does safety climate moderate the influence of staffing adequacy and work conditions on nurse injuries? *Journal of Safety Research, 38*(4), 431–446.

Marsh, P., & Kendrick, D. (1998). Injury prevention training: Is it effective? *Health Education Research, 13,* 47–56. doi:10.1093/her/13.1.47

Martyny, J. W., Buchan, R. M., Keefe, T. J., & Blehm, K. D. (1988). Impact of an OSHA onsite consultation program with an educational component on small businesses in Colorado. *Applied Industrial Hygiene, 3*(6), 12–14.

Mattila, M. (1990). Improving working practices and workplace safety through behavior analysis in the veneer industry. In B. Das (Ed.), *Advances in industrial ergonomics and safety* (pp. 957–961). London, UK: Taylor & Francis.

Mattila, M., & Hyodynmaa, M. (1988). Promoting job safety in building: An experiment on the behavior analysis approach. *Journal of Occupational Accidents, 9,* 255–267. doi:10.1016/0-376-6349(88)90017-X

Mayer, A. S., Brazile, W. J., Erb, S. A., Barker, E. A., Miller, C. M., Mroz, M. M., Maier, L. A., &Van Dyke, M. (2013). Developing effective health and safety training materials for workers in beryllium-using industries. *Journal of Occupational and Environmental Medicine, 55,* 746–751. doi:10.1097/JOM.0b013e3182972f1b

Mayer, J. A., Slymen, D. J., Clapp, E., Pichon, L., Eckhardt, L., Eichenfield, F., & Oh, S. (2007). Promoting sun safety among U.S. Postal Service letter carriers: Impact of a 2-year intervention. *American Journal of Public Health, 97,* 559–565. doi:10.2105/AJPH.2005.083907

Mayer, J. A., Slymen, D. J., Clapp, E. J., Pichon, L. C., Elder, J. P., Sallis, J. F., …, & Weinstock, M. A. (2009). Long-term maintenance of a successful occupational sun safety intervention. *Archives of Dermatology, 145*(1), 88.

McCauley, M. (1990). The effect of body mechanics instruction on work performance among young workers. *American Journal of Occupational Therapy, 44*(5), 402–407.

McGrath, J. M. (2011). The role of equipment warning labels in the industrial workplace. *International Journal of Occupational Safety and Ergonomics, 17*(1), 49–60.

McIntyre, L., Vallaster, L., Wilcott, L., Henderson, S. B., & Kosatsky, T. (2013). Evaluation of food safety knowledge, attitudes and self-reported hand washing practices in FOODSAFE trained and untrained food handlers in British Columbia, Canada. *Food Control, 30*(1), 150–156.

Melhorn, J. (1996). A prospective study for upper-extremity cumulative trauma disorders of workers in aircraft manufacturing. *Occupational & Environmental Medicine, 38*, 1264–1271.

Morrow, P. C., & Crum, M. R. (1998). The effects of perceived and objective safety risk on employee outcomes. *Journal of Vocational Behavior, 53*(2), 300–313.

Morrow, C. C., Jarett, M. Q., & Rupinski, M. T. (1997). An investigation of the effect and economic utility of corporate-wide training. *Personnel Psychology, 50*(1), 91–119.

Mujuru, P., Helmkamp, J. C., Mutambudzi, M., Hu, W., & Bell, J. L. (2009). Evaluating the impact of an intervention to reduce injuries among loggers in West Virginia, 1999–2007. *Journal of Agricultural Safety and Health, 15*(1), 75–88.

National Institute of Environmental Health Sciences (2010). *Safety and health awareness for oil spill cleanup workers.* Research Triangle Park, NC: National Institute of Environmental Health Sciences' Worker Education and Training Program. Published in cooperation with the Occupational Safety and Health Administration (OSHA).

Neal, A., & Griffin, M. A. (2004). Safety climate and safety at work. In J. Barling & M. R. Frone (Eds.), *The psychology of workplace safety* (pp. 15–34). Washington, DC: American Psychological Association.

Neal, A., Griffin, M. A., & Hart, P. M. (2000). The impact of organizational climate on safety climate and individual behavior. *Safety Science, 34*(1), 99–109.

Nielsen, D., Sigurdsson, S. O., & Austin, J. (2009). Preventing back injuries in hospital settings: The effects of video modeling on safe patient lifting by nurses. *Journal of Applied Behavior Analysis, 42*(3), 551–561.

Nieto-Montenegro, S., Brown, J. L., & LaBorde, L. F. (2008). Development and assessment of pilot food safety educational materials and training strategies for Hispanic workers in the mushroom industry using the Health Action Model. *Food Control, 19*(6), 616–633.

Nieuwenhuijsen, E. R. (2004). Health behavior change among office workers: An exploratory study to prevent repetitive strain injuries. *Work, 23*(3), 215–224.

Orr, T. J., Mallet, L. G., & Margolis, K. A. (2009). Enhanced fire escape training for mine workers using virtual reality simulation. *Mining Engineering, 61*(11), 41–44.

Parenmark, G., Engvall, B., & Malmkvist, A. K. (1988). Ergonomic on-the-job training of assembly workers: Arm–neck–shoulder complaints drastically reduced amongst beginners. *Applied Ergonomics, 19*(2), 143–146.

Park, S. H., Kwak, T. K., & Chang, H. J. (2010). Evaluation of the food safety training for food handlers in restaurant operations. *Nutrition Research and Practice, 4*(1), 58–68.

Parkinson, D. K., Bromet, E. J., Dew, M. A., Dunn, L. O., Barkman, M., & Wright, M. (1989). Effectiveness of the United Steel Workers of America Coke Oven Intervention Program. *Journal of Occupational Medicine, 31*(5), 464–472.

Pashler, H., Rohrer, D., & Cepeda, N. J. (2006). Temporal spacing and learning. *Observer, 19*(3).

Patros, S. (2001). *Healthcare worker compliance with standard precautions: A study of two small community hospitals* (Unpublished doctoral dissertation). University of Kentucky, Lexington.

Paul, P. S., & Maiti, J. (2007). The role of behavioral factors on safety management in underground mines. *Safety Science, 45*(4), 449–471.

Pedersen, B. H., Dyreborg, J., Kines, P., Mikkelsen, K. L., Hannerz, H., Andersen, D. R., & Spangenberg, S. (2010). Protocol for a mixed-methods study on leader-based interventions in construction contractors' safety commitments. *Injury Prevention, 16*(3), 1–7.

Pedersen, L. M., & Kines, P. (2011). Why do workers work safely? Development of safety motivation questionnaire scales. *Safety Science Monitor, 15*(1), 1–10.

Perry, M. J., & Layde, P. M. (2003). Farm pesticides: Outcomes of a randomized controlled intervention to reduce risks. *American Journal of Preventive Medicine*, 24, 310–315. doi:10.1016/ S0749-3797(03)00023-0

Peterson, E. L., McGlothlin, J. D., & Blue, C. L. (2004). The development of an ergonomics training program to identify, evaluate, and control musculoskeletal disorders among nursing assistants at a state run veterans home. *Journal of Occupational and Environmental Hygiene*, 1(1), 10–16.

Pidgeon, N. F. (1991). Safety culture and risk management in organizations. *Journal of Cross-Cultural Psychology*, 22, 129–140. doi:10.1177/0022022191221009

Porru, S., Donato, F., Apostoli, P., Coniglio, L., Piergiorgio, D., & Alessio, L. (1993). The utility of health education among lead workers: The experience of one program. *American Journal of Industrial Medicine*, 23, 473–481. doi:10.1002/ajim.4700230310

Probst, T. M. (2004). Safety and insecurity: Exploring the moderating effect of organizational safety climate. *Journal of Occupational Health Psychology*, 9(1), 3–10.

Probst, T. M., & Estrada, A. X. (2010). Accident under-reporting among employees: Testing the moderating influence of psychological safety climate and supervisor enforcement of safety practices. *Accident Analysis & Prevention*, 42(5), 1438–1444.

Rabøl, L., McPhail, M., Bjørn, B., Anhøj, J., Mogensen, T., Østergaard, D., & Andersen, H. (2012). Outcomes of a classroom-based team training intervention for multi-professional hospital staff. *Medical Teacher*, 34, 868–869. doi:10.3109/0142159X.2012.716182

Rasmussen, K., Carsrensen, O., Lauritsen, J. M., Glassock, D. J., Hansen, O. N., & Jensen, U. F. (2003). Prevention of farm injuries in Denmark. *Scandinavian Journal of Work, Environment, and Health*, 29(4), 288–296.

Ray, P. S., Bishop, P. A., & Wang, M. Q. (1997). Efficacy of the components of a behavioral safety program. *International Journal of Industrial Ergonomics*, 19, 19–29. doi:10.1016/0169-814 1(95)00067-4

Reber, R. A., Wallin, J. A., & Chhokar, J. S. (1984). Reducing industrial accidents: A behavioral experiment. *Industrial Relations*, 23, 119–125. doi:10.1111/j.1468-232X.1984.tb00881.x

Reddell, C. R., Congleton, J. J., Huchingson, R. D., & Montgomery, J. F. (1992). An evaluation of a weightlifting belt and back injury prevention training class for airline baggage handlers. *Applied Ergonomics*, 23(5), 319–329.

Reif, R. H., Fraser, L. A., & Liffers, M. L. (2013). Laser safety program at Woods Hole Oceanographic Institution. *Health Physics*, 104(2S), S37–S42.

Reiners, T., Teras, H., Chang, V., Wood, L., Gregory, S., Gibson, D., Petter, N., & Teras, M. (2014). Authentic, immersive, and emotional experience in virtual learning environments: The fear of dying as an important learning experience in a simulation. In *Transformative, innovative and engaging*. Presentation at the Teaching and Learning Forum 2014 held at the University of Western Australia, Perth, WA, Australia.

Rempel, D. M., Krause, N., Goldberg, R., Benner, D., Hudes, M., & Goldner, G. U. (2006). A randomized controlled trial evaluating the effects of two workstation interventions on upper body pain and incident musculoskeletal disorders among computer operators. *Occupational & Environmental Medicine*, 63(5), 300–306.

Rhoton, W. W. (1980). A procedure to improve compliance with coal mine safety regulations. *Organizational Behavior Management*, 2(4), 243–250.

Richardson, D. B., Loomis, D., Bena, J., & Bailer, A. J. (2004). Fatal occupational injury rates in southern and non-southern states, by race and Hispanic ethnicity. *American Journal of Public Health*, 94(10), 1756.

Robins, T. G., Hugentobler, M. K., Kaminski, M., & Klitzman, S. (1990). Implementation of the federal hazard communication standard: Does training work? *Journal of Occupational Medicine*, 32(11), 1133–1140.

Robson, L., Stephenson, C., Schulte, P., Amick, B., Chan, S., Bielecky, A., … , & Grubb, P. (2010). *A systematic review of the effectiveness of training & education for the protection of workers.* Toronto, ON, Canada: Institute for Work & Health.

Robson, L. S., Stephenson, C. M., Schulte, P. A., Amick, B. C., Irvin, E. L., Eggerth, D. E...., & Grubb, P. L. (2012). A systematic review of the effectiveness of occupational health and safety training. *Scandinavian Journal of Work and Environmental Health, 38*(3), 193–208.

Rundio, A. (1994). Understanding microbiological concepts and computerized surveillance: Enhancing professional practice. *Health Care Supervision, 12*(3), 20–27.

Saarela, K. L., Saari, J., & Alltonen, M. (1989).The effects of an informational safety campaign in the shipbuilding industry. *Journal of Occupational Accidents, 10*(4), 255–266.

Saari, J., & Nasanen, M. (1989). The effect of positive feedback on industrial housekeeping and accidents: A long-term study at a shipyard. *International Journal of Industrial Ergonomics, 4*, 201–211. doi:10.1016/0169-8141(89)90003-6

Sadler, O. W., & Montgomery, G. M. (1982). The application of positive practice overcorrection to the use of hearing protection. *American Industrial Hygiene Association Journal, 43*, 451–454. doi:10.1080/15298668291410026

Salas, E., Burke, C. S., Bowers, C. A., & Wilson, K. A. (2001). Team training in the skies: Does crew resource management (CRM) training work? *Human Factors, 43*(4), 641–674.

Salas, E., & Cannon-Bowers, J. A. (2001). The science of training: A decade of progress. *Annual Review of Psychology, 52*(1), 471–499.

Salas, E., DiazGranados, D., Klein, C., Burke, C. S., Stagl, K. C., Goodwin, G. F., & Halpin, S. M. (2008). Does team training improve team performance? A meta-analysis. *Human Factors: The Journal of the Human Factors and Ergonomics Society, 50*(6), 903–933.

Salas, E., Fowlkes, J. E., Stout, R. J., Milanovich, D. M., & Prince, C. (1999). Does CRM training improve teamwork skills in the cockpit? Two evaluation studies. *Human Factors, 41*, 326–343.

Samples, J., Bergstad, E. A., Ventura, S., Sanchez, V., Farquhar, S. A., & Shadbeh, N. (2009). Pesticide exposure and occupational safety training of indigenous farmworkers in Oregon. *American Journal of Public Health, 99*(S3), S581–S584

Schwartz, R. K. (1989). Cognition and learning in industrial accident injury prevention: An occupational therapy perspective. In J. A. Johnson & E. Jaffe (Eds.), *Health promotion and preventive programs: Model of occupational therapy practice* (pp. 67–85). New York, NY: Haworth Press.

Schwartz, S. H. (1999). A theory of cultural values and some implications for work. *Applied Psychology: An International Review, 48*(1), 23–47.

Seto, W. H., Ching, T. Y., Chu, Y. B., & Fielding, F. (1990). Reduction of the frequency of needle recapping by effective education: A need for conceptual alteration. *Infection Control and Hospital Epidemiology, 11*, 194–196. doi:10.1086/646149

Sinclair, R. R., Martin, J. E., & Sears, L. E. (2010). Labor unions and safety climate: Perceived union safety values and retail employee safety outcomes. *Accident Analysis & Prevention, 42*, 1477–1487. doi:10.1016/j.aap.2009.11.003

Smith, M. J., Anger, W. K., & Uslan, S. S. (1978). Behavioral modification applied to occupational safety. *Journal of Safety Research, 10*(2), 87–88.

Smith-Crowe, K., Burke, M. J., & Landis, R. S. (2003). Organizational climate as a moderator of safety knowledge–safety performance relationships. *Journal of Organizational Behavior, 24*(7), 861–876.

Stephens, S. D., & Ludwig, T. D. (2005). Improving anesthesia nurse compliance with universal precautions using group goals and public feedback. *Journal of Organizational Behavior Management, 25*, 37–71. doi:10.1300/J075v25n02_02

Strong, L. L., & Zimmerman, F. J. (2005). Occupational injury and absence from work among African American, Hispanic, and non-Hispanic white workers in the national longitudinal survey of youth. *American Journal of Public Health, 95*(7), 1226–1232.

Sulzer-Azaroff, B., & Austin, J. (2000). Does BBS work? Bahavior-based safety and injury reduction: A survey of the evidence. *Professional Safety, 45*(7), 19–24.

Sulzer-Azaroff, B., & de Santamaria, M. C. (1980). Industrial safety hazard reduction through performance feedback. *Journal of Applied Behavior Analysis, 13*(2), 287–295.

Symes, A. M., Graveling, R. A., & Campbell, S. J. (1992). *Risk training and materials handling.* Edinburgh, Scotland: Institute of Occupational Medicine.

Taylor, M. A., & Alvero, A. M. (2012). The effects of safety discrimination training and frequent safety observations on safety-related behavior. *Journal of Organizational Behavior Management*, *32*(3), 169–193.

Taylor, P. J., Russ-Eft, D. F., & Chan, D. W. L. (2005). A meta-analytic review of behavior modeling training. *Journal of Applied Psychology*, *90*, 692–709. doi:10.1037/0021-9010.90.4.692

Tompa, E., Dolinschi, R., de Oliverira, C., & Irvin, E. (2009). A systematic review of occupational health and safety interventions with economic analysis. *Journal of Occupational & Environmental Medicine*, *51*(9), 1004–1023.

Uwakwe, C. B. (2000). Systematized HIV/AIDS education for student nurses at the University of Ibadan, Nigeria: Impact on knowledge, attitudes and compliance with universal precautions. *Journal of Advanced Nursing*, *32*, 416–424. doi:10.1046/j.1365-2648.2000.01492.x

van Poppel, M. N., Koes, B. W., van der Ploeg, T., Smid, T., & Bouter, L. M. (1998). Lumbar supports and education for the prevention of low back pain in industry: A randomized controlled trial. *Journal of the American Medical Association*, *279*(22), 1789–1794.

Vaught, C., Brinch, M. J., & Kellner, H. J. (1988). *Instructional mode and its effect on initial self-contained self-rescuer donning attempts during training*. Pittsburgh, PA: US Bureau of Mines.

Videman, T., Rauhala, H., Asp, S., Lindstrom, K., Cedercreutz, G., Kamppi, M., & Troup, J. D. (1989). Patient-handling skill, back injuries, and back pain: An intervention study in nursing. *Spine*, *14*, 148–156. doi:10.1097/00007632-198902000-00002

Vinodkumar, M. N., & Bhasi, M. (2010). Safety management practices and safety behaviour: Assessing the mediating role of safety knowledge and motivation. *Accident Analysis & Prevention*, *42*(6), 2082–2093.

Wallace, C., & Chen, G. (2006). A multilevel integration of personality, climate, self-regulation, and performance. *Personnel Psychology*, *59*(3), 529–557.

Wallace, J. C., Little, L. M., & Shull, A. (2008). The moderating effects of task complexity on the relationship between regulatory foci and safety and production performance. *Journal of Occupational Health Psychology*, *13*(2), 95–104.

Wallerstein, N., & Weinger, M. (1992). Health and safety education for empowerment. *American Journal of Industrial Medicine*, *22*(5), 619–635.

Wang, H., Fennie, K., He, G., Burgess, J., & Williams, A. B. (2003). A training programme for prevention of occupational exposure to bloodborne pathogens: Impact on knowledge, behaviour and incidence of needlestick injuries among student nurses in Changsha, People's Republic of China. *Journal of Advanced Nursing*, *41*, 187–194. doi:10.1046/j.1365-2648.2003.02519.x

Weinstein, N. D. (2000). Perceived probability, perceived severity, and health-protective behavior. *Health Psychology*, *19*(1), 65–74.

West, C., Slatin, C., Sanborn, W., & Volicer, B. (2009). Computer-based simulation in blended learning curriculum for hazardous waste site worker health and safety training. *International Journal of Information and Communication Technology Education*, *5*, 62–73. doi:10.4018/jicte.2009010105

Whitby, M., Stead, P., & Najman, J. M. (1991). Needlestick injury: Impact of a recapping device and an associated education program. *Infection Control and Hospital Epidemiology*, *12*, 220–225. doi:10.1086/646328

Williams, J. H., & Geller, E. S. (2000). Behavior-based intervention for occupational safety: Critical impact of social comparison feedback. *Journal of Safety Research*, *31*, 135–142. doi:10.1016/S0022-4375(00)00030-X

Wong, E. S., Stotka, J. L., Chinchilli, V. M., Williams, D. S., Stuart, G., & Markowitz, S. M. (1991). Are universal precautions effective in reducing the number of occupational exposures among health care workers? *Journal of the American Medical Association*, *265*, 1123–1128. doi:10.1001/jama.265.9.1123

Wright, B. J., Turner, J. G., & Daffin, P. (1997). Effectiveness of computer-assisted instruction in increasing the rate of universal precautions-related behaviors. *American Journal of Infection Control*, *25*(5), 426–429.

Wynn, J. S., & Black, S. (1998). Evaluation of retention of safety and survival training content versus industry standard for training. *Air Medical Journal, 17*, 166–168. doi:10.1016/S1-067-991X(98)90044-X

Yao, W. X., Wu, Y. L., Yang, B., Zhang, L. Y., Yao, C., Huang, C. H., & Qian, Y. R. (2013). Occupational safety training and education for needlestick injuries among nursing students in China: Intervention study. *Nurse Education Today, 33*(8), 834–837.

Yarrall, M. (1986). Educating for hearing conversation. *Occupational Health, 10*, 333–335.

Yassi, A., Cooper, J., Tate, R., Gerlach, S., Muir, M., Trottier, J., & Massey, K. (2001). A randomized controlled trial to prevent patient lift and transfer injuries of health care workers. *Spine, 26*, 1739–1746. doi:10.1097/00007632-200108150-00002

Yu, W., Yu, I. T. S., Wang, X., Li, Z., Wan, S., Qiu, H., Lin, H., Xie, S., & Sun, T. (2013). Effectiveness of participatory training for prevention of musculoskeletal disorders: A randomized controlled trial. *International Archives of Occupational and Envrionmental Health, 86*(4), 431–440.

Zhang, X., Zhao, W., Jing, R., Wheeler, K., Smith, G. A., Stallones, L., & Xiang, H. (2011). Work-related pesticide poisoning among farmers in two villages of Southern China: A cross-sectional survey. *BMC Public Health, 11*(1), 429.

Zhao, D., & Lucas, J. (2014). Virtual reality simulation for construction safety promotion. *International Journal of Injury Control and Safety Promotion*. doi:10.1080/17457300.2013.861853.

Zohar, D. (2011). Safety climate: Conceptual and measurement issues. In J. C. Quick & L. E. Tetrick (Eds.), *Handbook of occupational health psychology* (2nd edn., pp. 141–164). Washington, DC: American Psychological Association.

Zohar, D., & Luria, G. (2005). A multilevel model of safety climate: Cross-level relationships between organization and group-level climates. *Journal of Applied Psychology, 90*(4), 616–628.

16

Safety Climate and Supervisory-Based Interventions

Gil Luria

Introduction

This study reviews recent directions in the growing body of literature on safety climate. The concept of safety climate was first introduced by Zohar (1980) to predict safety outcomes in organizations. Zohar provided first empirical results for the concept as well as an approach to understanding safety behavior in organizations. This has given rise to many studies since that time (see summary in Flin, Mearns, O'Connor, & Bryden, 2000; Guldenmund, 2000; Zohar, 2010, 2011; Zohar & Hofmann, 2012). Results concerning the validity of safety climate are supported in multiple studies across the globe and in meta-analytic tests of the relationship between safety climate, safety behavior, and objective safety outcomes such as injury (Beus, Payne, Bergman, & Arthur, 2010; Christian, Bradley, Wallace, & Burke, 2009; Clarke, 2006, 2010; Nahrgang, Morgeson, & Hofmann, 2011). The relationship between climate and outcome is not exclusive to safety research, and other facets of climate, such as service climate, were shown to be valid predictors of relevant outcomes (Kuenzi & Schminke, 2009; Ostroff, Knicki, & Muhammad, 2012; Schneider, Ehrhart, & Macey, 2011; Schneider, Macey, Lee & Young, 2009; Schulte, Ostroff, Shmulyian, & Kinicki, 2009).

This chapter reviews current knowledge about group-level safety climate, and discusses group processes from a multilevel perspective. First I explain the individual-level rationale of employee safety decision-making and behavior. In order to comprehend the need for safety climate, it is important to know why some employees behave in an unsafe manner, and why organizational practices are needed in order to correct such behavior. I also discuss organizational influence on groups or units within an organization. In sum, this is an attempt to explain how and which group-level processes create shared safety climate among members of the group (i.e., sense-making and sense-giving), and the relationship between organizational-level and group-level climates.

The Wiley Blackwell Handbook of the Psychology of Occupational Safety and Workplace Health, First Edition. Edited by Sharon Clarke, Tahira M. Probst, Frank Guldenmund, and Jonathan Passmore. © 2016 John Wiley & Sons Ltd. Published 2020 by John Wiley & Sons Ltd.

Safety climate is one of the few facet-specific climates that can influence safety and should be considered together. I present several facet-specific climates relevant to safety, and discuss models in which they can be studied together in order to predict safety outcomes. Based on safety climate theory, I enlarge on intervention studies whose intention is to improve safety by modifying managerial safety practices that are perceived by employees and influence their behavior.

Key questions are asked, such as: Why do employees behave in an unsafe manner? How do group processes create safe climates within groups? How do the safety activities of management at the organizational level influence group-level safety, and ultimately the employees' rates of safe behaviors and accidents? What actions should be taken to improve safety based on the safety climate approach?

Multilevel Safety Climate

Creating an organizational reality and atmosphere in which employees behave in a safe manner is a challenge confronting many organizations. Some managers are surprised that employees tend to behave in a way that endangers their own health and well-being so that organizations must invest many resources in promoting employees' safety compliance and safety participation. In order to understand the role of organizational-level and group-level practices in promoting safety behavior it is important to start with the individual psychological processes of employees. This is important because it is these decisions and behaviors that the organizational- and group-level processes try to influence. Furthermore, it is the individual behavior of employees that mainly determines an organization's injury and accident rates. For example, US National Safety Council (NSC) statistics have demonstrated that in about 40 percent of work accidents employees failed to use the safety gear provided. This is only one example of individual behavior of employees at the workplace (NSC, 1999).

Studies focusing on the reasons and mechanisms conducive to safety-related behaviors revealed an individual-level tendency to behave unsafely. This tendency was explained in several ways. For example, two psychological mechanisms that explain the cost–benefit analysis of human decision-making related to safe behavior are the melioration bias (Herrnstein, Loewnstein, Prelec, & Vaughan, 1993), and the rare-events bias (Plous, 1993). Melioration bias studies found that human beings tend to assign greater weight to short-term results when choosing among alternative actions. This is important for occupational psychology because many safety-related behaviors have undesirable short-term consequences (e.g., demand more time, reduce the level of comfort in performing a task) and therefore individuals avoid them. For example, frequent use of protective gear (safety glasses, helmet, ear plugs, etc.) necessitates bringing or carrying it, and decreases ease of work while using it. Rare-events studies demonstrate that individuals have a tendency to under-evaluate, or ignore the possibility of being adversely affected by occasional negative events (Barron & Erev, 2003; Erev, 1998; Schurr, Rodensky, & Erev, 2014; Yechiam, Erev, & Barron, 2006). Given that the negative outcome of unsafe behavior (i.e., an accident) is rare, many people adopt risky behaviors for which, in many cases, they have an immediate and certain reward. When considering these two attitudes in order to understand and predict employees' safety behavior, it would appear that, to an employee, the outcome of safe behavior is the non-event (i.e., decreased low-probability injury potential), whereas unsafe behavior leads to immediate reinforcement and tangible benefits (e.g., increased pace, greater comfort). Thus it is predictable that frequency of unsafe behaviors will increase, and frequency of safe behavior will decrease. Furthermore, it seems that when employees make decisions based on experience, rare events tend to receive less consideration than they deserve according to objective probability (Hertwig & Erev, 2009). Safety-related decisions are frequently based on experience because employees constantly perform the same actions and learn "firsthand" what happens when they behave unsafely. Since accidents are infrequent, when employees behave unsafely without experiencing undesirable outcomes, they believe they can continue unless confronted with other managerial reactions such as feedback or approval. Thus, individual safety psychology indicates that employees are predisposed to unsafe behavior. This is a basic human trait that is not exclusive to employees. Supervisors and group managers may also be affected by melioration bias (Herrnstein et al., 1993) and rare-events bias (Plous, 1993), and monitor and evaluate issues that give immediate measurable results, such as productivity rather than safety. For example, some supervisors (department-level management) compromised safety in order to improve productivity and mission accomplishment (Zohar & Luria, 2004). Group managers have discretion concerning emphasis on safety in their managerial practices, and studies documenting the frequency of safety interactions found differences between group-managers' safety-related interactions with their subordinates (Luria, Zohar, & Erev, 2008; Zohar, 2002a; Zohar & Luria, 2003). It is important to note that the tension between competing goals is not exclusive to safety decisions and behaviors. Productivity and speed, for example, seem to be central goals in organizations, influencing managers and employees to work faster and pay less attention to quality (Luria, Yagil, & Gal, 2014).

The "rare event" assumption concerning safety behavior that exists at the individual and group levels alike, is less valid at the organizational level. Here, a strong bias toward productivity and speed may create a reality in which the probability is that one or more of the members will participate in an accident (at a rate of several accidents per year, which is not an unusual organizational outcome). In other words, many employees working together in an unsafe manner can engender accumulated risk to themselves and to others, creating a strong probability of accidents and injuries at the organizational level. In many countries, managements are legally liable and responsible for the safety of their employees (Ridley & Channing, 2008), so that accidents have immediate financial consequences deriving from increased insurance costs. Organizational management should be less influenced by unsafe biases (Herrnstein et al., 1993; Plous, 1993), and should be prone to promote safety in their workplace.

The organizational safety climate concept captures the top-down pro-safety influences in the organization. It measures employee perceptions regarding safety policies, procedures, and practices in the work environment (Zohar, 1980). These key organizational attributes inform employees on the behaviors likely to be supported and rewarded (Ostroff et al., 2012; Zohar & Hofmann, 2012). The explained effect of climate on behavior is that climate perceptions reveal the underlying logic of actions in the work environment, pointing the employee toward better-rewarded role behavior (Zohar, 2010, 2011; Zohar & Hofmann, 2012). Individual employees perceive what is expected of them at the organizational and within the sub-organizational (group) levels. The importance of safety may differ between organizational and group levels, and employees are apparently able to sense these differences (Zohar, Livne, Tenne-Gazit, Admi, & Donchin, 2007; Zohar & Luria, 2005, 2010), understand how they are expected to behave regarding safety, and behave accordingly because of possible organizational consequences for improper behavior.

Safety climate scales focus on recurrent themes indicating the importance of safety, also known as safety climate dimensions (Kath, Marks, & Ranney, 2010). Kath et al. (2010) identified three dimensions: (1) management attitudes concerning safety that capture their awareness of safety issues, and their willingness to invest resources in addressing risks; (2) the tension between safety and work, assuming that when work demands interfere and compete with safety behavior it is harder for employees to behave in a safe manner; (3) pressure from coworkers to behave safely, indicating horizontal influence within groups also termed as peer safety pressure (Zohar, 1980). Flin et al. (2000) reviewed 18 safety-climate studies and identified a fourth dimension – the safety system, encompassing differ-ent aspects of organizational safety-management systems, including safety officials, permit to work systems, safety equipment, and others. Flin et al. (2000) also found an interest-ing fifth dimension occurring in less than half of the scales they reviewed. It focuses on competence in regard to safety related organizational activities such as selection, training, standards, and assessment.

The multilevel organizational analysis presented above suggests that organization man-agement should try to correct for individual-level biases against safety in order to reduce frequency of unsafe behavior; that is, they should generate safety policies, procedures, and practices in order to communicate organizational-level expectations of behaving safely, and to correct for the natural bias against safety. These perceptions of safety procedures, practices, and policies are defined as organizational safety climate (Zohar, 1980, 2010). Employees behave according to these perceptions, and middle managers also perceive them. Middle managers' behavior is related to safety practices that are also perceived by the employees as group-level climate. Due to individual differences between managers such as personality and values, some department managers may execute organizational policies and procedures differently from others, and communicate different levels of climate to their employees.

In regard to **measurement** of safety climate: it is assessed by aggregating individual perceptions to the required unit of analysis. *Climate level* (average of the climate percep-tions of group members), captures the "sense of imperative" – the perceived importance of safety to members of the group. The second safety climate measure, *climate strength*, represents homogeneity within a unit in regard to the importance of safety, and is often calculated by means of various homogeneity measures such as intra-class correlation (ICC1, ICC2: James, 1982), within-group correlation (e.g., James, Demaree, & Wolf, 1984, 1993), and standard deviation (Schneider, Salvaggio, & Subirats, 2002). The con-cept of climate strength is based on the classical notion of situational strength (Mischel, 1976), which has received renewed interest (Meyer, Kuenzi, & Greenbaum, 2010). Each level of analysis has its own safety climate level and agreement regarding this level. An accepted model of typology of composition models is that of Chan (1998). His refer-ent-shift consensus model is frequently used to explain multilevel climate phenomena (Kozlowski & Klein, 2000). The model suggests that employees can form and share con-current climate perceptions concerning both their immediate workgroup (group-level safety climate) and the organization at large (organizational-level safety climate).

Several studies focused on multilevel effects of safety climate in organizations (Jiang, Yu, Li, & Li, 2010; Zohar et al., 2007; Zohar & Luria, 2005, 2010), these studies found meaningful variance between departments within the same organization in group-level climate. In other words, not all groups interpret organizational policies and procedures similarly, giving rise to different group-level safety climates within the same organization. This is important because multilevel studies have demonstrated that organizational-level policies and procedures influence employees' behavior via the mediation of group-level safety climate (Zohar & Luria, 2005) rather than directly. Hence, group-level climate can better predict employees' safety behavior, so that even if organizational-level climate is high, some departments may have lower group-level safety climate in which employees are expected to behave unsafely due to the stronger effect of group-level climate on behavior. The study by Zohar et al. (2007) of health care climate demonstrated that safety is achieved when both unit and hospital climates are high. However, high unit safety climate can compensate for detrimental effects of low hospital (organizational) climate. Jiang et al. (2010) studied group-level safety climate and individual-level outcomes, and found that group-level climate moderates the relationship between employees' knowledge and their safety behavior.

Group-level Safety Climate and its Antecedents

Multilevel safety climate research has indicated that group-level safety climate perceptions emerge in each sub-unit of an organization. It is evident that these group-level climates can differ significantly from the organizational-level climate and from one another. That is, group safety climate is not necessarily aligned with organizational safety climate. Furthermore, it seems that the group-level perceptions have stronger influence on employees' behavior than those at the organizational level. So what creates the homogeneity in safety climate perceptions within groups, and/or heterogeneity between groups within the same organization?

Two main theories are presented in the climate literature of how safety climate emerges within groups. One is the interaction-based theory that processes between group members create shared understandings and safety perceptions (social sense-making). The other is the leadership perspective, suggesting that top-down processes between group leaders and group members (sense-giving) create shared safety perceptions within each group.

Group members' safety sense-making processes

Sense-making is how employees give meaning to their experiences (Klein, Moon, & Hoffman, 2006; Weick, 1993), and is important because the working environment is complex and may include many conflicting signals (Argyris & Schön, 1996). Some of these signals may concern the importance of safety (Zohar & Luria, 2004). Employees need to consider the many incidents they experience, and try to reach conclusions about the relative importance of safety in comparison with other goals. This can be difficult because there may be conflicting pieces of information and gaps between espousals and enactments (Zohar & Hofmann, 2012). For example, it is possible that the espoused priorities in an organization (i.e., written policies and declarations) will state that safety has the highest priority, while the enacted safety priorities (i.e., daily practices) compromise safety in order to improve operational requirements (Paté-Cornell, 1990).

Employees have to deduce a pattern from all these incidents in order to decide about the true priority of safety. Some sense-making processes involve internal individual-level processes (i.e., an employee summarizes the received information and reaches a decision) while others involve processes of social construction in which group members try to interpret confusing signals by interacting with each other (Isabella, 1990; Sackmann, 1991; Weick & Roberts, 1993). This involves creating short narratives of the experienced phenomena (Volkema, Farquhar, & Bergmann, 1996). Studies have shown that employees try to understand the motivation for safety, and differentiate between managerial commitment to employee well-being and compliance with external laws that are important in the understanding of the priority of safety (Luria & Rafaeli, 2008). Discussions within each group/organizational unit about their experiences and their interpretations of these experiences can explain why, in different groups within the same organization, different safety climates and different levels of consensus may emerge (Luria, 2008).

A meta-analysis indicated that group-level processes are central in the emergence of safety climate (Clarke, 2010). Such processes include coordination, cooperation, and communication (Kozlowski & Bell, 2003; Kozlowski & Ilgen, 2006; Stewart, 2006). It seems that there are two possible effects of these social interactions on safety climate. The first is building agreement and shared understanding through communication between group members (emergence of safety climate strength based on sense-making). The second is the effect of frequent interactions concerning the safety level within a group that may, in turn, influence perceptions about the importance of safety for that group (safety climate level). Studies have shown that frequent interaction has positive effects on both safety level in the unit and on its safety climate.

Group members who communicate more about safety are more likely to notice and prevent risks (Hofmann & Morgeson, 1999; Hofmann & Stetzer, 1996). This positive effect is not exclusive to safety-related interactions but can also be seen in group interactions that are not safety-specific. For example, variables that indicate high levels of social interaction between members of a group such as group cohesion, sense of belonging, and sharing information were found to predict safety performance (Zacharatos, Barling, & Iverson, 2005). Group interaction apparently results in improved shared understanding and coordination, both of which are important to safety-performance levels. Furthermore, group members who interact with one another are also likely to discuss safety issues because they are exposed to a risky environment (Tucker, Chmiel, Turner, Hershcovis, & Stride, 2008); and because coworkers are in their proximity when they are performing risky tasks (Roberts & Geller, 1995), it is hardly surprising that this can affect risk-taking (Westaby & Lowe, 2005).

A possible explanation for coworkers' safety protective effect is that of Geller (1991), who suggested the concept of "active caring," defined as actions intended to maintain coworker safety that are generated by caring for the coworker(s). Active caring is more likely to occur in cohesive groups (Geller, Roberts, & Gilmore, 1996); that is, coworkers who interact frequently and care about each other are likely to take safety-related actions (Burt, Howden, Worrall, & Whelan, 2008; Geller, 1991). A number of studies demonstrate that coworkers are influential conveyors of safety information (Laurence, 2005), and express their safety concerns (Tucker et al., 2008). Work groups with strong social support and quality relationships among coworkers were found to have a higher propensity to comply with safety rules (Simard & Marchand, 1997; Yagil & Luria, 2010), which was ultimately conducive to lower accident rates (Iverson & Erwin, 1997; Oliver, Cheyne, Tomás, & Cox, 2002). It is therefore reasonable to assume that in cohesive groups with high levels of interaction, the quality of relationships with coworkers was found to be related to safety climate perceptions (Luria, 2008).

Supervisors' safety sense-giving

Another explanation for the emergence of group-level safety climate is to be found in the first studies that refer to the climate concept, following Kurt Lewin's studies (Lewin, Lippitt, & White, 1939) focusing on the leader as the creator of group climate, and investigating his or her interaction with group members. Several studies connected leadership-related variables with safety climate perceptions and found significant links between different aspects of leadership and safety climate (Barling, Loughlin, & Kelloway, 2002; Clarke, 2006; Kapp, 2012; Luria, 2008, 2010; Thompson et al., 2011; Zohar, 2002b; Zohar & Luria, 2004, 2010; Zohar & Tenne-Gazit, 2008; Wu, Chen, & Li, 2008).

One explanation of how the leader of a group influences the safety climate perception of the group members is by sense-giving. Sense-giving is performed by managers with the intention of affecting the sense-making processes of their employees (Gioia & Chittipeddi, 1991). That is, managers interact with their employees, and frame the situation and the information they communicate to them in order to make the employees understand a situation in a certain way. Studies of sense-making have shown that managers utilize different strategies in order to reinforce their premises in the eyes of their subordinates (Bartunek, Krim, Necochea, & Humphries, 1999; Maitlis, 2005).

It has also been demonstrated that one role of the leader is as mediator between organizational features and subordinates' perceptions (Kozlowski and Doherty, 1989). González-Roma, Peiró, and Tordera (2002) found that by communicating with their followers, group leaders serve as interpretive filters of work-unit events and processes, thus creating similar climate perceptions among their subordinates. Similarly, Kozlowski and Doherty (1989) found that leaders that have close relationships with their subordinates also create stronger climates in their group. Evidence of the effect of the leader on levels of agreement in his/her group was also found in regard to safety climate. Luria (2008) found that transformational leadership is positively correlated with safety climate strength. Clarke and Ward (2006) studied leadership tactics as antecedents of safety climate, and found that leaders create safety climate by consultation, inspirational appeals, and rational persuasion; and that both directly and through the mediating role of safety climate, these tactics predict safety participation of employees.

Leaders do not only create strong safety climate in their group, they also influence the *level* of the climate. This is because group leaders who have a good relationship with their subordinates are genuinely concerned for their well-being, and consequently practice better safety. For example, active caring resists short-term production pressures in order to protect their employees (Paté-Cornell, 1990). Ultimately, therefore, leaders create safer work conditions for subordinates and the high quality of social relationships in the workgroup will promote safety (Geller, 1991) and health (Heaphy & Dutton, 2008).

Luria (2010) found that leaders who create relationships of higher trust with their subordinates also have higher levels of climate in their groups and fewer injuries. Zohar (2002b) found that transformational leadership is positively correlated with safety climate. Wu et al. (2008) reported a link between safety leadership and safety climate. Nielsen, Eid, Mearns, and Larsson (2013) found that authentic leadership is positively correlated with safety climate. Zohar and Luria's (2010) study demonstrated that transformational leaders act as safety "gate keepers" and, in organizations with low safety climate, develop high group safety climate. Apparently, managers with high leadership attributes care for the safety of their subordinates and try to make "safe sense" in their group to create a strong and high safety climate.

Moderators and Mediators of Safety Climate

Using mediation models

Central to climate research is the attempt to reveal the processes in which safety climate emerges and ultimately influences safety performance. Perhaps the most frequently studied process is the basic process that explains the link between safety perceptions and outcomes in the mediation of behavior. Safety climate was thought to influence safety outcomes (injury rate and accidents) in that members of groups with higher safety climate tend to behave more safely which, in turn, reduces the risk of accidents or injuries. Most studies relating to safety climate and behaviors focus on employees' compliance with safety procedures, such as the correct use of personal protective equipment. However, it has been suggested (Marchand, Simard, Carpentier-Roy, & Ouellet, 1998; Neal & Griffin, 1997) that this is only one example of safety behavior and that the subject requires more comprehensive study, for instance of safety participation, which would include behaviors such as helping to teach safety procedures to new crew members, and making safety-related recommendations (Neal & Griffin, 2006).

The two categories of behaviors are aligned with the literature about in-role and extra-role behaviors, also known as organizational citizenship behaviors (Podsakoff, MacKenzie, Paine, & Bacharach, 2000). Safety participation differs from compliance in that it extends beyond regular safety-role requirements (Clarke, 2006). The two categories of behavior are complementary. Organizations need their employees to both comply with safety procedures and to be more involved and proactive in order to avoid injury from the unexpected (Didla, Mearns, & Flin, 2009). Several safety climate studies that had tested the mediation model were aggregated together into meta-analytic studies. For example, Clarke (2006) found support for the link between safety climate and safety behavior (stronger relationships with safety participation than with safety compliance). The study offered only partial support for the mediation model because of weak links between safety climate and accidents. As Clarke explained: "Only prospective designs, in which accidents were measured **after** measurement of safety climate, demonstrated validity generalization" (Clarke, 2006, p. 315). Christian et al. (2009) tested the mediation of safety behavior on the relationship between safety climate and accidents. They aggregated data from 90 samples and found support for the suggested mediation. Safety climate predicted safety compliance and participation, which in turn predicted injuries. This meta-analytic study provided additional interesting comparisons between individual-level safety climate and group safety climate, and found that group safety climate was the strongest predictor of injuries and accidents.

In regard to the link between safety climate and safety outcomes, some studies also attempt to understand the psychological process through which safety climate influences behavior. Several such mediators have frequently been discussed in the literature. Neal and Griffin's (2004) study suggested that safety knowledge and safety motivation are two key variables that explain the link between safety climate and injuries. These variables are based on the theory of performance of Campbell, McCloy, Oppler, and Sager (1993), which explains an individual's performance according to three antecedents: knowledge, skills, and motivation. They suggested that, according to their model, in high safety climate employees understand that safety is important and therefore make more effort to behave safely (motivation) and learn more about safety due to their willingness to learn about it (knowledge). It is hypothesized that employees with safety knowledge and motivation understand how they should behave and are willing to behave safely even when it demands effort. Christian et al. (2009) aggregated all the relevant studies that tested these variables in their meta-analytic study, and found support for the mediation of safety motivation and safety knowledge in the relationship between safety climate and safety behavior.

Morrow and Crum (1998) described the "positive spill-over" process in which employees who perceive high safety climate believe that their managers protect them, and therefore increase their commitment to the organization and work satisfaction. Using meta-analysis Clarke (2010) found that commitment and satisfaction partially mediated the relationship between safety climate and safety behavior.

Thus, most studies and theories regarding the link between safety climate and outcomes suggest a linear model in which safety climate influences behavior which, in turn, influences injuries. These studies also explain the process that links safety climate with behavior. However, it is important to note that these studies are essentially cross-sectional, so that it is difficult to determine causality. For example, Beus et al. (2010) found that injuries were more predictive of safety climate scores than safety climate was predictive of injuries. Beus et al. (2010) demonstrate that although safety climate outcome relationships have been examined in multiple studies, there is still a need to study such relationships with better methodology in order to determine the direction and causality of links between safety climate and outcomes.

Boundary conditions

Several studies have examined boundary conditions for the emergence of climate and the effect of climate on outcomes. Zohar (2002b) found stronger relationships between leadership and group safety climate when safety priorities were high, in that managerial leadership qualities had greater influence on the emergence of high safety climate when they assigned high priority to safety. Zohar and Luria's (2005) multilevel study tested organizational safety climate as antecedent of group safety climate, and found that the level of formalized routine in a group gave rise to a stronger relationship between organizational and group safety climate levels. Organizational safety climate level and strength were shown to predict group safety climate level and strength (respectively), and routinization–formalization moderated both the multilevel relationship and the two climate levels and the two climate strengths. In a different study, Zohar and Luria (2010) found that transformational leadership moderated the relationship between organizational and group climates (concerning both level and strength). Results indicated that, under low level of organizational climate, transformational leaders promoted higher group climate level as compared with that of organizational climate level. Similarly, under weak organizational climate strength, transformational leaders promoted stronger group climate strength, reflecting greater consensus among group members. Zohar and Luria (2004) also found that a managerial safety script emphasizing the priority of safety is especially important as a safety climate antecedent under low levels of leadership and can correct for low leadership ability. Thus, even leaders with low leadership abilities can facilitate high levels of safety climate if they are oriented toward safety.

Other researchers identified moderators in the link between safety climate and outcomes. For example, Hoffman and Mark's (2006) study of the health industry indicated the moderating effect of patient complexity on the link between safety climate and two safety outcomes (medical errors and back injuries). It seems that safety climate safeguards strongly against incidents in conditions of high patient complexity, and less strongly in conditions of low patient complexity. Earlier studies of safety climate as a multidimensional concept pointed to yet another moderator. Katz-Navon, Naveh, and Stern (2005) found that perceived priority of safety moderated the relationship between managerial safety practices and errors in treatment (see also for explanations of the multi-dimensional approach). The perceived practices of unit managers are especially important in situations in which employees perceive low safety priority in their unit. Clarke's (2006) meta-analytic study aggregated data from 35 studies, and revealed that the study design moderated the relationship between safety climate and accident involvement, that is only prospective designs in which accidents were measured **after** measurement of safety climate, demonstrated validity generalization.

Multiple Group-level Climates and their Effects on Safety

Safety climate is a facet-specific climate perceived by employees in their work group. It is also important to consider other climates that may also influence safety-related outcomes. Yagil and Luria (2010) classify facet-specific climates into two main groups: the first consists of climates that are primarily designed to enhance employee performance for the profitability of the organization, by emphasizing a desired element of performance including, among others, productivity (Patterson, Warr, & West, 2004), service (Schneider et al., 2009), initiative (Baer & Frese, 2003), quality (Luria, 2008), and goal orientation (Gonzalez-Roma et al., 2002). The second category includes climates that focus on employee well-being, among which are safety (Zohar, 2010), psychological safety (Baer & Frese, 2003), supervisory support (Bacharach & Bamberger, 2007), coworker support (Bacharach, Bamberger, & Feigin-Vashdi, 2005), sharing concerns (Kossek, Colquitt, & Noe, 2001), and justice (e.g., Mayer, Nishii, Schneider, & Goldstein, 2007; Naumann & Bennett, 2000; Spell & Arnold, 2007). Schneider, Smith, Taylor, and Fleenor (1998) distinguished between foundational and facet-specific climates, explaining that some climates are more fundamental than others because they reflect basic contextual factors concerning resource-availability for performing the work, and managerial relationships with employees that may be related to various facet-specific climates. They proposed two foundational climates – work facilitation and internal organizational support – that predict facet-specific climate (service climate). The simultaneous existence of several facet-specific climates is relevant because it may affect the importance of a specific facet as perceived by employees. Under the assumption that organizational resources are limited, the relative importance of a facet should be determined not only at its own level but also in comparison to other facets. For example, a unit with high safety climate and low productivity (Patterson et al., 2004) may provide a safer working environment than one that has a similar high safety climate, but also has a high productivity climate. Such logic suggests that some facet-specific climates will interact with safety climate and moderate the relationships between safety climate and outcome. Facet-specific climates emphasize goals that may compete with safety and moderate the safety climate relationship with behavior, such as climates that directly compete with safety such as productivity (Patterson et al., 2004) that encourage employees to work faster. Facets such as quality or service, that are not in direct competition with safety, may also compete for the limited resources and attention of employees (Luria, 2008; Schneider et al., 2009).

Zohar and Hofmann (2012) present two additional theoretical models of how multiple climates coexist in organizations. The first is that each climate may independently affect employee behavior without interaction or relationship with other climates. For example, safety climate may give employees a sense of the importance of safety, and that safety behavior will be rewarded. Concurrently, psychological safety climate (Baer & Frese, 2003) may increase awareness about safety issues and hazard identification, which may also have a direct effect on the safety level of the unit.

The other theoretical model of relationships between climates is the causal relationship, in which one climate facet relates to another, leading to an outcome, that is, a mediation process. Wallace, Popp, and Mondore (2006) found that organizational support climate predicted safety climate which, in turn, mediated the relationship between organizational support and occupational accidents. Wallace et al. (2006) suggested that organizational support (and management–employee relations) are foundation climates conducive to safety climate. In units with high-foundation climates, greater care for the well-being of employees is expected. This may, in turn, evoke commitment to employees' safety and to safety climate. Other climates that can also be regarded as foundation climates include supervisory support (Bacharach & Bamberger, 2007), coworker support (Bacharach et al., 2005), and sharing concerns (Kossek et al., 2001), and should also create an atmosphere that enhances safety climate.

Context-specific Safety Climate: The Example of Road Safety

Tailored safety climate scales should be developed for specific contexts (Luria et al. 2014; Zohar, 2010). An example of this is "road safety climate." This is an important aspect of safety because of the large number of employees injured on the roads. The United States National Highway Traffic Safety Administration report of 2003 states that motor vehicle crashes cost employers $60 billion annually in medical care, legal expenses, property damage, and lost productivity. The 2013 IOSH statistics indicate that a large proportion of road casualties involve people driving in the course of their work, so that improving work-related road safety (WRRS) is vital.

Several papers have focused on organizational influences on road safety climate (Huang et al., 2013; Strahan et al., 2008; Wills, Watson, & Biggs, 2006, 2009; Zohar, Huang, Lee, & Robertson 2014). The road safety climate scale can measure safety climate in organizations or specific populations within organizations, to which the general safety climate is not applicable. The major differences between work within an organization and out of the organization is that safety climate scales for factory employees are not relevant in the context of driving. Transportation is a very dangerous occupation: for example, the rate of fatal accidents in the trucking industry is ten times higher than that of accidents among workers within an organization (US Bureau of Labor Statistics, 2012).

Road safety climate is a good predictor of road safety outcomes. The study by Wills et al. (2006) of road safety climate shows that it predicts employees' reports of work-related driving behaviors. Zohar et al. (2014) demonstrated the relationship between road safety climate and objective measures of driving behavior, using GPS-based truck deceleration data that measured the frequency of hard-braking (i.e., traffic "near-misses"). Their results indicated that road safety climate perceptions predicted hard-braking events. Huang et al. (2013) demonstrated predictive validity for the road safety climate variable, correlating it with self-reported driving safety behaviors and objective safety-performance measures of road injuries. Their study also supported the need for a more specific scale for road safety because the more-specific items offered stronger predictive value.

Road safety climate also predicts self-reported fatigue, near misses (Strahan et al., 2008), and safety motivation, which means greater investment of effort in driving safely (Newman et al., 2008). However not all the studies found significant correlations among all the variables. Indeed, some found no correlation with self-reported accidents and near misses (Morrow & Crum, 2004). These studies demonstrate that the safety climate measure is also valid for the specific case of road safety. The results align with several meta-analyses (Beus et al., 2010; Christian et al., 2009; Nahrgang et al., 2011) demonstrating the validity of the safety climate variable in organizations. Hundreds of studies, mostly of manufacturing industries, in which employees work within the border of an organization supervised by managers and other organizational safety personnel were analyzed. The results indicate that safety climate is also applicable in the specific context of transportation, in which climate predicts road safety behavior beyond the boundaries of an organization.

Supervisory Intervention and Improvement of Safety Climate

Climate modifies methods of improving safety in organizations because it focuses on perceptions. Managerial interventions that focus on improvement of group safety practices are likely to impact strongly on safety outcomes. Initially, climate theory was intended to explain the psychology of employees' safety behaviors. In numerous studies, safety climate was also shown to be a good predictor of safety outcomes, and ultimately to have the ability to control and change those outcomes in intervention studies. Several studies of managerial intervention provide support to climate theory by demonstrating that manipulation and improvement of group-level climate also improves safety climate and safety outcomes.

Climate theory provided a new approach to the field of safety intervention. Essentially, safety interventions were formerly based on the individual-level economic aspect known as "behavioral safety" (Geller et al. 1996; Krispin & Hantula, 1996; Lebbon, Sigurdsson, & Austin, 2012; McAfee & Winn, 1989; Myers, McSween, Medina, Rost, & Alvero, 2010; O'Hara, Johnson, & Beehr, 1985; see also Geller & Robinson, Chapter 14, this volume). Behavioral safety interventions focus on employees and modify their safety behavior by offering short-term rewards intended to outweigh the immediate costs of behaving safely. This is the "antecedent–behavior–consequence" (ABC) framework in regard to safety behavior (Luthans & Kreitner, 1985; Stajkovic & Luthans, 1997); employees are offered antecedents such as safety training and goals, and the approach is based on cost–benefit analyses of safe behavior (as described in the first section of this chapter).

The climate approach also suggests that top-down processes of sense giving from managers to employees influence how employees make sense and understand the importance of safety in their group (Zohar, 2010). Based on this theory, it is possible that by influencing the behavior of supervisors, the safety climate perceptions and safety behaviors of employees will change. This has been demonstrated in a number of studies (Luria et al., 2008; Zohar, 2002a; Zohar & Luria, 2003; Zohar & Polachek, 2014).

Interventions have focused on modifying the safety practices of middle managers and encouraging them to increase monitoring and interactions with employees regarding safety (feedback, training). Several studies (Luria et al., 2008; Zohar, 2002a; Zohar & Luria, 2003) measured the proportion of middle-managers' safety interactions with employees, using experience sampling methodology (ESM) with short questionnaires to collect factual data at random times during the workday, concerning work activities and work-related interactions (Alliger & Williams, 1993). The researchers then provided feedback to the managers about their levels of safety interaction with employees. Results indicated that this intervention increased the number of safety interactions between managers and their employees, and that safety climate levels were higher after the intervention, so that unsafe behaviors of employees decreased accordingly.

A study by Zohar and Polachek (2014) demonstrated that such interventions not only improve safety climate and safety behavior, but also decrease subjective workload and improve teamwork and (independently measured) safety audit scores. Luria et al. (2008) examined the boundary conditions of such interventions. Their results demonstrate that interventions are more effective in good visibility conditions than in poor visibility conditions. That is, because interventions are based on daily interactions between managers and employees, when a manager does not see his/her employees, monitoring and providing accurate feedback can be problematic.

Future Research

Studies presented in this chapter suggest that safety climate exists in organizations and in smaller groups, although the climate literature to date has focused mainly on the organizational level of analysis, demonstrating that groups within organizations provide stronger effects on employee behavior (see Guediri & Griffin, Chapter 13, this volume). A study also found evidence for safety climate in groups that are not part of a formal organizational structure, and introduced the family-level road safety climate (Taubman-Ben-Ari &

Katz-Ben-Ami, 2012). The study demonstrated that informal safety practices within the family – communication about safety, feedback, and reactions to safe and unsafe behaviors – and the behavior and role-model of parents create shared perceptions within the family about the importance of safety. Similarly, Luria, Boehm, and Mazor (2014) demonstrate that the community is also an informal group in which safety climate perceptions can emerge. It is important to expand the perspective of group safety climate by studying safety climate in informal groups because safety behavior also occurs when individuals are *not* actually working at their job. Many employees do not drive at/for work, so that organizational influence on their driving behavior is limited, and understanding the influence of informal groups outside formal organizational units is important in order to predict such behaviors.

Several intervention programs for increasing the frequency of safety-related interactions in organizations also target the participation of employees as well as that of managers. Erev et al. (2010) demonstrated that safety behavior can be improved if team members gently reprimand their coworkers each time they deviate from the safety norm. Similarly, Luria and Morag (2012) demonstrated that when employees and managers participate in safety tours, safety behavior is improved. A study of a participative-ergonomics intervention demonstrates the potential of employees and managers being involved in detecting and correcting ergonomic risks in their organization (Morag & Luria, 2013). These interventions were shown to improve safety behaviors but did not control for safety climate scores. It is also possible that group-level climate may be improved by initiating interactions between employees themselves, and not just with managers (due to the sense-making processes mentioned earlier in this chapter). It is important to note that these studies have not yet been widely replicated, so that these effects may be context-specific, that is national or regional.

Most studies of safety climate and safety behavior are at a single level of analysis. Studies at the multiple level have demonstrated the importance of multilevel perspectives, but are still rare due to the complexity of such analyses. Christian et al. (2009) aggregated some 100 samples in their meta-analytic study focusing on predictors of safety outcomes in the workplace. Only two of these samples had a multilevel perspective. Furthermore, some 80 percent of the papers focused on the individual level of analysis, about 15 percent on the group level, and less than 10 percent on the organizational level. Similarly, more than 80 percent of Clarke's (2006) meta-analyses of the link between safety climate and safety outcomes were at the individual level. Today, as more statistical tools and procedures for analyzing multilevel data are available, based on previously discovered significant effects, future studies should endeavour to improve understanding of integrative models that comprise analyses of organizational group-level effects together with individual-level variables. Future research should try to avoid the methodological limitations that frequently appear in many of the climate studies mentioned in this chapter, and adopt a longitudinal design using multiple sources and objective data.

Most climate studies point to direct relationships between climate and outcomes, while others also relate to processes with mediation models. Fewer studies have related to boundary conditions. There is a need to test the moderators between climate and its outcomes. Furthermore, methodological tools proposed by Edwards and Lambert (2007) use a bootstrap procedure to test the indirect effects of interaction (Edwards & Lambert, 2007; MacKinnon, Fairchild, & Fritz, 2007; Preacher, Rucker, & Hayes, 2007), which enables testing mediation and moderation together. This non-parametric procedure estimates effect sizes and constructs bias-corrected confidence intervals from 1000 random samples. This method allows comparisons between several mediators in the same model (e.g., between motivation and knowledge in the prediction of behavior) as well as testing moderated mediation (e.g., the interaction between safety climate and productivity climate as an independent variable, predicting both behavior as a mediator and, eventually, injuries). The different variables can thus be integrated into a statistical model that will shed light on a wider picture.

Conclusion

This review is summarized in Figure 16.1, though it is difficult to integrate all the variables in a single model. I have, however, tried to position all central variables in the model in the most logical places. It is important to note that a specific variable may also have been tested in another position in the climate literature (e.g., a variable presented as a mediator has been tested as a moderator elsewhere). However, it is my belief that the model below best illustrates the logic of this chapter.

The model presents the processes and variables that contribute to the emergence of group safety climate (above the group safety climate variable) and the outcomes of safety climate (below). Initially, organizational influences are perceived differently in each group due to sense-making and sense-giving processes that contribute to the emergence of safety climate. These perceptions influence individual members of the group by modifying the safety motivation and knowledge levels that determine their safety behavior. Ultimately, frequency of unsafe behavior leads to safety outcomes such as injuries and accidents.

The model also includes moderators that set boundary conditions for direct effects in the model. For example, the relationship between organizational and group safety climate can be moderated by routine formalization in the organization, leadership qualities of

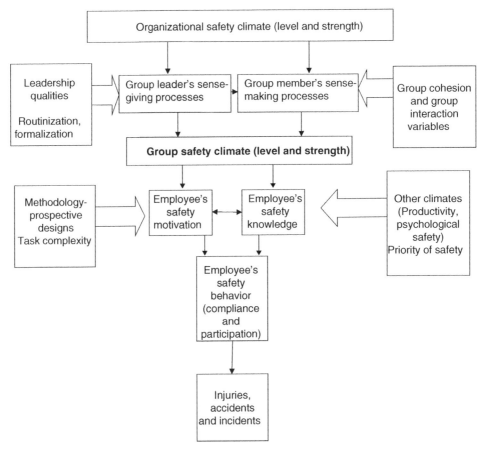

Figure 16.1 Conceptual model for safety climate.

group leaders, and cohesion of the group. The influence of group-level climate on behavior may be moderated by the level of competing climate facets such as productivity, by methodological design issues, and by the priorities of safety and task complexity.

The model does not represent the intervention studies described in the chapter, but its logic can be the foundation for managerial interventions that aim to change sensegiving processes in each group in order to influence the safety climate and eventually decrease the number of injuries and accidents. Nor does it include the informal group levels described in the chapter (family and community). Future multilevel studies should attempt to integrate safety influences from such informal groups with organizational and departmental influences, in order to understand how such influences contribute to the safety behavior of the individual.

References

Alliger, G. M., & Williams, K. J. (1993). Using signal-contingent experience sampling methodology to study work in the field: A discussion and illustration examining task perception and mood. *Journal of Occupational Psychology, 46*(3), 1–18.

Argyris, C., & Schon, D. A. (1996). *Organizational learning II: Theory, method, and practice.* Boston, MA: Addison-Wesley.

Bacharach, S., & Bamberger, P. (2007). Organizational context and post-event distress: 9/11 and the New York City firefighters. *Academy of Management Journal, 50*, 849–868.

Bacharach, S., Bamberger, P., & Feigin-Vashdi, D. (2005). Diversity and homophily at work: Supportive relations among White and African-American peers. *Academy of Management Journal, 48*(4), 619–644.

Baer, M., & Frese, M. (2003). Innovation is not enough: Climates for initiative and psychological safety, process innovations, and firm performance. *Journal of Organizational Behavior, 24*(1), 45–68.

Barling, J., Loughlin, C., & Kelloway, E. K. (2002). Development and test of a model linking safety-specific transformational leadership and occupational safety. *Journal of Applied Psychology, 87*(3), 488–496.

Barron, G., & Erev, I. (2003). Small feedback based decisions and their limited correspondence to description based decisions. *Journal of Behavioral Decision Making, 16*(3), 215–233.

Bartunek, J., Krim, R., Necochea, R., & Humphries, M. (1999). Sensemaking, sensegiving, and leadership in strategic organizational development. In J. Wagner (Ed.), *Advances in qualitative organizational research* (vol. 2, pp. 37–71). Greenwich, CT: JAI Press.

Beus, J., Payne, S., Bergman, M., & Arthur, W. (2010). Safety climate and injuries: An examination of theoretical and empirical relationships. *Journal of Applied Psychology, 95*(4), 713–727.

Bureau of Labor Statistics (2012). Census of fatal occupational injuries (CFOI) – Current and revised data. http://www.bls.gov/iif/oshcfoi1.htm (accessed June 14, 2015).

Burt, T. P., Howden, N. J. K., Worrall, F., & Whelan, M. J. (2008). Importance of long-term monitoring for detecting environmental change: Lessons from a lowland river in south east England. *Biogeosciences, 5*(3), 1529–1535.

Campbell, J. P., McCloy, R. A., Oppler, S. H., & Sager, C. E. (1993). A theory of performance. In N. Schmit & W. C. Borman (Eds.), *Personnel selection in organizations* (pp. 35–70). San Francisco, CA: Jossey-Bass.

Chan, D. (1998). Functional relations among constructs in the same content domain at different levels of analysis: A typology of composition models. *Journal of Applied Psychology, 83*(2), 234.

Christian, M. S., Bradley, J. C., Wallace, J. C., & Burke, M. J. (2009). Workplace safety: A meta-analysis of the roles of person and situation factors. *Journal of Applied Psychology, 94*(5), 1103.

Clarke, S. (2006). The relationship between safety climate and safety performance: A meta-analytic review. *Journal of Occupational Health Psychology, 11*(4), 315–327.

Clarke, S. (2010). An integrative model of safety climate: Linking psychological climate and work attitudes to individual safety outcomes using meta-analysis. *Journal of Occupational and Organizational Psychology, 83*(3), 553–578.

Clarke, S., & Ward, K. (2006). The role of leader influence tactics and safety climate in engaging employees' safety participation. *Risk Analysis, 26*(5), 1175–1185.

Didla, S., Mearns, K., & Flin, R. (2009). Safety citizenship behaviour: A proactive approach to risk management. *Journal of Risk Research, 12*(3–4), 475–483.

Edwards, J. R., & Lambert, L. S. (2007). Methods for integrating moderation and mediation: General analytical framework using moderated path analysis. *Psychological Methods, 12*(1), 1–22

Erev, I. (1998). Signal detection by human observers: A cut-off reinforcement learning model of categorization decisions under uncertainty. *Psychological Review, 105*(2), 280–298.

Erev, I., Rodensky, D., Levi, M. A., England-Hershler, M., Admi, H., & Donchin, Y. (2010). The value of "gentle reminder" on safe medical behavior. *Quality and Safety in Health Care, 19*(49), 1–3.

Flin, R., Mearns, P., O'Connor, P., & Bryden, R. (2000). Measuring safety climate: Identifying the common features. *Safety Science, 34*(1–3), 177–192.

Geller, E. S. (1991). The buckle-up promise card: A versatile intervention for large-scale behavior change. *Journal of Applied Behavior Analysis, 24*(1), 91–94.

Geller, E. S., Roberts, D. S., & Gilmore, M. (1996). Predicting propensity to activity care for occupational safety. *Journal of Safety Research, 27*, 1–8.

Gioia, D. A., & Chittipeddi, K. (1991). Sensemaking and sensegiving in strategic change initiation. *Strategic Management Journal, 12*(6), 433–448.

González-Roma, V., Peiró, J. M., & Tordera, N. (2002). An examination of the antecedents and moderator influences of climate strength. *Journal of Applied Psychology, 87*(3), 465–473.

Guldenmund, F. W. (2000). The nature of safety culture: A review of theory and research. *Safety Science, 34*(1–3), 215–257.

Heaphy, E. D., & Dutton, J. E. (2008). Positive social interactions and the human body at work: Linking organizations and physiology. *Academy of Management Review, 33*(1), 137–162.

Herrnstein, R. J., Loewnstein, G. F., Prelec, D., & Vaughan, W. (1993). Utility maximization and melioration: Internalities in individual choice. *Journal of Behavioral Decision Making, 6*(3), 149–185.

Hertwig, R., & Erev, I. (2009). The description–experience gap in risky choice. *Trends in Cognitive Sciences, 13*(12), 517–523.

Hoffman, D., & Mark, B. (2006). An investigation of the relationship between safety climate and medication errors as well as other nurse and patient outcomes. *Personnel Psychology, 59*(4), 847–869.

Hofmann, D. A., & Morgeson, F. P. (1999). Safety-related behavior as a social exchange: The role of perceived organizational support and leader–member exchange. *Journal of Applied Psychology, 84*(2), 286–296

Hofmann, D. A., & Stetzer, A. (1996). A cross-level investigation of factors influencing unsafe behaviors and accidents. *Personnel Psychology, 49*(2), 307–339.

Huang, Y. H., Zohar, D., Robertson, M. M., Garabet, A., Murphy, L. A., & Lee, J. (2013). Development and validation of safety climate scales for mobile remote workers using utility/electrical workers as exemplar. *Accident Analysis & Prevention, 59*, 76–86.

IOSH (2013) http://www.iosh.co.uk/roadsafety (accessed May 23, 2015).

Isabella, L. A. (1990). Evolving interpretations as a change unfolds: How managers construe key organizational events. *Academy of Management Journal, 33*(1), 7–41.

National Safety Council (NSC) (1999). Injury facts 1999 edition (pp. 9–12). Itasca, IL: National Safety Council.

Iverson, R. D., and Erwin, P. J. (1997). Predicting occupational injury: The role of affectivity. *Journal of Occupational and Organizational Psychology, 70*(2), 113–128

James, L. R. (1982). Aggregation bias in estimates of perceptual agreement. *Journal of Applied Psychology, 67*(2), 219–229.

James, L. R., Demaree, R. G., & Wolf, G. (1984). Estimating within-group interrater reliability with and without response bias. *Journal of Applied Psychology, 69(1)*, 85–98.

James, L. R., Demaree, R. G., & Wolf, G. (1993). Rwg: An assessment of within-group inter-rater agreement. *Journal of Applied Psychology, 78*(2), 306–309.

Jiang, L., Yu, G., Li, Y., & Li, F. (2010). Perceived colleagues' safety knowledge/behavior and safety performance: Safety climate as a moderator in a multilevel study. *Accident Analysis & Prevention, 42*(5), 1468–1476.

Kapp, E. A. (2012). The influence of supervisor leadership practices and perceived group safety climate on employee safety performance. *Safety Science, 50*(4), 1119–1124.

Kath, L. M., Marks, K. M., & Ranney, J. (2010). Safety climate dimensions, leader–member exchange, and organizational support as predictors of upward safety communication in a sample of rail industry workers. *Safety Science, 48*(5), 643–650.

Katz-Navon, T., Naveh, E., & Stern, Z. (2005). Safety climate in health care organization: A multi-dimensional approach. *Academy of Management Journal, 45*(6), 1075–1089.

Klein, G., Moon, B., & Hoffman, R. R. (2006). Making sense of sensemaking 1: Alternative perspectives. *Browse Journals & Magazines, 21*(4), 70–73.

Kossek, E. E., Colquitt, J. A., & Noe, R. A. (2001). Caregiving decisions, well-being, and performance: The effects of place and provider as a function of dependent type and work–family climates. *Academy of Management Journal, 44*(1), 29–44.

Kozlowski, S. W. J., & Bell, B. S. (2003). Work groups and teams in organizations. In W. C. Borman, D. R. Ilgen, & R. J. Klimoski (Eds.), *Handbook of psychology: Industrial and organizational psychology* (vol. 12, pp. 333–375). New York, NY: John Wiley and Sons, Inc.

Kozlowski, S. W. J., & Doherty, M. L. (1989). Integration of climate and leadership: Examination of a neglected issue. *Journal of Applied Psychology, 74*(4), 546–553.

Kozlowski, S., & Ilgen, D. (2006). Enhancing the effectiveness of work groups and teams. *Psychological Science in the Public Interest, 7*(3), 77–123.

Kozlowski, S. W. J., & Klein, K. J. (2000). A multilevel approach to theory and research in organizations: Contextual, temporal, and emergent processes. In K. J. Klein & S. W. J. Kozlowski (Eds.), *Multilevel theory, research and methods in organizations: Foundations, extensions, and new directions* (pp. 3–90). San Francisco, CA: Jossey-Bass.

Krispin, J. & Hantula, D. A. (1996). A meta-analysis of behavioral safety interventions in organizations, *Proceedings of the 1996 annual meeting of the Eastern Academy of Management*. Philadelphia, PA.

Kuenzi, M., & Schminke, M. (2009). Assembling fragments into a lens: A review, critique, and a proposed research agenda for the organizational work climate literature. *Journal of Management, 35*. doi:10.1177/0149206308330559

Laurence, D. (2005). Safety rules and regulations on mine sites – the problem and a solution. *Journal of Safety Research, 36*(1), 39–50.

Lebbon, A., Sigurdsson, S. O., & Austin, J. (2012). Behavioral safety in the food services industry: Challenges and outcomes. *Journal of Organizational Behavior Management, 32*(1), 44–57.

Lewin, K., Lippitt, R., & White, R. K. (1939). Patterns of aggressive behavior in experimentally created social climates. *Journal of Social Psychology, 10*(2), 271–299.

Luria, G. (2008). Climate strength: How leaders form consensus. *Leadership Quarterly, 19*(1), 42–53.

Luria, G. (2010). The social aspect of safety management: Trust and safety climate. *Accident Analysis and Prevention, 42*(4), 1288–1295.

Luria, G., Boehm, A., & Mazor, T. (2014). Conceptualizing and measuring community road safety climate. *Safety Science, 70*, 288–294.

Luria, G., & Morag, I. (2012). Safety management by walking around (SMBWA): A safety intervention program based on both peer and manager participation. *Accident Analysis and Prevention, 45*, 248–257.

Luria, G., & Rafaeli, A. (2008). Testing safety commitment in organizations through interpretations of safety artifacts. *Journal of Safety Research, 39*(5), 519–528.

Luria, G., Yagil, D., & Gal, I. (2014). Quality and productivity: Role conflict in the service context. *Service Industries Journal, 34*(12), 955–973.

Luria, G., Zohar, D., & Erev, I. (2008). The effect of workers' visibility on effectiveness of leadership development programs: The case of supervisory based safety interventions. *Journal of Safety Research, 39*(3), 273–280.

Luthans, F., & Kreitner, R. (1985). *Organizational behavior modification and beyond*. Glenview, IL: Scott, Foresman.

MacKinnon, D. P., Fairchild, A. J., & Fritz, M. S. (2007). Mediation analysis. *Annual Review of Psychology, 58*, 593–614.

Maitlis, S. (2005). The social processes of organizational sensemaking. *Academy of Management Journal, 48*(1), 21–49.

Marchand, A., Simard, M., Carpentier-Roy, M. C., & Ouellet, F. (1998). From a unidimensional to a bidimensional concept and measurement of workers' safety behavior. *Scandinavian Journal of Work, Environment & Health, 2*(4), 293–299.

Mayer, D., Nishii, L., Schneider, B., & Goldstein, H. (2007). The precursors and products of justice climates: Group leader antecedents and employee attitudinal consequences. *Personnel Psychology, 60*(4), 929–963.

McAfee, R. B., & Winn, A. R. (1989). The use of incentives/feedback to enhance workplace safety: A critique of the literature. *Journal of Safety Research, 20*(1), 7–19.

Meyer, D. M., Kuenzi, M., & Greenbaum, R. L. (2010). Examining the link between ethical leadership and employee misconduct: The mediating role of ethical climate. *Journal of Business Ethics, 95*(1), 7–16

Mischel, W. (1976). *Introduction to personality* (2nd edn.). New York, NY: Holt, Rinehart, & Winston.

Morag, I., & Luria, G. (2013). A framework for performing workplace hazard and risk analysis: A participative ergonomics approach. *Ergonomics, 56*(7), 1086–1100.

Morrow, P. C., & Crum, M. R. (1998). The effects of perceived and objective safety risk on employee outcomes. *Journal of Vocational Behavior, 53*(2), 300–314.

Morrow, P. C., & Crum, M. R. (2004). Antecedents of fatigue, close calls, and crashes among commercial motor-vehicle drivers. *Journal of Safety Research, 35*(1), 59–69.

Myers, W., McSween, T. E., Medina, R. E., Rost, K., & Alvero, A. M. (2010). The implementation and maintenance of a behavioral safety process in a petroleum refinery. *Journal of Organizational Behavior Management, 30*(4), 285–307.

Nahrgang, J. D., Morgeson, F. P., & Hofmann, D. A. (2011). Safety at work: A meta-analytic investigation of the link between job demands, job resources, burnout, engagement, and safety outcomes. *Journal of Applied Psychology, 96*(1), 71–94

Naumann, S. E., & Bennett, N. (2000). A case for procedural justice climate: Development and test of a multilevel model. *Academy of Management Journal, 43*(5), 881–889.

Neal, A., & Griffin, M. A. (1997). Perceptions of safety at work developing a model to link organizational safety climate and individual behavior. *Journal of Occupational Health Psychology, 5*(3), 347–358.

Neal, A., & Griffin, M. A. (2004). Safety climate and safety at work. In J. Barling, & M. R. Frone (Eds.), *The psychology of workplace safety* (pp. 15–34). Washington, DC: American Psychological Association.

Neal, A., & Griffin, M. A. (2006). A study of the lagged relationships among safety climate, safety motivation, safety behavior, and accidents at the individual and group levels. *Journal of Applied Psychology, 91*(4), 946.

Newman, S., Griffin, M. A., & Mason, C. (2008). Safety in work vehicles: A multilevel study linking safety values and individual predictors to work-related driving crashes. *Journal of Applied Psychology, 93*(3), 632–644.

Nielsen, M. B., Eid, J., Mearns, K., & Larsson, G. (2013). Authentic leadership and its relationship with risk perception and safety climate. *Leadership & Organization Development Journal, 34*(4), 308–325.

O'Hara, K., Johnson, C. M., & Beehr, T. A. (1985). Organizational behavior management in the private sector: A review of empirical research and recommendations for further investigation. *Academy of Management Review, 10*(4), 848–864.

Oliver, A., Cheyne, A., Tomás, J. M., & Cox, S. (2002) The effects of organizational and individual factors on occupational accidents. *Journal of Occupational and Organizational Psychology, 75*(4), 473–488.

Ostroff, C., Kinicki, A. J. & Muhammad, R. S. (2012). Organizational culture and climate. In I. B. Weiner, N. W. Schmitt, & S. Highhouse (Eds.), *Handbook of psychology: Industrial and organizational psychology* (vol. 12, pp. 643–676). Hoboken, NJ: John Wiley & Sons, Inc.

Paté-Cornell, M. E. (1990). Organizational aspects of engineering system safety: The case of offshore platforms. *Science, 250*, 1210–1217.

Patterson, M., Warr, P., & West, M. (2004). Organizational climate and company productivity: The role of employee affect and employee level. *Journal of Occupational and Organizational Psychology, 77*(2), 193–216.

Plous, S. (1993). *The psychology of judgment and decision-making.* Philadelphia, PA:Temple University Press.

Podsakoff, P. M., MacKenzie, S. B., Paine, B. J., & Bacharach, D. J. (2000). Organizational citizenship behavior: A critical review of the theoretical and empirical literature and suggestions for future research. *Journal of Management, 26*(3), 513–563.

Preacher, K. J., Rucker, D. D., & Hayes, A. F. (2007). Addressing moderated mediation hypotheses: Theory, methods, and prescriptions. *Multivariate Behavioral Research, 42*(1), 185–227.

Ridley, J., & Channing, J. (2008). *Safety at work* (7th edn.). London, UK: Routledge.

Roberts, D. S., & Geller, E. S. (1995). An "actively caring" model for occupational safety: A field test. *Applied and Preventive Psychology, 4*(1), 53–59.

Sackmann, S. A. (1991). *Cultural knowledge in organizations: Exploring the collective mind.* Newbury Park, CA: Sage.

Schneider, B., Ehrhart, M. G., & Macey, W. A. (2011). Organizational climate research: Achievements and the road ahead. In N. Ashkanasy, C. P. M. Wilderom, & M. F. Peterson (Eds.), *Handbook of organizational culture and climate* (2nd edn., pp. 29–49). Thousand Oaks, CA: Sage.

Schneider, B., Macey, W. H., Lee, W. C., & Young, S. A. (2009). Organizational service climate drivers of the American Customer Satisfaction Index (ACSI) and financial and market performance. *Journal of Service Research, 12*(1), 3–14.

Schneider, B., Salvaggio, A. M., & Subirats, M. (2002). Climate strength: A new direction for climate research. *Journal of Applied Psychology, 87*(2), 220–229.

Schneider, B., Smith, D. B., Taylor, S., & Fleenor, J. (1998). Personality and organizations: A test of the homogeneity of personality hypothesis. *Journal of Applied Psychology, 83*(3), 462–470.

Schulte, M., Ostroff, C., Shmulyian, S., & Kinicki, A. (2009). Organizational climate configurations: Relationships to collective attitudes, customer satisfaction, and financial performance. *Journal of Applied Psychology, 94*(3), 618–634.

Schurr, A., Rodensky, D., & Erev, I. (2014). The effect of unpleasant experiences on evaluation and behavior. *Journal of Economic Behavior & Organization, 106*, 1–9.

Simard, M., & Marchand, M. (1997). Workgroups' propensity to comply with safety rules: The influence of micro-macro organisational factors. *Ergonomics, 40*(2), 172–188.

Spell, C., & Arnold, T. (2007). A multi-level analysis of organizational justice climate, structure and employee mental health. *Journal of Management, 33*(5), 724–751.

Stajkovic, A. D., & Luthans, F. (1997). A meta-analysis of the effects of organizational behavior modification on task performance, 1975–95. *Academy of Management Journal, 40*(5), 1122–1149.

Stewart, G. L. (2006). A meta-analytic review of relationships between team design features and team performance. *Journal of Management, 32*(1), 29–55.

Strahan, E. J., Lafrance, A., Wilson, A. E., Ethier, N., Spencer, S. J., & Zanna, M. P. (2008). Victoria's dirty secret: How sociocultural norms influence adolescent girls and women. *Society for Personality and Social Psychology, 34*(2), 288–301.

Taubman-Ben-Ari, O., & Katz-Ben-Ami, L., (2012). The contribution of family climate for road safety and social environment to the reported driving behavior of young drivers. *Accident Analysis & Prevention, 47*, 1–10.

Thompson, D. N., Hoffman, L. A., Sereika, S. M., Lorenz, H. L., Wolf, G. A., Burns, H. K., Minnier, T. E., & Ramanujam, R. (2011). A relational leadership perspective on unit-level safety climate. *Journal of Nursing Administration, 41*(11), 479–487.

Tucker, S., Chmiel, N., Turner, N., Hershcovis, M.S., & Stride, C.B. (2008). Perceived organizational support for safety and employee safety voice: The mediating role of coworker support for safety. *Journal of Occupational Health Psychology, 13*(4), 319–330.

Volkema, R. J., Farquhar, K., & Bergmann, T. J. (1996). Third-party sensemaking in interpersonal conflicts at work: A theoretical framework. *Human Relations, 49*(11), 1437–1454.

Wallace, J. C., Popp, E., & Mondore, S. (2006). Safety climate as a mediator between foundation climates and occupational accidents: A group-level investigation. *Journal of Applied Psychology, 91*(3), 681–688.

Weick, K. E. (1993). Reprinted from "The collapse of sensemaking in organizations: The Mann Gulch disaster." *Administrative Science Quarterly, 38*, 628–652.

Weick, K. E., & Roberts, K. H. (1993). Collective mind in organizations: Heedful interrelating on flight decks. *Administrative Science Quarterly, 38*, 357–381.

Westaby, J. D., & Lowe, J. K. (2005). Risk taking orientation and injury among youth workers: Examining the social influence of supervisors, coworkers, and parents. *Journal of Applied Psychology, 90*(5), 1297–1305.

Wills, A. R., Watson, B., & Biggs, H. C., (2006). Comparing safety climate factors as predictors of work-related driving behavior. *Journal of Safety Research, 37*(4), 375–383.

Wills, A., Watson, B., & Biggs, H. (2009). An exploratory investigation into safety climate and work-related driving. *Work: A journal of prevention, assessment and rehabilitation, 32*(1), 81–94.

Wu, T. C., Chen, C. H., & Li, C. C. (2008). A correlation among safety leadership, safety climate and safety performance. *Journal of Loss Prevention in the Process Industries, 21*(3), 307–318.

Yagil, D., & Luria, G. (2010) Friends in need: The protective effect of social relationships under low organizational safety climate. *Group and Organization Management, 35*(6), 727–750.

Yechiam, E., Erev, I., & Barron, G. (2006). The effect of experience on using a safety device. *Safety Science, 44*(6), 515–522.

Zacharatos, A., Barling, J., & Iverson, R. (2005) High-performance work systems and occupational safety. *Journal of Applied Psychology, 90*(1), 77–93.

Zohar, D. (1980). Safety climate in industrial organizations: Theoretical and applied implications. *Journal of Applied Psychology, 65*(1), 96.

Zohar, D. (2002a). Modifying supervisory practices to improve subunit safety: A leadership-based intervention model. *Journal of Applied Psychology, 87*(1), 156.

Zohar, D. (2002b). The effects of leadership dimensions, safety climate, and assigned priorities on minor injuries in work groups. *Journal of Organizational Behavior, 23*(1), 75–92.

Zohar, D. (2010). Thirty years of safety climate research: Reflections and future directions. *Accident Analysis and Prevention, 42*(5), 1517–1522.

Zohar, D. (2011). Safety climate: Conceptual and measurement issues. In J. Quick, & L. Tetrick (Eds.), *Handbook of organizational health psychology* (2nd edn., pp. 141–164). Washington, DC: American Psychological Association.

Zohar, D., & Hofmann, D. (2012). Organizational culture and climate. In S. Kozlowski (Ed.), *Handbook of industrial and organizational psychology* (pp. 643–666). New York, NY: Oxford University Press.

Zohar, D., Huang, Y. H., Lee, J., & Robertson, M. (2014). A mediation model linking dispatcher leadership and work ownership with safety climate as predictors of truck driver safety performance. *Accident Analysis & Prevention, 62*, 17–25.

Zohar, D., Livne, Y., Tenne-Gazit, O., Admi, H., & Donchin, Y. (2007). Healthcare climate: A framework for measuring and improving patient safety. *Critical care medicine, 35*(5), 1312–1317.

Zohar, D., & Luria, G. (2003). The use of supervisory practices as leverage to improve safety behavior: A cross-level intervention model. *Journal of Safety Research, 34*(5), 567–577.

Zohar, D., & Luria, G. (2004). Climate as a social-cognitive construction of supervisory safety practices: Testing environmental and social-interaction factors. *Journal of Applied Psychology, 89*(2), 322–333.

Zohar, D., & Luria, G. (2005). A multilevel model of safety climate: Cross-level relationships between organization and group-level climates. *Journal of Applied Psychology, 90*(4), 616.

Zohar, D., & Luria, G. (2010). Group leaders as gatekeepers: Testing safety climate variations across levels of analysis. *Applied Psychology, 59*(4), 647–673.

Zohar, D., & Polachek, T. (2014). Discourse-based intervention for modifying supervisory communication as leverage for safety climate and performance improvement: A randomized field study. *Journal of Applied Psychology, 99*(1), 113.

Zohar, D., & Tenne-Gazit, O. (2008). Transformational leadership and group interaction as climate antecedents: A social network analysis. *Journal of Applied Psychology, 93*(4), 744.

17

Workplace Health Promotion

Arla Day and Thomas Helson

Introduction

Over 17 years ago, Cox (1997) argued that maintaining "health and the quality of life" was one "of the greatest challenges facing society in the next century" (p. 1). Chu et al. (2000) echoed these concerns, and stressed that as "we move into the 21st century the world's population will face enormous challenges to contain health care costs, on the one hand, and improve the quality of life on the other" (p. 166). Given the large presence that work plays in most people's lives, the workplace is a logical venue for addressing this challenge. That is, in efforts to promote physically and psychologically healthy workers, the workplace can play an important role in helping to create healthy behavior change (Conn, Hafdahl, Cooper, Brown, & Lusk, 2009).

Somewhat ironically, much has been written on the negative impact of work on employee health and well-being. Workplace factors, such as poor leadership (Kuoppala, Lamminpää, Liira, & Vainio, 2008) can create and exacerbate ill-health. The negative impact of job stressors on health and burnout has been well documented (Day & Livingstone, 2001; Day, Sibley, Scott, Tallon, & Ackroyd-Stolarz, 2009; Kivimäki et al., 2006; Nixon, Mazzola, Bauer, Krueger, & Spector, 2011; Sonnentag & Frese, 2003). Sustained computer use at work has been associated with upper limb musculoskeletal symptoms for both women and men (e.g., Blatter & Bongers, 2002). Similarly, having low physical job demands (Choi et al., 2010) or any type of sitting for prolonged periods (for a review, see Owen, Healy, Matthews, & Dunstan, 2010) is associated with obesity, low metabolic health, and premature mortality risk (see also O'Driscoll & Roche, Chapter 9; Nielsen et al., Chapter 10, this volume).

Despite these negative associations, given the amount of time spent at work, and given a supportive and collegial environment, work has the potential for being one of the best venues for improving one's mental and physical health. Workplaces have the infrastructure, social support, and motivators necessary for effective behavior change and maintenance.

The Wiley Blackwell Handbook of the Psychology of Occupational Safety and Workplace Health, First Edition. Edited by Sharon Clarke, Tahira M. Probst, Frank Guldenmund, and Jonathan Passmore. © 2016 John Wiley & Sons Ltd. Published 2020 by John Wiley & Sons Ltd.

Conn et al. (2009) argued that compared with programs in a more general social domain, workplace programs have some potential advantages. That is, workplace programs may be more convenient and accessible by employees on a daily basis. There are "existing patterns of formal and informal communication among employees in a worksite" (p. 330) that would aid in implementing and maintaining the programs. Because of existing workplace social networks, group support may be more readily accessible. Finally, organizational culture and behavior norms that are conducive to improved health behaviors may be potentially advantageous (Conn et al., 2009).

Therefore, we need to examine the entirety of workplace health promotion (WHP) by first defining health and health promotion, examining the WHP components, reviewing the literature on the effectiveness of WHP initiatives, and assessing the deterrents and facilitators of implementation, expectations and ethical issues, future research, and methodological issues to move the area forward, both in terms of research and practice. In this chapter, we will focus on psychosocial and physical health, examining both individually focused programs (i.e., cessation of unhealthy behaviors, promotion of healthy behaviors and lifestyles, health screening) and contextual/environmental programs that address health through changing the workplace. This focus is in line with WHP work arguing for a simultaneous application of health protection and health promotion to reduce risk and improve health (Sorensen, 2001). It has been argued, at least implicitly, that WHP should also involve a focus on safety (Hymel et al., 2011). That is, according to the definition of health promotion through the reduction of risk factors and engaging in health-promoting activities, it is feasible to suggest that safety involves both reducing risks and promoting safe activities. Although the inclusion of safety in such a model is essential, in this chapter, we focus on the components of psychological and physical health to avoid duplication with other chapters in this book that address safety in greater detail than would be possible in this chapter.

Workplace Health Promotion Definition and Components

We can view health in terms of physical health, mental health, social functioning, role functioning, and general health perceptions (Ware, 1987). The World Health Organization (WHO) defined health as "a state of complete physical, mental and social well-being and not merely the absence of disease or infirmity" (WHO, 2006, p. 1). Therefore, health promotion can be viewed as an interaction between reducing or avoiding risk factors and engaging in activities that promote health. According to the WHO (2015), health promotion is defined as "the process of enabling people to increase control over, and to improve, their health. It moves beyond a focus on individual behaviors toward a wide range of social and environmental interventions." This definition encompasses two critical elements of health promotion, by emphasizing the importance of both individual and contextual factors on health. Bringing the general health promotion definition into a work environment, we should focus both on the individual worker and the workplace as defining elements in improving or "promoting" worker health.

However, early workplace health promotion (WHP) programs originally focused on a single health concern (Chu et al., 2000), and the view of health promotion (especially in the Western world) focused responsibility to the individual to have "control" over his or her own health (Cox, 1997). These types of health promotion initiatives typically involved helping people quit bad habits or reduce unhealthy lifestyles, and helping people increase healthy lifestyles. Similarly, within this framework, health promotion also would involve screening for potential negative health indicators.

Further to the arguments above, it is equally important to recognize that health promotion can involve changing the environment that creates ill health and creating positive, healthy workplaces that promote well-being and health of employees (Chu et al., 2000; WHO, 2015). In fact, there are several criticisms of solely focusing on an individually oriented approach to stress management. It ignores the influence of adverse working conditions. The focus on individuals as opposed to organizations contravenes OSH legislation, and these types of interventions often fail to achieve any significant long-term health and/or productivity outcomes (Noblet & LaMontagne, 2006).

Therefore, it is important to examine WHP, both in terms of individual and contextual aspects and to distinguish between the target of the promotion efforts (i.e., efforts aimed directly at changing the individual or actions aimed at improving health by changing the environment). Therefore, models need to examine WHP efforts targeting the organization and the individual and aimed at both physical and psychosocial health.

Model of Workplace Health Promotion

Therefore, we should view WHP as a holistic concept, incorporating not only the individual, but also contextual aspects (e.g., the organization as a whole or the specific workplace), such that using a comprehensive approach of both individual and organizational interventions is the most effective at targeting health (Noblet & LaMontagne, 2006). Moreover, many WHP interventions explicitly or implicitly also take the social context into consideration, in terms of group-level processes (Partanen et al., 2002; Sorensen et al., 2011).

The WHP Model identifies these components, in terms of psychological, physical, and behavioral health indicators, and the multi-focus influences (individual, program, and context) of such approaches (see Figure 17.1). WHP initiatives may be characterized as either individual or environment focused. Within the individual focus, the initiatives may be loosely categorized as focusing on: (1) cessation of unhealthy behaviors and lifestyles; (2) promotion of positive health behaviors and lifestyle; and (3) screening. Most of these categories involve a health education component, and it is important to note that many initiatives target behavior change from more than one perspective, thus spanning several categories.

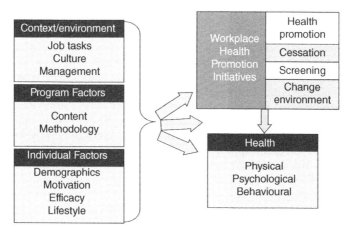

Figure 17.1 Model of workplace health promotion.

Cessation of unhealthy behaviors and lifestyles

Many initiatives have defined WHP in terms of stopping "bad" behaviors and lifestyles, such as smoking and drinking.

Smoking cessation   Given the increase in smoking bans in organizations and in public areas across countries, it is natural that one of the primary cessation programs introduced in organizations would be smoking cessation programs. Cessation programs may involve counseling (e.g., Cruse, Forster, Thurgood, & Sys, 2001); nicotine replacement therapy (e.g., Wallace et al., 2008); feedback, and targeted educational materials (Sorensen et al., 2007).

Although smoking cessation programs tend to have moderate success (Viswesvaran & Schmidt, 1992), counseling in combination with medically based interventions (e.g., nicotine patches) has been shown to be somewhat effective in smoking cessation. For example, using a smoking cessation program that included five one-on-one support and counseling sessions, nicotine replacement therapy (NRT) as well as a non-NRT treatment option, bupropion, approximately 20 percent of the 123 UK workers at GlaxoSmith Kline stopped smoking during a 12-month follow-up (Cruse et al., 2001). Similarly, the point-prevalence-quit rate for 935 US blue-collar workers was 27.5 percent for workers using phone-counseling sessions (25.5 percent for workers in the one-call session and 28.9 percent and for workers in the five-call session; Ringen, Anderson, McAfee, Zbikowski, & Fales, 2002). Sorensen et al. (2007) examined the effects of a tailored phone-based intervention, providing counseling, feedback, and educational materials to 582 construction workers who were members of the Laborers' International Union of North America. Compared with the control group, participants in the tailored intervention group were more likely to quit smoking. In their study examining the effects of a free nicotine replacement therapy for eight weeks on Australian health service staff, Wallace et al. (2008) found that 31 percent of the participants quit smoking. Of the 69 percent of participants who continued to smoke, 85 percent of them reduced their cigarette intake. Other participants in this study reported that nicotine replacement therapy would be an attractive option the next time they attempted to quit (Wallace et al., 2008).

Alcohol consumption   Given the impact of heavy episodic drinking on absenteeism (Bacharach, Bamberger, & Biron, 2010), excessive chronic drinking increases the risk of chronic health problems (e.g., liver, musculoskeletal, and cardiovascular problems; Hanebuth, Meinel, & Fischer, 2006; Jones, Casswell, & Zhang, 1995), and the impact of drinking on workplace safety (Webb et al., 1994), drinking behavior also has been the target of workplace cessation programs. Most of the programs involve educational components, and some have tailored feedback. For example, Doumas and Hannah (2008) designed two interventions to reduce high-risk drinking among 124 youths in five US companies. Both interventions involved a web-based personalized feedback program, and one intervention included an additional 15-minute motivational interviewing session to the web-based personalized feedback program. At the 30-day follow-up, the drinking habits of young workers in both intervention groups were significantly lower than the control group. The program appeared to be most effective for individuals who rated themselves as high-risk drinkers at baseline. The motivational interview did not improve the effectiveness of the web-based feedback program (Doumas & Hannah, 2008), supporting previous findings demonstrating that adding a motivational interview session to feedback does not improve outcomes (Murphy et al., 2004). Therefore, despite the efficacy of motivational interviews in many situations, these results suggest that they may not produce additional positive effects (beyond the effects of feedback) for younger workers.

Similarly, Matano et al. (2007) examined the effectiveness of an interactive web-based intervention aimed at reducing alcohol consumption in 145 moderate- to low-risk drinkers. Participants either received general information about alcohol use and feedback on their own stress levels ("limited" feedback group), or they received specific feedback about their own alcohol use, risks, and their levels of stress, use of coping strategies and risk for alcohol-related problems ("full" feedback group). For the moderate-risk participants, the frequency of beer binges decreased significantly more among the full feedback group (48 percent reduction) than compared with the limited feedback group (13 percent increase). For low-risk participants, the frequency of both beer and hard liquor binges decreased significantly for the full feedback group than compared with the limited feedback group (Matano et al., 2007).

Richmond, Kehoe, Heather, and Wodak (2000) examined the effectiveness of an intervention aimed to reduce excessive alcohol consumption in 1206 Australian postal workers. The intervention involved a four-week lifestyle campaign that was comprised of three components: a health promotion campaign to improve participation and awareness (via flyers about the barriers of participation, slogans, and incentives), employee health assessments (i.e., questionnaire), and brief interventions (i.e., 15 minute advice about the risk of excessive alcohol consumption and how to reduce consumption). The intervention was associated with a significant decrease in alcohol consumption among women, but not among men. Richmond et al. argued the non-significant findings for men may indicate that a stronger intervention is needed, and they also noted there was a large variation in men's drinking habits, which may have contributed to the non-significant findings.

Promotion of positive health behaviors and lifestyle

There is a strong link between positive lifestyle behaviors and overall good health. For example, individuals who engage in low-risk behaviors (e.g., sleeping 7–8 hours/night) tend to have a lower mortality risk factor (Djoussé, Driver, & Gaziano, 2009; Farquhar et al., 1977; Ford, Zhao, Tsai, & Li, 2011). Given these links, and the links between health and organizational outcomes, there has been a proliferation of organizations offering initiatives that focus on promoting healthy behaviors and lifestyles, such as physical health programs, creating space for fitness programs (e.g., yoga at lunch and after work; Hartfiel et al., 2012); promoting social fitness (e.g., competitive team-sports intervention; Staley, 2009); and promoting healthy eating (Plotnikoff, McCargar, Wilson, & Loucaides, 2005).

Yoga can be effective for reducing perceived stress, alleviating back pain, and improving psychological well-being. Gura (2002) argued that the benefits of practicing yoga in the workplace include increased muscle relaxation, and reduced heart rate, breath rate, and blood pressure. In one of the few studies to look at yoga's health effects in the workplace, Hartfiel et al. (2012) examined the ability of a workplace yoga intervention to reduce back pain and improve psychological well-being in 74 British local government workers who were randomized into a yoga group (an eight-week yoga session; DVD for home practice), and a control group (which received no intervention). In comparison to the control group, the yoga group reported significant reductions in perceived stress and back pain, sadness and hostility, and reported substantial improvements in feeling self-assured, attentive, and serene. Yoga also has been used as a means of relieving symptoms of carpal tunnel syndrome (Garfinkel et al., 1998).

In their meta-analysis of workplace physical activity interventions from 1969 to 2007, Conn et al. (2009) found that workplace fitness interventions can increase physical activity of employees, improve both health and workplace outcomes. They concluded that some physical activity interventions are capable of improving both health and worksite outcomes, which can potentially decrease job stress and improve work culture. However, they urged caution in interpreting their results because they had a limited number of studies that had sufficient data to include in the meta-analysis, the actual physical activity interventions varied widely, and they identified measurement issues (e.g., lack of objectively measured physical activity; wide variety in assessment and methodology across studies).

Sorensen et al. (2007) examined the effects of an intervention aimed at improving health behaviors, including increasing fruit and vegetable consumption. Participants in the tailored intervention group, which included telephone counseling, tailored feedback, and targeted educational materials, increased their fruit and vegetable consumption by 1.52 servings/day (p < .001), whereas the control group did not increase consumption. In reviewing three WHP studies from the USA, Canada, and Taiwan, Chan and Perry (2012) suggested that health behavioral interventions for nurses can be successful in weight reduction, improved diet quality, increased activity, reduced blood pressure, and smoking cessation among nursing populations. They noted that all of the interventions involved some sort of motivational support element (e.g., group members, research team, managers), which may be an important component of their success.

Plotnikoff et al. (2005) examined the effect of a program focusing on physical activity and nutrition on 2121 employees from five large workplaces in Alberta, Canada. Participants received two weekly emails that focused on physical activity and nutrition issues for 12 weeks. The control group did not receive e-mails. The intervention group increased their average physical activity level, whereas the control group saw an 11 percent decline. Campbell et al. (2002) examined the effectiveness of two interventions designed to improve the nutrition, physical activity, smoking, and cancer screening of female workers as part of the five-year Health Works for Women (HWW), which focused on rural, blue-collar women working in US manufacturing settings. Both interventions increased fruit and vegetable consumption and rates of exercise.

Despite the effectiveness of some of these programs targeting physical health and fitness, Erfurt, Foote, and Heirich (1992) noted that:

> It is ironic that many of the wellness programs in corporate America today are primarily fitness programs, and rely on the existence of well-equipped and staffed physical fitness facilities to promote healthy behaviors within the workforce. This limited wellness model is quite popular for two basic reasons: (a) the employees perceive the fitness facility as a valuable benefit, even though only a small percentage of employees may actually use the facility on a regular basis ... and (b) the model is easy to implement (though expensive) ... Despite the lack of evidence of effectiveness for this model, it is widely utilized and is high on the "wish list" of many companies that do not have such a fitness center. (pp. 22–23)

Erfurt et al. (1992) examined the effectiveness and annual direct costs of worksite wellness programs across four manufacturing plants. The first site was a "comparison" site, in that it only offered various forms of health education. The second site set up an in-house fitness facility. The third site had both health education and follow-up counseling, and the fourth site had the education, follow-up counseling, and organization-based initiatives (e.g., health events, a walking track, and some fitness equipment). Compared with the first site (offering health education only), programs at the second site were not associated with improved outcomes. However, programs at the last two sites were associated with higher participation in the exercise program, the blood pressure treatment program, the smoking cessation program, and the weight loss program (Erfurt et al., 1992), and they were more cost effective. Erfurt et al. go on to argue that data from their study demonstrated that having a fitness facility, without a "systematic, persistent outreach to employees with health risks and routine long-term follow-up to assist them in making health improvements is not effective in reducing health risks" (Erfurt et al., 1992, p. 23).

In addition to the promotion of physical health, a growing number of organizational initiatives are targeting workers' psychosocial well-being. For example, Goldgruber and Ahrens (2010) reviewed 17 meta-analyses or systematic reviews of health promotion and primary prevention intervention research. They reported that most stress reduction interventions examined tended to be effective. Of these interventions, cognitive behavior interventions were the most effective, and relaxation techniques tended to be the most common. Overall, only 69 percent of interventions were found to be effective. Of the studies reviewed, 91 percent of stress-related interventions were effective, whereas 69–78 percent of physical activity, organizational development interventions, and smoking interventions were effective. Interventions to reduce back pain and ergonomic interventions were effective less than half the time (48 percent; Goldgruber & Ahrens, 2010).

Health screening

In promoting the health and well-being of employees, employers have offered health services to provide education and/or provide screening assessments for several physical conditions, such as high blood pressure; cholesterol screening, spirometry for lung health assessment (Ferguson, Enright, Buist, & Higgins, 2000), cervical and breast cancer screening (Allen, Stoddard, Mays, & Sorensen, 2001), and for receiving general annual physical check-ups.

Screening and education may be important components of WHP initiatives for several reasons. Dunning, Heath, and Suls (2005) argued that people's self perceptions of their risk for health complications are unrealistically optimistic. Most people rate their likelihood of being afflicted by a disease or health problems and other health risks (e.g., cancer or HIV) as being average or less than average (see for example, Ji, Zhang, Usborne, & Guan, 2004; Weinstein, 1987). In a study of 7797 Dow Chemical workers in the USA, Collins et al. (2005) found that 65 percent (the majority of which were office and clerical workers) reported experiencing a chronic condition. Therefore, implementing screening practices may be beneficial, such that workplace screening may provide a standard of (perceived) objectivity to health assessment.

There is some evidence that screening can be effective for both the individual and organization. However, there are varying success rates in these types of programs. For example, Allen et al. (2001) used a random controlled trial with a large number of diverse worksites to examine the effect of a 16-month intervention aimed at increasing prevalence rate of mammograms, clinical breast examinations, and Pap tests in women over the age of 40. Despite the low response rate, they found that women at the intervention worksites (receiving information about screening and positive norms about testing) were more likely to report Pap tests (4.7 percent compared with 1.9 percent in the control groups). However, these rates are still very low, and there were no significant differences between these groups in terms of rates of obtaining mammograms and clinical breast exams.

Other types of screening may be appropriate in organizations. For example, in their review of health programs, Danna and Griffin (1999) noted that cancer screening programs that were combined with at-work educational sessions were shown to be effective not only for early detection but also for prevention of cancer. Ferguson et al. (2000) suggested that organizations offer spirometry (breathing) tests for adult smokers because spirometry may be able to detect Chronic Obstructive Pulmonary Disease before symptoms are prevalent.

Chu et al. (2000) reported on a study conducted by the Shanghai Health Education Institute, involving 21,613 workers in four Shanghai workplaces. Each of the four workplaces implemented and evaluated integrative WHP programs, addressing the organizational, environmental, and behavioral factors specific to their workplace and employees that contributed to poor health. Chu et al. (2000) reported very positive outcomes of these initiatives including: a 50 percent reduction in sick leave; a 10–20 percent reduction in work-related injuries; reduced diseases and related health-care costs; improved health and safety knowledge and practices (including an increase in the use of safety devices from 20–30 percent to 70–90 percent); and reduced risk behavior (e.g., cigarette smoking).

Changing the environment

Cox (1997) argued that the "broader concept of occupational health should both encompass traditional WHP and inject into it a proper concern for context, for organizational factors and for organizational-level prevention" (p. 4). To what extent has this integration and expansion occurred over the past 17 years?

Unfortunately, few studies have examined WHP programs involving environmental changes, and many of the studies that have been conducted have poor methodological quality (Engbers, van Poppel, Chin A Paw, & van Mechelen, 2005). In the stress-reduction literature, when comparing the effectiveness of individual and organizational based interventions to reduce stress, individual-focused interventions tend to be less effective at reducing stress (Caulfield, Chang, Dollard, & Elshaug, 2004) and may have shorter-term results (Giga, Noblet, Faragher, & Cooper, 2003). Therefore, organizational WHP interventions also may be an effective way of improving employee health.

Despite the lack of focus on how changing workplace factors (e.g., physical environment, organizational culture and policies, the social context) can promote workplace health, there has been a lot of research on the impact of organizational factors on employee well-being and health. For example, in a cross-sectional study on workplace flexibility to meet work and family demands and health behaviors (e.g., sleep, physical activity, lifestyle) in 3193 pharmaceutical company employees in the USA, flexibility was related to all of the health behaviors (with the exception of participation in health seminars; Grzywacz, Casey, & Jones, 2007). Major organizational change (e.g., change from being a government to private agency) is associated with significant increases in BMI and blood pressure increases (cf. Ferrie, Shipley, Marmot, Stansfeld, & Smith, 1998). Moreover, anticipation of change, or waiting to be transferred is positively associated with adverse sleep patterns and increases in the amount of people who rated their health as average or worse (Ferrie et al., 1998).

In their review of articles that looked at WHP programs involving environmental changes, Engbers et al. (2005) noted that there is evidence of an effect of organizational change (e.g., increasing availability of healthy products, providing promotional materials in the worksite) on dietary intake. There was inconclusive evidence of the effect of organizational change on physical activity, and there was no evidence of an effect of change on health-risk indicators. However, Engbers et al. argued that because of the lack of studies in this area, and because of the general poor methodological quality of the studies that do exist, the results pertaining to the effects of organizational change on employee health (in terms of dietary intake, physical activity, and health risk indicators) are difficult to interpret. Despite these weak and inconclusive findings, they still suggested that multi-component WHP programs that involve environmental changes may potentially benefit employees (Engbers et al., 2005).

Kahn-Marshall and Gallant (2012) conducted a literature review of peer-reviewed articles from 1995–2010 that focused on environment and/or policy change interventions in the workplace to improve health behaviors (diet and physical activity). They concluded that, in general, studies that implemented only environmental and/or policy changes yielded inconclusive evidence and methodological quality was often poor. They also argued that those studies that implemented both environment and individual health behavior change interventions averaged better methodological quality and were moderately effective in improving employee dietary and physical activity behaviors. Therefore, they would argue that multi-component interventions that targeted both dietary and physical activity behavior change proven to be the most effective form of intervention (Kahn-Marshall & Gallant, 2012).

Although the majority of smoking cessation programs focus on the individual smoker (in terms of education, counseling, providing nicotine patches), it also is important to look at contextual issues, such workplace policies, culture, and environment. For example, Fichtenberg and Glantz (2002) found that smoke-free workplaces lead to a 3.8 percent reduction in the prevalence of smoking, while additionally reducing the amount of cigarettes smoked in continuing smokers by 1.3 (on average) per day, resulting in an overall reduction of 29 percent. Similarly, in their five-year study of the impact of the work environment on smoking in Danish workers, Albertsen, Hannerz, Borg, and Burr (2004) examined the extent to which workplace factors contributed to the likelihood of smoking cessation. Smoking cessation was negatively correlated to noise and physical load and was positively correlated to work with high responsibility and high psychological demands.

Business case for WHP initiatives

To what degree are organizations actually using these WHP initiatives? Chu et al. (2000) argued that WHP is a relatively new concept in Europe: Although some European countries initiated some programs an early as the 1970s, it was not until the European Commission Framework Directive on health and safety in 1989 that the issue was readdressed, giving "rise to a widespread reorientation of occupational safety and health in Europe" (Chu et al., 2000, p. 156). In the 1980s, between 21.1 percent and 37.6 percent of American companies had health promotion programs in place (Danna & Griffin, 1999). In 2006, only 19 percent of companies in the USA with over 500 people offered some sort of wellness program, while in 2008, 77 percent of large manufacturing plants offered a formal health or wellness program (Baicker, Cutler, & Song, 2010). Moreover, 81% of firms offered a health risk assessment for employees, and 31 percent offered added incentives for participating in such programs (Baicker et al., 2010). In a study by the U.S. Department of Health and Human Services (2000; see Linnan et al., 2008), it was proposed that at least 75 percent of US worksites should be offering comprehensive health promotion programs yet only 6.9 percent of respondents did. In studying 873 faculty and staff across the United States, Eaton, Marx, and Bowie (2007) found that almost all schools surveyed offered at least one health promotion activity or service for faculty and staff. However, few schools offered coordinated services within a comprehensive employee wellness program.

Given the interest in WHP initiatives, the apparent effectiveness of some of these programs, coupled with the seemingly low implementation of these programs in organizations, it is interesting as to whether a business case for offering WHP initiatives be established, taking into consideration both impact of WHP initiatives on improved employee health and their financial impact for organizations. Witt, Olsen, and Ablah (2013) suggested that cost is the most significant factor when organizations are deciding to implement and select a health promotion program.

In establishing a business case, the outcomes and costs associated with psychological issues at work need to be examined. Bertera (1991) looked at employee health risks (smoking, excess alcohol consumption, obesity, elevated cholesterol, high blood pressure, lack of seatbelt use, and lack of exercise) from a sample of 45,976 employees from a large industrial organization in the USA. Employees who had at least one of these health risks had significantly higher absenteeism rates (10–32 percent), and they had significantly higher illness costs in terms of compensation, health care, and health care benefits compared with participants with none of these seven health risks. Bertera estimated costs associated with annual excess illness costs in terms of compensation, benefits, health care costs, and absenteeism costs over the past year for each risk factor, ranging from $130 (lack of exercise) to $960 (smoking), and noted that the company's total cost of excess illness was estimated at around $70.8 million dollars a year. In looking at the business case for WHP, Collins et al. (2005) found that employees that reported depression, anxiety, or emotional disorder as a primary condition had the highest total costs per worker per year ($18,864 in 2002; in terms of medical/pharmaceuticals, absenteeism, and work impairment; not just health care costs). Those with allergies had the lowest total cost per worker per year ($6947). In their meta-analysis of 17 studies evaluating the impact of on- or off-site organizational wellness programs, Parks and Steelman (2008) found that overall, participating in an organizational wellness program (fitness or comprehensive) tended to be associated with reduced absenteeism. When comparing the costs due to chronic health conditions, Collins et al. (2005) argued that absenteeism costs the organization $661 per employee, medical care cost $2278, and presenteeism (or work impairment) cost the organization $6721 per employee, emphasizing the importance of measuring presenteeism as well as absenteeism and medical costs.

Unfortunately, as with many attempts to put a dollar amount on organizational programs, the methodology of some studies that purport to examine the business case is lacking. For example, in their review of WHP literature from 1974 to 1986, Warner, Wickizer, Wolfe, Schildroth, and Samuelson (1988) concluded that hypertension control and programs that focused on smoking cessation tended to be cost effective. However, they noted that empirical evidence was noticeably absent in early health promotion literature and that programs did not utilize adequate research designs to support claims.

Several studies have calculated cost estimates and Return On Investment (ROI) information. In their meta-analysis of costs and savings of workplace disease prevention and wellness programs (in terms of health care costs and absenteeism) across 36 studies, Baicker et al. (2010) found the average decline in health care costs and absenteeism was approximately $3.27 and $2.73, respectively, for every dollar spent on employee wellness programs. Ringen et al. (2002) found that the annual cost of their smoking cessation initiative was $1025.28 per smoker who quit (which worked out to $11.78 per full-time employee). They further estimated the compounded savings in reduced medical costs for those who quit (based on reduced smoking across one's lifetime) to be 15 times the cost of the program, for an annual ROI of 27.6 percent for the program. Based on a simulation model to estimate the ROI of workplace obesity interventions using estimated annual savings in health care costs and absenteeism of a US company, Trogdon, Finkelstein, Reyes, and Dietz (2009) estimated that a 5 percent decrease in weight for overweight and obese employees would yield an annual reduction of $90 per person in total annual savings.

In a study of WHP costs, Mills, Kessler, Cooper, and Sullivan (2007) found that costs for the WHP were £70.00 for each of the 618 eligible employees of a multinational UK-based corporation. Based upon this cost and the decreases in absenteeism (4.3 fewer missed days/year), they calculated the ROI for the program to be almost 2 to 1 in salary costs alone. Although putting a monetary value on increased performance is difficult, based on an assumption that prior work performance was at 50 percent capacity, they estimated a $1364 return per employee, bringing the ROI of both reduced absenteeism and increased performance to over a 6 to 1 ratio.

Some of the costs may not be measurable in direct reduction to healthcare costs. In examining the financial impact of a comprehensive WHP program involving 6246 employees and retirees of a US school district, Aldana, Merrill, Price, Hardy, and Hager (2005) found that there were no significant differences in health care costs between employees who participated in any aspect of the wellness program and employees who did not participate. However, participation in the wellness program was associated with lower levels of absenteeism, such that each dollar spent on the wellness program was associated with cost savings due to reduced absenteeism of $15.60, translating into savings of over $3 million due to absenteeism (Aldana et al., 2005), highlighting the importance of targeting absenteeism. Despite no significant short-term health-care cost differences, program participation was associated with an estimated $3,041,290 difference in absenteeism costs compared with non-participation.

Interestingly, there is a trade-off between "intensity" (and presumably, cost) of program and its effectiveness. Saleh, Alameddine, Hill, Darney-Beuhler, and Morgan (2010) examined the effectiveness and cost effectiveness of rural employer-based wellness programs. More intense intervention exhibited the greater improvement in health. However, the less intense intervention had the best cost-effectiveness ratio, highlighting the challenge of creating valid programs with enduring effects, which are still economically feasible.

In an attempt to compare costs of WHP programs, Erfurt et al. (1992) examined the programs from three worksites (which had fitness center, follow-up counseling, and organizational components, respectively) to a "comparison" site, which had a less expensive and simpler program (i.e., health education only). Annual direct costs were based on salaries of the health educator and medical staff, the costs of programs, equipment, and fitness classes, and initial screening costs for the last two sites. These costs ranged from $28,892 to $156,850 for each of the three years of the study (Erfurt et al., 1992).

The comparison site (health education) costs were $17.68/employee/year. The second site (fitness facility) cost $39.28/ employee/year, but did not result in any significant increase in health benefits over the comparison site. However, the last two sites (which had education and follow-up counseling, and the fourth site also had organizational initiatives) had costs of $30.96 and $38.57, respectively, and they were "cost-effective in terms of both engaging employees at risk of cardiovascular disease in treatment or program participation, and reducing their risks and/or preventing relapse" (Erfurt et al., 1992, p. 6).

Deterrents and facilitators of WHP initiatives

Given the above review on the potential positive impact of WHP initiatives on health, and the positive ROI of such successful programs, we next need to examine the implementation of WHP initiatives, and in doing so, attempt to systematically explore the individual, program, and organizational factors that influence program success.

Individual factors Individual characteristics may influence one's choice to participate in programs, stay in WHP programs, and succeed in such programs. Demographics, such as age and gender, may influence participation in programs, health promoting behaviors, and thus, the success of the WHP program. Older employees may be more likely to resist employer involvement in personal health promotion initiatives (Robroek, van de Vathorst, Hillhorst, & Burdorf, 2012). Women, employees in higher occupational status, and non-English speakers may be more likely to attend health-risk assessment programs (Dobbins, Simpson, Oldenburg, Owen, & Harris, 1998). There are differences between the occupational statuses of people who use the health promotion resources. In their meta-analysis, Gebhardt and Crump (1990) found that although all employees were offered the same resources, 48 percent of white-collar employees took advantage of them, whereas only 3 percent of blue-collar workers did. Similarly, workers in lower-wage industries tend to have fewer WHP options and engage in more health risk behaviors than workers in higher-wage industries (Harris, Huang, Hannon, & Williams, 2011; Huang, Hannon, Williams, & Harris, 2011). In terms of effectiveness and "success" of WHP initiatives, WHP programs may tend to be more effective for younger workers than for older workers (Rongen, Robroek, van Lenthe, & Burdorf, 2013). Compared with men, women tend to report having better nutritional habits and more interpersonal support, and taking a greater responsibility for their own health compared with men (Martinelli, 1999).

Personality, behaviors, and beliefs can impact engagement and success in WHP initiatives. In her study of health promotion behaviors among 97 smoking and 142 non-smoking college students, Martinelli (1999) argued that self-efficacy is the strongest predictor of health promotion behaviors and may act as a buffer to protect young people from unhealthy behaviors as well as increase healthy behaviors. Pender, Walker, Sechrist, and Frank-Stromborg (1990) found that four factors accounted for 31 percent of the variance in health promoting lifestyles at work: self-efficacy in dealing with life situations, self-reported health status as high, low belief in the influence of fate on personal health, and a wellness-oriented view. Thus, workers who are high in self-efficacy and who value their own health are more likely to utilize health-promoting resources in the workplace.

Not surprisingly, the extent to which participants are ready for change impacts the success rate of any WHP program. Cruse et al. (2001) found that not being ready to stop smoking was one of the primary reasons for failure in their smoking cessation programs. Interestingly, however, instead of viewing change readiness as a necessary component for smoking cessation programs, they argued that this finding indicated the need for an ongoing smoking cessation intervention as opposed to a one-time offer (Cruse et al., 2001).

Ironically, several studies have suggested that those individuals who may have a greater need for WHP initiatives are the ones who do not use them. For example, current or past Australian smokers tend to be less likely to attend the health risk assessment seminars (Dobbins et al., 1998). Similarly, in their study of the prevalence and costs of chronic conditions of 7797 Dow Chemical workers in the USA, Collins et al. (2005) found that workers who agreed to be part of a WHP initiative were more likely to be non-smokers. Workers (n=3737) at a large agribusiness in North Carolina who had poorer health at the outset of intervention were significantly less likely to participate in a WHP program (Merrill, Aldana, Garrett, & Ross, 2011). Moreover, retaining employees in WHP programs may be even more problematic for employees who are deemed to be less healthy (Dobbins et al., 1998).

Klesges et al. (1988) identified a number of individual factors (e.g., attitudes toward workplace smoking policies; number of years smoking; beliefs about health impact of smoking; previous attempts to quit) that impact on participation in workplaces smoking cessation programs, attrition from program, and cessation "success." Although heavier smokers may be more likely to join a smoking cessation program, they tend to be less likely to quit smoking (Klesges et al., 1988).

Program factors   Several meta-analyses have identified program characteristics that can impact intervention success. In fact, Rongen et al. (2013) concluded that the study components, such as design and population characteristics, may be just as important as the intervention itself. For example, WHP programs tend to be more effective when there are at least weekly contacts (Rongen et al., 2013). The effectiveness of different types of contact (e.g., face-to-face, phone-based, web-based) has not been established and requires future research.

When examining the perceived quality and effectiveness of a cardiovascular health promotion program involving individual counseling sessions and seminars targeting five risk factors (i.e., obesity, physical inactivity, smoking, alcohol consumption, unhealthy diet), flexibility in the timing of counseling sessions, as well as the duration and location of sessions, were found to be important aspects of the intervention (Liau, Hassali, Shafie, & Ibrahim, 2014). Moreover, having frequent follow-ups, two-way communication, and individualized counseling sessions were identified as being effective strategies (Liau et al., 2014). The frequency of contact plays an important role in the effectiveness of the program and was four times more effective when contact was at least once a week, because high intensity keeps participants actively involved (Rongen et al., 2013).

When creating WHP programs, Liau et al. (2014) suggested that the language and degree of specificity of the education should be at a level suitable to the target audience. They also suggested that having visually appealing products (e.g., program booklets) beyond the actual program content may impact participant attitudes. Finally, having a high-quality counselor (in terms of positive communication and personality characteristics), articulating clear program goals, and having support from the upper levels in the organization are integral to program success.

To add to the confusion about the components that improve health, many studies have combined multiple WHP components into their programs, and they have targeted several health promotion behaviors. In one of the few studies to attempt to compare different programs components, Erfurt et al. (1992) looked at the effectiveness and annual direct costs of worksite wellness programs across four manufacturing plants. The sites differed in the programs they offered (e.g., health education, in-house fitness facility, follow-up counseling, and organization-based initiatives). Erfurt et al. compared the programs from the last three sites with the first "comparison" site, which had the less expensive and simpler program (health education only). They found differences in effectiveness and costs of the four programs, such that the two sites that both had education and follow-up counseling cost-effective in terms of both engaging workers and reducing their risks (Erfurt et al., 1992).

Erfurt et al.'s (1992) study provided an interesting comparison of different types of programs, and highlighted a component (i.e., follow-up measures) that may have contributed to the success of two worksites over the other two worksites, and it highlights the importance of identifying why the programs work in order to create sustainable and valid programs in different contexts.

Organizational factors In addition to directly influencing employee strain and well-being, the "context" can impact on the success of a program. Workplace factors may impact smoker outcomes in terms of program participation and attrition, and smoking cessation success (Klesges et al., 1988). For example, compared with program dropouts, workers in a workplace smoking cessation program who completed the program felt a higher degree of support from the workplace for worksite smoking restrictions (Klesges et al., 1988). Their study suggests that group-level (and social) factors influence individual behavior change, and thus, should be taken into consideration. Cruse et al. (2001) found that shift work interfered with one-on-one counseling support, contributing to a high rate of smoking relapse and failure to attend counseling sessions.

Another reason why it is important to take environment into consideration is that there may be some unique challenges in implementing WHP initiatives across different industries. For example, blue-collar workers may be exposed to a high degree of physical demands and hazards on the job (Sorensen, 2001). Blue-collar work is quite often very physically demanding, stressful, with long/unpredictable hours with a culture inadvertently promoting unhealthy lifestyles (e.g., drinking and smoking) and masculine stereotypes (Du Plessis, Cronin, Corney, & Greene, 2013). Compared with white-collar workers, blue-collar workers are more likely to be smokers (Sorensen, 2001). Therefore, the challenges associated with implementing WHP programs in blue-collar industries involve individual risk factors, such as masculine norms in refusing to seek help or wanting to appear independent, and low socioeconomic status, which is associated with morbidity and chronic disease. Other challenges involve structural issues, such as having to work long and/or unpredictable hours, having multiple employers (e.g., subcontractors who work with different bosses), and project-based work (Du Plessis et al., 2013). To effectively implement WHP, Du Plessis et al. (2013) argued that it is important to take a whole-industry approach to ensure sustainability.

Summary: Successful factors for WHP

How do we create successful and sustainable WHP initiatives? Based on the preceding review, and based on general organizational intervention and change literature, there are several factors that organizations should consider when developing and implementing WHP initiatives to ensure their success and sustainability.

1   **Individual factors**. Although many individual characteristics are not "changeable" per se, it is necessary to understand the context (including individual characteristics) to improve program success. Having a good understanding of individual characteristics will help to involve employees and tailor the program to the context and the individual employees. Involving employees in the WHP process (Chu et al., 2000), in terms of participating in redesign of work and improving communication (Goldgruber & Ahrens, 2010), can increase "ownership" of the process, increase its perceived relevance and benefits, and help ensure sustainability of the program. The Queensland Health (1996) guidelines for WHP programs state that programs should be managed internally (i.e., rather than by stakeholders external to the organization), re-emphasizing the importance of involving employees.

2   **Program characteristics**. Several suggestions about the scope and content of WHP programs have arisen from this review.

    a   **Scope of program**. Interestingly, although most programs may target a specific behavior, Partanen et al. (2002) advocate that WHP should not concern itself with attempting to target a specific disease or particular behavior such as smoking, but instead should focus on lifestyle changes and reducing workplace health hazards in order to effectively change the prevalence of major disease rates.

    b   **Focus of initiatives**. Many reviews of the WHP literature have noted the importance of including both individual- and environment-directed initiatives (Chu et al., 2000; Goldgruber & Ahrens, 2010; Larsson, Ljungblad, Sandmark, & Åkerlind, 2014; Secker & Membrey, 2003; Shain & Kramer, 2004; Sorensen et al., 2011). The choice of individual programs (i.e., cessation, promotion, education, and screening) tends to be a function of the specific workplace and employee needs. However, providing a multidisciplinary perspective in setting up initiatives and implementing programs is recommended (Chu et al., 2000; Wynne, 1997). "In practice, behavior-oriented measures [targeting risk factors] still dominate health promotion even though leading experts and international and national conference resolutions demand a holistic orientation for work-place health-promotion programs ... through which workers and management can collectively endeavor to change the workplace into a health-promoting set-ting" (Chu et al., 2000, p. 163). Therefore, "integrating health behavior change programs with work environment changes may be synergistic and enhance their effectiveness" (Sorensen et al., 2011, p. S197).

c **Program support and encouragement**. Based on their comparison of WHP at four worksites, Erfurt et al. (1992) concluded that "behavior change requires sustained support, encouragement, and assistance with problem solving, along with a variety of options for making changes" (p. 23). They encourage organi-zations to include wellness screening, follow-up outreach and counseling, and choices of several health programs.

3 **Organizational factors**. Several workplace factors were identified as significantly impacting not only employee health but also WHP program success.

   a As with any organizational change or intervention process, it is important to con-sider the structure and culture of a workplace in order to tailor WHP initiatives to the specific organizational needs (Goldgruber & Ahrens, 2010; Queensland Health, 1996). In addition to simply tailoring the programs, organizations need to take one step further by ensuring that the programs are integrated into the organization's "normal" practices and incorporated into the mission or corporate plan (Chu et al., 2000).

   b In addition to employee support and involvement, it also is necessary to have management support (Chu et al., 2000; Wynne, 1997) to ensure the necessary resources are made available to create and sustain the programs. Similarly, the in-fluence of social support and social norms at work on changing health behaviors has been demonstrated (Sorensen, 2001).

   c Based on many reviews and literature, organizational change seems to be an inte-gral part of WHP initiatives. Erfurt et al. (1992) found that although organiza-tion change reduced health risk and lowered recidivism, its ROI was not as good as another program. However, they argued that the "qualitative gains ... and the relatively low additional costs per person that are required, lead us to recommend that [organizational change] be included as a program component" (p. 24).

4. **Process and method issues**. Ensuring solid project management practices, in terms of a conducting a valid needs assessment, setting priorities based on employee needs, planning, implementation, and valid and ongoing monitoring and evaluation is an essential component of successful WHP initiatives (Chu et al., 2000; Queensland Health, 1996). For example, conducting a needs assessment (cf. Queensland Health, 1996) can identify the specific requirements of the employees and help to set up pro-grams to meet their needs to tailor it to the individual employees and organizational context (see points 1 and 3).

WHP expectations and ethical issues

Despite the evidence of the effectiveness of some WHP initiatives, the question of whether the workplace is a legitimate venue for health promotion largely rests on the perceptions of the employees. After finding that some employees had concerns about employers being involved in personal health outcomes, Robroek et al. (2012) argued that special attention toward moral considerations (e.g., violation of privacy) should be given in regard to com-munication, design, and implementation of WHP programs to accommodate employees.

This caution is especially important in light of some organizations requiring compulsory weigh-ins and health screenings. At best, these compulsory initiatives are intrusive and unpleasant. At the worst, they are serious breaches of privacy, creating stress, and developing a culture of distrust and low morale.

Interestingly, little information is known about employees' opinions about employer involvement in lifestyle and health (Robroek et al., 2012). For example, even though almost all participants and non-participants of a WHP program across five companies agreed that a healthy lifestyle is important, non-participation was often based on convictions of keeping personal life private from employers (Robroek et al., 2012). In fact, over a quarter of non-participants (26 percent) believed that employer interference in trying to improve employees' health and lifestyle was a violation of privacy.

Similarly, not all interventions, or topics of interventions, may be deemed suitable for all organizations. For example, in their study of health behaviors of 688 Australian postal workers, Richmond, Wodak, Bourne, and Heather (1998) found that respondents found that 63 percent of participants felt that employers should take steps to demonstrate an interest in the health of their employees, specifically as it pertains to drinking. However, substantially fewer people said that they would consider turning to their workplace for advice on body weight (25 percent) and smoking (16 percent percent; Richmond et al., 1998). Similarly, in their study of 718 workers from six companies in the Netherlands, Robroek et al. (2012) found that non-participation in WHP initiatives are often based on convictions of keeping personal life private from employers. About one quarter of non-participants believed that employers' attempts try to improve employees' health and lifestyle was a violation of privacy, even though 90 percent of participants and non-participants agreed that a healthy lifestyle is important.

So what do employees expect from WHP initiatives? Nöhammer, Schusterschitz, and Stummer (2013) examined this question using 237 employees from four Austrian organizations that had approved, high-quality WHP programs. Nöhammer et al. factored the responses into four types of expectations, in terms of cognitive (e.g., having an opportunity to try WHP), emotion (e.g., feeling appreciated), convenience/pleasure (being able to better afford prevention, enjoying participation in WHP, avoiding health problems becoming worse, and getting occupational medical assistance), and social (e.g., having better contact with colleagues).

It is possible that perceptions of organizational involvement in health promotion may be influenced by the degree of trust and respect in management, and the extent to which employees are involved in the WHP process. Interestingly, in their annual survey of employed adults in the USA, APA found that only 25 percent of the 1,562 respondents said that they trust their organization and feel valued (APA, 2014). The extent to which workers have control over WHP initiatives, feel respected, and perceive that their involvement and information from the process are confidential can increase the perceived legitimacy of the WHP initiatives. Based on results from their small study of healthy workplace practices of a Swedish organization, Eriksson, Axelsson, and Axelsson (2012) recommended that collaboration of management and organizations should begin on a small scale to gain trust. This increased trust, paired with adequate financial and human resources support, will help organizations develop successful WHP strategies to decrease sickness rates.

Future Research

There has been an increase not only in the amount of WHP initiatives developed in organizations, but also an increase in WHP literature. Based on this review, there are several directions for future research based on general methodological issues (in terms of validated programs, longitudinal designs, randomized controlled trials, and maintenance of effects); target populations and work industries (e.g., high-risk, blue collar, rural); organizational-based interventions; and technology.

Methodological issues

Validated WHP initiatives Even though there have been some exceptional studies examining the effectiveness of WHP initiatives, there have been concerns raised about a lack of validated programs (Conn et al., 2009; Goldgruber & Ahrens, 2010). The long-term effectiveness of many initiatives is unknown at this time because of the lack of studies looking at this issue (cf. Jepson, Harris, Platt, & Tannahill, 2010). Some of the studies claiming positive effects of WHP initiatives have not used longitudinal designs, do not have a control or comparison group, do not use random assignment, and do not take into account attrition from the program. Future research should examine the validity of specific programs as well as general areas of intervention using strong methodological designs, such as longitudinal interventions and wait-list control groups. Some researchers even argue that randomized controlled trials (RCTs) are the necessary standard to understand the efficacy of WHP programs (e.g., Hartfiel et al., 2012). The challenge in trying to validate many WHP initiatives is to isolate the effects of an individual program, when typically, many WHP initiatives are offered concurrently. For example, most studies that look at WHP in terms of organizational change also tend to include other initiatives in addition to the change (Engbers et al., 2005; Kahn-Marshall & Gallant, 2012). Therefore, not only should the RCTs compare an intervention group (for a single WHP program) to a control group, it would be beneficial to compare various programs with a control group to assess the relative effectiveness of different initiatives.

WHP criteria for "success" One of the ignored components of many validation studies is the criteria used to validate a program. Many of the WHP studies rely on self-report behavior change. Using more objective criteria, and multi-source data may increase the efficacy of the programs. Moreover, although some programs may not directly reduce health care costs, it may have indirect effects on other outcomes (e.g., absenteeism) that have important financial implications (see Aldana et al., 2005).

It also may be interesting to examine the multiple stakeholders of any WHP initiative. In their review of organizational change WHP programs, Kahn-Marshall and Gallant (2012) argued that despite the fact that environmental and policy changes yielded poor to inconclusive evidence in relation to improving nutrition and physical activity among the workplace, their continued use is important because these types of approaches can be implemented throughout a workplace and can potentially have an effect on all workers, not just those who agreed to participate. Their arguments not only highlight the often-cited suggestion of using strong methodologies to examine WHP initiatives (in this case, to study environmental changes), but more importantly, their arguments suggest that using more inclusive research designs and expanded health and well-being criteria for all workers may provide a more accurate representation of the effects of WHP initiatives. That is, according to their line of reasoning, there may be indirect effects from these types of organizational changes and policies on all workers that are not adequately measured by assessing specific behavior changes or attitudes for program participants only. Therefore, future research involving organization-wide change should look at both the direct effects (e.g., health indicators) and indirect effects (e.g., job satisfaction and engagement; attitudes toward organization) of both program participants and non-participants.

Retaining employees and maintaining effects   The challenge of achieving healthy out-comes through WHP is frequently overshadowed by the challenge of retaining employees in WHP programs, and maintaining any positive effects of the programs over an extended period. For example, Dobbins et al. (1998) noted that even though initial recruitment rates of employees for health-risk assessment programs have been reported to be as high as 80 percent, there is a problem with retaining participants. Ironically, they noted that those employees who are deemed to be less healthy (and therefore, may benefit most from the programs) may be more likely to drop out of the programs.

In several studies that do try to assess longer-term intervention effects, maintenance of positive health outcomes over time is a challenge. For example, in their 12-week health promotion program involving 566 employees from Nova Scotia, Makrides et al. (2008) found that even though participants demonstrated significant reductions in BMI (body mass index) and cholesterol levels, these reductions were not sustained. Similarly, Goldgruber and Ahrens (2010) concluded that the general consensus is that smoking ces-sation programs may be successful, but maintenance of effects is difficult.

Therefore, developing studies with strong research designs (e.g., longitudinal, control groups, randomization, etc.) is a first step in understanding the validity of programs. Research also must address methods of retaining participants and increasing mainte-nance effects. For example, involving workers in the design of the program may increase "buy-in" into the program. Creating efficient programs that are tailored to the individual, not only in terms of content, but also in terms of timing of the program, may increase participation (Day, Francis, Stevens, Hurrell, & McGrath, 2014). Finally, having sup-portive organizational cultures and systems that promote participation may be beneficial. Offering brief follow-up sessions with counselors and program coordinators after program completion may be an effective means of sustaining program effects (cf. Day et al., 2014; Erfurt et al., 1992).

Tailored vs. standardized initiatives   One of the core components of RCTs is having a standardized treatment or intervention. However, Sorensen (2001) argued tailoring a program to meet the needs of the individual worker may increase "the intensity of inter-ventions delivered" and enhance "the relevance of interventions" (p. 98) to the workers, thereby increasing the program's effectiveness. For example, Sorensen, Emmons, Hunt, and Johnston (1998) argued that there has been a trend for smoking cessation programs to use more tailored approaches to assist with cessation. Paradoxically, although it has been argued that tailored programs may be more effective (cf. Day et al., 2014; Sorensen et al., 2007), having a lack of consistency in the treatment across participants is a major critique of tailored types of intervention research. How can research resolve this seeming dilemma?

To complicate the area further, Goldgruber and Ahrens (2010) concluded that singular interventions tend to show limited effectiveness, whereas workplace interventions that are tailored to individual employee needs and target the organization as well tend to be more effective than interventions that target the general workforce as a whole. That is, even though more complex interventions have a greater probability of success, there are more difficulties in validating these types of complex programs (Goldgruber & Ahrens, 2010; Thomson et al., 2004).

Given Goldgruber and Ahren's (2010) perspective, future research needs to address the challenging task of validating more complex initiatives that involve tailoring the program to individual needs. Although this task may seem challenging, research on an incivility intervention (Civility, Respect, and Engagement in the Workplace; CREW) has dem-onstrated how programs can have both a standardized component (in order to make comparisons across groups) yet still involve tailored components to allow individual groups to adapt the program for the specific needs of their work group (Leiter, Laschinger, Day, & Gilin-Oore, 2011, 2012).

Populations   Even though the WHP literature has done a fairly good job of looking at various populations across countries, industries, and individual workforces, future research could focus on some pertinent populations and contexts (Chu et al., 2000; Conn et al., 2009). As with much of the work and organizational research, workers in rural areas and isolated areas, migrant workers, seasonal workers, and the informal sector tend to be understudied (Chu et al., 2000). Given that many of these workers may have higher health risks, and that some of the industries may be less regulated, these workers seem to be particularly important populations to study. Although high-risk industries have been studied in terms of safety factors, more research could examine WHP issues within these types of industries.

WHP initiatives may be more prevalent in large worksites (Linnan et al., 2008). However, because a large majority of worksites in the USA and elsewhere are small businesses, research needs to examine how to make WHP programs possible for small businesses. Even though Linnan et al. (2008) argued that small businesses may be less likely or less capable of implementing these programs and supporting worker health, Day (2012) argued that small workplaces actually may have better opportunities to create a healthy workplace, if they have a positive health-oriented culture and supportive leadership. Because of their flexibility, adaptability, and responsiveness to employees, small businessess may be able to create and implement healthy workplace practices more effectively and in a timely manner. Similarly, Clarke (2014) identified recommendations for creating healthy small businesses, in terms of developing a positive health and safety climate, increasing the commitment of owners to health and safety, promoting positive communication, and using participative approaches to foster employee involvement.

Technology   DeVries (2010) suggested new tools to improve employer opportunities to provide a healthier workplace for their employees, including wireless technology, integrated wellness solutions, and telephone health coaching. Research has begun to develop looking at using the web both for training, measurement, and feedback (e.g., QuitNet; a quit-smoking on-line program; Bialous et al., 2009). Telephone health coaching, such as the ABLE program (a 10–12 week job stress and work–life balance phone-based health promotion program; Day et al., 2014) and such as a short-term smoking cessation program (consisting of one or five phone counseling sessions; Ringen et al., 2002), has shown some promise in terms of addressing various stress and health issues. Other stress and wellness programs have been offered using web-based programs and assessment. Future research should compare the relative effectiveness of various forms of technology to offer, support, and assess WHP initiatives. Effectiveness may be defined solely in terms of improving worker health and well-being, or it may include other criteria, such as cost effectiveness, perceived convenience and accessibility by participant, and perceived confidentiality (cf. Day et al., 2014).

Conclusion

Although health promotion has become a major social issue, initiatives to improve general health and increase healthy behaviors have been labeled as only marginally successful (Maes et al., 2012), and there is a paucity of research in this area (Chan & Perry, 2012).

There has been increasing support to consider the workplace as a viable context in which to study, and change, health behavior. Indeed, failure to consider the workplace, in which full-time workers spend almost one quarter of their lives, as an environment for lifestyle improvement, is a great oversight.

Interestingly, health promotion in organizations has traditionally focused on the individual level, emphasizing reductions in unhealthy behaviors and lifestyles. Through repeated calls (cf. Cox, 1997; Ilgen, 1990), the focus has expanded from this individual focus, to taking into consideration the impact of the environment/organization (e.g., Engbers et al., 2005; Klesges et al., 1988; Shain & Kramer, 2004; Sorensen et al., 2011). It has moved beyond a focus on reducing negative factors (cessation; screening) to include increasing positive health factors (promotion of both physical and psychosocial health). A model of WHP initiatives was developed incorporating both these individual components and contextual factors. We have summarized the current literature on health promotion interventions, identifying the sample, industry, goal of the research, type, and duration of interventions used, the aspect of the model the research tended to focus on (cessation of negative health behaviors, promotion of positive behaviors, and/or screening), and the main findings of the research (see Table 17.1).

To summarize the current research on WHP, it appears that some programs work some of the time, with some people, for some criteria. Effectiveness of WHP initiatives depends on the specific program components. It depends on the specific health issue studied. It depends on the specific populations. It depends on the implementation. Finally, it depends on how we define "effective." We can look both to the WHP literature as well as to the general organizational change/intervention literature for practical suggestions for practitioners in implementing WHP initiatives. The support of workers and management is integral to the success of WHP programs. Involving workers in the process may help ensure the relevance of programs and their acceptance across workers. Tailored programs may make the intervention personally relevant to the participant, increasing its power for change (Sorensen et al., 2007), and adopting a holistic approach to health increases success (Sorensen et al., 2011). Integrating individual factors, program factors, and the environment (in terms of workplace, industry, management, etc.) into WHP initiatives is a critical step for future WHP research and organization programs.

There are several other avenues for future research in the WHP literature. Most notably has been the consistent call for more stringent methodological designs to examine the validity of WHP initiatives, using longitudinal designs, RCTs, and comparative programs. More research using specific populations (e.g., rural and migrant workers) not only may provide greater generalizability of program effectiveness, but may also provide information on specific contexts that promote or inhibit program success. Consideration also should be given to the criteria used in evaluating WHP programs: Although worker health and well-being has been the primary criterion, studies should also consider the ROI of such programs (including absenteeism and health cost data), the attitudes of participants, and the potential indirect effects of organizational initiatives on non-participants.

In examining how to implement effective WHP initiatives, the challenge for practitioners is to identify and implement valid initiatives that work for their specific employees and environments. The challenge for researchers is to clearly identify and communicate the effectiveness of WHP initiatives, as well as the specific drivers or barriers to their success. Continuing to bring both practitioners and researchers together to develop, implement, and study effective WHP initiatives is the ongoing goal of WHP.

Table 17.1 Summary of workplace health promotion programs

Reference	Sample and industry	Research objectives	Intervention and initiatives used	Focus	Duration and contact	Main findings
Aldana et al. (2005)	N=6,246 Washoe County School District (WCSD) employees and retirees (USA)	Examine the impact of a wellness program on health care costs and absenteeism rates	WCSD Wellness Program Involved 11 different wellness programs to encourage employees to engage in healthy behaviors.	Promotion	1-year or 2-year participation in program Online or in person enrolment	No significant difference in health care costs between participants and non-participants. However, participants averaged three fewer missed days of work which equated to cost savings of US$15.60 for every dollar spent on the program.
Allen et al. (2001)	N=2,943 (baseline) N=2,747 (follow-up) women from 25 worksites (e.g., private and public hospitals, state universities, chronic care facilities; 25 worksites in total).	Assess an intervention designed to increase breast cancer and cervical cancer screening use	Female employees were recruited and trained as peer health advisors (PHA) who acted as role models, disseminated information, fostered positive norms, and organized six discussion sessions to discuss, educate, and promote cancer screening. PHAs also provided counseling and social support. Other initiatives were also offered.	Screening and promotion	16-month intervention with six small-group discussion sessions	Intervention participation produced a significant increase in cervical cancer screening (Pap tests). The increase in breast cancer screening (mammography or clinical breast examinations) was not significant.

(Continues)

Table 17.1 (Continued)

Reference	Sample and industry	Research objectives	Intervention and initiatives used	Focus	Duration and contact	Main findings
Bialous et al. (2009)	N=1,790 nurses and nursing students	Describe registrants, observe relationships between demographics and smoking characteristics, and assess program strategies and use	Internet-Based Nurses QuitNet Online smoking cessation program that offers resources, online support systems, tailored resources, a quitting plan tool, individual counseling with an expert, and pharmacotherapy guidance and information.	Cessation	No specified duration. Participants accessed program as they felt necessary	Most registrants were female, 45–54 years old, Caucasian, and had college educations. Registrants smoked on average 10–20 cigarettes a day (more than 68 percent) and smoked within 30 minutes of waking up (66.4 percent). Of the registrants with previous quit attempts, half did not use evidence-based methods and a third had not attempted to quit in the past year. The most frequently used resource was the "Read-only" social support system.
Campbell et al. (2002)	N=538 rural female blue-collar employees from nine small to midsize workplaces in the USA	Assess the effects of the Health Works for Women (HWW) intervention on improving nutrition, physical activity, and other health behaviors	Health Works for Women (HWW) intervention Involved two computer-tailored magazines and a natural helpers support program.	Promotion, cessation, and screening	18-month intervention with a survey at baseline, 6 months, and 18 months	Program participation was associated with increased vegetable and fruit consumption of 0.7 servings per day, significant decreases in fat intake at 6 months, and improved strengthening and flexibility exercise frequency. Smoking and cancer screening rates did not differ between groups.
Conn et al. (2009)	N=approx. 38,231 participants across all studies	Meta-analysis of workplace physical activity interventions	Multiple interventions across different studies.	Promotion and environment	Duration varied across studies in the meta-analysis.	Significant effects were found for physical activity, fitness (oxygen consumption), lipids, anthropometric measure, job stress, and absenteeism.

Cruse et al. (2001)	N=123 (at follow up) UK manufacturing, research and development, and corporate worksites	Assess the effectiveness of a 10-week smoking cessation program	One-on-one support sessions with an occupational health advisor and access to nicotine replacement therapy patches.	Cessation	10-week/5 session program with bi-weekly support sessions and a 12 month follow-up	At follow-up, 20 percent of participants were non-smokers and more than half (52 percent) of participants commented on the particularly useful regular face-to-face contact and progress monitoring in helping them quit smoking.
Day et al. (2014)	Study 1=63 health-care workers (N=23 at Time 2) Study 2=103 employees from 15 organizations	Assess the validity of a workshop (Study 1) and 12-week phone-based coaching program (ABLE; Study 2) to help employees improve health, and reduce stress and work–non-work conflict.	Study 1: Workshop-based program to achieve physical and psychological health goals. Study 2: Tailored phone-based coaching program, involving weekly phone meetings, manual, and web resources to set and achieve health goals, learn coping strategies, and identify demands and resources.	Cessation and promotion	Study 1: 1 workshop/ 1 month for 6 months Study 2: weekly phone meetings over 12 weeks	Study 1: There were significant increases in positive mood and decreases in stress, strain, negative mood, exhaustion, workers compensation claims, and absenteeism. Study 2: Compared with the contrast group, coaching group reported increases in life satisfaction, and decreases in negative mood, stress, and hassles from Time 1 to Time 2.
Doumas & Hannah (2008)	N=124 (at follow-up) young adults (18–24 years) from five local companies in the northwest USA	Evaluate the effectiveness of an alcohol personalized web-based feedback program for young adults.	A web-based intervention either alone or in combination with a 15-minute motivational interview session to target high-risk drinking.	Cessation	30-day follow-up after completion of intervention.	Participants of the intervention reported significantly lower levels of drinking than the control group at follow-up that was especially true for high-risk drinkers at baseline. The motivational interview session did not improve the

(Continues)

Table 17.1 (Continued)

Reference	Sample and industry	Research objectives	Intervention and initiatives used	Focus	Duration and contact	Main findings
Engbers et al. (2005)	13 WHP programs Various industries	Systematic review of environment-focused WHP programs on physical activity, nutrition, and health risk indicators	All studies focused on healthy dietary intake and three of the 13 focused on physical activity. Examples of environment modifications included raising awareness, education, changes in offered food, labeling of food, and offering exercise space and equipment.	Environment	Follow-up occurred on average after 1 year	Methodological quality was often poor however there was significant evidence for an effect of environment modifications on dietary intake and inconclusive and no evidence for physical activity and health risk indicators.
Erfurt et al. (1992)	N=1,374, 2,448, 2,089, and 1,893 (T1 Screened) and N=493, 505, 482, and 403 (re-screened) from four US automotive manufacturing plants	Assess the cost and effectiveness of four wellness programs using various initiatives. Health risks assessed included hypertension, obesity, cigarette smoking, and physical inactivity	Four different workplace wellness programs (one for each worksite): 1 health education; 2 physical fitness facility; 3 health education combined with support and counseling every 6 months; and 4 health education combined with support, counseling, and environmental changes.	Promotion, cessation, environment	15-minute screening session followed by the 3-year program	The physical fitness facility was the most costly per employee and did not produce significant benefits over the health education program. This program reported the lowest percentage of employees exercising regularly at follow-up. The two programs involving support and counseling were the most cost-effective at engaging at-risk employees in treatment and participation as well as preventing and reducing health risks.
Fichtenberg & Glantz (2002)	US, Australian, Canadian, and German smoke-free workplaces	Systematic review of 26 studies on the effects of smoke-free workplaces on smoking habits	Smoke-free workplaces	Environment	Duration varied across studies in the review	Smoke-free workplaces are associated with a decrease in smoking prevalence by 3.8 percent and 3.1 fewer cigarettes per day per continuing smoker.

Grzywacz et al. (2007)	N=3,193 US pharmaceutical company employees	Examine the relationship between workplace flexibility and health behaviors	No interventions used. Cross-sectional and longitudinal study of workplace flexibility and health behaviors (hours of sleep, physical activity frequency, health education seminar attendance, frequency of practicing resilience techniques, and self-appraised lifestyle).	Environment	1 year (for longitudinal study)	All examined health behaviors except health education seminar attendance were positively related to perceived flexibility in cross-sectional analyses. In longitudinal analyses, only sleep and self-appraised lifestyle were related to perceived flexibility.
Hartfiel et al. (2012)	N=59 British government authorities	Assess the effectiveness of a yoga-based intervention targeting stress and back pain at work	A 50-minute Dru Yoga session each week with a 20-minute home practice DVD.	Promotion	8 weeks of weekly yoga sessions at lunch or after work	The workplace yoga intervention group reported significantly lower levels of perceived stress and back pain as well as an increase in psychological well-being when compared with the control group.
Kahn-Marshall & Gallant (2012)	Varied across the study	Review of 27 studies examining the effectiveness of worksite health promotion programs using environment, policy changes, and individual health behavior change strategies	Environment and/or policy changes	Promotion, environment	Duration varied across studies in the meta-analysis	Limited evidence was found for the effectiveness of environment and policy changes alone to change employee behavior (n=11) however there was moderate evidence for the effectiveness of interventions that combined environment and policy changes with individual-level strategies (n=16).

(Continues)

401

Table 17.1 *(Continued)*

Reference	*Sample and industry*	*Research objectives*	*Intervention and initiatives used*	*Focus*	*Duration and contact*	*Main findings*
Klesges et al. (1988)	N=194 (at baseline), 44 (enrolled in program), 24 (completed program) cigarette smokers from two worksites (glass manufacturer and media services business)	Assess factors (demographics, interpersonal/ organizational variables) related to continuing smoking and smoking cessation during and after the intervention	Smoking cessation program involving six weekly meetings that focused on making brand changes, reducing number of cigarettes smoked, negotiating a "quit date," and education on maintenance and relapse-prevention. Participants were offered cognitive and behavioral coping strategies.	Cessation	Baseline 1 month before program; 6 weekly meetings during work hours followed by a 6-month follow-up	Predictive factors of smoker participation included the number of years smoking, length of previous cessation attempts, and perception of smoking-related disease vulnerability. Cessation was associated with attitudes related to post-cessation weight gain. Long term cessation (6 months) was predicted by the number of coworkers that smoked and weight gain concerns.
Larsson et al. (2014)	N=60 managers and 8,082 employees from 60 Swedish municipal social care organizations	Investigate employers' management characteristics, provision of WHP measures, satisfaction with WHP, employee health	Health promotion programs	Promotion	Duration varied across studies in the meta-analysis	Individual and organizational WHP measures and employee satisfaction with WHP were associated with employee health. General organizational and management characteristics were not significantly related to employee health.
Leiter et al. (2011)	N=1,173 (Time 1) N=907 (Time 2) Health care workers in Nova Scotia and Ontario, Canada	Assess the impact of a civility-based intervention that focused on reducing incivility and improving employee outcomes	CREW (Civility, Respect, and Engagement at Work) intervention	Promotion	6 months of unit-based intervention to improve interpersonal interactions	Compared with the contrast groups, the intervention groups reported significantly greater improvements in coworker civility and supervisor incivility, cynicism, job satisfaction, management trust, respect, and absenteeism.

402

Study	Sample	Purpose	Intervention	Focus	Duration	Findings
Leiter et al. (2012)	N=1,957 health care workers in Nova Scotia and Ontario, Canada	Assess the sustainability of a civility-based intervention on reducing incivility and improving employee outcomes	CREW (Civility, Respect, and Engagement at Work) intervention	Promotion	6 months of unit-based intervention to improve interpersonal interactions (with a 1 year follow-up)	When examining outcomes at a 1-year follow-up, workplace civility, supervisor incivility, and distress continually improved, work attitude improvements were maintained, and absences returned to pre-intervention levels.
Maes et al. (2012)	European organizations	Systematic review of 37 articles examining WHP interventions involving a healthy diet and/or increasing physical activity	Various health promotion programs	Promotion	Duration varied across studies in the review	Overall, low to moderate evidence was found for positive effects of nutrition interventions (with or without physical activity) in the workplace.
Makrides et al. (2008)	N=566 employees in Nova Scotia, Canada	Assess the efficacy of a health promotion program at reducing coronary risk factors for employees with a minimum of two modifiable risk factors	Health promotion program involving exercise, education seminars, nutritional analysis and smoking cessation counseling.	Cessation, promotion	12-week program, follow-up at 3 and 6 months	There were significant differences in coronary risk score, smoking cessation, physical activity levels, BMI and serum cholesterol at 3 months. At 6 months, improvements were maintained across all outcomes except cholesterol. Intervention participants showed significant improvements in both cardiac and stroke risk at both follow-ups when compared with the control group.

(Continues)

Table 17.1 (Continued)

Reference	Sample and industry	Research objectives	Intervention and initiatives used	Focus	Duration and contact	Main findings
Matano et al. (2007)	N=145 employees in California with a low to moderate risk of alcohol problems	Testing the effectiveness of a web-based intervention (limited vs. full individualized feedback) on reducing alcohol consumption	Web-based intervention for reducing alcohol consumption that offered feedback on employee stress levels and coping strategies.	Cessation	90 days	Study offered preliminary evidence supporting the use of an interactive web-based intervention to provide individualized feedback for those at risk of alcohol problems. Greater decreases in alcohol consumption were observed in the full individualized feedback group than in the limited feedback group.
Merrill et al. (2011)	N=3,737 employees at a large agri-business in the USA	Testing the effectiveness of a program in which employees were compensated for healthy behaviors (e.g., regular physical exams, healthy eating, physical activity)	"Reaping Rewards Program" Rewards were offered in the form of monetary incentives for "good-health behaviors."	Promotion	3 years	Significant improvements in biometric scores (e.g., reductions in BMI, blood pressure, cholesterol) were observed for those in poor health; improvements were also noted in ability to cope with stress, amount of physical energy, sleep, fruit and vegetable consumption, as well as an increase in job satisfaction.
Mills et al. (2007)	N=266 in intervention group) and 1242 (control group) employees from a multinational corporation based in the UK	Examine the effectiveness of a multi-component health promotion program on the number of health risk factors, work performance, and work absenteeism	Multicomponent health promotion program involving a health risk appraisal questionnaire, offering access to a web-based tailored health improvement portal, wellness literature, and wellness-focused seminars and workshops.	Promotion, screening	12 months	Significant improvements were found in all outcome variables for those in the intervention group compared with those in the control group.

404

	Sample	Aim	Intervention	Type	Duration	Findings
Parks & Steelman (2008)	N=7,705 (measured on absenteeism); N=2,480 (measured on job satisfaction) participants of organizational wellness programs	Meta-analysis of 17 studies examining the effect of organizational wellness program participation on absenteeism and job satisfaction.	Various organizational wellness programs	Promotion	Duration varied across studies in the meta-analysis	Organizational wellness program participation was associated with decreased absenteeism and increased job satisfaction.
Plotnikoff et al. (2005)	N=2,121 (with 1,566 of them in the intervention group and 555 in the control group) from five large workplaces in Alberta, Canada	Determine the effectiveness of weekly physical activity and nutrition messages delivered via email on related knowledge, attitudes, and behaviors	Email intervention for the promotion of physical activity and nutrition behavior in the workplace.	Promotion	Baseline 1 week before; 12-week intervention; follow-up 1 week after	The intervention group showed improvements on self-efficacy, intentions, and behaviors related to physical activity, and reported more favorable changes in healthy eating habits, balancing food intake with activity level, cooking low-fat meals, and avoiding high-fat foods. However, effect sizes were small.
Richmond et al. (2000)	N=67 worksites; 1,206 employees from eight Australia Post networks	Assess the effectiveness of a broad lifestyle program on alcohol consumption	Broad-spectrum lifestyle campaign involving screening, managerial support, employee health awareness, brief interventions for high-risk behaviors, and focus groups to address cultural factors.	Screening, cessation	Baseline screening followed by the 4-week program; follow-up 10 months after baseline	Women in the experimental condition showed a significant decline in alcohol consumption from baseline to follow-up compared with the control group.

(Continues)

Table 17.1 *(Continued)*

Reference	*Sample and industry*	*Research objectives*	*Intervention and initiatives used*	*Focus*	*Duration and contact*	*Main findings*
Ringen et al. (2002)	N=325 smokers of the Carpenters Health and Security Trust of Western Washington	Assess the effectiveness of a smoking cessation program for blue-collar workers	Smoking cessation program. Involved a 1-call or 5-call counseling session program with access to medication (nicotine patches, nicotine gum, or Bupropion).	Cessation	12 months; program evaluated participants 6 and 12 months after quit date	Quit rates were at least 25 percent for both programs. The 5-call counseling session program was selected by most participants (61 percent) and 75 percent of all participants used medication. The highest quit rate was observed in the 5-call group that used bupropion. Over 90 percent of participants were satisfied with the program.
Rongen et al. (2013)	18 workplaces	Meta-analysis of 18 studies involving 21 workplace health promotion programs (e.g. physical activity, nutrition, weight, and lifestyle)	Programs varied across the 18 studies	Promotion	Duration varied across studies in the meta-analysis	The overall effectiveness of workplace health promotion programs was small however the effects of the programs depended on intervention, study, and population characteristics.
Saleh et al. (2010)	N=673 employee from six rural US organizations (1 control group and 2 intervention groups)	Examine the effectiveness (outcome and cost) of rural employee wellness programs on wellness scores,	Wellness programs with 3 degrees of wellness activity intensity (i.e., health risk assessment (HRA) only; HRA and year-round wellness messages; HRA, high-risk referral/case	Promotion, screening	4 years; yearly health risk assessments	The most intense wellness program (coaching and referral) exhibited the most favorable results. However, the HRA and year-round wellness messages intervention was the most

Study	Sample	Purpose	Intervention	Focus	Duration/Follow-up	Results
		good health indicators, and risk factors	management and year-round wellness messages).			cost effective. A total of six wellness areas improved: nutrition, tobacco use, LDL cholesterol, heart health, cancer, and happiness.
Sorensen et al. (2007)	N=582 construction workers	Test a behavioral intervention to promote smoking cessation and increase fruit and vegetable consumption	Tailored telephone-delivered and mailed intervention.	Cessation, promotion	3 month intervention; Follow-up 6 months after baseline	A significant difference in cessation of smoking and a significant increase in fruit and vegetable consumption were observed among intervention participants when compared with the control group.
Wallace et al. (2008)	N=385 (enrolled) and 244 (at follow-up) Sydney South West Area Health service staff	Test the effectiveness of a nicotine replacement therapy program on smoking cessation	Smoke-free environment policy (SFEP) with free nicotine replacement therapy.	Cessation	8-week intervention; 90-day follow-up	Overall, 31 percent of staff in the program had quit smoking after 3 months. Of those that continued to smoke, 85 percent had reduced the amount they smoked.

References

Albertsen, K., Hannerz, H., Borg, V., & Burr, H. (2004). Work environment and smoking cessation over a five-year period. *Scandinavian Journal of Public Health, 32*(3), 164–171.

Aldana, S. G., Merrill, R. M., Price, K., Hardy, A., & Hager, R. (2005). Financial impact of a comprehensive multi-site workplace health promotion program. *Preventive Medicine, 40*(2), 131–137.

Allen, J. D., Stoddard, A. M., Mays, J., & Sorensen, G. (2001). Promoting breast and cervical cancer screening at the workplace: Results from the Woman to Woman Study. *American Journal of Public Health, 91*(4), 584–590.

American Psychological Association (2014). *2014 Work and Well-Being Survey.* http://www.apaexcellence.org/assets/general/2014-work-and-wellbeing-survey-results.pdf (accessed May 25, 2015).

Bacharach, S. B., Bamberger, P., & Biron, M. (2010). Alcohol consumption and workplace absenteeism: The moderating effect of social support. *Journal of Applied Psychology, 95*(2), 334–348.

Baicker, K., Cutler, D., & Song, Z. (2010). Workplace wellness programs can generate savings. *Health Affairs, 29*(2), 304–311.

Bertera, R. L. (1991). The effects of behavioral risks on absenteeism and health-care costs in the workplace. *Journal of Occupational and Environmental Medicine, 33*(11), 1119–1124.

Bialous, S. A., Sarna, L., Wells, M., Elashoff, D., Wewers, M. E., & Froelicher, E. S. (2009). Characteristics of nurses who used the internet-based nurses QuitNet for smoking cessation. *Public Health Nursing, 26*(4), 329–338.

Blatter, B. M., & Bongers, P. M. (2002). Duration of computer use and mouse use in relation to musculoskeletal disorders of neck or upper limb. *International Journal of Industrial Ergonomics, 30*(4), 295–306.

Campbell, M. K., Tessaro, I., DeVellis, B., Benedict, S., Kelsey, K., Belton, L., & Sanhueza, A. (2002). Effects of a tailored health promotion program for female blue-collar workers: Health works for women. *Preventative Medicine, 34*(3), 313–323.

Caulfield, N., Chang, D., Dollard, M. F., & Elshaug, C. (2004). A review of occupational stress interventions in Australia. *International Journal of Stress Management, 11*(2), 149–166.

Chan, W. C. & Perry, L. (2012). Lifestyle health promotion interventions for the nursing workforce: A systematic review. *Journal of Clinical Nursing, 21*(15–16), 2247–2261.

Choi, B., Schnall, P. L., Yang, H., Dobson, M., Landsbergis, P., Israel, L., Karasek, R., & Baker, D. (2010). Sedentary work, low physical job demand, and obesity in US workers. *American Journal of Industrial Medicine, 53*(11), 1088–1101.

Chu, C., Breucker, G., Harris, N., Stitzel, A., Gan, X., Gu, X., & Dwyer, S. (2000). Health-promoting workplaces–international settings development. *Health Promotion International, 15*(2), 155–167.

Clarke, S. (2014). Creating a healthy small business. In A. Day, K. E. Kelloway, & J. J. Hurrell, Jr., (Eds.), (*Workplace well-being: How to build psychologically healthy workplaces* (pp. 281–298). Chichester, UK: John Wiley & Sons, Ltd.

Collins, J. J., Baase, C. M., Sharda, C. E., Ozminkowski, R. J., Nicholson, S., Billotti, G. M., … , &Berger, M. L. (2005). The assessment of chronic health conditions on work performance, absence, and total economic impact for employers. *Journal of Occupational and Environmental Medicine, 47*(6), 547–557.

Conn, V. S., Hafdahl, A. R., Cooper, P. S., Brown, L. M., & Lusk, S. L. (2009). Meta-analysis of workplace physical activity interventions. *American Journal of Preventive Medicine, 37*(4), 330–339.

Cox, T. (1997). Workplace health promotion. *Work & Stress, 11*(1), 1–5.

Cruse, S. M., Forster, N. J. D., Thurgood, G., & Sys, L. (2001). Smoking cessation in the workplace: Results of an intervention programme using nicotine patches. *Occupational Medicine, 51*(8), 501–506.

Danna, K., & Griffin, R. W. (1999). Health and well-being in the workplace: A review and synthesis of the literature. *Journal of Management, 25*(3), 357–384.

Day, A. (2012). Small and medium sized enterprises as healthy workplaces. In E. K. Kelloway, & C. L. Cooper (Eds.), *Occupational health and safety in small and medium sized enterprises* (pp. 159–188). Cheltenham, UK: Edward Elgar.

Day, A. L., & Livingstone, H. A. (2001). Chronic and acute stressors among military personnel: Do coping styles buffer their negative impact on health? *Journal of Occupational Health Psychology, 6*(4), 348–360.

Day, A. L., Sibley, A., Scott, N., Tallon, J. M., & Ackroyd-Stolarz, S. (2009). Workplace risks and stressors as predictors of burnout: The moderating impact of job control and team efficacy. *Canadian Journal of Administrative Sciences, 26*(1), 7–22.

Day, A., Francis, L., Stevens, S., Hurrell, J. J., Jr, & McGrath, P. (2014). Improving employee health and work–life balance: Developing and validating a coaching-based ABLE (Achieving Balance in Life and Employment) Program. In C. L. Cooper, R. Burke, & C. Biron (Eds.), *Creating healthy workplaces: Stress reduction, improved well-being, and organizational effectiveness* (pp. 67–90). London, UK: Gower.

DeVries G. T. III, (2010). Innovations in workplace wellness: Six new tools to enhance programs and maximize employee health and productivity. *Compensation and Benefits Review, 42*(1), 46–51.

Djoussé, L., Driver, J. A., & Gaziano, J. M. (2009). Relation between modifiable lifestyle factors and lifetime risk of heart failure. *Journal of American Medical Association, 302*(4), 394–400.

Dobbins, T. A., Simpson, J. M., Oldenburg, B., Owen, N., & Harris, D. (1998). Who comes to a workplace health risk assessment? *International Journal of Behavioral Medicine, 5*(4), 323–334.

Doumas, D. M., & Hannah, E. (2008). Preventing high-risk drinking in youth in the workplace: A web-based normative feedback program. *Journal of Substance Abuse Treatment, 34*(3), 263–271.

Du Plessis, K., Cronin, D., Corney, T., & Green, E. (2013). Australian blue-collar men's health and well-being: Contextual issues for workplace health promotion interventions. *Health Promotion Practice, 14*(5), 715–720.

Dunning, D., Heath, C., & Suls, J. M. (2005). Flawed self-assessment implications for health, education, and the workplace. *Psychological Science in the Public Interest, 5*(3), 69–106.

Eaton, D. K., Marx, E., & Bowie, S. E. (2007). Faculty and staff health promotion: Results from the School Health Policies and Programs Study 2006. *Journal of School Health, 77*(8), 557–566.

Engbers, L. H., van Poppel, M. N., Chin A Paw, M. J., & van Mechelen, W. (2005). Worksite health promotion programs with environmental changes: A systematic review. *American Journal of Preventive Medicine, 29*(1), 61–70.

Erfurt, J. C., Foote, A., & Heirich, M. A. (1992). The cost-effectiveness of worksite wellness programs for hypertension control, weight loss, smoking cessation, and exercise. *Personnel Psychology, 45*(1), 5–27.

Eriksson, A., Axelsson, S. B., & Axelsson, R. (2012). Collaboration in workplace health promotion –a case study. *International Journal of Workplace Health Management, 5*(3), 181–193.

Farquhar, J., Wood, P., Breitrose, H., Haskell, W., Meyer, A., Maccoby, N., Alexander, J., Brown, B., Mcalister, A., Nash, J., & Stern, M. (1977). Community education for cardiovascular health. *The Lancet, 309*(8023), 1192–1195.

Ferguson, G. T., Enright, P. L., Buist, A. S., & Higgins, M. W. (2000). Office spirometry for lung health assessment in adults: A consensus statement from the National Lung Health Education Program. *CHEST Journal, 117*(4), 1146–1161.

Ferrie, J. E., Shipley, M. J., Marmot, M. G., Stansfeld, S., & Smith, G. D. (1998). The health effects of major organisational change and job insecurity. *Social Science & Medicine, 46*(2), 243–254.

Fichtenberg, C. M., & Glantz, S. A. (2002). Effect of smoke-free workplaces on smoking behaviour: Systematic review. *BMJ, 325*(7357), 188–194.

Ford, E. S., Zhao, G., Tsai, J., & Li, C. (2011). Low-risk lifestyle behaviors and all-cause mortality: Findings from the National Health and Nutrition Examination Survey III Mortality Study. *American Journal of Public Health, 101*(10), 1922–1929.

Garfinkel, M. S., Singhal, A., Katz, W. A., Allan, D. A., Reshetar, R., & Schumacher H. R. Jr, (1998). Yoga-based intervention for carpal tunnel syndrome: A randomized trial. *Journal of American Medical Association, 280*(18), 1601–1603.

Gebhardt, D. L., & Crump, C. E. (1990). Employee fitness and wellness programs in the workplace. *American Psychologist*, 45(2), 262–272.

Giga, S., Noblet, A., Faragher, B., & Cooper, C. (2003). Organisational stress management interventions: A review of UK-based research. *Australian Psychologist*, 38(2), 158–164.

Goldgruber, J., & Ahrens, D. (2010). Effectiveness of workplace health promotion and primary prevention interventions: A review. *Journal of Public Health*, 18(1), 75–88.

Grzywacz, J. G., Casey, P. R., & Jones, F. A. (2007). The effects of workplace flexibility on health behaviors: A cross-sectional and longitudinal analysis. *Journal of Occupational and Environmental Medicine*, 49(12), 1302–1309.

Gura, S. T. (2002). Yoga for stress reduction and injury prevention at work. *Work: A Journal of Prevention, Assessment and Rehabilitation*, 19(1), 3–7.

Hanebuth D., Meinel M., & Fischer J. E. (2006). Health-related quality of life, psychosocial work conditions, and absenteeism in an industrial sample of blue- and white-collar employees: A comparison of potential predictors. *Journal of Occupational and Environmental Medicine*, 48(1), 28–37.

Harris, J. R., Huang, Y., Hannon, P. A., & Williams, B. (2011). Low-socioeconomic status workers: Their health risks and how to reach them. *Journal of Occupational and Environmental Medicine*, 53(2), 132–138.

Hartfiel, N., Burton, C., Rycroft-Malone, J., Clarke, G., Havenhand, J., Khalsa, S. B., & Edwards, R. T. (2012). Yoga for reducing perceived stress and back pain at work. *Occupational Medicine*, 62(8), 606–612.

Huang, Y., Hannon, P. A., Williams, B., & Harris, J. R. (2011). Workers' health risk behaviors by state, demographic characteristics, and health insurance status. *Preventing Chronic Disease*, 8(1), 1–13. http://www.cdc.gov/pcd/issues/2011/jan/10_0017.htm (accessed June 14, 2015).

Hymel, P. A., Loeppke, R. R., Baase, C. M., Burton, W. N., Hartenbaum, N. P., Hudson, T. W., … , & Larson, P. W. (2011). Workplace health protection and promotion: A new pathway for a healthier – and safer – workforce. *Journal of Occupational and Environmental Medicine*, 53(6), 695–702.

Ilgen, D. R. (1990). Health issues at work: Opportunities for industrial/organizational psychology. *American Psychologist*, 45(2), 273–283.

Jepson, R. G., Harris, F. M., Platt, S., & Tannahill, C. (2010). The effectiveness of interventions to change six health behaviours: A review of reviews. *BMC Public Health*, 10(1), 1–16.

Ji, L. J., Zhang, Z., Usborne, E., & Guan, Y. (2004). Optimism across cultures: In response to the severe acute respiratory syndrome outbreak. *Asian Journal of Social Psychology*, 7(1), 25–34.

Jones, S., Casswell, S., & Zhang, J. F. (1995). The economic costs of alcohol-related absenteeism and reduced productivity among the working population of New Zealand. *Addiction*, 90(11), 1455–1461.

Kahn-Marshall, J. L., & Gallant, M. P. (2012). Making healthy behaviors the easy choice for employees: A review of the literature on environmental and policy changes in worksite health promotion. *Health Education & Behavior*, 39(6), 752–776.

Kivimäki, M., Virtanen, M., Elovainio, M., Kouvonen, A., Väänänen, A., & Vahtera, J. (2006). Work stress in the etiology of coronary heart disease—a meta-analysis. *Scandinavian Journal of Work, Environment & Health*, 32(6), 431–442.

Klesges, R. C., Brown, K., Pascale, R. W., Murphy, M., Williams, E., & Cigrang, J. A. (1988). Factors associated with participation, attrition, and outcome in a smoking cessation program at the workplace. *Health Psychology*, 7(6), 575–589.

Kuoppala, J., Lamminpää, A., Liira, J., & Vainio, H. (2008). Leadership, job well-being, and health effects: A systematic review and a meta-analysis. *Journal of Occupational and Environmental Medicine*, 50(8), 904–915.

Larsson, R., Ljungblad, C., Sandmark, H., & Åkerlind, I. (2014). Workplace health promotion and employee health in Swedish municipal social care organizations. *Journal of Public Health*, 22(3), 235–244.

Leiter, M. P., Laschinger, H. K. S., Day, A., & Gilin-Oore, D. (2011). The impact of civility interventions on employee social behavior, distress, and attitudes. *Journal of Applied Psychology, 96*(6), 1258–1274.

Leiter, M. P., Laschinger, H. K., Day, A., & Gilin-Oore, D. (2012). Getting better and staying better: Assessing civility, incivility, distress, and job attitudes one year after a civility intervention. *Journal of Occupational Health Psychology, 17*(4), 425–434.

Liau, S. Y., Hassali, M. A. A., Shafie, A. A., & Ibrahim, M. I. M. (2014). Assessing quality of a worksite health promotion programme from participants' views: Findings from a qualitative study in Malaysia. *Health Expectations, 17*(1), 116–128.

Linnan, L., Bowling, M., Childress, J., Lindsay, G., Blakey, C., Pronk, S., Wieker, S., & Royall, P. (2008). Results of the 2004 national worksite health promotion survey. *American Journal of Public Health, 98*(8), 1503–1509.

Maes, L., Van Cauwenberghe, E., Van Lippevelde, W., Spittaels, H., De Pauw, E., Oppert, J. M., ..., & De Bourdeaudhuij, I. (2012). Effectiveness of workplace interventions in Europe promoting healthy eating: A systematic review. *European Journal of Public Health, 22*(5), 677–683.

Makrides, L., Dagenais, G. R., Chockalingam, A., LeLorier, J., Kishchuck, N., Richard, J., ..., & Veinot, P. (2008). Evaluation of a workplace health program to reduce coronary risk factors. *Clinical Governance: An International Journal, 13*(2), 95–105.

Martinelli, A. M. (1999). An explanatory model of variables influencing health promotion behaviors in smoking and non-smoking college students. *Public Health Nursing, 16*(4), 263–269.

Matano, R. A., Koopman, C., Wanat, S. F., Winzelberg, A. J., Whitshell, S. D., Westrup, D., ..., & Taylor, C. B. (2007). A pilot study of an interactive website in the workplace for reducing alcohol consumption. *Journal of Substance Abuse Treatment, 32*(1), 71–80.

Merrill, R. M., Aldana, S. G., Garrett, J., & Ross, C. (2011). Effectiveness of a workplace wellness program for maintaining health and promoting healthy behaviors. *Journal of Occupational and Environmental Medicine, 53*(7), 782–787.

Mills, P. R., Kessler, R. C., Cooper, J., & Sullivan, S. (2007). Impact of a health promotion program on employee health risks and work productivity. *American Journal of Health Promotion, 22*(1), 45–53.

Murphy, J. G., Benson, T. A., Vuchinich, R. E., Deskins, M. M., Eakin, D., Flood, A. M., McDevitt-Murphy, M. E., & Torrealday, O. (2004). A comparison of personalized feedback for college student drinkers delivered with and without a motivational interview. *Journal of Studies on Alcohol, 65*(2), 200–203.

Nixon, A. E., Mazzola, J. J., Bauer, J., Krueger, J. R., & Spector, P. E. (2011). Can work make you sick? A meta-analysis of the relationships between job stressors and physical symptoms. *Work & Stress, 25*(1), 1–22.

Noblet, A. & LaMontagne, A. D. (2006). The role of workplace health promotion in addressing job stress. *Health Promotion International, 21*(4), 346–353.

Nöhammer, E., Schusterschitz, C., & Stummer, H. (2013). Employee perceived effects of workplace health promotion. *International Journal of Workplace Health Management, 6*(1), 38–53.

Owen, N., Healy, G. N., Matthews, C. E., & Dunstan, D. W. (2010). Too much sitting: The population-health science of sedentary behavior. *Exercise and Sport Sciences Reviews, 38*(3), 105–113.

Parks, K. M., & Steelman, L. A. (2008). Organizational wellness programs: A meta-analysis. *Journal of Occupational Health Psychology, 13*(1), 58–68.

Partanen. T., Johansson, M., Ahrens, W., Sala, M., Wesseling, C., Boffetta, P., ..., & Neuvonen, K. (2002). Assessment of feasibility of workplace health promotion. *Preventative Medicine, 35*(3), 323–240.

Pender, N. J., Walker, S. N., Sechrist, K. R., & Frank-Stromborg, M. (1990). Predicting health-promoting lifestyles in the workplace. *Nursing Research, 39*(6), 326–332.

Plotnikoff, R. C., McCargar, L. J., Wilson, P. M., & Loucaides, C. A. (2005). Efficacy of an e-mail intervention for the promotion of physical activity and nutrition behavior in the workplace context. *American Journal of Health Promotion, 19*(6), 422–439.

Queensland Health (1996). *Better health for working people: Guiding principles*. Brisbane, Australia: QLD Health.

Richmond, R., Kehoe, L., Heather, N., & Wodak, A. (2000). Evaluation of a workplace brief intervention for excessive alcohol consumption: The Workscreen Project. *Preventative Medicine, 30*(1), 51–63.

Richmond, R., Wodak, A., Bourne, S., & Heather, N. (1998). Screening for unhealthy lifestyle factors in the workplace. *Australian and New Zealand Journal of Public Health, 22*(3), 324–331.

Ringen, K., Anderson, N., McAfee, T., Zbikowski, S. M., & Fales, D. (2002). Smoking cessation in a blue-collar population: Results from an evidence-based pilot program. *American Journal of Industrial Medicine, 42*(5), 367–377.

Robroek, S. J., van de Vathorst, S., Hilhorst, M. T., & Burdorf, A. (2012). Moral issues in workplace health promotion. *International Archives of Occupational and Environmental Health, 85*(3), 327–331.

Rongen, A., Robroek, S. J. W., van Lenthe, F. J., & Burdorf, A. (2013). Workplace health promotion: A meta-analysis of effectiveness. *American Journal of Preventative Medicine, 44*(4), 406–415.

Saleh, S. S., Alameddine, M. S., Hill, D., Darney-Beuhler, J., & Morgan, A. (2010). The effectiveness and cost-effectiveness of a rural employer-based wellness program. *Journal of Rural Health, 26*(3), 259–265.

Secker, J., & Membrey, H. (2003). Promoting mental health through employment and developing healthy workplaces: The potential of natural supports at work. *Health Education Research, 18*(2), 207–215.

Shain, M., & Kramer, D. M. (2004). Health promotion in the workplace: Framing the concept; reviewing the evidence. *Occupational and Environmental Medicine, 61*(7), 643–648.

Sonnentag, S., & Frese, M. (2003). *Stress in organizations*. Hoboken, NJ: John Wiley & Sons.

Sorensen, G., Emmons, K., Hunt, M. K., & Johnston, D. (1998). Implications of the results of community intervention trials. *Annual Review of Public Health, 19*(1), 379–416.

Sorensen, G. (2001). Worksite tobacco control programs: The role of occupational health. *Respiration Physiology, 128*(1), 89–102.

Sorensen, G., Barbeau, E. M., Stoddard, A. M., Hunt, M. K., Goldman, R., Smith, A., Brennan, A. A., & Wallace, L. (2007). Tools for health: The efficacy of a tailored intervention targeted for construction laborers. *Cancer Causes & Control, 18*(1), 51–59.

Sorensen, G., Landsbergis, P., Hammer, L., Amick III, B. C., Linnan, L., Yancey, A., …, & Pratt, C. (2011). Preventing chronic disease in the workplace: A workshop report and recommendations. *American Journal of Public Health, 101*(S1), 196–207.

Staley, J. A. (2009). "Get Firefighters Moving": Marketing a physical fitness intervention to reduce sudden cardiac death risk in full-time firefighters. *Social Marketing Quarterly, 15*(3), 85–99.

Thomson, H., Hoskins, R., Petticrew, M., Craig, N., Quinn, T., Lindsay, G., & Ogilvie, D. (2004). Evaluating the health effects of social interventions. *BMJ, 328*(7434), 282–285.

Trogdon, J., Finkelstein, E. A., Reyes, M., & Dietz, W. H. (2009). A return-on-investment simulation model of workplace obesity interventions. *Journal of Occupational and Environmental Medicine, 51*(7), 751–758.

US Department of Health and Human Services (2000). *Healthy people 2010: Understanding and improving health*. Washington, DC: US Government Printing Office.

Viswesvaran, C., & Schmidt, F. L. (1992). A meta-analytic comparison of the effectiveness of smoking cessation methods. *Journal of Applied Psychology, 77*(4), 554–561.

Wallace, C., Bedford, K., Rissel, C., Carroll, T., Hua, M., & Maunsell, T. (2008). The effectiveness of the provision of free nicotine replacement therapy on quit rates among health staff. *Australian and New Zealand Journal of Public Health, 32*(2), 184–185.

Warner, K. E., Wickizer, T. M., Wolfe, R. A., Schildroth, J. E., & Samuelson, M. H. (1988). Economic implications of workplace health promotion programs: Review of the literature. *Journal of Occupational and Environmental Medicine, 30*(2), 106–112.

Ware J. Jr, (1987). Standards for validating health measures: Definition and content. *Journal of Chronic Diseases, 40*(6), 473–480.

Webb, G. R., Redman, S., Hennrikus, D. J., Kelman, G. R., Gibberd, R. W., & Sanson-Fisher, R. W. (1994). The relationships between high-risk and problem drinking and the occurrence of work injuries and related absences. *Journal of Studies on Alcohol and Drugs, 55*(4), 434–446.

Weinstein, N. D. (1987). Unrealistic optimism about susceptibility to health problems: Conclusions from a community-wide sample. *Journal of Behavioral Medicine, 10*(5), 481–500.

Witt, L. B., Olsen, D., & Ablah, E. (2013). Motivating factors for small and midsized businesses to implement worksite health promotion. *Health Promotion Practice, 14*(6), 876–884.

World Health Organization (WHO) (2006). Constitution of the World Health Organization. *Basic documents*, Forty-fifth edition, Supplement, October 2006. www.who.int/governance/eb/who_constitution_en.pdf (accessed June 14, 2015).

World Health Organization (WHO) (2015). *Health promotion*. http://www.who.int/topics/health_promotion/en/ (accessed May 25, 2015).

Wynne, R. (1997). The challenge of workplace health promotion: New roles are needed. *Work & Stress, 11*(4), 301–303.

18

Psychosocial Safety Climate

Amy Zadow and Maureen F. Dollard

Introduction

Demographic shifts, increased economic globalization, and accelerated technological change have led to a range of emerging workplace psychosocial hazards such as precarious contracts, job insecurity, lean production and outsourcing, long working hours, work intensification and high emotional demands (European Agency for Safety and Health at Work, 2012). Work-related stress affects more than 40 million individuals across the European Union costing an estimated 3–4 percent of GNP (World Health Organization, 2008). Stress, depression, or anxiety are considered the second most frequently reported work-related health problem after musculoskeletal health problems (European Agency for Safety and Health at Work, 2012). Therefore psychosocial hazards and their health and safety risks are a significant challenge for contemporary managers, employees, and policymakers alike (Biron, Karanika-Murray, & Cooper, 2012).

Recent evidence suggests that the causes of work stress are more distal than initially assumed and are influenced by the organizational context (Dextras-Gauthier, Marchand, & Haines, 2012; see also Guediri & Griffin, Chapter 13, this volume). Previously, work stress theory and research has emphasized job design, or the individual work conditions that cause work stress such as work pressure, job control, and social support, highlighted in models such as the Job Demands-Resources (JD-R) model (Bakker & Demerouti, 2007; Demerouti, Bakker, Nachreiner, & Schaufeli, 2001; Schaufeli & Bakker, 2004), the Job Demands-Control (JD-C) model (Karasek, 1979), the Job Demands-Control-Support (JDCS) model (Johnson & Hall, 1988), and the Effort-Reward Imbalance (ERI) model (Siegrist, 1996) (see also Taris & Schaufeli, Chapter 8, this volume). Growing evidence suggests that multilevel systems or comprehensive organizational approaches in combination with individual-level job

The Wiley Blackwell Handbook of the Psychology of Occupational Safety and Workplace Health, First Edition.
Edited by Sharon Clarke, Tahira M. Probst, Frank Guldenmund, and Jonathan Passmore. © 2016 John Wiley & Sons Ltd. Published 2020 by John Wiley & Sons Ltd.

design changes are required to make sustainable change to levels of workplace stress (LaMontagne, Noblet, & Landsbergis, 2012).

Multilevel system approaches to manage physical safety at work have been used for more than 30 years (Law, Dollard, Tuckey, & Dormann, 2011). The development and operation of high-risk organizations such as nuclear power plants, hospitals, petrochemical plants, aircraft, and modern defense systems entail significant potential harm to people and the environment and have prompted organizations to proactively identify, measure, mitigate, and monitor organizational risk (Bloomfield et al., 2012). For instance the nuclear power industry clearly recognized the importance of organizational climate in safety performance following the Chernobyl accident (European Agency for Safety and Health at Work, 2011; International Atomic Energy Agency, 2002). The assessment of "leading indicators" such as the measurement of safety climate reduces the need to wait for the system to fail in order to identify weaknesses and to take remedial action (Flin, Mearns, O'Connor, & Bryden, 2000). Yet the research literature has been markedly silent in identifying a climate construct related to psychological health and safety (Idris, Dollard, Coward, & Dormann, 2012). Two separate research and practice literatures have developed in the fields of work, health and safety, and occupational health psychology. On the one hand work health and safety research, has focused on workplace climate, management systems, the physical work environment, physical health (mainly referred to in terms of injuries), and accidents; on the other hand occupational health psychology literature has focused on work-related stress research linking job characteristics to psychological health (Dollard & Bakker, 2010). Within these two bodies of literature a clear gap in safety research knowledge has developed that has hampered prevention efforts particularly in relation to psychosocial hazards. In the work health and safety literature there is evidence that physical safety climate is related to physical injury risk, safety behaviors, and physical accidents and injuries such as musculoskeletal pain and hearing loss (e.g., Huang, Ho, Smith & Chen, 2006; Neal & Griffin, 2006; Snyder, Krauss, Chen, Finlinson, & Huang, 2008). Work related stress, burnout, depression, and anxiety represent an immense growing cost for organizations due to productivity loss, staff turnover, absenteeism, and workers' compensation claims, yet until recently managers had little available research theory and evidence to structure organizations to prevent the development of the work conditions that lead to poor psychological health (Law et al., 2011). This chapter chronicles the development of the safety climate construct in psychosocial terms, that is, psychosocial safety climate. The elaboration of this construct draws together the two fields of research and helps us address the question: What is the role of the organization or system factors in the creation of the psychosocial work characteristics that are risk factors for poor psychological health?

Psychosocial safety climate theory (Dollard & Bakker, 2010; Dollard & Karasek, 2010; Dollard & McTernan, 2011; Hall, Dollard, & Coward, 2010; Idris, Dollard, & Winefield, 2011) defines the organizational context preceding the development of risky work conditions that lead to poor psychological health. Psychosocial safety climate is conceptualized as the "cause of the causes" of workplace stress (Dollard, 2012). Psychosocial safety climate theory proposes that the origin of stress begins at the organizational level via management practices, priorities and values, supervisory methods, production methods, budgets, and resource allocation, before the development of the specific job level characteristics such as high job demands and low resources emphasized in dominant work stress theories (Dollard, 2012; Dollard & Karasek, 2010; Law et al., 2011). Since psychosocial safety climate is proposed as a precursor to these workplace stressors the theory challenges the conception of the individual as responsible for monitoring and managing psychological health, proposing instead that a broader systems level approach will promote more effective sustainable change (Law et al., 2011).

Psychosocial safety climate theory, as it links to both areas, brings together these two unconnected areas of research; the safety climate research and the work stress literature, filling an abysmal gap in safety research (Dollard & Karasek, 2010). This chapter further outlines psychosocial safety climate as an extension of current work stress frameworks, expounds its predictive and ameliorating or moderating roles, its multilevel characteristics, and role in interventions to improve workplace psychological health. The evidence-base for psychosocial safety climate theory is examined and potential future research directions are explored.

Psychosocial Safety Climate

Psychosocial safety climate is a specific aspect of organizational climate relating to psychological health and safety (Dollard & Bakker, 2010). Psychosocial safety climate may be conceptualized as the organizational policies, practices, and procedures for the protection of worker psychological health and safety (Dollard & Neser, 2013). Workers reporting high levels of psychosocial safety climate feel that their psychological safety and well-being is protected and supported by senior management (Bond, Tuckey, & Dollard, 2010). To promote a strong psychosocial safety climate, senior management value worker psychological health, prioritize the psychological health of workers over profit and productivity, and commit to and support psychological health protection (Hall et al., 2010). General measures of safety climate are defined in this chapter as measures of physical safety climate. Both psychosocial safety climate and physical safety climate measure worker perceptions of organizational policies, procedures, and practices with regard to safety (Cox & Cheyne, 2000; Reichers & Schneider, 1990), reflect the properties of a group or organization (Hall et al., 2010), and precede safety behavior (Hall et al., 2010). The distinction between the two constructs is that general measures of safety climate emphasize physical health and injuries while measures of psychosocial safety climate prioritize psychological health and safety.

The Psychosocial Safety Climate tool has 12 items (PSC-12) that reflect the four main theoretical domains of PSC (Hall et al., 2010). These domains were developed by Dollard and Bakker (2010) following a review of stress prevention interventions (Dollard & Bakker, 2010; Dollard & Kang, 2007; Jordan et al., 2003; Kompier & Cooper, 1999; Kompier & Kristensen, 2001). After a further review of the safety climate literature the management priority for safety was included as a further domain (Cheyne, Cox, Oliver, & Tomás, 1998; Zohar, 1980). The four specific domains are defined in Table 18.1.

Together these domains depict what an organization, unit, or team would need to develop in order to create a strong psychosocial safety climate (Dollard, Tuckey, & Dormann, 2012). The construct validity (Hall et al., 2010), predictive validity (Dollard, 2012; Dollard & Bakker, 2010; Law et al., 2011) and conceptual distinctiveness (Idris, et al., 2012) of the psychosocial safety climate measure have been established in research. Psychosocial safety climate items have recently been included in the Job Content Questionnaire-2 (JCQ-2), a highly cited measure of workplace psychosocial factors used in a wide range of languages (Karasek et al., 1998).

In delineating a new construct it is important to verify that it differs from related constructs. Using confirmatory factor analysis, Idris and colleagues demonstrated that psychosocial safety climate is uniquely different from a measure of physical safety climate when operationalized in matching domains (Idris et al., 2012). There is an extensive range of physical safety climate measures that have accumulated over 30 years (Zohar, 2010). Measures such as the Loughborough Safety Climate Assessment Toolkit (LSCAT) (Cox & Cheyne, 2000), the Multilevel Safety Climate Scale (MSC) (Zohar & Luria,

Table 18.1 The organizational psychosocial safety climate framework (a new work stress theory).

Domain	Key processes	Example item
Management commitment and support	Senior management show **support and commitment** to psychological health through involvement and commitment. Senior management take quick and decisive action to correct problems or issues that affect psychological health.	Senior management acts decisively when a concern of an employee's psychological status is raised.
Management priority	**Priority** management give to psychological health and safety versus productivity goals. Demonstrated by the enacted policies, procedures, and practices of an organization and the priority of psychological health policies relative to policies promoting productivity goals.	Senior management considers employee psychological health to be as important as productivity.
Organizational communication	Extent and effectiveness of organizational **communication.** An organization communicates with employees about issues that may affect psychological health and safety, and brings these issues to the attention of the employees. Part of this is the way employees communicate occupational health and safety concerns and how this process is reflected in policies and procedures.	There is good communication around here about psychological safety issues that affect me.
Organizational participation	Organizational **participation and involvement**. Involves the integration of stakeholders including employees, unions, and health and safety representatives in the occupational health and safety process, through participation and consultation involving all levels of the organization.	Employees are encouraged to become involved in psychological safety matters.

2005), the Nordic Safety Climate Questionnaire (NOSACQ-50) (Kines et al., 2011), the Safety Awareness Questionnaire (SAQ) (Grote & Kunzler, 2000; Grote, 2008) and the Organizational and Safety Climate Inventory (OSCI) (Silvia, Lima, & Baptista, 2004) to help managers and researchers develop and identify safety climates that reduce physical injury risk, and promote safety behaviors to predominantly protect physical health, physical accidents, and injuries. Idris et al. (2012) identified that psychosocial safety climate makes a unique and important contribution to measures of workplace psychological health (psychological distress and emotional exhaustion) outcomes over and above that of physical safety climate. Levels of psychosocial safety climate were also significantly lower than those of physical safety climate indicating a lack of attention to workplace psychological health in Australian and Malaysian samples in comparison to physical health and safety.

Idris et al. (2012) also identified that the psychosocial safety climate construct is distinct from other related climate measures and is superior to other team-level climate measures such as *perceived organizational support* (Eisenberger, Huntington, Hutchison, & Sowa, 1986), and *team psychological safety* (Edmonson, 1999) in its negative relationship to both job demands and psychological health problems. Perceived organizational support measures the extent workers feel that their organization values their contribution and well-being, resulting in perceived productivity outcomes (Eisenberger et al., 1986). Psychosocial safety climate goes further than perceived organizational support by focusing specifically on psychological health, employee psychological status, and stress prevention (Idris et al., 2012). Another similar construct, team psychological safety, reflects a belief that a work team is safe to engage in new interpersonal behaviors necessary for learning and performance (Edmonson, 1999). Psychosocial safety climate is more strongly related to psychological health than team psychological safety as it is not limited to interpersonal behaviors but rather affects a range of workplace stressors (Idris et al., 2012).

Another construct that should not be confused with psychosocial safety climate is psychological climate. Psychological climate defines individual perceptions and beliefs about the work environment measured at the *individual level* (Clarke, 2006, 2010; Parker et al., 2003) while psychosocial safety climate measures individual perceptions of organizational policies, practices and procedures to protect psychological health and safety which are *aggregated to the level of the team, organization, or even at a sociopolitical level*; for example, large databases such as the European Working Conditions Survey (2010) and the European Survey on New and Emerging Risks (2009) enabled comparisons of organizational psychosocial safety climate levels between countries (Dollard & Neser, 2013).

Psychosocial Safety Climate: An Extension of Current Work Stress Frameworks

An important aspect of the psychosocial safety climate construct is that it fits to and extends current models of workplace stress. Most existing models of workplace stress begin with job design and explain how psychosocial work conditions affect psychological health. Currently the most highly cited models of workplace stress seen in the literature are defined in Table 18.2.

The JD-R model (Bakker & Demerouti, 2007; Demerouti et al., 2001; Schaufeli & Bakker, 2004) is widely used by researchers because of its broad scope and flexibility, and has been cited more than 24,000 times (de Jonge, Demerouti, & Dormann, 2014; Schaufeli & Taris, 2014; see Taris & Schaufeli, Chapter 8, this volume). The JD-R model describes two processes. The first process is a health impairment process whereby job demands such as work overload, cognitive or emotional demands can exhaust mental and physical resources, contributing to emotional exhaustion and in turn chronic health problems (Bakker & Demerouti, 2007). The second process is a motivational process whereby job resources promote high work engagement and in turn greater work performance (Bakker & Demerouti, 2007), greater productivity and profit (Harter, Schmidt, & Hayes, 2002). There are cross-links between the processes whereby poor psychological health is associated with reduced productivity (McTernan, Dollard, & LaMontagne, 2013; Sanderson, Tilse, Nicholson, Oldenburg, & Graves, 2007), and has even been related to accidents and errors (Clarke, 2010; Nahrgang, Morgeson, & Hofmann, 2011).

Table 18.2 Workplace stress models.

Model	Key processes	Evidence
Job Demands-Resources framework (JD-R model) (Bakker & Demerouti, 2007; Demerouti et al., 2001; Schaufeli & Bakker, 2004).	Proposes two processes: (1) poorly designed jobs or chronic job demands (e.g. work overload, emotional demands) exhaust employees' mental and physical resources leading to a state of exhaustion (health impairment process); (2) workers with high levels of job resources have high work engagement (motivational process). Proposes that high demands require sufficient resources to offset the negative effects of the job demands.	Supports the additive effects of stressors and resources on job strain (Crawford, Le Pine, & Rich, 2010; de Jonge et al., 2014; Demerouti & Bakker, 2011; Schaufeli & Taris, 2014). Evidence for combined effects of demands and resources shown through moderating effects has received mixed support. For example, some studies have failed to confirm the moderating role of personal resources in predicting psychological health outcomes (e.g., Xanthopoulu, Bakker, Demerouti, & Schaufeli, 2007).
Job Demands-Control model (JD-C model) (Karasek, 1979; Karasek & Theorell, 1990) and the Job Demands-Control-Support model (JDCS) (Johnson & Hall, 1988).	The JD-C model proposes that employees working in a high-strain job (high demands-low control) experience the poorest psychological health. Control can moderate the negative effects of high demands on well-being. The expanded JDCS model predicts the worst psychological health outcomes among workers when they experience high demands-low control-low social support work. The JDCS model proposes that social support can moderate the negative impact of high demands and low control on psychological health.	Supports the additive effects of demands, control, and social support on general psychological well-being although this relationship is more consistently supported in cross-sectional studies than in longitudinal data suggesting reversed causation might account for part of the association and evidence for interactive effects is weak (Häusser, Mojzisch, Niesel, & Schulz-Hardt, 2010; Van der Doef & Maes, 1999).
Effort-Reward Imbalance (ERI) model (Siegrist, 1996).	Workers expend effort at work and expect rewards as part of a socially negotiated organized exchange process. When an imbalance occurs between the level of effort and rewards obtained, psychological strain develops. Extrinsic (job demands) and intrinsic (over-commitment) efforts are differentiated and it is proposed that over-commitment could moderate or mediate the relationship between job demands and rewards.	Most studies support the proposition that high effort and low reward impairs employee health (Van Vegchel, de Jonge, Bosma, & Schaufeli, 2005). While most studies find evidence that high-overcommitted employees have impaired health compared with less overcommitted counterparts, the interaction hypothesis between ERI and OVC lacks evidence (Van Vegchel et al., 2005).

(Continues)

Table 18.2 *(Continued)*

Model	Key processes	Evidence
Demand-Induced Strain Model (DISC) (de Jonge & Dormann, 2003, 2006).	Based on the Triple Match principle (TMP) proposing that job demands, job resources, and job related outcomes may contain cognitive, emotional, and physical dimensions where the strongest interactive relations between job demands and job resources are observed when demands, resources, and outcomes are based on similar dimensions. The TMP is a probabilistic principle so while TMP effects are considered to be more likely non-matching effects are also anticipated.	This is a relatively new model with recent DISC studies showing support for the TMP (de Jonge et al., 2014; Van den Tooren, de Jonge, & Dormann, 2011; Van de Ven, de Jonge, & Vlerick, 2014).

Psychosocial safety climate extends JD-R theory and is conceived as trigger for both the health erosion and motivational hypotheses of the JD-R model, as shown in Figure 18.1 (Dollard & Bakker, 2010; Idris et al., 2011; Law et al., 2011). Psychosocial safety climate defines the organizational context and management practices that precede the individual job demands and job resources articulated in the JD-R model. This clarification provides an opportunity to intervene at an organizational level to proactively identify and mitigate psychosocial risk by establishing organizational and management systems to create and sustain healthy work conditions with associated health and productivity benefits. By contrast, targeting individual-level job demands and resources defined in the JD-R, as they arise, is a complex, time consuming, and potentially less effective process for organizations.

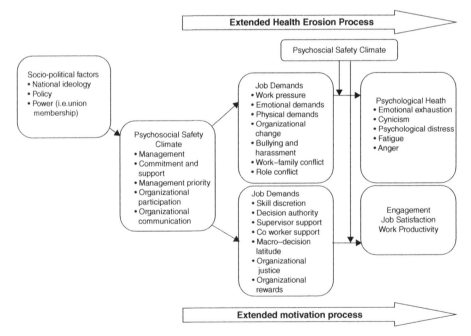

Figure 18.1 Psychosocial safety climate theoretical framework

Longitudinal studies show that psychosocial safety climate negatively predicts psychosocial risk factors (e.g., emotional demands, bullying, harassment), that are subsequently positively related to psychological health problems in the so-called extended health impairment pathway (Bond et al., 2010; Dollard & Bailey, 2014; Dollard & Bakker, 2010; Dollard, Opie, et al., 2012; Idris & Dollard, 2011; Idris et al., 2012; Law et al., 2011). There is also evidence for the extended motivational pathway as resources mediate the relationship between psychosocial safety climate and engagement (Dollard & Bailey, 2014; Dollard & Bakker, 2010; Idris & Dollard, 2011; Idris et al., 2012). These findings provide evidence for a multilevel model of psychosocial safety climate as a lead indicator of work conditions, psychological health, and employee engagement (Law et al., 2011). More broadly psychosocial safety climate extends all stress theories that elaborate job design as the starting point for psychological health problems, such as the JD-R model (Bakker & Demerouti, 2007; Demerouti et al., 2001; Schaufeli & Bakker, 2004), the JD-C model (Karasek, 1979), the JDCS model (Johnson & Hall, 1988), and the ERI model (Siegrist, 1996). A summary of these models of workplace stress including a description of the processes involved and associated research evidence is provided in Table 18.2.

Psychosocial Safety Climate: Predicting and Moderating Function

Psychosocial safety climate exerts a *primary* and *secondary function* in the development of workplace psychological health. As a *primary predictor*, psychosocial safety climate directly prevents adverse work conditions leading to poor psychological health (see Figure 18.1). In its primary role, psychosocial safety climate predicts job demands such as work pressure and emotional demands, and subsequent change in psychological health problems, as well as job resources such as skill discretion and decision authority and subsequent changes in engagement (Dollard & Bakker, 2010).

Psychosocial safety climate also has a *secondary function* as an ameliorator or moderator of the impact of the negative work conditions when they are present in an organization. Several longitudinal studies have found that psychosocial safety climate is a buffer to moderate the effects of job demands and bullying on psychological health outcomes (Bond et al., 2010; Dollard & Bakker, 2010; Dollard, Tuckey, & Dormann, 2012; Law et al., 2011). In particular the impact of job demands on psychological health are reduced when psychosocial safety climate is high (Dollard & Bakker, 2010; Dollard, Tuckey, & Dormann, 2012; Law et al., 2011). In its secondary role psychosocial safety climate acts as a safety signal indicating to workers when it is safe to use personal (e.g., coping strategies) and organizational (e.g., autonomy) resources to manage job demands (Dollard, Tuckey, & Dormann, 2012).

The secondary function of psychosocial safety climate may explain the variability in empirical findings testing interaction effects proposed in work stress models. Several work stress theories are based on an interaction hypothesis, that is, a high level of job demands will lead to psychological distress and this relationship will be moderated when there are high job resources such as job control and social support. For instance the JD-C model (Karasek, 1979) proposes that the positive relationship between demands and psychological health problems will be reduced when job control is high. The JDCS model (Johnson & Hall, 1988) proposes that higher levels of social support may moderate that negative impact of high job demands and limited job resources on psychological health. While the literature has found substantial evidence to support main effects, reviews have found limited or mixed evidence to support interactive effects. Van der Doef and Maes (1999) found that job control moderated the negative effect of job demands on psychological health in only 15 of the 31 studies reviewed and that there was insufficient evidence to assess the impact of social support. De Lange, Taris, Kompier, Houtman, and Bongers (2003) selected 19 longitudinal studies of perceived high methodological quality for analysis finding that only eight studies demonstrated the expected combination of additive and multiplicative effects. Finally, Häusser, Mojzisch, Niesel, and Schulz-Hardt (2010) identified that only 29 of 97 studies supported the demand–control interaction and that only seven of 52 studies supported the interaction between demand, control, and social support. An explanation for the inconsistent interaction effects could be that the organizational context, and the role of management, influences when and how job resources are used (Dollard, Tuckey, & Dormann, 2012). Poor psychosocial safety climate may negatively influence the proposed beneficial interaction between job demands and control and consequent psychological health, and therefore may account for the inconsistent findings of the job demand–job control interaction between studies (de Lange et al., 2003; Häusser et al., 2010; Van der Doef & Maes, 1999).

Dollard, Tuckey, and Dormann (2012) proposed that the demand–resource interaction depends on the organizational context; in particular high levels of psychosocial safety climate will enable the safe utilization of resources to reduce demands. Dollard, Tuckey, and Dormann (2012) found that high emotional resources moderated the positive relationship between emotional demands and change in workgroup distress *only* when there were high levels of unit psychosocial safety climate. For example, employees may only feel comfortable to report violence or bullying, or seek additional supervisor or coworker support, when they are working in an environment where their psychological health is valued above productivity concerns and communication practices are in place to raise and address these issues. The practical implication of these findings suggest that the provision of resources alone to counter high demands may be insufficient to improve psychological health in an environment where senior management support, commitment, and priority of psychological health is not evident, and when communication and participation strategies to manage psychological health issues are not clearly structured and understood. Resources may only be utilized when the climate is right.

Psychosocial Safety Climate: Multilevel Characteristics

Evidence supports psychosocial safety climate as a multilevel theory combining organizational, job, and individual level aspects (Dollard & Bakker, 2010; Dollard, Tuckey, & Dormann, 2012; Idris et al., 2012; Law et al., 2011). General measures of safety climate have also been recently redefined as multilevel to contrast the priorities of senior management with those of work group supervisors (Zohar, 2008). Theoretical rationale and empirical data indicate significant variation between organization and group-level priorities (Zohar, 2008). For example, a supervisor who directs workers to disregard safety procedures when production falls behind schedule creates a distinction between the organizational goals dictated by senior management and their own work group practices (Zohar, 2008). Psychosocial safety climate research has also demonstrated climate properties at the work group level (Dollard & Bakker, 2010; Idris et al., 2012) and at the level of the organization (Law et al., 2011). Psychosocial safety climate at the group level may be a property of the higher, organizational level, but may have distinct components as well.

Recent research has shown that psychosocial safety climate assessed by one group of workers can predict work conditions (e.g., workload, control) and psychological health at a later time in different workers in the same work unit, supporting the premise that psychosocial safety climate is the property of the organization and not the individual (Dollard, Opie, et al., 2012). Dollard, Opie, et al. (2012) used two unrelated samples of remote area nurses from two separate time periods matched at the work unit level. Unit psychosocial safety climate assessed by nurses predicted work conditions (workload, control, supervisor support) and psychological strain in different nurses in the same work unit 24 months later. The research design used also overcame a problem in longitudinal research of workers in high-stress industries where matching data over time is a problem because of high turnover and sickness absence. Multilevel modeling enabled the aggregated data, in this case psychosocial safety climate at the work unit level, to be combined with the individual data of other workers in the same unit. The research design enabled the examination of an under resourced, remote group of employees facing high work demands and turnover, and demonstrated that the assessment of psychosocial safety climate can predict the future work conditions and the health of other employees (Dollard, Opie, et al., 2012; Wakerman & Davey, 2008). In this highly complex work environment primary prevention of negative psychological health outcomes may be achieved by targeting organizational and management practices, and the development of a strong psychosocial safety climate, rather than the individual employee's specific job design which, given the high turnover, would only constitute a temporary solution (Dollard, Opie, et al., 2012).

Extending beyond the multilevel structure of organizational, work group, and individual characteristics, recent research has identified that external or macro-level factors affect workplace psychological health (Dollard, Osborne, & Manning, 2012). A recent study of psychosocial safety climate levels across 31 countries has identified that macro-level union density and organizational psychosocial safety climate are important predictors of worker self-reported health (Dollard & Neser, 2013). Dollard and Neser suggest that sociopolitical mechanisms of countries such as national ideology, policy, and power (e.g., union density) influence organizational levels of psychosocial safety climate and the subsequent health of the workforce across nations (Dollard & Neser, 2013). Notably it was not the quality of work conditions, but rather, workplace protective factors at both the macro (union density) and organizational level (psychosocial safety climate) that were most important in terms of national differences in worker health. Importantly the measure of psychosocial safety climate used in the research was reported by work health and safety managers, and not the workers themselves, yet it was still related to self-reported worker health at a national level. Worker self-reported health was also related to population health and gross domestic product (GDP) at a national level. Dollard and Neser (2013) propose that the nature of society, its fundamental ideology regarding labor market legislation, policies and welfare regimes, influenced by and in combination with unions and management, give rise to important protective structures and functions within the workplace that influence worker health. For instance, countries that are social democratic in nature (i.e., Sweden, Finland, Denmark, Norway) reported high levels of psychosocial safety climate, but so too did a few neo-liberal economies (e.g., UK, Ireland). Dollard and Neser (2013) argued that acknowledgement of the sheer economic costs of work stress to organizations and production may be an effective strategy to trigger change in organizations in neo-liberal economies that are driven by economic rationalist principles (Dollard & Bailey, 2014). This research also showed that the health of workers is higher, as is the national gross domestic product, in countries that take action to develop higher levels of psychosocial safety climate within their organizations by using consultation and participatory processes, and implementing procedures to address stress, bullying, and violence (Dollard & Neser, 2013).

Psychosocial Safety Climate: Role in Interventions

Workplace stress interventions can be classified in terms of the approach (i.e., primary, secondary, tertiary) and the target population (i.e., individual, organization, individual/organization interface) (Pignata, Biron, & Dollard, 2014). *Primary interventions* are long-term approaches that attempt to eliminate the source of the stressors (e.g., reducing staff workloads). *Secondary interventions* try to reduce the effects of stress in employees who are showing signs of stress by modifying their reaction to the existing stressor (e.g., relaxation training). Finally, *tertiary interventions* focus on managing employees with stress-related health problems (e.g., anxiety and depression) by providing professional treatment for the identified health problem (Kompier & Cooper, 1999).

Stress management interventions may also be classified in terms of the *targets* of interventions (Pignata et al., 2014). Interventions to reduce stress in the workplace may target the individual, the organization, or the interface between the individual and the organization (De Frank & Cooper, 1987). Interventions targeted at the individual seek to help the individual adapt to the stressful work condition while organizational interventions aim to modify certain aspects of the organization such as leadership structure (Pignata et al., 2014). Actions taken within a team or a department may focus on the interface between the individual and the organization. An example would be setting up coworker support groups to improve relationships at work (Pignata et al., 2014).

While stress interventions are usually categorized within these classification systems the boundaries between these levels are not mutually exclusive and may overlap (Giga, Noblet, Faragher, & Cooper, 2003; Pignata et al., 2014). Most approaches to reduce anxiety, depression, burnout, and workplace stress use secondary approaches to target the *individual* (Biron, Karanika-Murray, & Cooper, 2012). Individual-level interventions often use external trainers to provide cognitive behavioral training, mindfulness training, or relaxation and communication skills exercises to assist participants to adapt to the taxing aspects of the job design (Marine, Ruotsalainen, Serra, & Verbeek, 2006; Richardson & Rothstein, 2008; Van Wyk & Pillay-Van Wyk, 2010; see also Day & Helson, Chapter 17, this volume). Positive psychology interventions, such as self-help interventions and individual therapy, can be classified as secondary approaches targeted at the individual level and are primarily aimed at raising positive feelings, cognitions, or behavior. These approaches are currently widely used and show some limited enhancement of subjective well-being among individuals (Bolier et al., 2013). Psychosocial safety climate theory challenges the orthodoxy of monitoring and managing psychological health by an individual worker, proposing that interventions need to address the cause of the adverse work conditions using a primary prevention approach to target the organizational context and management practices that create and sustain unhealthy work environments (Rickard et al., 2012). These organizational responses may be more effective and sustainable (Law et al., 2011). Targeting psychosocial safety climate for intervention will ensure that the adverse work conditions will be ameliorated at the source providing a more reliable, efficient, and sustainable control strategy than addressing existing work conditions (Dollard, 2012).

Psychosocial safety climate theory is consistent with evidence suggesting that individually focused approaches are effective at the individual level but high-level system approaches combining individual and organization directed approaches (i.e., working conditions and management practices) provide broader benefits for both the individual and organization (LaMontagne, Keegel, Louie, Ostry, & Landsbergis, 2007; see also Day & Helson, Chapter 17, this volume). Sustainable change can be achieved by shifting management values, attitudes and actions for short-term profit to the long-term protection of psychological health and associated productivity benefits (Idris et al., 2012). Psychosocial safety climate theory suggests that interventions to improve workplace conditions and psychological health should be tailored to the level of the organization with a socially coordinated approach including management commitment and priority, organizational communication, participation and involvement (Dollard & Karasek, 2010). Interventions pitched at the level of the organization using socially collective structures provide an opportunity for social dialogue, empowerment, and democratic engagement. These features are best practice elements identified in psychosocial risk management intervention evaluations (Dollard & Karasek, 2010).

Interventions to develop a strong psychosocial safety climate in organizations will ensure that senior managers and leaders create and enact policies, practices, and procedures that protect worker psychological health and well-being (Bond et al., 2010). Empirical data indicates that leaders have a significant role in the development of worker health and well-being (e.g., Arnold, Turner, Barling, Kelloway, & McKee, 2007; Tuckey, Bakker, & Dollard, 2012; Skogstad, Einarsen, Torsheim, Aasland, & Hetland, 2007). By developing clear practices and policies, management establishes a protocol for the type of behaviors that are valued and encouraged within the workplace (Bond et al., 2010). The psychosocial safety climate domains can be used as guidance for building psychosocial safety climate and should be viewed as a continuous organizational development strategy (Law et al., 2011). Dollard and Karasek (2010) proposed the *Healthy Conducive Production Model* to use as a guide to structure organizational intervention processes. The main steps involve the development of management or political will to facilitate the change, to build a social-level controller (e.g., a tripartite committee) to resource incoming demands, to provide social dialogue between stakeholders to promote democratic engagement, and to design and develop well-coordinated policies, practices and procedures (e.g., action plans). These steps are also consistent with international best practice, established work, health, and safety methods, and continuous improvement processes (Bailey, Pignata, & Dollard, 2014).

It is important to consider the levels of PSC in organizations and work units where interventions are planned. Dollard (2012) found significantly better intervention implementation in work units with higher starting levels of psychosocial safety climate. Nielsen and Randall (2012) also identified that employees' participation in intervention processes was significantly related to levels of pre-intervention autonomy and job satisfaction. Nielsen (2013) argued that the role of employees in interventions needs to be reconsidered as employees are not passive recipients and actively shape the intervention process and context. Organizational stress management interventions are typically complex, long term, and require significant resources. Pre-intervention work to build strong management support and an organizational environment with effective communication and stakeholder consultation processes, using the psychosocial safety climate theoretical framework, may strongly influence how employees shape and develop the intervention process, and the ultimate efficacy of the project.

Some interventions have been accomplished using a socially coordinated approach consistent with psychosocial safety climate theory, with strong senior management support, the active participation of employees, the development and implementation of policies and procedures based on the intervention findings, and the coordination of strategies to ensure that the intervention impact is sustainable, with evaluations showing improvement in either work conditions or psychological health measures. However, the number of these organizational interventions is currently very limited (Dollard & Gordon, 2014; Dollard & Karasek, 2010; Halbesleben, Osburn, & Mumford, 2006; Le Blanc, Hox, Schaufeli, Taris, & Peeters, 2007; Leiter, Laschinger, Day, & Oore, 2011). Dollard and Gordon

(2014) recently completed an intervention following best practice principles including top management commitment and support provided through a written statement to employees from the chief executive officer and resourcing of the project. The study made use of existing workgroup structures and organizational data (i.e., annual organization development survey, sick leave, and grievance data) to generate change plans modifying policies, procedures, and norms. The organization enlisted external facilitators to convene capacity-building workshops and an expert researcher to supply workgroup reports that specifically highlighted stress risks as determined from the organization development survey. The intervention used a participatory approach, with inputs from employees and a tripartite health and safety committee, with an upward communication system. A fundamental premise of the intervention was that workgroups developing action plans were part of an overall socially coordinated workplace stress reduction system connected to higher-level committees and power structures. Job design, training and development, and morale improved following the intervention compared to the control group. Marginal improvements for quality and positive performance management were also seen in the intervention group. Organizational sickness absence duration decreased in the intervention group consistent with an intervention effect.

Evidence Base for Psychosocial Safety Climate

Dollard and Bakker (2010) first tested the psychosocial safety climate framework using a sample of teachers. They found that psychosocial safety climate predicted changes in work characteristics (skill discretion, work pressure, and emotional demands) leading to individual psychological health problems (psychological distress and emotional exhaustion) (see Figure 18.1). When senior management failed to value psychological well-being, this was evident in terms of increased demands, perhaps because of a lack of attentiveness to work scheduling and adjustments of workload, leading to an erosion of health (Dollard & Bakker, 2010). Psychosocial safety climate also moderated the impact of emotional demands on psychological health problems while skill discretion mediated the effect of psychosocial safety climate on work engagement (Dollard & Bakker, 2010). This research was the first to define the organizational conditions leading to the adverse work characteristics articulated in the JD-R framework (Dollard & Bakker, 2010). The comprehensive research design of this study used an aggregated measure of psychosocial safety climate, and a longitudinal design that controlled for baseline measures, added to the strength of the findings (Dollard & Bakker, 2010).

Using a sample of police officers, Bond et al. (2010) identified that workplace bullying was predicted by psychosocial safety climate, and psychosocial safety climate also moderated the impact of workplace bullying on post-traumatic health symptoms. Psychosocial safety climate aggregated to the level of the police station predicted future levels of bullying. These findings highlight psychosocial safety climate as a crucial intervention target in not only preventing the development of workplace bullying, but also in moderating the impact of this form of organizational crisis on psychological outcomes for victims.

Law et al. (2011) extended the findings of Dollard and Bakker (2011) operationalizing other sources of stress (e.g., workplace bullying and harassment) and job resources (e.g., rewards) that could carry the effects of psychosocial safety climate on to psychological health outcomes. Law et al. (2011) used data from telephone interviews of 220 employees in 30 organizations. They demonstrated that psychosocial safety climate was negatively associated with workplace bullying and harassment (i.e., emotional demands) and in turn psychological health problems. Psychosocial safety climate was also positively associated with work rewards (job resources) and in turn work engagement. Accordingly, the researchers concluded that psychosocial safety climate triggers the health impairment and motivational pathways justifying the extension of the JD-R model in a multilevel way.

Law et al. (2011) identified that psychosocial safety climate, as an organization-based resource, also moderated the positive relationship between bullying/harassment and psychological health problems, and the negative relationship between bullying/harassment and engagement (Law et al., 2011). Importantly, the research found a significant relationship between organizational-level psychosocial safety climate and bullying/ harassment and further tests showed this was over and above within-group effects of psychosocial safety climate (i.e., individual self-reports of psychosocial safety climate) (Bond et al., 2010; Law et al., 2011). This illustrates that the link between climate and bullying and harassment cannot be dismissed as purely subjective (Law et al., 2011). This result is important as it indicates that we can predict reports of bullying/harassment from knowing about organizational levels of psychosocial safety climate (Bond et al., 2010; Law et al., 2011). The study used population-based sampling telephoning individuals at home and then grouped individuals within the same organizations. The advantage of this design was that organizations did not have the power to veto the participation of employees therefore ensuring a more diverse and potentially representative sample of organizations participating in the research (Law et al., 2011). Furthermore, socioeconomic effects were addressed in the study by controlling for income level.

Idris and Dollard (2011) found that psychosocial safety climate had an indirect effect on negative emotions (e.g., anger and depression) via job demands (emotional demands, role conflict). Psychosocial safety climate also related to job resources (supervisor support, coworker support), which correlated with engagement. Idris, Dollard, and Winefield (2011) went further and identified that psychosocial safety climate was negatively related to job demands that in turn were associated with burnout (emotional exhaustion and cynicism). Psychosocial safety climate was also positively related to resources and subsequent levels of engagement. This suggests that psychosocial safety climate can be perceived as antecedent to the health erosion and motivational pathways articulated in the JD-R model (Bakker & Demerouti, 2007; Demerouti et al., 2001; Schaufeli & Bakker, 2004), or as an extension of these pathways. A further Malaysian-Australian study (Idris et al., 2012) identified that psychosocial safety climate related to demands and in turn to psychological health problems in a Malaysian sample but not an Australian sample. It was acknowledged that these results were limited by restricted sample sizes.

Dollard, Opie, et al. (2012) determined that work unit-level measures of psychosocial safety climate predicted work conditions (workload, control, and supervisor support) and psychological strain in different nurses in the same work unit 24 months later. There was evidence that the between-group relationship between unit psychosocial safety climate and psychological strain was mediated by Time 2 work conditions (workload, job control) as well as Time 1 emotional demands. The results supported a multilevel work stress model with psychosocial safety climate as a plausible primary cause, or "cause of the causes" of work-related psychological strain.

Dollard, Tuckey, and Dormann (2012) demonstrated that high emotional resources moderated the positive relationship between emotional demands and change in work-group psychological distress when there were high levels of unit psychosocial safety climate. The results supported psychosocial safety climate as a property of the organization and a target for higher order controls to reduce work stress suggesting that the "right" climate enables resources to do their job. A major strength of this study was that support was found for the three-way-interaction even when data relating to psychosocial safety climate was derived from a different source (i.e., split-samples). Split-samples overcame the problem of common method variance of single source studies. A limitation of the study was low power due to the small number of upper level units. Although effects were small they were consistent with theoretical predictions and it is widely acknowledged in social science research that effect sizes are typically small and in the order of 1–3 percent (Champoux & Peters, 1987; Chaplin, 1991; Evans, 1985).

The Australian Workplace Barometer (AWB) project also tested the relationship between psychosocial safety climate, job demands, and psychological health (Dollard, Bailey, et al., 2012; Dollard & Bailey, 2014). The final multi-occupational sample comprised 5743 interviews from individual participants representing a wide range of occupations and industries. Researchers identified that organizational psychosocial safety climate (in this large population-based study psychosocial safety climate was assessed at the individual level since most interviewees came from different organizations – a limitation in this study is it is not possible to determine if effects are due to perceived psychosocial safety climate or organizational-level psychosocial safety climate) was negatively associated with demands (in particular work–family conflict, work pressure, emotional demands, and workplace bullying and harassment) that in turn related to poor psychological health including psychological distress, emotional exhaustion, depression, and fatigue (Dollard, Bailey, et al., 2012). Psychosocial safety climate was also positively associated with resources (job control and social support) as well as macro-decision latitude, work rewards, organizational justice, and in turn work engagement (Dollard, Bailey, et al., 2012). The research indicated that a 10 percent increase in psychosocial safety climate within organizations would lead to a 4.5 percent decrease in bullying, a 4 percent decrease in demands, and an 8 percent increase in resources (Dollard & Bailey, 2014). Using hierarchical multiple regression psychosocial safety climate explained 9 percent of the variance in psychological health outcomes and 13 percent of the variance in engagement (Dollard & Bailey, 2014). The AWB project also identified that people with only mild symptoms of depression took twice as many sick days as those with no symptoms of depression (McTernan et al., 2013). These results suggest that psychosocial safety climate is a logical upstream target, not just for injury prevention but also for productivity outcomes such as absenteeism (McTernan et al., 2013). The AWB project provides a compelling evidence base for the creation of adequately resourced work environments that stimulate problem solving, creativity, and innovation, underpinned and maintained by a strong psychosocial safety climate (Dollard & Bailey, 2014).

Hall, Dollard, Winefield, Bakker, and Dormann (2013) used a general population sample of 2343 workers (an earlier AWB sample) and identified that psychosocial safety climate moderated the effects of job demands (psychological and emotional demands) on depression and further moderated the effects of depression on positive organizational behaviors (engagement and job satisfaction). Zimmerman, Haun, Dormann, and Dollard (2009) also found, in a study of 50 car sales employees, that high levels of psychosocial safety climate protected employees from the negative consequences of difficult customer behavior, by reducing their negative emotional reactions.

Yulita, Idris, and Dollard (2014), using a sample of 909 police personnel from 58 departments, examined how team-level psychosocial safety climate affects job demands, specifically challenge demands and hindrance demands (Cavanaugh, Boswell, Roehling, & Boudreau, 2000). Hindrance demands were considered to be demands that could be perceived as a threat to personal growth and mastery such as role conflict and job insecurity while challenge demands were defined as those that can be perceived to lead to personal growth, creativity, and innovative performance such as high workload and job complexity (LePine, Podsakoff, & LePine, 2005). Yulita et al. (2014) identified that psychosocial safety climate at the team level was negatively related to hindrance demands.

Hindrance demands were also positively related to emotional exhaustion and physical health problems (Yulita et al., 2014). This study used cross-sectional data so further exploration of the hindrance and challenge job demand differentiation using longitudinal data is needed.

Bailey, Dollard, and Richards (2015) identified benchmark levels of psychosocial safety climate that would signify risk of job strain (jobs with high levels of demands and low levels of resources), and subsequent levels of adverse workplace psychological health in organizations. Using the AWB data set (N = 1081) and interview data from Australian employees matched at two time points 12 months apart, psychosocial safety climate was a significant predictor of job strain (determined by combining two separate measures of psychological demands and job control), and in turn depression. Using additional data (N = 3,140) benchmarks of organizational psychosocial safety climate (range 12–60) were established for low-risk (41 or above) and high risk (37 or below) for employee job strain and depressive symptoms. Finally, population attributable risk was assessed finding that improving psychosocial safety climate in organizations to 37 or above could reduce 14 percent of job strain and 16 percent of depressive symptoms in the Australian working population.

Future Research

An extended four-level framework incorporating sociopolitical, organizational, work group, and individual factors is warranted in further research to explain the multifaceted causes of work-related psychological health across a wider range of sociopolitical contexts (Dollard & Neser, 2013). Future research should try to maximize the number of upper-level groups in the sample to examine between-organization relationships (Idris et al., 2012).

To manage problems associated with common method variance and subjective bias, future studies could triangulate evidence from a variety of sources (e.g., injury rates, sickness absence, near miss reports, work stress compensation claims, focus groups, situational audits, hospital records, or levels of patient readmission or mortality rates) (Idris et al., 2012; Law et al., 2011). Psychosocial safety climate could be measured in alternative ways, for example, as actual awareness of organizational policies, practices, and procedures, or by assessing whether the monitoring or assessment of psychosocial hazards actually occurs (Dollard, Bailey, et al., 2012) For example, Dollard and Neser (2013) operationalized psychosocial safety climate in terms of policies and procedures for stress, bullying, and violence. Specific labor policies and their direct effect on worker health could also be assessed (see Dragano, Siegrist, & Wahrendorf, 2011), and the impact of external policy influences on internal workplace policy development (Dollard & Neser, 2013).

Item response analysis to verify that items and scales carry the same meaning across different cultures should be completed (Shimazu, Schaufeli, Miyanake, & Iwata, 2010). Knowledge development in Eastern and emerging economies in the field of work stress is especially scarce (Kang, Staniford, Dollard, & Kompier, 2008; Kortum, Leka, & Cox, 2008). Despite the adoption of Western-style working practices in developing countries most Western-derived theoretical models of stress have not been tested in these populations (Brough, Dollard, & Tuckey, 2014). The Asia Pacific, in particular, is the world's most populous region, yet many workers experience poor work conditions and insecure employment (Dollard, Shimazu, Nordin, Brough, & Tuckey, 2014). Greater research attention needs to be directed toward understanding the nature and influence of psychosocial factors in this region (Dollard et al., 2014).

Longitudinal data collection at three separate time points to test mediation is recommended for future research (Idris et al., 2012). Psychosocial safety climate strength and its correlates could also be examined (Dollard, Tuckey, & Dormann, 2012). Future studies could differentiate between permanent and temporary employees as Luria and Yagil (2010) found differences between the two groups in relation to safety perceptions.

Leaders are largely responsible for psychosocial safety climate and it is likely that different leadership styles influence levels of psychosocial safety climate (e.g., Barling, Loughlin, & Kelloway, 2002; Zohar, 2002). Future research could compare the effects of psychosocial safety-specific leadership training on psychosocial factors and psychological health, in comparison with work groups where leaders are trained in general transformational leadership practices (Dollard, Tuckey, & Dormann, 2012). It is expected that training in leadership for psychosocial safety climate will be superior than training in other kinds of leadership for predicting psychosocial safety climate, work conditions, and health outcomes.

Conclusion

Work related stress, burnout, depression, and anxiety create workers' compensation claims, absenteeism, productivity loss, and staff turnover, yet until recently managers have had little available research theory and evidence to structure organizations to prevent the development of the work conditions that lead to poor psychological health (Law et al., 2011). Key stakeholder groups (such as trade unions, employer organizations, government agencies, occupational health services, researchers and academics), and non-traditional intervention groups (such as social security agencies, health insurers, families and partners, non-government organizations, health care institutions, customers or clients, shareholders, communities, employment agencies, media, judiciary system employees, and business consultants; World Health Organization, 2008) can use the psychosocial safety climate framework to proactively identify, measure, and monitor organizational psychosocial risk, design and evaluate targeted interventions at multiple levels, develop and set priorities for policies and interventions, benchmark progress, and monitor changing trends to improve work conditions, engagement, psychological health, and the productivity of employees (Hall et al., 2010). Organizations are complex multi-layered systems (Mathieu & Taylor, 2007) with dynamic interplay between levels (e.g., the organization, work unit and/or individual) (Dollard, Tuckey, & Dormann, 2012). Additional multi-level, longitudinal research using triangulated evidence, and interventions to evaluate the efficacy of psychosocial safety specific leadership training will assist our understanding of the mechanisms involved to promote the development of healthy workplaces.

References

Arnold, K. A., Turner, N., Barling, J., Kelloway, E. K., & McKee, M. C. (2007). Transformational leadership and psychological well-being: The mediating role of meaningful work. *Journal of Occupational Health Psychology, 12*, 193–203.

Bailey, T. S., Dollard, M. F., & Richards, P. A. M. (2015). A national standard for psychosocial safety climate (PSC): PSC 41 as the benchmark for low risk of job strain and depressive symptoms. *Journal of Occupational Health Psychology, 20*, 15–26.

Bailey, T. S., Pignata, S., & Dollard, M. F. (2014). Programmes and interventions for psychosocial risk and worker well-being: The psychosocial safety climate (PSC) framework. In R. J. Burke & A. M. Richardson (Eds.), *Corporate wellness programmes: Linking employee and organizational health* (pp. 101–119). Cheltenham, UK: Edward Elgar.

Bakker, A. B., & Demerouti, E. (2007). The Job Demands-Resources model: State of the art. *Journal of Managerial Psychology, 22,* 309–328

Barling, J., Loughlin, C., & Kelloway, E. K. (2002). Development and test of a model linking safety-specific transformational leadership and occupational safety. *Journal of Applied Psychology, 87,* 488–496.

Biron, C., Karankia-Murray, M., & Cooper, C. L. (2012). Organizational interventions for stress and well-being – an overview. In C. Biron, M. Karanika-Murray, & C. L. Cooper (Eds.), *Managing psychosocial risks in the workplace: The role of process issues.* New York, NY: Routledge Psychology Press.

Bloomfield, R., Chozos, N., Embrey, D., Henderson, J., Kelly, T., Koornneef, F., … , & Sujan, M. A. (2012). *Using safety cases in industry and healthcare: A pragmatic review of the use of safety cases in industry – lessons and prerequisites for their application in healthcare.* London, UK: Health Foundation.

Bolier, L., Haverman, M., Westerhof, G. J., Riper, H., Smit, F., & Bohlmeijer, E. (2013). Positive psychology interventions: A meta-analysis of randomized controlled studies. *BMC Public Health, 13,* 119.

Bond, S. A., Tuckey, M. R., Dollard, M. F. (2010). Psychosocial safety climate, workplace bullying, and symptoms of post-traumatic stress. *Organization Development Journal, 28,* 37–56.

Brough, P., Dollard, M. F., & Tuckey, M. R. (2014). Theory and methods to prevent and manage occupational stress: Innovations from around the globe. *International Journal of Stress Management, 21,* 1–6.

Cavanaugh, M. A., Boswell, W. R., Roehling, M. V., & Boudreau, J. W. (2000). An empirical examination of self-reported work stress among US managers. *Journal of Applied Psychology, 85,* 65–74.

Champoux, J. E., & Peters, W. S. (1987). Form effect size and power in moderated regression. *Journal of Occupational Psychology, 60,* 243–255.

Chaplin, W. E. (1991). The next generation of moderator research in personality psychology. *Journal of Personality, 59,* 143–178.

Cheyne, A., Cox, S., Oliver, A., & Tomás, J. M. (1998). Modelling safety climate in the predictions of levels of safety activity. *Work & Stress, 12,* 255–271.

Clarke, S. (2006). The relationship between safety climate and safety performance: A meta-analytic review. *Journal of Occupational Health Psychology, 11,* 315–327.

Clarke, S. (2010). An integrative model of safety climate: Linking psychological climate and work attitudes to individual safety outcomes using meta-analysis. *Journal of Occupational and Organizational Psychology, 83,* 553–578.

Cox, S. J., & Cheyne, A. J. T. (2000). Assessing safety culture in offshore environments. *Safety Science, 34,* 111–129.

Crawford, E. R., LePine, J. A., & Rich, B. L. (2010). Linking job demands and resources to employee engagement and burnout: A theoretical extension and meta-analytic test. *Journal of Applied Psychology, 95,* 834–848.

De Frank, R. S., & Cooper, C. L. (1987). Worksite stress management interventions: Their effectiveness and conceptualisation. *Journal of Managerial Psychology, 2,* 4–10.

De Jonge, J., Demerouti, E., & Dormann, C. (2014). Current theoretical perspectives in work psychology. In M. C. W. Peeters, J. de Jonge, & T. W. Taris (Eds.), *An introduction to contemporary work psychology* (pp. 89–113). Chichester, UK: John Wiley & Sons, Ltd.

De Jonge, J., & Dormann, C. (2003). The DISC model: Demand-Induced Strain Compensation mechanisms in job stress. In M. F. Dollard, H. R. Winefield, & A. H. Winefield (Eds.), *Occupational stress in the service professions* (pp. 43–74). Abingdon, UK: Taylor & Francis.

De Jonge, J., & Dormann. (2006). Stressors, resources, and strain at work: A longitudinal test of the Triple-Match Principle. *Journal of Applied Psychology, 91,* 1359–1374.

De Lange, A. H., Taris, T. W., Kompier, M. A. J., Houtman, I. L. D., & Bongers, P. M. (2003). The very best of the millennium: Longitudinal research and the demand-control-support model. *Journal of Occupational Health Psychology, 8,* 282–305.

Demerouti, E., & Bakker, A. B. (2011). The job demands-resources model: Challenges for future research. *SA Journal of Industrial Psychology, 37,* 1–9.

Demerouti, E., Bakker, A. B., Nachreiner, F., & Schaufeli, W. B. (2001). The job demands-resources model of burnout. *Journal of Applied Psychology, 86*(3), 499–512.

Dextras-Gauthier, J., Marchand, A., & Haines, V. (2012). Organizational culture, work organization conditions, and mental health: a proposed integration. *International Journal of Stress Management, 19*, 81–104

Dollard, M. F. (2012). Psychological safety climate: A lead indicator of work conditions, workplace psychological health and engagement and precursor to intervention success. In C. Biron, M. Karanika-Murray, & C. L. Cooper (Eds.), *Managing psychosocial risks in the workplace: Addressing process and context* (pp. 77–101). New York, NY: Routledge Psychology Press.

Dollard, M. F., & Bailey, T. S. (2014). *The Australian Workplace Barometer: Psychosocial safety climate and working conditions in Australia.* Samford Valley, Australia: Australian Academic Press.

Dollard, M. F., Bailey, T., McLinton, S., Richards, P., McTernan, W., Taylor, A., & Bond, S. (2012). *The Australian Workplace Barometer: Report on psychosocial safety climate and worker health in Australia.* Canberra, Australia: Safe Work Australia.

Dollard, M. F., & Bakker, A. B. (2010). Psychosocial safety climate as a precursor to conducive work environments, psychological health problems, and employee engagement. *Journal of Occupational and Organisational Psychology, 83*, 579–599.

Dollard, M. F. & Gordon, J. A. (2014). Evaluation of a participatory risk management work stress intervention. *International Journal of Stress Management, 21*, 27–42.

Dollard, M. F., & Kang, S. (2007). *Psychosocial safety climate measure.* Adelaide, Australia: Work & Stress Research Group, University of South Australia.

Dollard, M. F., & Karasek, R. (2010). Building psychosocial safety climate: Evaluation of a socially coordinated PAR risk management stress prevention study. In J. Houdmont & S. Leka, (Eds.), *Contemporary occupational health psychology: Global perspectives on research and practice,* (pp. 208–234). Oxford, UK: Wiley-Blackwell.

Dollard, M.F., & McTernan, W. (2011). Psychosocial safety climate: A multilevel theory of work stress in the health and community sector. *International Journal for Epidemiology and Psychiatric Services, 20*, 1–7.

Dollard, M. F., & Neser, D. (2013). Worker health is good for the economy: Union density and psychosocial safety climate as determinants of country differences in worker health and productivity in 31 European countries. *Social Science and Medicine, 92*, 114–123.

Dollard, M. F., Opie, T., Lenthall, S., Wakerman, J., Knight, S., Dunn, S., Rickard, G., & McLeod, M. (2012). Psychosocial safety climate as an antecedent to work characteristics and psychological strain: A multilevel model. *Work & Stress, 26*(4), 385–404.

Dollard, M. F., Osborne, K., & Manning, I. (2012). Organization-environment adaptation: A macrolevel shift in modeling work distress and morale. *Journal of Organizational Behavior, 34*, 629–647.

Dollard, M. F., Shimazu, A., Nordin, R. B., Brough, P., & Tuckey, M. R. (2014). *Psychosocial factors at work in the Asia Pacific.* Dordrecht, the Netherlands: Springer.

Dollard, M. F., Tuckey, M. R., & Dormann, C. (2012). Psychosocial safety climate moderates the job demand-resource interaction in predicting workgroup distress. *Accident Analysis and Prevention, 45*, 694–704.

Dragano, D., Siegrist, J., & Wahrendorf, M. (2011). Welfare regimes, labour policies and unhealthy psychosocial working conditions: A comparative study with 9917 older employees from 12 European countries. *Journal of Epidemiology and Community Health, 65*, 793–799.

Edmonson, A. (1999). Psychological safety and learning behaviour in work teams. *Administrative Science Quarterly, 44*, 350–383.

Eisenberger, R., Huntington, R., Hutchison, S., & Sowa, D. (1986). Perceived organisational support. *Journal of Applied Psychology, 71*, 500–507.

European Agency for Safety and Health at Work (2011). *Occupational safety and health culture assessment – A review of main approaches and selected tools.* Luxembourg: Publication Office of the European Union, 2011. doi:10.2802/53184

European Agency for Safety and Health at Work (2012). *Management of psychosocial risks at work: An analysis of the findings of the European survey of enterprises on new and emerging risks (ESENER).* Luxembourg: Publication Office of the European Union, 2011. doi:10.2802/92077

Evans, M. G. (1985). A Monte Carlo study of the effects of correlated method variance in moderated multiple regression analysis. *Organisational Behaviour and Human Decision Processes, 36,* 305–323.

Flin, R., Mearns, K., O'Connor, P., & Bryden, R. (2000). Measuring safety climate: Identifying the common features. *Safety Science, 34,* 177–192.

Giga, S. I., Noblet, A. J., Faragher, B., & Cooper, C. L. (2003). The UK perspective: A review of research on occupational stress management interventions. *Australian Psychologist, 38,* 158–164.

Grote, G. (2008). Diagnosis of safety culture: A replication and extension towards assessing "safe" organizational change processes. *Safety Science, 46,* 450–460.

Grote, G., & Kunzler, C. (2000). Diagnosis of safety culture in safety management audits. *Safety Science, 34,* 131–150.

Halbesleben, J. R. B., Osburn, H. K., & Mumford, M. D. (2006). Action research as a burnout intervention. *Journal of Applied Behavioral Science, 42,* 244–266.

Hall, G. B., Dollard, M. F., & Coward, J. (2010). Psychosocial safety climate: Development of the PSC-12. *International Journal of Stress Management, 17,* 353–383.

Hall, G. B., Dollard, M. F., Winefield, A. H., Bakker, A. B., & Dormann, C. (2013). Psychosocial safety climate buffers effects of job demands on depression and positive organisation behaviours. *Anxiety, Stress & Coping, 26,* 355–377.

Harter, J. K., Schmidt, F. L., & Hayes, T. L. (2002). Business-unit-level relationship between employee satisfaction, employee engagement, and business outcomes: A meta-analysis. *Journal of Applied Psychology, 87,* 268–279.

Häusser, J. A., Mojzisch, A., Niesel, M., & Schulz-Hardt, S. (2010). Ten years on: A review of recent research on the Job Demand-Control-Support model and psychological well-being. *Work & Stress, 24,* 1–35.

Huang, Y., Ho, M., Smith, G. S., & Chen, P. Y. (2006). Safety climate and self-reported injury: Assessing the mediating role of employee safety control. *Accident Analysis & Prevention, 38,* 425–433.

Idris, M. A., & Dollard, M. F. (2011). Psychosocial safety climate, work conditions and emotions in the workplace: A Malaysian population-based work stress study. *International Journal of Stress Management, 18,* 324–347.

Idris, M. A., Dollard, M. F., Coward, J., & Dormann, C. (2012). Psychosocial safety climate: Conceptual distinctiveness and effect on job demands and worker psychological health. *Safety Science, 50,* 19–28.

Idris, M. A., Dollard, M. F., & Winefield, A. H. (2011). The effect of globalization on employee psychological health and job satisfaction in Malaysian workplaces. *Journal of Occupational Health, 53,* 447–454.

International Atomic Energy Agency (2002). *Key practical issues in strengthening safety culture,* Report 15. Vienna, Austria: International Nuclear Safety Advisory Group (INSAG).

Johnson, J. V., & Hall, E. M. (1988). Job strain, work place social support, and cardiovascular disease: A cross sectional study of a random sample of the Swedish working population. *American Journal of Public Health, 78,* 1336–1342.

Jordon, J., Gurr, E., Tinline, G., Giga, S. I., Faragher, B., & Cooper, C. L. (2003). *Beacons of excellence in stress prevention.* Manchester, UK: Robertson Cooper and UMIST.

Kang, S. Y., Staniford, A., Dollard, M. F., & Kompier, M. (2008). Knowledge development and content in occupational health psychology: A systematic analysis of the *Journal of Occupational Health Psychology* and *Work & Stress,* 1996–2006. In J. Houdmont & S. Leka (Eds.), *Occupational health psychology: European perspectives on research, education and practice* (pp. 27–63). Maia, Portugal: ISMAI Publishers.

Karasek, R. A. (1979). Job demands, job decision latitude, and mental strain: Implications for job redesign. *Administration Science Quarterly, 224,* 285–307.

Karasek, R. B., Kawakami, C., Houtman. N., Bongers, I., & Amick, P. (1998). The Job Content Questionnaire (JCQ): An instrument for internationally comparative assessments of psychosocial job characteristics. *Journal of Occupational Health Psychology, 3,* 322–355.

Karasek, R., & Theorell, T. (1990). *Healthy work: Stress, productivity, and the reconstruction of working life*. New York, NY: Basic Books.

Kines, P., Lappalainen, J., Mikkelsen, K. L., Olsen, E., Pousette, A., Tharaldsen, J., Tomasson, K., & Torner, M. (2011). Nordic Safety Climate Questionnaire (NOSACQ-50). *International Journal of Industrial Ergonomics, 41*, 634–646.

Kompier, M., & Cooper, C. L. (Eds.) (1999). *Preventing stress, improving productivity: European case studies in the workplace*. London, UK: Routledge.

Kompier, M. A. J., & Kristensen, T. S. (2001). Organizational work stress interventions in a theoretical, methodological and practical context. In J. Dunham (Ed.), *Stress in the workplace: Past, present and future* (pp. 164–190). London, UK: Whurr.

Kortum, E., Leka, S., & Cox, T. (2008). Understanding the perception of occupational psychosocial risk factors in developing countries: Setting priorities for action. In J. Houdmont & S. Leka (Eds.), *Occupational health psychology, European perspectives on research, education and practice* (vol. 3, pp. 191–228). Nottingham, UK: Nottingham University Press

Le Blanc, P. M., Hox, J. J., Schaufeli, W. B., Taris, T. W., & Peeters, M. C. W. (2007). Take care! The evaluation of a team-based burnout intervention program for oncology care providers. *Journal of Applied Psychology, 92*, 213–227.

LaMontagne, A. D., Keegel, T., Louie, A. M., Ostry, A., & Landsbergis, P. A. (2007). A systematic review of the job-stress intervention evaluation literature 1990–2005. *International Journal of Occupational and Environmental Medicine, 13*, 268–280.

LaMontagne, A. D., Noblet, A. J., & Landsbergis, P. A. (2012). Intervention development and implementation: Understanding and addressing barriers to organizational-level interventions. In C. Biron, M. Karanika-Murray, & C. L. Cooper (Eds.), *Managing psychosocial risks in the workplace: The role of process issues* (pp. 21–38). New York, NY: Routledge Psychology Press.

Law, R., Dollard, M., Tuckey, M., & Dormann, C. (2011). Psychosocial safety climate as a lead indicator of workplace bullying and harassment, job resources, psychological health and employee engagement. *Accident Analysis and Prevention, 43*, 1782–1793.

Leiter, M. P., Laschinger, H. K. S., Day, A., & Oore, D. G. (2011). The impact of civility interventions on employee social behaviour, distress, and attitudes. *Journal of Applied Psychology, 96*, 1258–1274.

LePine, J. A., Podsakoff, N. P., & LePine, M. A. (2005). A meta-analytic test of the challenge stressor-hindrance stressor framework: An explanation for inconsistent relationships among stressors and performance. *Academy of Management Journal, 48*, 764–775.

Luria, G., & Yagil, D. (2010). Safety perception referents of permanent and temporary employees: Safety climate boundaries in the industrial workplace. *Accident Analysis & Prevention, 42*, 1423–1430.

Marine, A., Ruotsalainen, J. H., Serra, C., & Verbeek, J. H. (2006). Preventing occupational stress in healthcare workers. *Cochrane Database of Systematic Reviews, 4*. doi:10.1002/14651858. CD002892.pub2

Mathieu, J., & Taylor, S. (2007). Framework for testing meso-mediational relationships in organizational behaviour. *Journal of Organizational Behavior, 28*, 141–172

McTernan, W. P., Dollard, M. F., & LaMontagne, A. D. (2013). Clinical and sub-clinical depression in Australian workplaces: An economic cost analysis of depression-related productivity loss attributable to job-strain and bullying. *Work & Stress, 27*, 321–338.

Nahrgang, J. D., Morgeson, F. P., & Hofmann (2011). Safety at work: A meta-analytic investigation of the link between job demands, job resources, burnout, engagement, and safety outcomes. *Journal of Applied Psychology, 96*, 71–94.

Neal, A., & Griffin, M. A. (2006). A study of the lagged relationships among safety climate, safety motivation, safety behaviour, and accidents at the individual and group levels. *Journal of Applied Psychology, 91*, 946–953.

Nielsen, K. (2013). Review Article: How can we make organizational interventions work? Employees and line managers as actively crafting interventions. *Human Relations, 66*, 1029–1050.

Nielsen, K., & Randall, R. (2012). The importance of employee participation and perceptions of changes in procedures in a teamworking intervention. *Work & Stress, 26*, 91–111.

Parker, C. P., Baltes, B. B., Young, S. A., Huff, J. W, Altmann, R. A., LaCost, H. A., & Roberts, J. E. (2003). Relationships between psychological climate perceptions and work outcomes: A meta-analytic review. *Journal of Organizational Behavior, 24,* 389–416.

Pignata, S., Biron, C., & Dollard, M. F. (2014). Managing psychosocial risks in the workplace prevention and intervention. In M. C. W. Peeters, J. de Jonge, & T. W. Taris (Eds.), *An introduction to contemporary work psychology* (pp. 393–413). Chichester, UK: John Wiley & Sons, Ltd.

Reichers, A. E., & Schneider, B. (1990). Climate and culture: An evolution of constructs. In B. Schneider (Ed.), *Organizational climate and culture* (pp. 5–39). San Franscisco, CA: Jossey-Bass.

Richardson, K. M., & Rothstein, H. R. (2008). Effects of occupational stress management intervention programs: A meta-analysis. *Journal of Occupational Health Psychology, 13,* 69–93.

Rickard, G., Lenthall, S., Dollard, M., Opie, T., Knight, S., Dunn, S., Wakerman, J., MacLeod, M., Seiler, J., & Brewester-Webb, D. (2012). Organisational intervention to reduce occupational stress and turnover in hospital nurses in the Northern Territory, Australia. *Collegian, 165,* 1–11.

Sanderson, K., Tilse, E., Nicholson, J., Oldenburg, B., & Graves, N. (2007). Which presenteeism measures are more sensitive to depression and anxiety? *Journal of Affect Disorders, 101,* 65–74.

Schaufeli, W. B., & Bakker, A. B. (2004). Job demands, job resources, and their relationship with burnout and engagement: A multi-sample study. *Journal of Organizational Behavior, 25,* 293–315.

Schaufeli, W. B., & Taris, T. W. (2014). A critical review of the job demands-resource model: Implications for improving work and health. In G. Bauer & O. Hamming (Eds.), *Bridging occupational, organizational and public health: A transdisciplinary approach* (pp. 43–68). Dordrecht, the Netherlands: Springer.

Schimazu, A., Schaufeli, W. B., Miyanake, D., & Iwata, N. (2010). Why Japanese workers show low work engagement: An item response theory analysis of the Ultrecht Work Engagement Scale. *BioPsychoSocial Medicine, 4,* 1–6

Siegrist, J. (1996). Adverse health effects of high-effort/low-reward conditions. *Journal of Occupational Health Psychology, 1,* 27–41.

Silvia, S., Lima, M. L., & Baptista, C. (2004). OSCI: An organisational and safety climate inventory. *Safety Science, 42,* 205–220.

Skogstad, A., Einarsen, S., Torsheim, T., Aasland, M. S., & Hetland, H. (2007). The destructiveness of laissez-faire leadership behaviour. *Journal of Occupational Health Psychology, 12,* 80–92.

Snyder, L. A., Krauss, A. D., Chen, P. Y., Finlinson, S., & Huang, Y. (2008). Occupational safety: Application of the job-demand-control-support model. *Accident Analysis & Prevention, 40,* 1713–1723.

Tuckey, M. R., Bakker, A. B., & Dollard, M. F. (2012). Empowering leaders optimize working conditions for engagement: A multilevel study. *Journal of Occupational Health Psychology, 17,* 15–27.

Van der Doef, M., & Maes, S. (1999). The Job Demand-Control (-Support) Model and psychological well-being: A review of 20 years of empirical research. *Work & Stress, 13,* 87–114.

Van den Tooren, M., de Jonge, J., & Dormann, C. (2011). The Demand-Induced Strain Compensation Model: Background, key principles, theoretical underpinnings, and extended empirical evidence. In A. Caetano, S. A. Silvia, & M. J. Chambel (Eds.), *New challenges for a healthy workplace in human services* (pp. 13–59). Mering: Rainer Hampp Verlag.

Van Vegchel, N., de Jonge, J., Bosma, H., & Schaufeli, W. (2005). Reviewing the effort-reward imbalance model: Drawing up the balance of 45 empirical studies. *Social Science and Medicine, 60,* 1117–1131.

Van de Ven, B., de Jonge, J., & Vlerick, P. (2014). Testing the Triple-Match Principle in the technology sector: A two-wave longitudinal panel study. *Applied Psychology: An International Review, 63,* 300–325.

Van Wyk, B. E., & Pillay-Van Wyk, V. (2010). Preventative staff-support interventions for health workers. *Cochrane Database of Systematic Reviews, 3.* doi:10:1002/14651858.CD003541.pub2

Wakerman, J., & Davey, C. (2008). Rural and remote health management: "The next generation is not going to put up with this." *Asia Pacific Journal of Health Management, 3,* 13–18.

World Health Organization (WHO) (2008). PRIMA-EF Guidance on the European framework for psychosocial risk management (Protecting Workers' Health 9). Geneva, Switzerland: WHO.

Xanthopoulou, D., Bakker, A. B., Demerouti, E., & Schaufeli, W. B. (2007). The role of personal resources in the job demands-resources model. *International Journal of Stress Management, 14,* 121–141.

Yulita, Idris, M. A., & Dollard, M. F. (2014). A multi-level study of psychosocial safety climate, challenge and hindrance demands, employee exhaustion, engagement and physical health. In M. F. Dollard, A. Shimazu, R. B. Nordin, P. Brough, & M. R. Tuckey (Eds.), *Psychosocial factors at work in the Asia Pacific* (pp. 127–143). Dordrecht, the Netherlands: Springer.

Zimmerman, B. K., Haun, S., Dormann, C., & Dollard, M. (2009). Stress and reciprocity in service interactions: Main and moderating effects of psychosocial safety climate. In P. H. Langford, N. J. Reynolds, & J. E. Kehoe (Eds.), *Meeting the future: Promising sustainable organisational growth, 8th Industrial and Organisational Psychology Conference proceedings* (pp. 150–155). Sydney, Australia: Australian Psychological Society.

Zohar, D. (1980). Safety climate in industrial organizations: Theoretical and applied implications. *Journal of Applied Psychology, 65,* 96–102.

Zohar, D. (2002). The effects of leadership dimensions, safety climate and assigned priorities on minor injuries in work groups. *Journal of Organizational Behaviour, 23,* 75–92.

Zohar, D. (2008). Safety climate and beyond: A multi-level multi-climate framework. *Safety Science, 46,* 376–387.

Zohar, D. (2010). Thirty years of safety climate research: Reflections and future directions. *Accident Analysis and Prevention, 42,* 1517–1522.

Zohar, D., & Luria, G. (2005). A multilevel of safety climate: Cross-level relationships between organisation and group-level climates. *Journal of Applied Psychology, 90,* 616–628.

19

Organizational Safety Culture

Frank Guldenmund

Introduction

Safety culture has become an important entry in both the safety scientist's and safety practitioner's handbook. This has not always been the case, on the contrary. The focus on group interaction and shared understanding is a more recent development in the history of Safety Science, which was preceded by eras where the primary focus was, firstly, on technology (First Age of Safety) and, secondly, on human factors, that is, behavior and competence (Second Age) respectively (Hale & Hovden, 1998). According to Hale and Hovden, we currently find ourselves in the Third Age of Safety, characterized by a strong focus on the formal organization surrounding safety, the safety management systems. The attention on safety culture in this third era could be considered an offshoot of the latter, with the additional remark that safety management is concerned with the more formal aspects of (organizational) safety, whereas safety culture, as will become clearer later in this chapter, pertains to the informal side of organizational life.

The notion of culture relating to safety was first introduced in the 1970s by Turner in his sociological account of man-made disasters (Turner, 1976, 1978).[1] However, at the time, neither the academic world nor safety practitioners took up the term for further exploration. In 1986, after the Chernobyl disaster, the term again was used to describe the failing organizational, but also political, circumstances surrounding the nuclear catastrophe. Yet, once more, the term remained largely untouched in academia and the applied safety field. Instead, after Chernobyl, the term started to reappear in various accident investigation reports as a causal mechanism underlying mishap and disaster. In the mean time, research focused on the concept of safety *climate* (Guldenmund, 2000), a psychological construct that is described in detail in other parts of this book (see Guediri & Griffin, Chapter 13; Luria, Chapter 16, this volume) and which is typically considered the "measurable aspect" of safety culture (Zohar, 2008).

In aforesaid accident reports the term safety culture was used mostly as a characteristic of an organization, a trait that the organization under investigation was obviously lacking,

The Wiley Blackwell Handbook of the Psychology of Occupational Safety and Workplace Health, First Edition. Edited by Sharon Clarke, Tahira M. Probst, Frank Guldenmund, and Jonathan Passmore. © 2016 John Wiley & Sons Ltd. Published 2020 by John Wiley & Sons Ltd.

or not having enough of. This is a particular interpretation of the term safety culture, which can be contrasted with the viewpoint that cultures emerge where people interact and have to accomplish something together. Such interaction requires some shared understanding, which ultimately leads to, at least partly, shared patterns of meaning that go by the name of culture (Smircich, 1985). If such understanding takes place within the context of an organization, the emergent culture is called an organizational culture. If this organization has risk on its agenda, because of occupational hazards or process hazards or any other physical or social threat the organization might face, safety will be a subject around which shared understandings develop. Through these understandings, members of the organization make sense of the (organizational) world and their activities therein. This, in a nutshell, is the position opposite the viewpoint taken in many accident reports and which will be discussed extensively later on.

Finally, at the end of the 1990s, safety culture started to become a topic for discussion and research, as exemplified by two thematic issues of *Work & Stress* (1998) and *Safety Science* (2000) on the subject (Glendon, 2008b; Guldenmund, 2007). Overall, one could say that the term *safety culture* was born out of a need to use contextual data surrounding a disaster to explain its manifestation. How culture can play a role in such events, and what culture basically is, are the topics of this chapter. First I will provide a critical perspective on the concept of culture and its use for organizational purposes. Next is a section on the different levels of culture (culture, organizational culture, and safety culture), followed by a section discussing models of (organizational safety) culture. How safety culture can be assessed through research will then be reviewed. Influencing safety culture applying the model proposed in a previous section, and which is often the goal of a safety culture assessment, is taken up next. The chapter ends with a future outlook on safety culture research.

Understanding Organizational Culture: A Critical Perspective

The scientific study of culture shows great variety and various disputes and scholars often differ on what culture actually "is" (Bouwhuijsen, Claes, & Derde, 1995; Keesing, 1981). According to Geertz there is no culture without humans but, also, "more significantly, without culture no men" (Geertz, 1973, p. 49). As early as 1952 anthropologists Kroeber and Kluckhohn (1952) had already compiled a list of 164 definitions of culture. Adding another definition to this extensive list seems rather pointless, but nevertheless I will need to provide a description of what I mean by culture and safety culture in this chapter. In talking about culture I will avoid treating culture as if it is a physical object in the world ready for us to observe and measure. I consider culture a phenomenon that has to be deciphered from these observables and measurables, hence primarily belonging to Habermas' practical knowledge interest (1987), which is aimed at understanding human reality by producing knowledge through interpretation (Alvesson, 2012). The definition of Richter and Koch (2004) seems to fit this take on safety culture well: "the shared and learned meanings, experiences and interpretations of work and safety – expressed partially symbolically – which guide peoples' actions towards risks, accidents and prevention" (p. 705).

The managerial interest for organizational culture emerged in the early 1980s, seeing the publication of books such as *In Search of Excellence* (Peters & Waterman, 1982), *Organizational Cultures* (Deal & Kennedy, 1982), and *Theory Z* (Ouchi, 1981). The emergence coincides with an apparent decline of US corporate efficiency and the rise of Japanese management methods. Indeed, Japanese corporations were at the time commonly associated with "strong" organizational cultures, and the early management literature made passionate claims about the connection between strong, homogeneous organizational cultures and organizational performance. Organizational culture in the 1980s became a recipe for success promoted by management consultants like McKinsey, who also sponsored the publication of two of the above-mentioned books (Alvesson, 1993). While many of the claims made by this early literature were overstated, the interest for organizational culture heralded an interest for the non-rational and symbolic dimension of organizational life.

The rise of culture as a means of control was particularly important in so-called knowledge-intensive organizations (Alvesson, 2004), dominated not by formal bureaucratic structures but rather by "loose couplings" (Weick, 1976). In a context where work processes as well as results are difficult to analyze, measure, and manage, directing the organizational control efforts toward norms and values becomes an efficient way of managing the workforce. As put by Ouchi (1979, p. 844):

> [I]f it is not possible to measure either behavior or outputs and it is therefore not possible to "rationally" evaluate the work of the organization, what alternative is there but to carefully select workers so that you can be assured of having an able and committed set of people, and then engaging in rituals and ceremonies which serve the purpose of rewarding those who display the underlying attitudes and values which are likely to lead to organizational success, thus reminding everyone of what they are supposed to be trying to achieve, even if they can't tell whether or not they are achieving it?

The management of organizational culture thus suggests a solution to a fundamental control problem in many organizations. This view has, however, met rather fierce critique. This critique can be divided into three groups: (1) critique regarding the empirical foundation for the claims made by proponents of "culture management," (2) critique regarding the ethics of cultural control, and (3) critique regarding the underlying conceptualization of "culture" within culture management. I will briefly discuss the first two critiques, and develop the third more thoroughly.

The first critique addresses the proposed link between strong and homogeneous organizational cultures, based on simple values and meanings, and organizational performance (for an overview see Alvesson, 1993). A core problem here is the reductionism involved in measuring organizational culture. This involves simplifying a richness of symbols, values, and meanings in order to relate these to performance measures. Such an approach will exclude many of those aspects considered to be the very reason culture is important. Moreover, there are problems of distinctly connecting symbolic action, for example, managerial attempts at influencing culture, to organizational performance (Pfeffer, 1981). While management and leadership certainly aim to influence meanings and symbols in an organization, the effects of such attempts are rarely unambiguous or easily evaluated (Smircich & Morgan, 1982). As summarized by Alvesson (1993, p. 42), "The general conclusion which can be drawn from these investigations of the link between organizational culture and performance is that the idea of culture very often promises more than it delivers."

The second critique regards the ethical foundation of cultural management. Here, drawing from critical theories from such diverse theorists as Foucault, Habermas, Horkheimer, Derrida, Marx, and Adorno, the underlying reason for cultural control is challenged. Cultural control is seen as less benign. Efforts at culture management are understood as colonizing the everyday life of employees, often without their prior consent. As a manager in Kunda's (1992, p. 5) seminal case study expresses it: "The idea is to educate people without them knowing it. Have the religion and not know how they even got it!" Culture management means imposing a corporate ideology on the employees and should therefore be analyzed from a power perspective (for an example in the field of safety culture, see Antonsen, 2009a). Accordingly, Axtell Ray (1986) identifies this as "the last frontier of control," arguing that management is no longer confined to managing time and bodies, but also souls.

In relation to the third critique, one should first note that the notion of culture implies a "depth" dimension, that is, culture exists at various levels. As argued by Schein (2010), culture manifests itself in terms of visible artifacts and espoused values but is fundamentally grounded in basic assumptions that "tend to be non-confrontable and non-debatable, and hence are extremely difficult to change" (Schein 2010, p. 28). In a more critical vein, then, it can be noted that cultural change often refers to superficial phenomena, such as slogans or participation in (ritualistic) behaviors, while the actual change in culture, that is, basic assumptions, is limited, or even absent. Indeed, the "recipients" of cultural change are often able to maintain distance and resist such change initiatives (e.g., Alvesson & Sveningsson, 2008; Fleming & Spicer, 2007; Kunda, 1992).

Secondly, culture is a multi-faceted phenomenon. There are different ways of approaching culture, and those approaching it from an anthropological perspective, influenced by authors such as Geertz (1973), often emphasize the indeterminacy and ambiguity of culture. Here, culture is not understood as some objective property of an organization, but rather as a particular perspective from which an analyst can approach an organization in order to attempt to understand its cultural and symbolic dimension. Put shortly, culture is considered not something an organization *has*, but something it *is* (Smircich, 1983). This also highlights the inherent ambiguity of cultural manifestations, and the potential of several, and conflicting, interpretations of cultural phenomena. Meyerson and Martin (1987) argue that from an ambiguity perspective "[d]ifferences in meaning, values, and behavioural norms are seen as incommensurable and irreconcilable" and that "[c]onsensus, dissensus, and confusion coexist, making it difficult to draw cultural and subcultural boundaries" (p. 637). Thus, while cultural manifestos and corporate slogans may appear clear and unambiguous, especially when interpreted by those responsible for creating them, in reality "organizational life seldom lives up to the facade of order it presents" (Batteau, 2001, p. 728). In fact, even organizational members may develop a competency in rehearsing slogans and manifestos, while at the same time not really internalizing them. Often, organizational cultures are "hypercultures, a carved-out set of positive-sounding statements about values, often decoupled from everyday-life thinking and practices" (Alvesson & Sveningsson, 2008, p. 119).

From what we might call a critical-anthropological view then, there are some important aspects of culture that influence how we could conceptualize and understand culture. Firstly, culture is not understood as something objectively accessible. Rather, manifestations of culture, such as ceremonies, artifacts, slogans, or change programs, should be understood in terms of their meaning to organizational members. This view on culture has a clear focus on interpretation, acknowledging the richness and symbolic dimension of meanings (Alvesson, 1993). It thereby also acknowledges both the "situated-ness" of meanings as well as the potentially ambiguous character of culture, inviting a broad understanding of how culture is received in the organization. Secondly, culture is viewed as contested and meaning-formation, and as a constant struggle, where different actors (e.g., top management, change agents, employees of different professions) may have different ideas of what culture means and different ways of relating to it. Thirdly, culture is viewed as a multilevel phenomenon, where different aspects of culture may have different meanings, and that these meanings may be more or less prone to change. As such, paying lip service to "customer is king" or "safety first" is something entirely different from embracing it as a core belief.

Approached from this perspective, culture becomes less interesting as a management tool but more interesting as a way of trying to understand organizational everyday life. Following Habermas' (1987) differentiation between human interests, we can see that the early adaptation of "culture" in management writing largely conformed to a technical-cognitive interest, approaching culture from an objectivist ontology with the aim of improving organizational performance. An anthropological view on culture, on the contrary, draws more on a practical and emancipatory knowledge interest. Here, the emphasis is primarily on understanding the meaning(s) held by actors in a particular organizational setting, and potentially identifying "ideologically frozen relations of dependence that can in principle be transformed" (Habermas, 1987, p. 310). In relation to the notion of safety culture, an inherently normative concept (Guldenmund, 2000), this perspective poses some distinct challenges (see further below).

As described above, much controversy existed on paradigms, ontologies, and epistemologies in the two final decades of the last century, often described as paradigm wars. However, while these issues may not have been resolved indefinitely, the dust has settled and the hatchet appears to have been buried. In an attempt to reconcile positions, Cunliffe (2011) proposes a rather pragmatic approach toward the study of organizational phenomena, including culture. She considers qualitative research a "craft" that may call for different perspectives for different challenges. All approaches bring a unique perspective on organizational issues, which might not be covered in the other perspectives and neither perspective can hold a claim of providing the most comprehensive, let alone the "right" view. Although I support this view on organization studies, I nevertheless think that researches should seriously reflect on issues of ontology and epistemology when embarking on culture study. I will pick this issue up again in a later section.

Culture, Organizational Culture, and Safety Culture

As stated previously, culture can be studied at several levels of aggregation of which national culture is considered to be the highest level (Hofstede, 1991). Although other groups can be defined at even higher levels (e.g., based on religion or profession), according to Hofstede the culture of such groups or categories of people are more determined by local (i.e., national or lower level) conditions. One person often belongs to a number of groups and can therefore share several cultures with different people.[2]

Overall, there are two analytical perspectives from which culture can be studied and both are well established within the scientific literature. The *functional* perspective considers culture a variable that can be *operationalized* like any other variable (Glendon, 2008a; Nævestad, 2009; Smircich, 1983), as well as manipulated and changed, and which is often managed from the top of the organization. This perspective is best illustrated by the statement: Object x *has* culture characteristics y, which have been *measured* by using method z. This is the perspective that was, and still is, dominant in much normative management literature on cultural change and culture management. It can be contrasted with the *interpretative* perspective, which considers culture a system of meanings and symbols that have to be (partly) fathomed to truly understand the people maintaining them (Alvesson, 2012; Haukelid, 2008; Richter & Koch, 2004). From the interpretive perspective, culture is *a way of looking* at particular groups, like organizations, departments, or teams. This is the perspective that has emerged from the critical-anthropological approach to organizational culture in the early 1990s and it largely conforms to the practical knowledge interest, mentioned above. The difference between these two perspectives is quite fundamental and it will reappear in several places in this chapter.

An assumed function of culture is reduction of uncertainty (Van Hoewijk, 1988) or even anxiety (Schein, 2010), which should lead to more continuity, because less time is spent on various mutual adjustments within a group. The fact that people know what to expect in a variety of situations, for example, with regard to particular rituals (like celebrations, meetings, appointments, etc.), the expression of emotions, dress codes, behaviors, and so on, makes life more predictable and hence more fluent (Alvesson, 2012; Smircich, 1985). Culture has also been linked to adaptation (Schein, 2010) and habituation. Adaptation is important for learning, for continuity, and therefore for survival. Forces from outside the organism that demand its adaptation will initiate change;[3] in this view, cultures are considered both functional and well-adapted to their environment, which is the basic premise of functionalism.

Culture should be distinguished from human nature (our genes) and personality (our character) in that it is shared by a defined group of people, whereas human nature and personality are not. Culture is sometimes considered the "collective memory"[4] of a group and is therefore thoroughly intertwined with the history of that group (Hofstede, 1991; Schein, 2010). Moreover, the term "memory" also implies that culture is learned, not inherited, unlike our human nature.

The distinction between the functional and interpretive approach toward culture is present in organizational culture studies and safety culture studies, although in the latter field the functional approach dominates (Glendon, 2008a; Guldenmund, 2007). One reason for this could be that establishing a causal link between (safety) culture and (safety) performance is problematic. When following a functional approach toward safety culture – this often implies administering a questionnaire and, hence, collecting semi-quantitative data – establishing such causal links is often attempted. Quantitative data clearly lend themselves to the modeling and testing of various statistical relationships between survey data and safety output data, like incidents, accidents, or any other type of relevant numerical data. From an interpretist viewpoint, however, the whole point of a culture study is understanding, not establishing, a nomothetic framework that can be applied everywhere. Moreover, from an interpretist's viewpoint most functionalist approaches do not study culture, they study attitudes at best (Guldenmund, 2007).

For some, safety culture is a specific kind of organizational culture, something an organization either has or does not have (e.g., Geller, 1994; International Atomic Energy Agency, 2002; Reason, 1997). The view here is primarily normative in that a culture is compared with a norm or standard of "safety culture." These standards are usually based on expert opinion (e.g., International Atomic Energy Agency, 2002) or experience (e.g., Energy Institute, undated). Other well-known conceptualizations of safety culture come from Reason (1997), Pidgeon and O'Leary (2000), and the International Nuclear Safety Advisory Group (1991, 1992). All of these have the normative flavor that often comes with the concept. However, stating what is desirable does not mean these desirabilities are easily established, let alone internalized.[5]

For functionalists, safety culture often defaults to *patterns of behavior* (e.g., Cooper, 2000; Cooper & Phillips, 2004; Furnham, 1997) whereas interpretists propose *patterns of meaning* and try to "read between and behind the lines" of the people of a cultural unit (Alvesson, 2012). In this chapter I consider safety culture that part of organizational culture that is concerned with safety; concerned with implying that organization members have developed specific meanings, symbols, and behaviors around safety through interaction and communication. Their behaviors can and sometimes will be symbolic in nature and hence have to be interpreted to understand their cultural meaning, that is, the meaning they have for the people within the cultural unit. Most scholars do not believe that raw data like words and deeds offer an unobstructed view on an underlying (organizational, safety) culture.

Another important aspect of culture, especially of organizational culture, is its integrity or wholeness. Regarding this wholeness there are three competing views: the *integration view*, the differentiation view, and the *fragmentation view* (Haukelid, 2008; Martin, 2002; Nævestad, 2009; Richter & Koch, 2004). Looking at culture from an integrated view implies looking for the homogeneity in a culture, the meanings and symbols shared by most. This view was particularly popular in the 1980s when researchers and consultants looked for the essence of "successful" organizational cultures, as this essence might hold the key for success (cf. Peters & Waterman, 1982). The assumption was that this essence permeated the whole of the organization, causing its success; see also the section on the genesis of organizational culture above. Subsequent research, however, revealed differentiation rather than integration, implying that "the" organizational culture might break down into multiple subcultures. Later, next to differentiation, fragmentation was also pinpointed in organizations, suggesting even less coherence than differentiation already implied. Richter and Koch (2004) develop fragmentation further in terms of ambiguity and conflict, following Alvesson (2012). However, as the latter explains, such ambiguity exists within certain boundaries, otherwise the notion of culture as a shared understanding is rendered useless. Moreover, Alvesson considers all three perspectives as analytical tools rather than descriptions of a fixed state of affairs. That is, when looking at a culture from an integrative (differentiation, fragmentation) perspective, how does it look?

To summarize, culture is a complex social-scientific phenomenon that allows multiple perspectives on its nature. Its manifestations do not offer a window upon its underlying meanings; these should be treated as symbols instead and interpreted further. These meanings emerge through people communicating and interacting within a particular context, yet they are influenced also by larger contexts like those governed by politics, economics, religion, or any other power exercised at the societal or even global level (Alvesson, 2012). Organizational and safety culture share many of the characteristics of culture but emerge in the particular context of an organization, or other social categories, like professions, with safety culture pertinent for organizations that face (significant) physical or social threats. Safety culture has been conceptualized both as an either/or characteristic – organizations either have it or not – or as symbols and meanings all organizations develop and which provide a framework to the people of a cultural unit (an organization, a department, a team) for understanding risk and safety. This framework is itself a subject for considerable discussion, and it will be taken up in the next section.

Models of Safety Culture

A unifying theory has always posed a stumbling block to scholars concerned with culture (Bouwhuijsen et al., 1995; Haukelid, 2008) and the same goes for safety culture (Guldenmund, 2000). Moreover, as Bouwhuijsen et al. write, "in order to talk about cultural differences sensibly you must have a theory specifying what makes human groups into cultures to begin with" (1995, p. 166). With regard to the latter, both a functionalist and an interpretist view can be put forward. A functionalist will look for a common denominator, an underlying structure that applies to all cultures. This structure will be found to some extent with all members of the culture (Hofstede, Hofstede, & Minkov, 2010; Cameron & Quinn, 2011). An interpretist will approach every culture anew, although it might acknowledge that the culture itself is the outcome of a process comparable across cultures.

A primary assumption that underlies much cultural thinking is that thought precedes action (Geertz, 1973; Nævestad, 2009). And, as we have seen in a previous paragraph, shared understanding influences human thought and cognition. Moreover, shared understanding emerges through interaction and communication within groups of people in a specific context. For functionalists, this process of construction of culture is driven by survival instincts and the need to adapt to a dynamic and sometimes intimidating environment. Such a viewpoint also opens a door to possible manipulation and steering from management, which has already been observed above. For interpretative researchers this process takes place anyway, is unpredictable, and does not have to lead to optimal results but rather results in coordinated and more fluent and informed work processes.

Hofstede presents a functionalist model in which (national) culture is the product of various conditions in which a society finds itself. Firstly, *outside influences* – forces of nature and forces of man like trade, domination, and scientific discovery – provide the conditions for *ecological factors* – geography, history, demography, hygiene, nutrition, economy, technology, and urbanization. These ecological factors specify the context for the development of *societal norms* or *value systems*. Hofstede's societal norms have subsequent *consequences* for the structure and functioning of local institutions, like family patterns, role differentiation, education, and political systems, that is, the ultimate manifestations of a national culture. The various conditions Hofstede mentions – that is, ecological factors, societal norms, and various institutions – both reinforce each other and provoke gradual change within each other (Hofstede, 2001, Exhibit 1.5, p. 12).

Berger and Luckman's 1966 model of the social construction of reality has been a major influence on social constructionism (Burr, 2003; Gergen, 2009) and can be proposed as a model for the formation of culture from an interpretive perspective (Antonsen, 2009b; Blazsin & Guldenmund, 2015). Their process model has five consecutive steps, running from "subjective reality," "externalization," "institutionalization/objectification," and "objective reality" to "internalization" (Berger & Luckmann, 1966). According to Berger and Luckmann, people's impression of an objective reality is actually shaped through a continuous process based on interaction, adjustment, and agreement resulting in formalization and institutionalization of those agreements. In other words, what we consider objective and truthful in society is the result of a long process of interaction, mutual adaptation, and agreement, but internalized to the extent that we cannot see "reality" any other way. And this is exactly how culture has been defined by many scholars (e.g., Hofstede et al., 2010; Schein, 2010).

Regarding the structure of culture, many authors have put forward a layered concept, sometimes using an onion or an iceberg as a metaphor (e.g., Hofstede, 1991; Rousseau, 1990; Sanders & Neuijen, 1987; Schein, 2010; Spencer-Oatey, 2000). Whereas the core is something (deeply) hidden, the culture projects itself gradually through and onto the outer layers. The more remotely a layer is located from the core, the more easily it can be observed but also the more indirect, or interpretive, its relation with the core becomes. This model again emphasizes that it is not straightforward to understand a culture from observing its manifestations, that is, its outer layer(s). With regard to influencing a culture a similar rule is put forward: the more deeply a layer is located, the more difficult it becomes to actually change it (Sanders & Neuijen, 1987; Meijer, 1999). Hofstede, citing Bem (1970), argues that a particular culture can be more effectively influenced by starting with the practices of the outer layers, not the values of the core (Hofstede, 2001). The latter change gradually, with different time estimates for different levels of culture. For instance, a substantial change in national culture might take no less than a century (Hofstede, 2001), whereas an organizational culture some 25 years (Schein, 2010), but different time estimates are offered by other authors as well.

When talking about organizational and safety culture, several authors point out the relevance of the context in which culture formation takes place (Alvesson, 2012; Guldenmund, 2000; Richter & Koch, 2004). Similar notions were expressed in the field of safety climate, when researchers started to administer a questionnaire developed in one industry or company in another (e.g., Brown & Holmes 1986). The triangle of social reality is a basic model (Figure 19.1) proposed by sociologists Boudreau and Newman (1993). It describes the interplay between organizational culture, social structure, and interaction, from which a particular social reality is constructed.

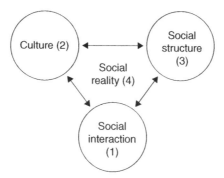

Figure 19.1 The triangle of social reality (adapted from Boudreau and Newman, 1993).

According to Boudreau and Newman, social interaction (1) is the primary basis for the construction of a social reality (4). Culture (2) also develops from social interaction as well as (social) structure (3), which pertains to the more stable features of culture. This model is employed by both Antonsen (2009b) and Guldenmund (2010a) in their studies of safety culture. Using this model Antonsen links organizational culture with safety culture, which then impacts safety, yet safety in his model is also influenced by the structure and (social) interaction. In his model, structure not only refers to social structure but also to hardware, like technology. A similar notion is found with Guldenmund (2010a).

It is possible to combine the model of Berger and Luckmann (1966) with the model above of Boudreau and Newman (1993) to describe two currents throughout the organization supporting the social construction of safety; a cultural flow resulting in symbols and implicit meanings about safety and a structural flow resulting in explicit formal rules and regulations. This model is shown in Figure 19.2.

In the first stage of Figure 19.2 "Sensemaking, enacting," a member of a group experiences a specific situation, of which he or she develops his or her own perceptions and makes specific sense. With regard to risk and safety, these individual perceptions will partly determine the sense-maker's subsequent enactment, that is, what is risky or safe behavior. The result of this process is an individual's understanding of reality. Or, quoting Berger and Luckmann, the stage of "reality . . . interpreted by men and subjectively meaningful to them as a coherent world" (1966, p. 33). The second stage corresponds to the "Interacting, exchanging" stage, which may be defined as "objectivations of subjective processes

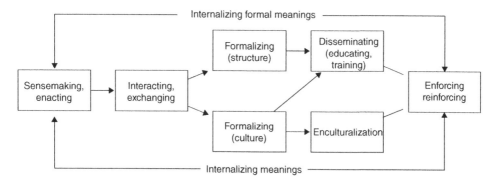

Figure 19.2 The development of organizational (safety) culture.

(and meanings) by which the *inter*subjective common-sense world is constructed" (Berger and Luckmann, 1966, p. 34, emphasis in original). This is the stage where members of a group interact and exchange meanings through formal and informal dialogue, giving rise to mutual adjustments, agreements, and expectations with regard to each other's behaviors. While not drawn explicitly in the figure, there is significant iteration between stages one and two as subjective and intersubjective understandings influence, and are influenced by, each other. Stage two eventually results in partly shared understandings, both as meanings (of risk, of safety) and as rules accompanying those meanings; for example, standards for behavior (procedures and rules), roles and responsibilities, and norms. The two formalization boxes of the third stage introduce the (formal) establishment of norms and meanings and the institutionalization of behavior and expectations. Here the current splits in two: one flow representing the formalization of structure, as advocated by Boudreau and Newman (1993), and the other flow representing the development of culture (symbols and meanings), as proposed by, for instance, Alvesson (2012) and Schein (2010). At this stage a specific set of shared representations and actions becomes explicit and official, and may be formalized so that, among other things, they can be taught to newcomers. This stage may be considered as one of "organizational consciousness," that is, "the reality of everyday life appears already objectified, that is, constituted by an order of objects that have been designated *as* objects before my appearance on the scene" (Berger & Luckmann 1966, p. 35, emphasis in original). In the fourth stage, the two currents remain separated, although the dissemination of formal structure and informal meanings often go hand in hand. Formal structure is usually institutionalized in organizational structures ("organograms"), rules, and procedures and instructed in various forms of education. Meanings are often disseminated "between and behind the lines" of spoken and written language (Alvesson, 2012) and acquired through various socialization processes, called enculturalization. Such enculturalization takes places in the classroom as well as on the shop floor, hence the arrow going from the lower stage three to the upper stage four. Finally, the fifth stage, titled "Enforcing, reinforcing," pictures the situation in which meanings, standards, and expectations are accepted to the extent that they are considered the "best" or, perhaps, the "only" way of doing things. Now, members of the group will share a comparable understanding of reality, at least with regard to the part of reality the group acts on, and structures and meanings are enforced and reinforced through various organizational processes.[6] Both structures and meanings are then internalized by the members of the group and woven into existing patterns of thought and action, through which individuals within the group understand and cope with reality. This, in turn, influences their perception of reality and subsequently, the way they make sense of and act on situations they experience.[7]

Equipped with this model we can describe several features of culture discussed above. Firstly, the development process of an organizational culture takes time to complete as it has to go through a number of stages where each stage takes time in its own right. It is continuous, as new experiences may be added to the process of mutual adjustment and will impact the other stages. Another feature which results from this iterative process and appears as characteristic of both organizational and safety culture, is its articulation of both cognitive and symbolic (cultural flow) as well as practical and behavioral (structural flow) aspects. Moreover, the structural flow does not have to be limited to the development of only social structures, but can result also in agreement on technology and hardware (cf. Antonsen, 2009b; Guldenmund, 2010a).

Secondly, the process depends on the composition of the group, its internal dynamics, the particular context in which the group operates, and so on. Therefore, the outcome is more arbitrary than intentional. It can be influenced, though, either by internal or by external forces. For instance, regarding the safety culture of a specific organization, corporate headquarters may try to influence local cultures through such means as organizational design, recruitment of new personnel, and the employment of new norms and standards. Yet, considering the importance of meanings developed by the group, the outcome of such measures is difficult to predict. Such measures may also include the implementation of standards that do not result from a consensus between group members, who, because of that, do not recognize them as their standards, and are therefore not internalized as meanings and understandings but rather as "obligations," that is, "the way we *have to do* things around here" instead of "the way we *do* things around here." Furthermore, the model can describe the emergence of integrated, differentiated, and fragmented features of culture. Integrated features pertain to meanings shared organization-wide, which might have their roots in the history of the organization (e.g., Boudreau & Newman, 1993; Schein, 2010) or might have been established through enforcement and coercion (see the fifth stage of the model). Differentiation follows straightforwardly from the model, in that shared understandings of reality develop in local contexts. Fragmentation and ambiguity are the result of lack of interaction, or unresolved disagreement (see the second stage of the model).

Thirdly, the model is a process model, describing how organizational culture, in principle, develops, comparable to the way the Plan-Do-Check-Act (PDCA) cycle (in principle) describes quality control and the empirical cycle (in principle) describes how empirical scientific research is carried out. This does not mean that in practice steps are skipped, poorly executed, or changed and such deviations might lead to the phenomena described above. Moreover, the model does not lead to predictions of outcomes as this is not what interpretists aim for.

On a final note, when using models or metaphors one should be aware of any underlying assumptions and limitations of a model.[8] For instance, the rationale underlying many models developed from a functionalist perspective, and the methodologies that accompany these, is the notion of uniform structure or framework that can be applied to most or all cultures, also known as nomothetic approaches. This line of thinking can be found with Hofstede and workers on both national and organizational cultures (Hofstede, 2001; Hofstede et al., 2010), Cameron and Quinn and their Competing Values Framework for organizations (Cameron & Quinn, 2011), Trompenaars and Hampden-Turner (1997) and the Hearts & Minds method (Energy Institute, undated), to name just a few examples. The latter approach is a model with hierarchically ordered metaphors referring to levels of safety culture maturity or development (Westrum, 2004). It will be discussed in the next section.

Assessing Safety Culture

Not so long ago, functionalist and interpretist approaches were entrenched in opposing camps disputing paradigms and research strategies. A researcher had to choose one or the other before embarking on a study. This controversy has largely been replaced by a more pragmatic approach in which methodologies are considered possibilities on a continuum of research perspectives (Creswell, 2009; Cunliffe, 2011; Fuchs, 2001). Any one of these could be employed when deemed appropriate. However, this does not discharge the researcher who should still think about the nature of her or his research object (i.e., its ontology), and how any knowledge can be acquired about it (i.e., its epistemology).[9] Below, the three most common approaches in safety culture research are discussed, the interpretive, the analytical and the pragmatic approach. As will become clear later on, the last approach is pragmatic in another sense than the "craft" (Cunliffe, 2011) of qualitative research itself, as mentioned above.

Interpretative or anthropological approach

The primary research methodology of cultural anthropology is ethnography, which is qualitative in nature. Its purpose is to describe and understand a culture and its members' worldview rather than evaluate it and, hence, it is non-normative, or value free. Moreover, the data collected are never fitted onto some researcher's pre-existing notions – like dimensions, facets, or archetypes – but rather used to identify such notions as they emerge in the analysis. Because of these characteristics, this approach is not well suited for a comparative research as no comparative framework is assumed to exist. Applied to organizations, culture is considered as something an organization *is*, rather than *has*. This approach is labeled "academic" because, until recently, it was employed almost exclusively by academic researchers and hardly used outside the scientific realm (Hofstede, 1991, p. 180). However, the International Atomic Energy Agency (IAEA) is currently advocating a safety culture self-assessment (SCSA) for its member states, involving just such an approach.

Schein has adopted this approach in what he calls "clinical research" (Schein, 1987). The term clinical seems to refer to a diagnostic, that is, evaluative, activity but this is more in terms of a discrepancy between a given organization's ambitions or intentions and what it actually accomplishes. In terms of safety this can become pertinent when a company claims to put safety as its number one priority, but nevertheless has many accidents.

The research method can be narrative research, a phenomenological study, a study using grounded theory, an ethnography or case study, or various combinations thereof (Creswell, 2007). Ideally, the research starts with a problem definition or an issue turned into a problem to focus the investigation; for instance, a discrepancy in priority between safety and production. Research techniques include interviews, observations, document studies, and whatever else the company brings forth that may hold clues for its underlying assumptions (e.g., see Guldenmund, 2010b, for an overview). What is important, however, is that information is collected with sufficient context, so that it can be interpreted accurately.

Whatever research method is chosen (case study, grounded theory, etc.) the results are (almost) never quantified because it is meaning and interpretation and not numerical abstractions and calculations that drive the research. Moreover, numbers are never taken as data abstracted from an objective world, which would be in conflict with the research paradigm. The result is "thick descriptions" (Geertz 1973), a "theory" of the culture of an organization (cf. Glaser & Strauss, 1967), or a set of metaphors sufficiently rich to invoke (parts of) the world lurking behind them (cf. Haukelid, 2008; Richter & Koch, 2004). Furthermore, different lenses can be applied to the material, to explore what the application of various lenses delivers in terms of more or deeper understanding. That is, the material can be studied through an integration lens, a differentiation lens, and a fragmentation lens to see what is actually shared within the entire company, shared within subunits, or what is a clear cause for ambiguity, or even conflict, respectively. In this approach (safety) culture is considered to be a nominal variable.

After the analysis or description phase is completed the academic approach might be used for a safety culture assessment or evaluation in two ways: (1) the organization itself (e.g., the management team, a dedicated safety culture self-assessment team, or whatever team the organization deems fit for this purpose) reflects on the assessment results and compares this with, for instance, its mission, its ambitions, its expectations, and so on; and (2), the description is compared with some external norm or standard. Several organizations in the field of nuclear safety have developed quite detailed norms, like the International Atomic Energy Agency (IAEA) and the US Institute of Nuclear Power Operations (INPO). Another candidate for a comparison exercise could be the Hearts & Minds matrix, which will be discussed in some detail below.

Given the more intense involvement of the researcher(s) with its subject (an organization, a department, a team) and the sheer amount of data a qualitative study can produce, an interpretive approach takes time to complete. This issue should be kept in mind before embarking on an academic, interpretive study. Often, such time is not available, which is why other approaches seem more attractive. These will be discussed in the next two sections.

While current safety culture literature is still not well endowed with qualitative studies (e.g., Zou, Sunindijo, & Dainty, 2014, calculate they form less than 25 percent of research in the construction industry), gradually more such studies start to appear in the literature. However, methods are often limited to either studies building on grounded theory (Stave & Törner, 2007; Walker, 2008) or case studies (Brooks, 2008; Farrington-Darby, Pickup, & Wilson, 2005; Guldenmund, 2008; Richter & Koch, 2004; Walker, 2010).

Analytical or psychological approach

The analytical approach is a research methodology that can be employed in either a case study or a (comparative) survey encompassing several organizations. Its research technique is a standardized questionnaire that is typically self-administered. It can be administered either group-wise, for instance at the start of a company training session or a lunch break, or sent to the workers' home addresses. These days, Internet-administered questionnaires have also gained much popularity. The approach is analytical in that it attempts to break down a complex construct into its constituent parts, often called dimensions, factors, or components. It is psychological because it assumes it is these dimensions that drive people's behaviors and perceptions and therefore one needs to canvass their views on pertinent topics. This approach often requires less time from both the researcher and the subject, and the involvement of the two can be limited as well.

Viewed from the analytical perspective culture is a multidimensional construct and different cultures can be positioned at diverse positions in that space. These dimensions are either given beforehand or determined through multivariate data analysis. An organization's position in this culture space is calculated using questionnaire responses, typically by using the mean as a common descriptor for a particular group on a dimension. Integration, differentiation, and fragmentation views are easily explored within this approach. The notions of integration and differentiation can be tested using various indices of within-group agreement (e.g., Bliese, 1998, 2000) at different levels of aggregation (e.g., Zohar & Luria, 2005). Fragmentation follows from a lack of agreement, at whatever level of aggregation.

Relationships with behavioral outcomes are equally easily examined within the analytical approach as indicators like accident and injury rates, self-reported accidents, incidents, and so on are readily available as frequencies or ratios. These can be plugged into statistical equations or models and subsequently tested. Richter and Koch (2004) acknowledge that these numbers are complex outcomes of the systems and processes underlying them if, indeed, they are the result of such complex cause and effect relationships. These are issues users of this approach should ponder, especially in terms of ecological validity.

There is abundant literature about research applying the analytic approach, which is extensively discussed in other chapters of this volume. While this research is sometimes referred to as safety culture research, it is more appropriately denominated as safety climate, the more "measurable aspect of safety culture" (cf. Zohar, 2008, 2010).

Pragmatic or experience-based approach

From an academic, interpretative point of view a culture can be neither "good" nor "bad," that is, cultures develop when people interact and have to accomplish something together. Therefore, cultures have significance and meaning in relation to their context, past history and (initial) group composition, not in comparison to some norm or notion of cultures in general, and safety cultures in particular. An organizational culture could be considered dysfunctional regarding its future, for instance, when compared with expressed ambitions or goals. Such ambitions can be about many things, so they could also be expressed about safety. For example, an organization's ambition might be to have "zero" accidents but serious accidents might still occur occasionally. Knowledge of its current cultural status might result in dissatisfaction with top management, which can be helpful in providing the organization with a sense of urgency to change.

The analytical approach does not deliver evaluations of culture either but, again, descriptions, although when scores can be compared to some norm, evaluations become possible. Such norms can be derived from means obtained from large aggregates. That is, a company's score on a scale or dimension can be compared to the mean score on this scale or dimension, which might be obtained by calculating the mean of all scores in a database. It is up to the analyst if this is a meaningful comparison and provides useful directions for possible interventions.

There is yet another approach that has produced methods which currently flourish as safety culture diagnostic and improvement "tools." While the previous approaches could be considered descriptive, the pragmatic approach is normative. This approach has been labeled "pragmatic" because its content is not so much the result of empirical research on cultures but rather based on experience and expert judgment. In practice, the pragmatic approach concentrates on both the structure and interactions of an organization, which, because of their dynamic interplay, will influence the culture in their wake (see also Figure 19.1 above).

Applied approaches concentrating on processes or interactions often focus on desired behavior and the correction of deviations. It is thought that a change in behavior will result in subsequent cultural adjustments. According to, for instance, cognitive dissonance theory (Eagly & Chaiken, 1993, p. 469 ff.), attitudes and thoughts about particular behaviors will change in the long run when the two are incongruent and the desired behavior is rewarded.

Typically, within this approach it is prescribed in detail what an organization should do to obtain an advanced or mature status; that is, what processes should be implemented supported by an accompanying structure. Geller's Total Safety Culture (Geller, 1994) is a prime example of this approach, and the IAEA requirements and characteristics for nuclear power plants are of a similar nature (International Atomic Energy Agency, 2002). Descriptive approaches toward culture such as the ones already discussed are of less relevance here, because it is not the organization's current status but deviations from a predefined norm that are assessed and considered.

Lately, stages or levels of organizational maturity with regard to safety management are becoming popular (Energy Institute, undated; Lardner, Fleming, & Joyner, 2001; Parker, Lawrie, & Hudson, 2006; Westrum, 2004). Each level describes common local attitudes and behaviors in relation to safety, especially in relation to incident and accident prevention, reporting, investigation, and solutions. An initial diagnosis of the current organizational status relating to these attitudes and behaviors might be prepared, which is often done by running multiple workshops using the accompanying questionnaire. However, the main objective is to ascend the safety maturity hierarchy. This might be accomplished by following the behavioral approach above, that is, an emphasis on organizational processes and behaviors in these, or with more structural adaptations. It is again assumed that culture will follow in the wake of these interventions. This approach assumes, rather implicitly, that safety culture is something an organization has, or does not have; that is, mature "generative" or "cooperating" organizations have "it," whereas immature "pathological" or "emerging" organizations do not (Energy Institute, undated; Lardner, Fleming, et al., 2001; Westrum 2004).

The level of development of an organization is assessed through behaviorally anchored rating scales, with either overt or covert ordinal scales that come with the package. These assessments are always done in groups for two important reasons. Firstly, it is a group's shared opinions one is after, not the "mean score" of a group of employees. Secondly, it is not so much the rating but the ensuing discussion that follows because of this rating process that is considered the most important outcome. Nevertheless, scores are often calculated and reported back to the organization, without the context in which they were obtained.

From the point of view of the interpretative academic approach, the inferences that are made about an underlying culture solely based on descriptions of behavior are committing a mortal sin. According to this approach it is impossible to infer such meanings only based on observed behavior. Geertz, quoting the philosopher Ryle, illustrates this nicely by comparing a wink, with a twitch, with a parody of a wink: all three look much the same, but have quite different meanings indeed (1973, p. 6 ff.).

While interpretation, understanding, and description are part and parcel of the job of culture researchers, evaluation does not come naturally to them. However, it is often this evaluation that is expected when safety comes into play. In conclusion, regarding the matter of safety culture and its appraisal, there are several aspects that require attention when assessing organizational safety culture:

1. From the interpretive and analytical viewpoints, culture is a descriptive, value-free concept, a nominal variable, whereas safety is not. Safety has a distinct normative flavor, pertaining to a state of being or feeling "safe" as opposed to an "unsafe" state of affairs. Moreover, safety is often embedded in cause-effect pathways, which are, albeit complex, ultimately deterministic. Again, culture is not. What both concepts have in common, though, is that they are, in the end, socially constructed, that is, both emerge from group interaction and consensus (Rochlin, 1999).

2. The purpose of organizational safety culture assessments is more often than not evaluation, not description, preferably with recommendations on how an underlying culture can be improved to support safety (more). This latter demand is again at odds with an interpretive take on organizational safety culture, which does not maintain the notion that culture can be managed, or changed as desired (Alvesson, 2012; Antonsen, 2009b).

3. Only the pragmatic approach merges the concept of culture with that of safety smoothly. However, as argued above, this approach focuses more on either safety behavior or on more formal aspects of organizational safety, like the formal processes of safety management.

4. Within the interpretive approach, safety and culture are both social constructs, influencing them both would mean influencing the social construction of both constructs. This is the topic of the next section.

Influencing Organizational Safety Culture

Most organizational safety culture assessments are not carried out for their own sake. Management is either interested in a diagnosis to compare it with a previous one or to benchmark with peer organizations, or the diagnosis is followed by a so-called gap analysis, where the present status of culture is compared with an ideal or optimal one, resulting in recommendations to improve the current status. Enough has been said about safety culture assessment in the previous section. With regard to influencing culture, some further remarks will be made.

When discussing Figure 19.2, it was already observed that the output of the development process is never an intended outcome, but rather the product of many different forces influencing the group at various points in time. In that sense, the resulting culture is not so much an optimal "textbook culture," but rather something that seems to work, in this group, under these conditions. When the group remains successful in its accomplishments, the accompanying set of symbols and meanings is reinforced and, thus, strengthened.

This does not mean that any attempts can be made to influence the current safety culture by influencing, for instance, its development process. To choose particular influences, Figure 19.2 can be taken as a starting point and interventions can be chosen that might influence the several stages within the model. In the following points, generic types of interventions are suggested, that might influence these various stages. Carrying out multiple interventions at the same time does seem to be more effective in influencing this process, rather than doing a single one or a few in succession (Hale, Guldenmund, van Loenhout, & Oh, 2010).

1. Harmonizing physical and social realities throughout the organization. The first stage in the model describes the exploring and sense-making processes of individual members of the group, their attempts in understanding organizational reality. Possible influences that might affect this process are aimed at ensuring that parts of the physical and social reality are comparable across the organization. With regard to the physical reality this would mean, for example, similar (information) technology, instruments, personal protection equipment, workplace layout, campaigns, posters, slogans, and so on. With regard to social reality possible influences are leadership styles, rituals (e.g., meetings, gatherings, celebrations, initiating practices), (systems for) recognition, and so on. The aim of these interventions would be to create similar meanings and understandings, a comparable "reality" across the organization.

2. Performing open dialogue. This is a crucial step in the development of culture (cf., Schein, 2013) and influences should be aimed at performing this dialogue across the organization to ensure that consensus is reached to the extent that most people in the organization have a comparable understanding of the reality they act on. Possible examples of interventions are STOP-GO cards or Last Minute Risk Assessments, briefing and debriefing rituals, rules for approaching and correcting people, reporting of unsafe situations, and so on. It should be noted that Stages 1 and 2 of the culture development process are actually iterative and remain so until a particular degree of consensus is reached (or a consensus is enforced, but this usually means that the ensuing rules are not sufficiently supported by the majority and therefore will also not be recognized nor internalized).

3. Developing norms, rules, and procedures based on consensus. At this stage the consensus on (parts of) reality that has been reached at Stage 2 will be formalized and institutionalized. Because of this shared consensus, the ensuing rules are recognized

and understood by the majority of the group. Importantly, some rules are not formalized to the extent that they are not written down, yet they function as such within a group. Rules developed elsewhere without the involvement of the group for whom they are written will not be recognized by the group as matching their understanding of reality and, hence, should be avoided.

4. Educating, training of shared rules. After formalizing the rules, they will be trained or otherwise disseminated among the members of the group. New members will often start at this step, although when things do not make sense to them, they might also speak up and processes at Stages 1 and 2 might become pertinent too. When an organization is operating for some time, new members will have less and less impact on institutionalized rules and practices, so they will either agree with the rules (or pretend they agree), or leave the company. This situation can change in the face of various threats or challenges the groups finds itself in, which implies the groups starts at Stage 1 again.

5. Reinforcing or correcting what is considered meaningful. To secure the shared understandings of a culture they have to be reinforced for some time. After a while, they become self-explanatory and objective to the extent that members of the organization cannot imagine understanding or approaching reality otherwise (Schein, 2010). This basic understanding is again influencing the sense-making of step one.

The process described above follows an overall integrative approach. That is, it is aimed at developing an integrated culture with common symbols and meanings throughout the organization. However, differentiation and fragmentation approaches might be applied also. For instance, interventions might allow for local subcultures to develop, or might even promote a certain degree of conflict and ambiguity, that is, bounded ambiguity (Alvesson, 2012). As scholars advocating high reliability organizing (HRO) might argue, conflict and ambiguity support a degree of organizational mindfulness that is required to spot "weak signals," that is, signals that often precede mayhem and disaster (Weick & Sutcliffe, 2007).

Future Research

The role organizational safety culture (research) might play in the development of an organizational mindfulness that supports safety seems obvious but, as yet, unclear. Moreover, defining a set of characteristics for such mindful organizations does not mean these can be easily adopted or implemented: "identification of the characteristics of highly reliable organizations is not the same thing as knowing how to make them so" (La Porte, 2006, p. 151). Even more basic, there is hardly any research available on the effect of organizational safety culture interventions and what have turned out to be the working ingredients in these endeavors. The model proposed above could function as a framework in such research. And research could contribute to identifying those working ingredients.

Linear representations of safety (management) make way for more complex, relational notions of safety (management) (Haavik, 2014; Reiman, Rollenhagen, Pietikäinen, & Heikkilä, 2015). Again, relations are important as well in high-reliability visions on safety in keeping teams heedful and persistently informed, in searching for local expertise in case of imminent threat or disaster (Weick & Sutcliffe, 2007). These new developments put other, different demands on safety management systems and its managers. Establishing and maintaining relations are central to the concept of culture and, hence, such developments will impact organizational (safety) culture, which will in turn impact management and leadership roles. And as culture will change, the meaning of safety will change accordingly, perhaps fundamentally. Again, future research should contribute to the shape of safety yet to come.

Conclusions

Organizational safety culture seems to follow the same route of theoretical development that organizational culture has followed. Initially coined as a variable explaining large-scale organizational performance (in case of organizational culture: organizational success; in case of organizational safety culture: disaster) the construct has now been adopted by many to streamline and fine-tune organizational members' behaviors. However, this is not the position taken in this chapter, not least because culture is not as malleable as suggested by the culture designers.

The approach in this chapter has been to treat culture as a lens, as a way of looking at organizations and everything that is happening in them. Furthermore, different types of lenses have been introduced to provide a multifocal view on culture, to be able to account for the many expressions of culture and to provide depth to a construct that otherwise so easily defaults to patterns of behavior. In following this approach, an organization can learn to unpack these patterns and gain an understanding in their symbolism, their fundamental reasons of being and, possibly, develop counter mechanisms that might influence their status quo. Such insight might even lead to "enlightenment," to fundamental insights into organizing (Alvesson, 2012; Weick, 1979) and how to develop characteristics that are deemed crucial for a level of safety that is able to cope with the mayhem and disaster mentioned previously (Weick & Sutcliffe, 2007). However, as Hopkins (2014) argues, organizations entertaining such levels of safety currently do not exist, unfortunately.

Acknowledgement

I am indebted to Johan Alvehus for his contributions to these pages, especially to the section "Understanding Organizational Culture: A Critical Perspective."

Notes

1. Interestingly, Barry Turner does not claim the term for himself as he also refers to the INSAG's report on the Chernobyl nuclear disaster as the original source of the construct of safety culture (Turner, 1992, p. 198).
2. It must be noted, however, that from a critical-anthropological view, these levels – e.g., nation or ethnicity, organizations, group – are analytical constructs. Identification with such groups does not necessarily mean internalization (Ashforth & Mael, 1989), and overarching concepts such as national culture may be of only limited relevance when understanding a particular group within a nation.
3. Please note that Schein (2010, pp. 298ff.) follows a similar reasoning about culture change.
4. Human nature is shared by everybody and a personality is held by one person. Additionally, Hofstede (1991) considers culture the "personality" of a group.
5. This view on culture often fails to appreciate the difficulty of changing culture and the possibility for organizational members to play along in performing a "hyperculture" rather than in fact internalizing the values and beliefs promoted by the normative framework. Again, interpretists would question whether these approaches are dealing at all with culture in any profound sense.

6. It should be noted that this process describes an ideal flow. This process could be disturbed in many different ways, not leading to a subsequent shared understanding of reality, but in quite different understandings and equal disagreement. It could also be argued that such a lack of common understanding lies at the root of many disasters (Rochlin, 1999; Weick & Sutcliffe, 2007). Moreover, it could also be the cause for differentiation and, ultimately, the formation of sub-cultures.

7. This development process has significant overlap with Weick's individual process of sense-making, i.e., natural selection, enactment, selection, and retention (Weick, 1979).

8. The development model outlined in this chapter does not make strong assumptions about one underlying framework, although it does assume that various social patterns develop through social interaction. In this respect it might be a product of Western thinking.

9. Some pragmatists, however, would rather 'change the subject' instead of keeping discussing worldviews and paradigms (Creswell, 2009).

References

Alvesson, M. (1993). *Cultural perspectives on organizations.* Cambridge, MA: Cambridge University Press.

Alvesson, M. (2004). *Knowledge work and knowledge intensive firms.* Oxford, UK: Oxford University Press.

Alvesson, M. (2012). *Understanding organizational culture* (2nd edn.). London, UK: Sage.

Alvesson, M., & S. Sveningsson (2008). *Changing organizational culture: Cultural change work in progress.* New York, NY: Routledge.

Antonsen, S. (2009a). Safety culture and the issue of power. *Safety Science, 47*(2), 183–191.

Antonsen, S. (2009b). *Safety culture: Theory, method and improvement.* Farnham, UK: Ashgate.

Ashforth, B. E., & Mael, F. (1989). Social identity theory and the organization. *Academy of Management Review, 14*(1), 20–39.

Axtell Ray, C. (1986). Corporate culture: The last frontier of control? *Journal of Management, 23*(3), 287–298.

Batteau, A. (2001). Negations and ambiguities in the cultures of organizations. *American Anthropologist, 102*(4), 726–740.

Bem, D. J. (1970). *Beliefs, attitudes and human affairs.* Belmont, CA: Brooks/Cole.

Berger, P. L., & Luckmann, T. (1966). *The social construction of reality: A treatise in the sociology of knowledge.* Garden City, NY: Anchor Books.

Blazsin, H., & Guldenmund, F. W. (2015). The social construction of safety: Comparing three realities. *Safety Science, 71*, Part A(0), 16–27.

Bliese, P. D. (1998). Group size, ICC values, and group-level correlations: A simulation. *Organizational Research Methods, 1*(4), 355–373.

Bliese, P. D. (2000). Within-group agreement, non-independence, and reliability. In K. J. Kline & S. W. Kozlowski (Eds.), *Multilevel theory, research, and methods in organizations* (pp. 349–381). San Francisco, CA: Jossey-Bass.

Boudreau, F. A., & Newman, W. M. (1993). *Understanding social life: An introduction to sociology.* Minneapolis, MN: West Publishing Company.

Bouwhuijsen, H. v. d., Claes, T., & Derde, W. (1995). Recovering culture. *Cultural Dynamics, 7*(2), 163–186.

Brooks, B. (2008). The natural selection of organizational and safety culture within a small to medium sized enterprise (SME). *Journal of Safety Research, 39*(1), 73–85.

Brown, R. L., & Holmes, H. (1986). The use of a factor-analytic procedure for assessing the validity of an employee safety climate model. *Accident Analysis & Prevention, 18*(6), 455–470.

Burr, V. (2003). *Social constructionism.* London, UK: Routledge.

Cameron, K. S., & Quinn, R. E. (2011). *Diagnosing and changing organizational culture based on the Competing Values Framework.* San Francisco, CA: Jossey-Bass.

Cooper, M. D. (2000). Towards a model for safety culture. *Safety Science, 36*(2), 111–136.

Cooper, M. D., & Phillips, R. A. (2004). Exploratory analysis of the safety climate and safety behavior relationship. *Journal of Safety Research, 35*(5), 497–512.

Creswell, J. W. (2007). *Qualitative inquiry and research design: Choosing among five traditions.* Thousand Oaks, CA: Sage.

Creswell, J. W. (2009). *Research design: Qualitative, quantitative, and mixed methods approaches.* Thousand Oaks, CA: Sage.

Cunliffe, A. L. (2011). Crafting qualitative research: Morgan and Smircich 30 years on. *Organizational Research Methods, 14*(4), 647–673.

Deal, T. E., & Kennedy, A. A. (1982). *Corporate cultures: The rites and rituals of corporate life.* Reading, MA: Addison-Wesley.

Eagly, A. H., & Chaiken, S. (1993). *The psychology of attitudes.* Fort Worth, TX: Harcourt Brace Jovanovich.

Energy Institute (Undated). Hearts and Minds programme. http://www.eimicrosites.org/heartsandminds/ (accessed June 3, 2015).

Farrington-Darby, T., Pickup, L., & Wilson, J. R. (2005). Safety culture in railway maintenance. *Safety Science, 43*(1), 39–60.

Fleming, P., & Spicer, A. (2007). *Contesting the corporation: Struggle, power and resistance in organizations.* New York, NY: Cambridge University Press.

Fuchs, S. (2001). *Against essentialism: A theory of culture and society.* Cambridge, MA: Harvard University Press.

Furnham, A. (1997). *The psychology of behaviour at work.* London, UK: Psychology Press.

Geertz, C. (1973). *The interpretation of cultures.* New York, NY: Basic Books.

Geller, E. S. (1994). Ten principles for achieving a Total Safety Culture. *Professional Safety,* September, 18–24.

Gergen, K. J. (2009). *An invitation to social construction.* London, UK: Sage.

Glaser, B. G., & Strauss, A. L. (1967). *The discovery of grounded theory: Strategies for qualitative research.* Chicago, IL: Aldine.

Glendon, A. I. (2008a). Safety culture and safety climate: How far have we come and where could we be heading? *Journal of Occupational Health and Safety – Australia and New Zealand, 24*(3), 249–271.

Glendon, A. I. (2008b). Safety culture: Snapshot of a developing concept (Editorial). *Journal of Occupational Health and Safety – Australia and New Zealand, 24*(3), 179–189.

Guldenmund, F. W. (2000). The nature of safety culture: A review of theory and research. *Safety Science, 34*(1–3), 215–257.

Guldenmund, F. W. (2007). The use of questionnaires in safety culture research – an evaluation. *Safety Science, 45*(6), 723–743.

Guldenmund, F. W. (2008). Safety culture in a service company. *Journal of Occupational Health and Safety – Australia and New Zealand, 24*(3), 221–235.

Guldenmund, F. W. (2010a). (Mis)understanding safety culture and its relationship to safety management. *Risk Analysis, 30*(10), 1466–1480.

Guldenmund, F. W. (2010b). *Understanding and exploring safety culture.* Oisterwijk, The Netherlands: BOX Press.

Haavik, T. K. (2014). On the ontology of safety. *Safety Science, 67,* 37–43.

Habermas, J. (1987). *Knowledge and human interests.* Cambridge, UK: Polity Press.

Hale, A. R., Guldenmund, F. W., van Loenhout, P. L. C. H., & Oh, J. I. H. (2010). Evaluating safety management and culture interventions to improve safety: Effective intervention strategies. *Safety Science, 48*(8), 1026–1035.

Hale, A. R., & Hovden, J. (1998). Management and culture: The third age of safety. A review of approaches to organizational aspects of safety, health, and environment. In A. M. Feyer & A. Williamson (Eds.), *Occupational injury: Risk, prevention and intervention* (pp. 129–165). London, UK: Taylor-Francis.

Haukelid, K. (2008). Theories of (safety) culture revisited: An anthropological approach. *Safety Science, 46*(3), 413–426.

Hofstede, G. R. (1991). *Cultures and organisations: Software of the mind.* London, UK: McGraw-Hill.

Hofstede, G. R. (2001). *Culture's consequences.* London, UK: Sage.

Hofstede, G. R., Hofstede, G. J., & Minkov, M. (2010). *Cultures and organisations: Software of the mind* (3rd edn.). New York, NY: McGraw-Hill.

Hopkins, A. (2014). Issues in safety science. *Safety Science, 67*, 6–14.

International Atomic Energy Agency (2002). *Safety culture in nuclear installations: Guidance for use in the enhancement of safety culture.* Vienna, Austria: IAEA.

International Nuclear Safety Advisory Group (1991). *Safety culture.* Vienna, Austria: IAEA.

International Nuclear Safety Advisory Group (1992). *INSAG-7. The Chernobyl accident: updating of INSAG-1.* Vienna, Austria: IAEA.

Keesing, R. M. (1981). *Cultural anthropology: A contemporary perspective.* Fort Worth, TX: Holt, Rinehart, and Winston.

Kroeber, A., & Kluckhohn, C. (1952). *Culture: A critical review of concepts and definitions.* New York, NY: Meridian Books.

Kunda, G. (1992). *Engineering culture: Control and commitment in a high-tech corporation.* Philadelphia, PA: Temple University Press.

La Porte, T. M. (2006). Organizational strategies for complex system resilience, reliability, and adaptation. In P. E. Auerswald, L. M.Branscomb, T. M. LaPorte, & E. O. Michel-Kerjan (Eds.), *Seeds of disaster, roots of response: How private action can reduce public vulnerability* (pp. 135–153). Cambridge, UK: Cambridge University Press.

Lardner, R., Fleming, M., & Joyner, P. (2001). Towards a mature safety culture. *IChemE Symposium Series, 148*, 635–642.

Martin, J. (2002). *Organizational culture: Mapping the terrain.* Thousand Oaks, CA: Sage.

Meijer, S. D. (1999). *The Gordian knot of organisational and safety culture (in Dutch).* PhD thesis, Eindhoven University of Technology, the Netherlands.

Meyerson, D., & Martin, J. (1987). Cultural change: An integration of three different views. *Journal of Management Studies, 24*(6), 623–647.

Nævestad, T. O. (2009). Mapping research on culture and safety in high-risk organizations: Arguments for a sociotechnical understanding of safety culture. *Journal of Contingencies and Crisis Management, 17*(2), 126–136.

Ouchi, W. G. (1979). A conceptual framework for the design of organizational control mechanisms. *Management Science, 25*(9), 833–848.

Ouchi, W. G. (1981). *Theory Z.* New York, NY: Avon Books.

Parker, D., Lawrie, M., & Hudson, P. T. W. (2006). A framework for understanding the development of organisational safety culture. *Safety Science, 44*(6), 551–562.

Peters, T., & Waterman, R. H. (1982). *In search of excellence.* New York, NY: Harper and Row.

Pfeffer, J. (1981). Management as symbolic action: The creation and maintenance of organizational paradigms. In L. L. Cummings & B. M. Staw (Eds.), *Research in organizational behaviour* (vol. 3, pp. 1–52). Greenwich, CT: JAI Press.

Pidgeon, N. F., & O'Leary, M. (2000). Man-made disasters: Why technology and organizations (sometimes) fail. *Safety Science, 34*(1), 15–30.

Reason, J. T. (1997). *Managing the risks of organizational accidents.* Aldershot, UK: Ashgate.

Reiman, T., Rollenhagen, C., Pietikäinen, E., & Heikkilä, J. (2015). Principles of adaptive management in complex safety-critical organizations. *Safety Science, 71*, Part B, 80–92.

Richter, A., & Koch, C. (2004). Integration, differentiation and ambiguity in safety cultures. *Safety Science, 42*, 703–722.

Rochlin, G. I. (1999). Safe operation as a social construct. *Ergonomics, 42*(11), 1549–1560.

Rousseau, D. M. (1990). Assessing organisational culture: The case for multiple methods. In B. Schneider and K. M. Barbera (Eds.), *Organisational climate and culture* (pp. 153–192). Oxford, UK: Jossey-Bass.

Sanders, G., & Neuijen, B. (1987). *Organisational culture: Diagnosis and influencing* (in Dutch). Assen, the Netherlands: Van Gorcum.

Schein, E. H. (1987). *The clinical perspective in fieldwork.* Newbury Park, CA: Sage.

Schein, E. H. (2010). *Organizational culture and leadership* (4th edn.). San Francisco, CA: Jossey-Bass.

Schein, E. H. (2013). *Humble inquiry: The gentle art of asking instead of telling.* San Francisco, CA: Berrett-Koehler.

Smircich, L. (1983). Concepts of culture and organizational analysis. *Administrative Science Quarterly, 28*(3), 339–358.

Smircich, L. (1985). Is the concept of culture a paradigm for understanding organizations and ourselves? In P. J. Frost, L. F. Moore, M. R. Louis, C. C. Lundberg, & J. Martin (Eds.), *Organizational culture* (pp. 55–72). Newbury Park, CA, Sage.

Smircich, L., & Morgan, G. (1982). Leadership: The management of meaning. *Journal of Applied Behavioral Science, 18*(3), 257–273.

Spencer-Oatey, H. (2000). *Culturally speaking: Managing rapport through talk across cultures.* London, UK: Continuum.

Stave, C., & Törner, M. (2007). Exploring the organisational preconditions for occupational accidents in food industry: A qualitative approach. *Safety Science, 45*(3), 355–371.

Trompenaars, F., & Hampden-Turner, C. (1997). *Riding the waves of culture: Understanding cultural diversity in business* (2nd edn.). London, UK: Nicholas Brieley.

Turner, B. A. (1976). The development of disasters – a sequence model for the analysis of the origins of disasters. *Sociological Review, 24*(4), 753–774.

Turner, B. A. (1978). *Man-made disasters.* London, UK: Wykeham.

Turner, B. A. (1992). The sociology of safety. In D. Blockley (Ed.), *Engineering safety* (pp. 186–201). London, UK: McGraw-Hill Book Company.

Van Hoewijk, R. (1988). The meaning of organisational culture: An overview of the literature (in Dutch). *M&O, Tijdschrift voor Organisatiekunde en Sociaal Beleid, 1, 4–46.*

Walker, A. (2008). A qualitative investigation of the safety culture of two organisations. *Journal of Occupational Health and Safety – Australia and New Zealand, 24*(3), 201–212.

Walker, G. W. (2010). A safety counterculture challenge to a "safety climate." *Safety Science, 48*(3), 333–341.

Weick, K. E. (1976). Educational organizations as loosely coupled systems. *Administrative Science Quarterly, 21*(1), 1–19.

Weick, K. E. (1979). *The social psychology of organizing.* Reading, MA: Addison-Wesley.

Weick, K. E., & Sutcliffe, K. M. (2007). *Managing the unexpected: Assuring high performance in an age of complexity.* San Francisco, CA: Jossey-Bass.

Westrum, R. (2004). A typology of organisational cultures. *Quality and Safety in Health Care 13*(Suppl II), ii22–ii27.

Zohar, D. (2008). Safety climate and beyond: A multi-level multi-climate framework. *Safety Science, 46*(3): 376–387.

Zohar, D. (2010). Thirty years of safety climate research: Reflections and future directions. *Accident Analysis and Prevention, 42*(5), 1517–1522.

Zohar, D., & Luria, G. (2005). A multilevel model of safety climate: Cross-level relationships between organization and group-level climates. *Journal of Applied Psychology, 90*(4), 616–628.

Zou, P. X. W., Sunindijo, R. Y., & Dainty, A. R. J. (2014). A mixed methods research design for bridging the gap between research and practice in construction safety. *Safety Science, 70,* 316–326.

20

Patient Safety Culture

Andrea Bishop, Mark Fleming, and Rhona Flin

Introduction

With the publication of the Institute of Medicine's report *To Err Is Human* in 1999, the full extent of harm associated with seeking medical care in the USA was quantified and a worldwide movement toward improving patient safety was launched. The report found that at least 44,000, and as many as 98,000 people, die in US hospitals each year as a result of preventable medical errors (Institute of Medicine, 1999). Reports in other jurisdictions, including Canada, England, Scotland and Australia, have found similar results, suggesting that 5–10 percent of all hospital admissions result in adverse events (Baker, Norton, Flintoft, & Blais, 2004; Vincent, Neale, & Woloshynowych, 2001; Wilson et al., 1995), defined as "unexpected and undesired incidents directly associated with the care or services provided to the patient" (Davies, Hebert, & Hoffman, 2003, p. 39). Furthermore, nearly half of these adverse events were found to be preventable, with roughly a third leading to further disability or death. With the increasing knowledge that being hospitalized came with significant risks, patient safety experts sought to learn from other industries (e.g., nuclear energy and aviation) where examples of high reliability organizations, had been identified. The importance of creating a positive safety culture was identified as a key factor in minimizing risk and learning from failure. This has resulted in significant researcher and practitioner interest in patient safety culture (see Waterson, 2014, for recent reviews).

Patient safety culture can be considered as a subset of an organization's overall safety culture (see Guldenmund, Chapter 19, this volume, for a discussion of organizational safety culture). As such, the importance of patient safety culture to improving patient safety lies at the intersection between organizational objectives and patient care. Essentially, it is important to understand health care from a systems perspective – the sum of all policies, procedures, and individuals collectively contribute to whether or not patient safety is considered a priority within the organization. This chapter explores how these two concepts, patient safety and organizational culture, are interrelated and it emphasizes the importance of a systems approach to patient safety in identifying and implementing quality improvement.

The Wiley Blackwell Handbook of the Psychology of Occupational Safety and Workplace Health, First Edition. Edited by Sharon Clarke, Tahira M. Probst, Frank Guldenmund, and Jonathan Passmore. © 2016 John Wiley & Sons Ltd. Published 2020 by John Wiley & Sons Ltd.

The content is intended to provide the reader with a basic understanding of the importance of organizational safety culture within health care and its development and relation
with the global patient safety movement. The first section explores what patient safety culture is and why it is important. The second section investigates the development of patient
safety culture within an organization and some of the common barriers to patient safety
culture implementation. The third section introduces various tools that have been developed to measure patient safety culture and discusses their strengths and weaknesses with
regard to measurement. The fourth section aims to contextualize patient safety within a
health care systems perspective and provides examples of how systems influence safe care.
Finally, the fifth section explores differences between patient safety culture findings across
countries and provides an international perspective on patient safety culture.

What is Patient Safety Culture?

Organizational culture

The exploration of patient safety culture first has to start with an understanding of its relation to an organization's overall culture. Every organization has a culture which speaks to
how things are done within the organization, including shared beliefs and values, and what
influences people who work there (Schein, 1990). In many ways, organizational culture
refers to "how things are done here" (Claridge & Sanders, 2007). The most widely accepted definition of organizational culture comes from Schein (1985) and is described as

> a pattern of basic assumptions – invented, discovered, or developed by a group as it learns to
> cope with its problems of external adaptation and internal integration – that has worked well
> enough to be considered valid and therefore, to be taught to new members as the correct
> way to perceive, think and feel in relation to those problems. (p. 17)

Organizational culture is often most clear when one first joins a new organization and
begins to learn what that organization values, how people work together, and what individuals within that organization deem as the "right" way to do things. Organizational
culture manifestations can range from the very tangible, such as an organization's mission
and vision statements, to the very abstract, such as basic assumptions held by employees.
Table 20.1 describes the three different levels of organizational culture.

All three of these levels ultimately influence what employees value within the workplace
and how they work together to achieve the goals of the organization. With regard to patient
safety, underlying assumptions could include never challenging a physician's clinical diagnosis, espoused values could include employee perceptions regarding how committed senior
leadership is to putting patient safety first, and artifacts could include patient safety checklists

Table 20.1 Levels of organizational culture.

Level	Description
Artifacts and behaviors	Visible, tangible, and identifiable elements of the organization
Espoused values	Philosophies held by the organization, stated values and rules of behavior, and strategies for the future
Underlying assumptions	Deeply embedded, taken-for-granted behaviors

Source: Guldenmund, 2000; Schein, 2004

used by health care teams to improve safety. Organizational culture can also be contextualized at different levels of the organization and subunits. At the very top of an organization, cultural factors will set the tone for how things are done, such as ensuring patient safety is a cornerstone of the vision statement for the organization. However, at the unit or team level within health care, behaviors, values, and assumptions may be more distinct and relate to the functions of the unit. As such, these "subcultures" may be present within a larger overarching organizational culture (Phipps & Ashcroft, 2012). There can also be competing subcultures within an organization, where values may be different between units. For example, within a hospital, one unit may value patient engagement and involvement in treatment decisions while another might not. As such, while it may appear that an organization has one overarching organizational culture, some organizations can have many cultures that can have common elements (Richter & Koch, 2004). In fact, in many large organizations, such as hospitals, it may be necessary to have more than one culture as it relates to the provision of care.

Safety culture

In organizations and industries that are considered high hazard, such as nuclear energy and aviation, an organizational safety culture is important to ensuring that the job gets done safely. The Advisory Committee on the Safety of Nuclear Installations (1993) has defined safety culture as:

> the product of individual and group values, attitudes, perceptions, competencies, and patterns of behaviour that determine commitment to, and the style and proficiency of, an organization's health and safety management. Organizations with a positive safety culture are characterized by communications founded on mutual trust, by shared perceptions of the importance of safety and by the efficacy of preventive measures. (p. 23)

Safety culture, therefore, points to the important beliefs and structures that are present in an organization that ensures the value of a safe work environment. If we use the levels of organizational culture discussed above (see Table 20.1), in an organization with a positive safety culture there would be reference to the importance of safety in all three levels (see Box 20.1). For instance, an organization that values safety would ensure that safety is found in their organizational mission statement, that values and rules of behavior would support a safe workplace, and that employees would have a deep concern for the safety of their coworkers. Other characteristics of a positive safety culture can be found in Box 20.1.

Box 20.1 Characteristics of a positive safety culture

- Open communication founded on mutual trust
- Good flow of information
- Shared perceptions of the importance of safety
- Recognition that errors are inevitable
- Proactive identification of potential threats to safety
- A focus on organizational learning
- Leadership that is committed to safety
- A "no-blame" approach to incident reporting and learning

Source: Claridge & Sanders, 2007; Kirk, Marshall, Claridge, Esmail, & Parker, 2006

While the definition of safety culture provided above helps to explain what it is, what many definitions lack is how safety culture is created and how it specifically relates to the broader concept of organizational culture. Safety culture has been contextualized in a number of different ways within the literature, including as a type of organizational culture, a subset of organizational culture, as well as resulting from an organization's culture (Guldenmund, 2000; Institute of Medicine, 1999; Singer, Gaba, & Geppert, 2003). Fleming and Hartnell (2007) suggest that the ways in which the terms "safety" and "culture" are used within the literature can create confusion, and, with little theoretical direction in the area, it is important to understand the many ways in which the term "safety culture" can be used. For the purposes of this chapter and to better understand the further term of "patient safety culture," the authors conceptualize safety culture as a result of organizational cultural influences. In essence, an organization's culture determines what will be a priority for that organization. For organizations with a strong safety culture, safety is a top priority of their endeavours which then becomes embedded as a requirement in all operations.

While research on safety culture has been relatively recent, it is very similar to Turner's man-made disaster theory that gained prominence in the 1970s (Turner, 1978). He theorized that organizational failures and disasters directly stemmed from cultural assumptions about how to do things. As a result, organizations are often unaware of potential failures in the system and therefore do not manage potential risks. Turner's theory is particularly relevant to health care organizations as often there is agreement that patient safety should be foremost, but they can find it difficult to conceptualize risks and scenarios that can lead to patient harm (Fleming & Hartnell, 2007). As such, understanding employee perceptions of safety and identifying possible conditions for disasters to occur are important foundations for health care organizations wishing to implement or improve their patient safety culture.

It is also important at this point to differentiate between the terms of safety culture and safety climate. Many people might use the terms culture and climate interchangeably, despite a body of research that has aimed to disentangle the two (Cox & Flin, 1998; Guldenmund, 2000; see also Guediri & Griffin, Chapter 13, this volume). There are some key differences to note. While patient safety culture refers to the norms, beliefs, and values of the organization, patient safety climate most commonly refers to the employees' perception of the organization's priorities regarding safety (Gershon, Stone, Bakken, & Larson, 2004; Guldenmund, 2000; Zohar & Luria, 2005). As such, safety climate most often refers to the espoused values and artifact levels of organizational culture in that safety climate is tangible and measurable, whereas the underlying assumptions of the culture are not easily measured. As such, safety climate is fundamentally related to what people think or how they act, whereas safety culture explains *why* people think or act in a particular way (Fleming & Hartnell, 2007). Because underlying assumptions are often very difficult to measure, as they are unconscious, it is therefore argued that safety culture questionnaires only tap into safety climate, as they do not assess these deeper aspects of culture. Meta-analyses have demonstrated a link between better safety climate scores and lower archival worker accident data and self-reported accident/injuries (Christian, Bradley, Wallace, & Burke, 2009a), as well as worker safety behaviors (Clarke, 2006).

Patient safety culture

With the realization that the health care encounter presents a number of risks to patients, safety culture has become an important facet of delivering safe care. With the release of *To Err is Human* in 1999 in the USA and *An Organization with a Memory* (Department of Health, 2000) in the UK, health care organizations around the world were tasked with the need to understand and assess their organizational safety culture. The unique challenge faced by health care organizations, however, is that their safety culture must not only relate to the safety of their employees, but it must also translate to the interaction between the patient and the organization (Kaufman & McCaughan, 2013). Patient safety culture has been defined as an integrated pattern of individual and organizational behavior, based upon shared beliefs and values, that continuously seeks to minimize patient harm that may result from the processes of care (Kizer, 1999). As such, patient safety culture refers to a health care organization's ability to incorporate and value the safety of the patient experience in all aspects of the organization.

Given the above definition, one of the grounding principles of patient safety culture is continuous improvement. While we explore ways to measure patient safety culture in the section *Measuring Safety Culture in Health Care*, the underlying assumption within this is that patient safety can and will ultimately be improved. For example, a health care organization that has a positive safety culture will strive to improve the quality of care provided to patients and reduce the number of adverse events (Baker et al., 2004). The use of quality improvement frameworks within the health care setting, therefore, is an important component of patient safety culture. Two of the most commonly used improvement frameworks in health care are total quality management (TQM) and continuous quality improvement (CQI) (Schmele, 1993). The emergence of TQM and CQI in health care started in the 1980s (McLaughlin & Kaluzny, 2006) and many of its guiding principles and tools are hallmarks of positive patient safety cultures in health care. Tools such as the plan-do-check-act cycle, root cause analysis, failure modes and effect analysis, and risk assessments are becoming increasingly used in health care organizations in order to proactively identify possible patient safety risks and implement and evaluate quality improvement changes (Carayon, 2011). As patient safety culture ultimately influences not only the outcomes of the health care organization, but also the health outcomes of each individual patient, the need to identify possible hazards and proactively remove them is an important step in minimizing harm experienced by patients when they enter the health care system.

As with organizational safety culture, a positive patient safety culture is characterized in a number of ways within an organization. These dimensions, as well as other important determinants of patient safety culture, are presented in the next section.

Development of and Barriers to Patient Safety Culture

Patient safety culture is generally viewed as a multi-dimensional construct, yet there is less agreement about the dimensions that make up the culture. In a comprehensive review of safety culture measurements used in health care (Flin, Burns, Mearns, Yule, & Robertson, 2006), a total of ten dimensions of patient safety culture were identified (Box 20.2).

Box 20.2. Dimensions of patient safety culture

1. Management and supervision
2. Safety systems
3. Risk perception
4. Job demands
5. Reporting and speaking up
6. Safety attitudes and behaviors
7. Communication and feedback
8. Teamwork
9. Personal resources
10. Organizational factors

Source: Flin et al., 2006

In a later review of additional papers, the most frequently cited dimensions across all literature include: (1) leadership and commitment to safety, (2) open communication founded on trust, (3) organizational learning, (4) a non-punitive approach to adverse event reporting and analysis, (5) teamwork, and (6) a shared belief in the importance of safety (Halligan & Zecevic, 2011). These dimensions help to frame the determinants of patient safety culture and describe the necessary structures, supports, and processes that can be assessed, evaluated, and improved. We next consider several of the key dimensions.

Research has identified perceptions of management support and actions as an important indicator of whether employee behavior and organizational performance uphold a safety culture (Griffiths, 1985; Zohar, 1980). As such, it is important for management action and communication to be consistent in delivering the message that safety is an important issue within the organization. However, mistrust of management may ultimately undermine goals to improve the adoption of safety beliefs and behaviors within an organization (Clarke, 1999). It is imperative that the development of a patient safety culture goes hand-in-hand with the promotion of a trusting and accountable organizational culture. Furthermore, the development of improvement of organizational safety culture can be used to help encourage greater knowledge of and support for patient safety practices (Institute of Medicine, 1999; Nieva & Sorra, 2003). Engaged management helps to ensure greater alignment between an organization's safety culture and patient safety strategies at the frontlines of care. Research has shown that patient safety culture is correlated with employee safety behaviors and patient and employee injuries, with the dimension of perceived managerial support also predicting safety behaviors and injuries (Agnew, Flin, & Mearns, 2013). The commitment of first line managers, such as ward charge nurses (Agnew & Flin, 2014), is a key component of establishing and maintaining a strong culture for patient safety. But this has to be fully supported by senior managers, who have a key influence on a hospital's safety culture (Dixon-Woods et al., 2014). Quality improvement interventions, such as leadership walkarounds in hospitals, need to be carefully designed and properly executed, otherwise they may diminish the safety culture rather than enhance it, as a recent English study demonstrates (Martin et al., 2014).

While commitment from management is a keystone of a positive patient safety culture, support and commitment from those providing direct care to patients is equally as important. Research has shown that patient safety culture can heavily influence provider likelihood to perform patient safety practices, such as hand washing and encouraging patients to ask questions (Bishop & Boyle, 2014). Perceptions of safety culture can therefore be changed or enhanced through the use of strong and consistent communication throughout an organization, as well as developing opportunities for employees to voice concerns and report incidents. In fact, even the act of surveying health care providers on their perceptions of patient safety culture can help to positively impact perceptions of risk and safety within an organization (Nolan, 2000). In some instances, the relationship between patient safety culture and patient safety improvements may not be readily seen (van Noord, de Bruijne, & Twisk, 2010). Closing the feedback loop after reporting by communicating action plans and clearly linking changes made to specific incidents has also been shown to be important when raising employee awareness of patient safety (Benn et al., 2009).

While demonstrating organizational commitment to patient safety through consistent messaging is important, equally as important is to ensure that communication during the provision of care creates a safe environment. Communication strategies such as the WHO Surgical Safety Checklist (Haynes et al., 2009), read backs, and time outs are all strategies that can be used within health care teams to ensure that all members understand their role during a procedure, have the necessary information to perform the procedure safely, and can safely speak up if there is a disagreement regarding care (Sammer, Lykens, Singh,

Mains, & Lacken, 2010). Teamwork across all levels of the organization and an emphasis on using teamwork as a "checks and balance" approach to improving organizational safety is an important step in the development of a positive patient safety culture in this age. With increasing use of multidisciplinary health care teams to carry out complex treatments and utilizing team-based care for chronic conditions, effective teamwork is essential to providing safe and high-quality health care (Sammer et al., 2010).

A team approach to ensuring that safety attitudes and behaviors are positively rein-forced can also be beneficial when developing or improving patient safety culture. Patient safety culture ultimately influences how employees interpret what is safe or unsafe and employee expectations of what safety should look like. As such, the patient safety culture of an organization can influence whether these provider-based strategies are being used to perform the job better or whether they are merely being paid "lip service" in order to ful-fill organizational or accreditation standards. In organizations where patient safety culture is poor, even the use of the Safety Surgical Checklist will not be effective if team members do not see the advantage to improving communication within the operating room (Levy et al., 2012). Motivation for involvement in these team-based tools needs to come from within the team itself to be truly effective. As such, peer-approval and modeling of posi-tive patient safety behaviors has been identified as an important construct of patient safety culture (Singer et al., 2007). Further discussion regarding system design, job demands, and organizational factors is presented in the next section.

While we have discussed some of the major dimensions of patient safety culture, these can vary as health care organizations move through different levels of patient safety cul-ture. The maturity model (Westrum, 1992), adapted for patient safety by Parker et al. (2008), describes five levels of organizational safety culture: (1) pathological, (2) reactive, (3) calculative, (4) proactive, and (5) generative (Table 20.2). This is focused primarily on how errors and accidents are reported and analyzed.

While many organizations look to reporting and learning from near misses and errors in order to improve, the ultimate goal is to create a generative patient safety culture whereby possible failures are actively sought out, identified, and corrected. Therefore, in order for an organization to advance from a pathological culture to a generative one, organizations must look thoughtfully at potential barriers. Potential barriers to the implementation of a generative patient safety culture are listed in Box 20.3.

Table 20.2 Patient safety maturity model.

Safety Maturity Level	Characteristics
1 Pathological	No systems or processes in place to promote a positive patient safety culture
2 Reactive	Systems and processes are in place but are only used in response to an error or as needed for regulatory requirements
3 Calculative	A systems approach to patient safety is evident but identification of possible risks is not performed
4 Proactive	Near misses and errors are resolved systematically and learning occurs to prevent recurrences
5 Generative	A positive patient safety culture is evident throughout all operations and formalized as a central mission of the organization. The organization is active in seeking out potential threats.

Source: Ashcroft, Morecroft, Parker, & Noyce, 2005; Fleming & Wentzell, 2008; Parker et al., 2008

Box 20.3 Patient safety culture barriers

- Fear of blame
- Fear of reporting
- Belief in the inevitability of error
- Lack of systematic analysis of failures
- Inadequate teamwork
- Complexity of work
- Provider desire for autonomy
- Divergent occupational responsibilities

Source: Kalisch & Aebersold, 2006; Waring, 2005

A common barrier health care organizations face is that of a "blame and shame" culture indicative of the pathological level of maturity (Institute of Medicine, 1999). A culture of blame assigns guilt to the individual clinician, often with damaging consequences (Dekker, 2013), rather than seeking a systems perspective in order to recover and learn from an event. In this case, individuals within the organization might tend to deny that errors occur due to the negative consequences of reporting them. Alternatively, employees may feel that trial and error is a necessary part of the provision of medical care and that risk is an inherent part of practicing medicine (Waring, 2005). Essentially, in an environment of ever-expanding complexity of work, health care providers might also expect a certain degree of error to occur and might not feel that it is important to report frequent errors. Health care is also unique as a high hazard organization in that many of the employees of the organization act autonomously. Most health care professions have their own regulatory body, governing structure, and codes of ethics and these may be more influential on provider behavior than management actions.

Classen and Kilbridge (2002) provide further detail on these concepts, suggesting seven essential components for safe health care delivery based on high-performing organizations: (1) governance and leadership, (2) a culture of safety, (3) creating a learning environment, (4) defining patient safety program objectives, (5) designing safe processes, (6) implementing processes, and (7) measuring and monitoring. It is clear from these seven components that promotion and enhancement of patient safety must come from a variety of sources and levels within an organization, with input and support required from frontline health care providers and senior leadership. As such, patient safety cannot be achieved through the introduction of stand-alone behaviors and practices, but rather must be integrated into everyday operations and culture. This is shown clearly in recent attempts to introduce Crew Resource Management courses, adapted from aviation, to train non-technical skills (Flin, Glavin, Patey, & Maran, 2010; Flin, O'Connor, & Crichton, 2008; Yule, Flin, Paterson-Brown, & Maran, 2006) in healthcare professionals (West et al., 2012). Essentially as culture reflects the norms of behavior, changing behavior is a key way to alter the associated norms and there are indications that this can be effective (Verbeek-van Noord et al., 2014). However, one study in London hospitals showed the importance of the prevailing culture in determining whether behavioral changes from this type of training were maintained in the longer term (McCulloch et al., 2009). Furthermore, a recent review of Crew Resource Management training in the health care sector suggests that strategies like this can only be one piece of the puzzle in order to achieve successful culture change (Verbeek-van Noord et al., 2014). Therefore, it can be helpful to assess the "toxicity" of an organization's safety culture before safety interventions are introduced.

The interplay between the myriad of actors and processes trying to achieve the same goal of patient safety necessitates the use of a systems perspective of patient safety culture. The next section will explore a systems perspective to patient safety and highlight some of the unique characteristics of this approach to safety in health care, including the need to incorporate the role of the patient within the system.

A Systems Perspective to Patient Safety Culture

Organizational system problems, such as gaps in the continuity of care, have been highlighted a as primary cause of safety issues within health care (Gosbee, 2002; Institute of Medicine, 1999; Nolan, 2000). Nadler and Hibino (1994) describe a system as a set of related activities or objects designed to achieve a specific purpose by receiving inputs and transforming them into outputs.

Within health care, systems theory provides a framework for understanding the complexity of health care organizations and identifying opportunities for failures to occur. Given the consequences of failure in health care are often high, such as harm to the patient or even death, using a holistic approach to understanding failures is important. A systems argument for patient safety suggests that incidents are more likely to occur when organizational safeguards that are normally in place fail. These safeguards can include processes such as handoff procedures between practitioners, trigger alerts for medication interactions, or policies and procedures for shift changes.

While these safeguards are important, it is also important to see how patient safety culture can influence the use of them. As stated earlier, patient safety culture influences all outcomes in a health care organization, including individual patient health outcomes. Within a health care systems perspective, this means that patient safety culture influences perceptions and motivations behind learning from past mistakes and errors, employee commitment to comply with practices aimed at improving patient safety, and the need to put patient safety first over efficiency. Patient safety culture influences how well the systems put in place within an organization uphold patient safety as a priority and closely mirror their intended use. For example, while many health care organizations have recently begun to utilize adverse event reporting systems as a means to identify areas of improvement, if the organization's culture does not see merit in providing feedback on these events back to health care providers, there may be a lack of willingness to comply with reporting (Handler et al., 2007; Hartnell, MacKinnon, Sketnis, & Fleming, 2012), thereby decreasing the ability of the organization to learn and improve safeguards.

While many times failures in safeguards are attributed to human error, such as an individual failing to follow specified procedures, focusing on why these policies, procedures, and systems are failing to detect and prevent errors from occurring is more useful. Take, for example, the issue of patient handoffs between health care providers. Gaps of care between health care providers are common occurrences in health care and are often bridged through policies and procedures mandated by an organization, such as shift change protocol (Cook, Render, & Woods, 2003). Most of the time these bridges are successful; however, they also create opportunities for patient safety incidents to occur. Patient information may be lost or lapses in continuity of care may present themselves when organizational conditions create obstacles to bridging. Cook et al. (2003) suggest that incidents occur because of conditions that overwhelm or nullify practitioner abilities to cope with gaps, such as improper staffing levels. While we often think of patient safety culture as being positive, it is also important to see how culture can hinder efforts to improve patient safety. In the case of handoffs between shifts, if employees perceive that the organization values efficiency over patient safety, such handoffs might not be formalized and greater emphasis will be placed on efficiency rather than comprehensiveness. When there are significant gaps within a health care system this speaks to a culture that does not value good communication among health care providers and does not aim to improve cooperation among systems.

Strategies that help to understand practitioner abilities to detect and cope with distractions and hazards may be useful in reducing patient safety incidents. For instance, studies of handover practices between shifts (Raduma, Flin, Yule, & Close, 2012) or between departments (Manser, Foster, Flin, & Patey, 2013) indicate that methods are not standardized and practitioners may not realize that this is a high-risk activity. Gaps in continuity of care during and following hospital discharge have also been noted as a significant source of patient safety incidents and unnecessary hospital readmission (Dhalla, O'Brien, Ko, & Laupacis, 2012). System policies, therefore, not only need to be established for bridging gaps within the hospital setting, but must also ensure that gaps between health care settings are adequately prevented. This speaks to the complexity of patient safety culture within health care, as not only must it exist within a singular health care organization, but it must also exist within the larger health care system that encompasses hospitals and care received within the community through family physicians and long-term care organizations.

One of the most widely accepted models of systems failures in health care is the Swiss Cheese Model of Accident Causation (Reason, 2000). This model posits that there are both active failures and latent conditions within a system that lead to incidents occurring. Active failures refer to unsafe acts that can be directly linked to the error that has occurred. Latent conditions are already present in the organization and can make system barriers less effective at preventing the error from occurring. Both active failures and latent conditions can occur in four domains: (1) organizational influences, (2) supervision, (3) preconditions, and (4) specific acts. Using the example of patient handoffs, organizational influences such as budget cuts to personnel, inadequate training of new employees on handoff policies, accepted shortcuts to handoff procedures, and the possibility of consulting the wrong patient chart could all lead to ineffective barriers. Within this model, culture has the ability to affect all four of the domains (Reason, 1998). This is because organizational culture can either uphold a culture of patient safety or undermine barriers put in place to prevent adverse events by communicating to employees that safety is not important. Culture can also direct health care providers and hospital administrators to consistently turn a blind eye to potential failures if they are seen as part of how things are done in an organization or have become accepted shortcuts. An example of this might be to always override medication error prompts when filling a prescription because they are so frequent, and ignoring them does not often result in negative consequences. The accident causation model also highlights that many incidents have a long causal history of latent conditions that predispose a system to failures and allow active failures to occur (Reason, 2000). In a generative patient safety culture, this is what the organization would be focused on. Rather than looking to the individual, generative patient safety cultures seek out potential latent conditions that could result in a hazard reaching the patient. However, in a pathological or reactive safety culture the organization would be more likely to blame individuals when a failure occurs and to implement "band-aid" solutions in the hope that the incident will not occur again.

Both active failures and latent conditions are important when considering system design, as they are often identifiable and manageable. There has been some critique of this model, however, that points to its lack of specificity regarding relationships between causal factors and how to practically apply it to organizational conditions when a failure does occur (Dekker, 2002; Luxhoj & Kauffeld, 2003). Management of incidents should, therefore, be based on creating safe systems that can proactively mitigate incidents from occurring by identifying and correcting unsafe conditions. It has also been proposed, by the high reliability organization theorists (Weick & Sutcliffe, 2001), that in order to maintain this attention to latent conditions, along with learning from active failures, managers need to be mindful, and have a sense of chronic unease. That is, they need to avoid complacency and have a level of vigilance, coupled with a clear understanding of the prevalent culture and an awareness of how risks might be realized (Fruhen et al., 2014).

Nolan (2000) expands on the concepts raised by Reason and argues that when designing systems of health care to be safer, organizations should focus on three main tasks: (1) designing the system to prevent errors, (2) designing procedures to make errors visible when they do occur so that they may be intercepted, and (3) designing procedures for mitigating the adverse effects of errors when they are not detected and intercepted. This research also provides examples of how to effectively perform these three tasks, including improving organizational and work environments, using patients as a resource for information and "double checking," and implementing processes that can help to halt and reverse harm to patients.

Finally, the Systems Engineering Initiative for Patient Safety (SEIPS) model provides an overarching framework for systems design within patient safety (Carayon et al., 2006). The SEIPS model attempts to explain the interactions between health care providers and patients within a health care environment that includes technology, tools, tasks, processes, and outcomes (Figure 20.1). According to this model, a person (e.g., employee of a health care organization) performs their job tasks using a number of tools and technologies, with the performance of such tasks taking place within a physical environment and under certain conditions to produce different outcomes (Carayon et al., 2006). Elements measured within this model, therefore, include things such as employee skills and demographics, work schedules, organizational culture, human factor characteristics (i.e., how easy it is to use an IV machine), job demands, and physical layout to identify their effect on organizational and patient outcomes.

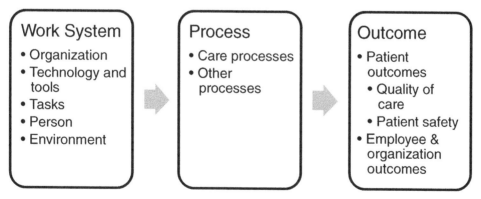

Figure 20.1 Systems engineering design for patient safety (adapted from Carayon et al., 2006).

As such, the model emphasizes how a system should be designed around individuals in order to facilitate performance and reduce negative consequences. This particular model also includes the patient as a key component of the interaction between individuals and their environment, acknowledging that patients often play a role in the provision of their treatment. This is a unique characteristic of patient safety culture when compared with safety cultures in other organizations. As patients are ultimately the end-user of a health care system, they are in a unique position to be included as an important dimension of patient safety culture. For example, if we think of safety culture within a manufacturing facility, often negative consequences of being unsafe will affect the employee(s) involved but will not affect the safety of the individual who will be purchasing the product. However, within health care not only are patients at the receiving end when an adverse event occurs, they are also present throughout the entire process of providing care. As such, this model posits that greater understanding of these interactions between individuals and their work system, and the impact on patient and provider processes and outcomes better equips system designers to improve the likelihood of obtaining a safe work environment where patient safety is enhanced.

Measuring Safety Culture in Health Care

Now that we have closely examined patient safety culture and its role in systems-level thinking and design in health care organizations, we move into an examination of the broader concept of organizational safety culture and how it can be measured. Investigations into failures in the delivery of safe health care have identified poor organizational safety culture as a significant contributing factor (Francis, 2013; Institute of Medicine, 2001). Within health care, tools have been developed as a means to better understand the role that the broader organizational safety culture plays in promoting and sustaining patient safety. Nieva and Sorra (2003) have identified a number of uses of safety culture assessment in health care organizations, including, (1) diagnosing safety culture to identify areas for improvement and raise awareness, (2) evaluating interventions and changes over time, (3) conducting benchmarking, and (4) fulfilling regulatory requirements. Safety culture can be measured in a number of ways, including individual health centre audits, questionnaires, and focus groups. Generally the best approach is to combine two or more of these methods, for example, hold focus groups to aid in the interpretation of survey findings (Mearns et al., 2013). While some researchers question the usefulness of using (solely) perception questionnaires to measure safety culture (Guldenmund, 2007), this method is currently the most widely accepted and utilized form of patient safety culture measurement to date.

The relationship of safety climate questionnaire scores to better patient safety outcomes is not as clear as the link between climate and worker safety in the industrial sector (Christian, Bradley, Wallace, & Burke, 2009b). However, studies generally show a positive relationship. For example, Haugen et al. (2010), in 30 ICU units, found that poorer safety climate scores related to increased length of stay for patients, and less favourable perceptions of management by staff were related to higher patient mortality rates. Staff perceptions of generic safety climate (without a specific focus on patient care) were related to treatment errors in one Israeli acute hospital (Naveh, Katz-Navon, & Stern, 2005).

Zohar, Livne, Tenne-Gazit, Admi, and Donchin (2007) observed 955 Israeli hospital nurses' safety behaviors and showed that both unit and hospital-level safety climates (using both generic and patient focused items) were predictors of workers' safety behaviors. Likewise, a study in the USA of 789 hospital workers found that when senior management support for worker safety, safety feedback and training were perceived favorably, workers had fewer blood and body fluid exposure incidents (Gershon et al., 2000). In Japan, a more positive safety climate was associated with safety of workers, with reduced needlestick and sharp injuries (Smith et al., 2010). However, in a survey of staff from 30 hospitals in the USA, no evidence of relationships between perceptions of senior management's engagement or unit managers' support for patient safety and patient safety indicators (e.g., hospital discharge data) were found (Rosen et al., 2010).

Few studies have measured both patient iatrogenic injuries and staff occupational injuries, but where they have, similar associations have been reported. A survey of 1127 nurses from 42 hospitals in the USA found that safety climate predicted both patient outcomes (medication errors, urinary tract infections) and nurse outcomes (back and needlestick injuries). The complexity of patient conditions exerted a moderating effect (Hofmann & Mark, 2006).

Taylor et al. (2012) studied 723 nurses from 29 units in one hospital and found that two safety climate factors were associated with nurse injuries and patient adverse events (decubitus ulcer). A staffing factor (turnover) was found to be a particular risk factor. Therefore, it appears that when safety climate is associated with safer patient care, it may also be associated with better safety for workers.

A brief description of the most widely used patient safety culture survey tools is provided below. A synopsis of the tools and their characteristics is presented in Table 20.3.

The Hospital Survey on Patient Safety Culture was developed by the Agency for Healthcare Research and Quality (AHRQ) in 2004 and is used to collect voluntary data submitted by US hospitals to allow for comparisons. The survey is divided into three sections and utilizes 14 different dimensions to measure patient safety culture at both the unit and hospital levels. Given the large publicly available database reports, and the widespread use of the survey in jurisdictions around the world (Sorra & Battles, 2014), the survey excels in its ability to provide organizations with comparative and benchmarking data. Examples of the use of this survey in other jurisdictions and comparisons between survey findings internationally are discussed in the next section.

The Safety Attitudes Questionnaire (SAQ), developed by the University of Texas (Sexton, Helmrich, & Neilands, 2006), incorporates constructs from Vincent's (1998) framework for analyzing safety and Donabedien's (1988) model for assessing quality. The SAQ has been adapted in a number of areas, including intensive care units (ICU) and ambulatory care, and can be used to compare safety cultures across different units. Furthermore, the SAQ includes open-ended questions that can help to elicit provider feedback on recommendations for how to improve safety culture (Etchegary & Thomas, 2014).

Singer et al. (2003) conducted a safety culture assessment of 15 hospitals in California using their Stanford/PSCI culture survey. This tool was created through the analysis and compilation of a number of previously validated and reliable tools that were unit or sector specific. The survey is aimed at assessing organizations on a number of dimensions of safety culture, including rewards and punishment, risk perception, fatigue, and stress (planning), employee training, and time and resources. In addition, the survey is divided into five different factors of safety culture: (1) organization, (2) department, (3) production, (4) reporting/seeking help, and (5) shame/self-awareness. The questionnaire is constructed entirely of close-ended questions and has been extensively piloted and tested on a large sample size of respondents. A modified version of this questionnaire was developed by Ginsburg and colleagues (Ginsburg, 2006; Ginsburg et al., 2009) using four dimensions that were found to be the most valid, reliable, and meaningful. The modified instrument also includes two questions from the Hospital Survey on Patient Safety Culture that allow respondents to grade their unit and region on overall patient safety.

Table 20.3 Patient safety culture survey tools.

	Hospital Survey on Patient Safety Culture[1]	Safety Attitudes Questionnaire[2]	Stanford Instrument[3]	Modified Stanford Instrument[4]	Canadian Patient Safety Climate Survey[5]
Constructs/ Dimensions Measured	• Teamwork within units • Supervisor/ manager expectations • Organizational learning • Management support • Overall perceptions • Feedback and communication • Communication openness • Frequency of events reported • Teamwork across units • Staffing • Handoffs and transitions • Nonpunitive response to errors	• Teamwork • Safety climate • Job satisfaction • Stress recognition • Perceptions of management • Working conditions	• Organization • Department • Production • Reporting • Shame/self-awareness	• Valuing safety • Fear of repercussions • Perceived state of safety • Supervisory leadership	• Management commitment • Supervisory com-mitment • Response to error • Open communication
Questionnaire Length	79 items	60 items	30 items	36 items	38 items
Scale	5-point Likert scale	5-point Likert scale	5-point Likert scale	5-point Likert scale	5-point Likert scale
Reliability	alpha = .63–.83	alpha = .65–.83	Not published	alpha = .66–.86	alpha = .70–.80

Strengths	• Tested on large sample size • Inclusion of many patient safety culture dimensions • Supporting documentation for tool available • Good psychometric properties	• Tested on large sample size • Detailed report describing survey tool available • Good psychometric properties	• Tested on large sample size • Literature available detailing tool development and factor structure • Good psychometric properties	• Relatively short length • Prioritization of most important survey questions • Good psychometric properties	• Tested on large sample size
Challenges	• Length of questionnaire	• Limited number of dimensions • Not specifically intended to measure safety culture	• No published reliability data • Limited number of dimensions	• Limited number of dimensions	• No published data from other jurisdictions

Source: Adapted from Colla, Bracken, Kinney, & Weeks, 2005; Fleming, 2005

[1] Blegen et al., 2009

[2] Sexton et al., 2006

[3] Singer et al., 2003

[4] Ginsburg, 2006; Ginsburg et al. 2009

[5] Ginsburg, Tregunno, Norton, Mitchell, & Howley, 2014

The Canadian Patient Safety Climate Survey was developed in response to the identification of persistent challenges faced when trying to measure patient safety culture, namely: (1) the large number of dimensions associated with patient safety culture, (2) the need to create context-specific factors for use within different settings and countries, (3) the inability to achieve reliable internal consistency, and (4) limited evidence of psychometric rigor (Ginsburg, Tregunno, Norton, Mitchell, & Howley, 2014). One of the strengths of this survey is the ability to capture a number of dimensions using a relatively small number of survey items. The testing and use of the survey within a universal health care system also increases its suitability for use within Europe and other similar jurisdictions.

While the previous examples target direct provider and clinician input for measuring safety culture, another approach incorporates feedback from all levels of an organization, including managers and high-level administration. The Strategies for Leadership tool developed by the Voluntary Hospitals of America (VHA) (2000) aims to provide a report card on an organization's safety culture based on seven dimensions (Box 20.4).

Box 20.4 VHA strategies for leadership dimensions

1   Leadership
2   Strategic planning
3   Information and analysis
4   Human resources
5   Process management
6   Patient and family involvement
7   Summary of key safety aspects

Source: Voluntary Hospitals of America, 2000

Team members are instructed to review each dimension themselves and then discuss their findings with the rest of the team. Each member is asked to assign a grade from A to E, indicating the level of implementation and discussion of each dimension within the organization. Hospitals are also able to compare their results with other organizations due to the inclusion of demographic information at the end of the tool. Dimensions are then scored and teams are instructed to identify three to five low scoring activities and develop improvement plans to be implemented throughout the organization, with annual measurements encouraged to evaluate progress. As with the Manchester tool (see below), the strength of the VHA audit is that it is solutions-based, with the aim to assess deficiencies and correct them. Furthermore, it provides the opportunity for discussion across the spectrum of health care personnel with the inclusion of both clinicians and administrators.

Qualitative methods have also been used to develop a framework to analyze safety culture within organizations. The Manchester Patient Safety Assessment Framework (Parker et al., 2008) was developed to be used in a workshop setting, providing discussion points on a number of dimensions, including (1) commitment to patient safety, (2) perceptions of the causes of incidents and their reporting, (3) investigating incidents, (4) learning following an incident, (5) communication, (6) staff management and safety issues, (7) staff education and training about risk management, and (8) team work. Participants are asked to rate their organizational safety culture individually based on a five-point scale that ranges from a pathological culture to a generative culture. Scores are then brought to the rest of the group for discussion. This approach works very well for targeting interventions and engaging clinical staff; however, there is a lack of data regarding the validity and reliability of this approach (Fleming & Hartnell, 2007).

With the range of tools available to health care organizations to assess patient safety culture, the onus is on the organization to select the right tool, analyze the data correctly, and then use the results to implement improvements. Prior to that, building capacity within the organization to ensure internal expertise is essential. Garnering support from all stakeholders within the organization, including administrative and clinical staff, helps to lay the foundation for change to occur and ensures there is a team-based approach to identifying and implementing strategies. Fleming (2005) provides a ten-step process for successful safety measurement and implementation in health care through a comparison and analysis of patient safety culture instruments (Figure 20.2).

These ten elements aim to ensure greater success of the application of safety culture to health care through lessons gleaned in other high-risk sectors, such as nuclear energy and aviation. The Patient Safety Culture Improvement Tool (PSCIT) can also be used by organizations during the cultural improvement process (Fleming & Wentzell, 2008). This encourages health care organizations to assess how well the structures and processes they use contribute to a positive patient safety culture by using a multidisciplinary team to assign scores to a number of patient safety indicators and to consider barriers that may be preventing improvement (Fleming & Wentzell, 2008). The PSCIT directly maps onto the maturity model, thereby allowing organizations to track their progress toward a generative patient safety culture. It is important to note that while safety culture assessments are important to assessing organizational culture and can result in positive changes, improper measurement and implementation can have negative impacts on the organization as well.

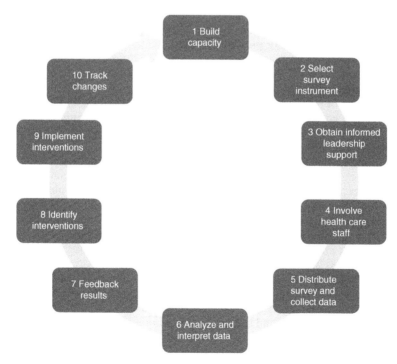

Figure 20.2 Ten-step process to successful safety culture measurement and improvement (Fleming, 2005).

As such, it is important for organizations to carefully consider safety culture measurement and to ensure ongoing support from staff and management throughout the process.

As patient safety culture differs widely within and between institutions (Huang et al., 2007; Singer et al., 2009), and indeed between jurisdictions and countries (Fugita et al., 2013), in the next section we explore the use of patient safety culture tools in a variety of settings. Differences in patient safety culture survey results across a number of jurisdictions are also considered.

International Comparisons

While the significant reports that have launched the patient safety movement have mainly come from the western world, such as *To Err is Human* and *An Organization with a Memory*, the patient safety movement has extended globally in the last decade. The widespread use of patient safety culture tools in a variety of jurisdictions has allowed for increased sharing of ideas and improved the ability for organizations to benchmark their data. As mentioned above, the Hospital Survey on Patient Safety Culture (HSOPSC) developed and distributed by AHRQ is one of the most widely utilized patient safety culture tools around the globe, with published research results from the UK (Sarac, Flin, Mearns, & Jackson, 2010; Waterson, Griffiths, Stride, Murphy, & Hignett, 2010); Europe (Pfeiffer & Manser, 2010; Smits, Dinglehoff, Wagner, Wal, & Groenewegen, 2008; Vlayen, Hellings, Claes, Peleman, & Schrooten, 2012); Scandinavia (Hedskold et al., 2013); the Middle East (Alahmadi, 2010; El-Jardali, Dimassi, Jamal, Jaafar, & Hemadeh, 2011; Najjar et al., 2013); Asia (Fujita et al., 2013), and the USA (Blegan, Gearhart, & Sehgal, 2009; Handler et al., 2006; Sorra & Dyer, 2010). The dimensions of the HSOPSC are shown above in Table 20.3. While many jurisdictions have adapted the HSOPSC somewhat to be better tailored to health care provision in their country, the results from around the world nevertheless allow for comparisons in relative strengths and weaknesses in patient safety culture between different health care systems (Waterson, 2014). Testing has also been done in these jurisdictions as to the psychometric properties of the survey and to determine predictors of patient safety culture using dimensions of HSOPSC. It is important to note that while comparisons are made between international examples, the HSOPSC measures differences at the unit level where culture is more localized, rather than at the organizational level (Zohar & Luria, 2005).

Results from Saudi Arabia found that the health care providers from 13 general hospitals perceive an overall positive patient safety culture, with the overall patient safety grade rated as excellent or very good by 60 percent (n=223) of respondents (Alahmadi, 2010). Overall strengths of this patient safety culture were found to be organizational learning and continuous improvement, teamwork within hospital units, and feedback and communication about error. Areas for improvement were found to be supervisor/manager expectations, under-reporting of events, non-punitive response to error, staffing, and teamwork across hospital units. In a comparison between survey results from Japan, Taiwan, and the USA, results found that US respondents were more likely to rate patient safety culture higher (Fujita et al., 2013). Respondents from Japan were more likely to rate organizational learning/continuous improvement as low, whereas the dimension of non-punitive response to error and lack of communication was found to be low in Taiwan. In comparison to both Japan and Taiwan, the dimension of staffing was found to be highest in the USA due to the relative high number of health care professionals there. However, even with less staffing, Japan rated highest in number of event reports. While these international differences are interesting, they need to be treated with caution as there may be differences across cultures in the way these questionnaires are responded to, such as willingness to criticize hospital management.

Application of the HSOPSC to the nursing home sector was performed in the USA and found differences between the hospital and long-term sectors in the dimensions of non-punitive response to errors, teamwork within units, communication openness, feedback and communication about error, and organizational learning, with nursing homes scoring significantly worse (Handler et al., 2006). Vlayen et al. (2012) also found differences between health care settings in their research across Belgium, with psychiatric and long-term hospitals having higher positive dimensional scores. The authors suggest this could stem from a greater emphasis on patient safety in these settings or a greater occurrence of unsafe acts occurring in the acute care setting.

While the use of the HSOPSC in predictive models has been cautioned due to psychometric properties (Blegan et al., 2009), this is another area of international research which has allowed for comparisons between regions. Researchers in Lebanon employed the HSOPSC throughout 68 hospitals in order to capture baseline data in the country and to create a prediction model based on the survey dimensions (El-Jardali et al., 2011). The research found that five dimensions predicted a positive patient safety culture grade by respondents, measured as a score out of 100, including (1) event reporting, (2) communication, (3) patient safety leadership and management, (4) staffing, and (5) accreditation. However, one weakness in this type of study is that the outcome measure is just another item on the questionnaire rating. Interestingly, predictors of positive safety culture dimensions have also been found to be different between physicians and nurses, indicating that further stratification of survey results based on professional groups may be warranted (Pfeiffer & Manser, 2010). Wagner, Smits, Sorra and Huang (2013), in an assessment of safety cultures across three countries, suggest that one common area of weakness that may see significant gains in many countries is in the area of handoffs and transitions.

Another important area of international research is the psychometric testing of the HSOPSC, with and without country-specific modifications, to ensure acceptable fit and measurement of the survey dimensions. The use of confirmatory factor analysis (CFA) and exploratory factor analysis (EFA) and measurements of internal consistency have been used by a number of researchers around the globe to better understand the appropriateness of use of the HSOPSC in other jurisdictions and suggest amendments and improvements in the survey tool. Research in the USA has found acceptable validity and reliability of the survey tool for use within the hospital setting (Blegan et al., 2009), with greater fit found when two items were removed from the questionnaire (Sorra & Dyer, 2010). An international study in Sweden measured a country-specific version of the HSOPSC and found acceptable validity of 12 factors when used in both the hospital and primary care settings using confirmatory factor analysis (Hedskold et al., 2013), speaking to potential applications of the survey tool in other health care settings besides hospitals. Application of the survey tool in Dutch hospitals also found acceptable validity and reliability with minor modifications of dimension factors (Smits et al., 2008). Acceptable validity and reliability has been established in Scotland using the original 12 factor model without need for modification (Sarac et al., 2010). However, results from Germany and England suggest that the use of the HSOPSC without any modifications for individual jurisdictions may be limited, with CFA in these studies failing to replicate the dimensions proposed by the tool (Pfeiffer & Manser, 2010; Waterson et al., 2010).

The ability to test and implement patient safety culture tools across countries is a positive step in better understanding the myriad of factors and structures that can influence hospital patient safety culture. It also is important in achieving greater validity and reliability in future patient safety culture tools allowing for improved comparisons and benchmarking between jurisdictions (Jackson, Sarac, & Flin, 2010). Perhaps one of the greatest lessons learned thus far is the awareness that health care organizations need to better understand survey tools before implementing them to ensure they are appropriate and will provide meaningful results. International results also speak to the importance of promoting positive cultures in which reporting is encouraged and celebrated and leaders are actively involved in promoting open communication and teamwork across units.

Future Research

As has been demonstrated in this chapter, the emphasis on patient safety culture within health care organizations has steadily been increasing over the last decade. While many health care organizations and regulatory bodies currently look to patient safety culture survey results to better understand areas for improvement and change, overall there is often a broken link between measuring patient safety culture and using those results to implement cultural change. For many organizations, this is simply due to a lack of awareness regarding cultural change and how to translate survey results into actionable implementation items. For many organizations, especially those who are exploring culture for the first time, the most difficult question following the collection of patient safety culture survey data is "now what?" (Guldenmund, 2000). Future research is needed to provide practical implementation strategies for health care organizations who wish to use these results to improve their culture.

While we have made reference in this chapter to the importance of patients in the discussion of patient safety culture, little research has focused on how patient involvement should be measured. Since patients are ultimately at the receiving end of health care and are often those affected by harm when failures in health care occur, the role of patients and the importance of patient involvement in supporting a positive patient safety culture should be explored. Existing literature shows that while many patients are involved in their care in varying ways, such as asking questions and helping to make treatment decisions, many barriers still exist for patients because of the way health care is delivered and perceptions of power imbalances between patients and their health care providers (Bishop & Macdonald, 2014). While a positive patient safety culture should strive to engage patients at all health care encounters, many patients are still wary to ask challenging questions of their health care providers and to speak up if they feel something is wrong (Bishop & Macdonald, 2014; Davis, Koutantji, & Vincent, 2008; Waterman et al., 2006). Patients are also in a unique position to help health care organizations measure how well their patient safety culture is being translated to the frontline of care. While most patient safety culture surveys, as described in this chapter, focus mainly on provider (employee) perceptions of safety, patients also experience patient safety culture when they receive care in a health care organization. Hence, patient experience and involvement could and perhaps should be incorporated as a dimension of patient safety culture moving forward to ensure that this important dimension is not overlooked.

Finally, whenever we talk about culture, we are inevitably talking about a context in which people interact. While there have been great strides at adapting and developing safety culture tools for use within health care, many current strategies employ a "one-size-fits-all" approach to measuring patient safety culture. While this provides some advantages with regard to being able to benchmark and compare data across organizations, the context of the organization can sometimes become diluted or lost. Strategies outlined by Fleming (2005) in Figure 20.2 can be used by organizations to ensure that they have internal expertise, strong management support, involved stakeholders in setting priorities and developing strategies, gather information to better understand areas for improvement, and feed back results to the organization. In addition, the ability to capture organizational readiness for change and organization-specific data for use in conjunction with patient safety culture instruments could greatly enhance the ability of health care organizations to implement changes to improve their culture (Burnett et al., 2010). While current strategies focus on finding areas of weakness, identifying areas of convergence and divergence of employee perceptions may help to indicate where change strategies may be more successful. Ultimately, although employee perceptions may indicate a need for change, current instruments do not identify whether change is likely to be successful. Future research should aim to provide organizations with further tools to better assess the context for cultural change.

Conclusion

The recognition of the unsafe nature of providing health care over the past two decades has led to greater interest and investment in understanding organizational safety culture. The identification of patient safety culture as a subset of an organization's safety culture has given rise to the application of safety culture principles from other high reliability industries to the study of health care. The application of a systems perspective to patient safety culture has helped health care organizations to move away from cultures of individual error and "blame and shame" to the proactive identification of failures and improvement of systems. Overcoming barriers, such as provider autonomy and fear of reporting, necessitates that health care organizations invite all stakeholders to the table when attempting to improve patient safety culture and provide safe and effective ways of gathering cultural data. Ensuring informed management support has repeatedly been shown to improve the success of implementing cultural improvement strategies and is also necessary to ensure that organizations provide timely feedback to employees and initiate action plans and changes in a timely manner.

As James Reason notes, "the best people can sometimes make the worst mistakes" (Reason, 1997). In health care, where the Hippocratic Oath of "never do harm" is alive and well, the sentiment is not lost. In an increasingly complex age, health care organizations have to look beyond provision of care to the provision of evidence-based and safe care. While we have come a long way in understanding and overcoming many of the safety challenges faced by health care organizations, we hope that further research will continue on this path to help organizations and their employees implement patient safety cultures which emphasize the role of the system and actively seek areas for improvement.

References

Advisory Committee on Safety of Nuclear Installations, Health and Safety Committee. (1993). *Human factors study group 3rd report: Organising for safety.* London, UK: ACSNI.

Agnew, C., & Flin, R. (2014). Senior charge nurses' leadership behaviours in relation to hospital ward safety: A mixed method study. *International Journal of Nursing Studies, 51*(5), 768–780.

Agnew, C., Flin, R., & Mearns, K. (2013). Patient safety climate and worker safety behaviours in acute hospitals in Scotland. *Journal of Safety Research, 45*(0), 95–101.

Alahmadi, H. A. (2010). Assessment of patient safety culture in Saudi Arabian hospitals. *BMJ Quality & Safety, 19*(5), e17.

Ashcroft, D. M., Morecroft, C., Parker, D., & Noyce, P. R. (2005). Safety culture assessment in community pharmacy: Development, face validity and feasibility of the Manchester patient safety framework. *Quality and Safety in Health Care, 14*(6), 417–421.

Baker, G. R., Norton, P. G., Flintoft, V., & Blais, R. (2004). The Canadian adverse events study: The incidence of adverse events among hospital patients in Canada. *Canadian Medical Association Journal, 170*(11), 1678–1686.

Benn, J., Koutantji, M., Wallace, L., Spurgeon, P., Rejman, M., & Healey, A. (2009). Feedback from incident reporting: Information and action to improve patient safety. *BMJ Quality & Safety, 18*(1), 11–21.

Bishop, A. C., & Boyle, T. A. (2014). The role of safety culture in influencing provider perceptions of patient safety. *Journal of Patient Safety,* Advance online publication.doi:10.1097/PTS.0000000000000092

Bishop, A. C., & Macdonald, M. (2014). Patient involvement in patient safety: A qualitative study of nursing staff and patient perceptions. *Journal of Patient Safety.* Advance online publication. doi:10.1097/PTS.0000000000000123

Blegan, M. A., Gearhart, S., & Sehgal, N. L., B. K. (2009). AHRQ's hospital survey on patient safety culture: Psychometric analyses. *Journal of Patient Safety, 3*(139), 144.

Burnett, S., Benn, J., Pinto, A., Parand, A., Iskander, S., & Vincent, C. (2010). Organisational readiness: Exploring the preconditions for success in organisation wide patient safety programmes. *Quality and Safety in Health Care, 19*(4), 313–317.

Carayon, P. (Ed.). (2011). *Handbook of human factors and ergonomics in health care and patient safety* (2nd edn.). Boca Raton, FL: CRC Press.

Carayon, P., Schoofs Hundt, A., Karsh, B., Gurses, A. P., Alvarado, C. J., Smith, M., & Flatley Brennan, P. (2006). Work system design for patient safety: The SEIPS model. *Quality and Safety in Health Care, 15*(suppl 1), i50–i58.

Christian, M. S., Bradley, J. S., Wallace, J. C., & Burke, M. J. (2009a). Workplace safety: A meta-analysis of the roles of person and situation factors. *Journal of Applied Psychology, 94*(5), 1103–1127.

Christian, M. S., Bradley, J. S., Wallace, J. C., & Burke, M. J. (2009b). Workplace safety: A meta-analysis of the roles of person and situation factors. *Journal of Applied Psychology, 94*(5), 1103–1127.

Claridge, T., & Sanders, J. (2007). Patient safety culture. In J. Sandars, & G. Cook (Eds.), *ABC of patient safety* (pp. 20–23). Oxford, UK: Blackwell.

Clarke, S. (1999). Perceptions of organizational safety: Implications for the development of safety culture. *Journal of Organizational Behavior, 20*(2), 185–198.

Clarke, S. (2006). The relationship between safety climate and safety performance: A meta-analytic review. *Journal of Occupational Health Psychology, 11*(4), 315–327.

Classen, D. C., & Kilbridge, P. M. (2002). The roles and responsibilities of physicians to improve patient safety within health care delivery systems. *Academic Medicine, 77*(10), 963–972.

Colla, J. B., Bracken, A. C., Kinney, L. M., & Weeks, W. B. (2005). Measuring patient safety climate: A review of surveys. *BMJ Quality & Safety, 14*(5), 364–366.

Cook, R. I., Render, M., & Woods, D. D. (2003). Gaps in the continuity of care and progress on patient safety. *British Medical Journal, 320*(7237), 791–794.

Cox, S., & Flin, R. (1998). Safety culture: Philosopher's stone or man of straw? *Work Stress, 12*(3), 189–201.

Davies, J. M., Hebert, P., & Hoffman, C. (2003). *The Canadian patient safety dictionary.* Ottawa, Canada: Royal College of Physicians and Surgeons.

Davis, R. E., Koutantji, M., & Vincent, C. A. (2008). How willing are patients to question healthcare staff on issues related to the quality and safety of their healthcare? An exploratory study. *Quality and Safety in Health Care, 17*(2), 90–96.

Dekker, S. (2002). *The field guide to human error investigations.* Burlington, VT: Ashgate.

Dekker, S. (2013). *Second victim: Error, guilt, trauma and resilience.* London, UK: CRC Press.

Department of Health (2000). *An organization with a memory: Report of an expert group on learning from adverse events in the NHS.* Chaired by the Chief Medical Officer. London, UK: The Stationery Office. http://www.aagbi.org/sites/default/files/An%20organisation%20with%20a%20memory.pdf (accessed June 20, 2015).

Dhalla, I. A., O'Brien, T., Ko, F., & Laupacis, A. (2012). Toward safer transitions: How can we reduce post-discharge adverse events? *Healthcare Quarterly, 15*, 63–67.

Dixon-Woods, M., Baker, R., Charles, K., Dawson, J., Jerzembek, G., Martin, G., . . . , & West, M. (2014). Culture and behaviour in the English National Health Service: Overview of lessons from a large multimethod study. *BMJ Quality & Safety, 23*(2), 106–115.

Donabedian, A. (1988). The quality of care: How can this be assessed? *Journal of the American Medical Association, 260*(12), 1743–1748.

El-Jardali, F., Dimassi, H., Jamal, D., Jaafar, M., & Hemadeh, N. (2011). Predictors and outcomes of patient safety culture in hospitals. *BMC Health Services Research, 11*, 45.

Etchegary, J., & Thomas, E. (2014). The safety attitudes questionnaire: Recent findings and future areas of research. In P. E. Waterson (Ed.), *Patient safety culture: Theory, methods, and application* (pp. 285–298). Aldershot, UK: Ashgate.

Fleming, M. (2005). Patient safety culture measurement and improvement: A "how to" guide. *Healthcare Quarterly, 8*(Special Issue), 14–19.

Fleming, M., & Hartnell, N. (2007). Measurement and improvement of safety culture. In N. J. MacKinnon (Ed.), *Safe and effective: The eight essential elements of an optimal medication-use system* (pp. 41–58). Ottawa, ON: Canadian Pharmacists Association.

Fleming, M., & Wentzell, N. (2008). Patient safety culture improvement tool: Development and guidelines for use. *Healthcare Quarterly, 11*(3, Special Issue), 10–15.

Flin, R., Burns, C., Mearns, K., Yule, S., & Robertson, E. M. (2006). Measuring safety climate in health care. *Quality and Safety in Health Care, 15*(2), 109–115.

Flin, R., Glavin, R., Patey, R., & Maran, N. (2010). Anaesthetists' non-technical skills. *British Journal of Anaesthesia, 105*(38), 44.

Flin, R., O'Connor, P., & Crichton, M. (2008). *Safety at the sharp end: A guide to non-technical skills*. Aldershot, UK: Ashgate.

Francis, R. (2013). *Final report of the Mid Staffordshire NHS foundation trust public inquiry*. London, UK: The Stationery Office.

Fujita, S., Seto, K., Ito, S., Wu, Y., Huang, C. C., & Hasegawa, T. (2013). The characteristics of patient safety culture in Japan, Taiwan and the United States. *BMC Health Services Research, 13*, 20.

Gershon, R. R. M., Karkashian, C. D., Grosch, J. W., Murphy, L., Escamilla-Cejudo, A., Flanagan, P., . . . , & Martin, L. (2000). Hospital safety climate and its relationship with safe work practices and workplace exposure incidents. *American Journal of Infection Control, 28*(3), 211–221.

Gershon, R. R. M., Stone, P. W., Bakken, S., & Larson, E. (2004). Measurement of organizational culture and climate in healthcare. *Journal of Nursing Administration,, 34*(1), 33–40.

Ginsburg, L. (2006). *Perceptions of patient safety culture in four health regions*. York, UK: York University.

Ginsburg, L., Gilin, D., Tregunno, D., Norton, P. G., Flemons, W., & Fleming, M. (2009). Advancing measurement of patient safety culture. *Health Services Research, 44*(1), 205–224.

Ginsburg, L., Tregunno, D., Norton, P. G., Mitchell, J. I., & Howley, H. (2014). "Not another safety culture survey": Using the Canadian patient safety climate survey (can-PSCS) to measure provider perceptions of PSC across health settings. *BMJ Quality & Safety, 23*(2), 162–170.

Gosbee, J. (2002). Human factors engineering and patient safety. *BMJ Quality & Safety, 11*(4), 352–354.

Griffiths, D. K. (1985). Safety attitudes of management. *Ergonomics, 28*(1), 61–67.

Guldenmund, F. W. (2000). The nature of safety culture: A review of theory and research. *Safety Science, 34*(1–3), 215–257.

Guldenmund, F. W. (2007). The use of questionnaires in safety culture research – an evaluation. *Safety Science, 45*(6), 723–743.

Halligan, M., & Zecevic, A. (2011). Safety culture in healthcare: A review of concepts, dimensions, measures and progress. *BMJ Quality & Safety, 20*(4), 338–343.

Handler, S. M., Castle, N. G., Studenski, S. A., Perera, S., Fridsma, D. B., Nace, D. A., & Hanlon, J. T. (2006). Patient safety culture assessment in the nursing home. *BMJ Quality & Safety, 15*(6), 400–404.

Handler, S. M., Perera, S., Olshansky, E. F., Studenski, S. A., Nace, D. A., Fridsma, D. B., & Hanlon, J. T. (2007). Identifying modifiable barriers to medication error reporting in the nursing home setting. *Jounral of the American Medical Directors Association*, 8(9), 568–574.

Hartnell, N., MacKinnon, N., Sketris, I., & Fleming, M. (2012). Identifying, understanding and overcoming barriers to medication error reporting in hospitals: A focus group study. *BMJ Quality & Safety*, 21(5), 361–368.

Haugen, A., Softeland, E., Eide, G., Nortvedt, M., Aase, K., & Harthug, S. (2010). Patient safety in surgical environments: Cross-countries comparison of psychometric properties and results of the Norwegian version of the hospital survey on patient safety. *BMC Health Services Research*, 10, 279. http://www.biomedcentral.com/content/pdf/1472-6963-10-279.pdf (accessed June 20, 2015).

Haynes, A. B., Weiser, T. G., Berry, W. R., Lipsitz, S. R., Breizat, A., Dellinger, P., . . . , & Gawande, A. A. (2009). A surgical safety checklist to reduce morbidity and mortality in a global population. *New England Journal of Medicine*, 360, 491–499.

Hedskold, M., Pukk-Harenstam, K., Berg, E., Lindh, M., Soop, M., Ovretveit, J., & Sachs, M. A. (2013). Pscyhometric properties of the hospital survey on patient safety culture, HSOPSC, applied on a large Swedish health care sample. *BMC Health Services Research*, 13, 332.

Hofmann, D., & Mark, B. (2006). An investigation of the relationship between safety climate and medication errors as well as other nurse and patient outcomes. *Personnel Psychology*, 59, 847–869.

Huang, D. T., Clermont, G., Sexton, J. B., Karlo, C., Miller, R., Weissfeld, A., Rowan, K., & Angus, D. (2007). Perceptions of safety culture vary across intensive care units of a single institution. *Critical Care Medicine*, 35(1), 165–176.

Institute of Medicine (1999). *To err is human: Building a safety health system*. L. T. Kohn, J. M. Corrigan, & M. S. Donaldson (Eds.).Washington, DC: National Academy Press.

Institute of Medicine (2001). *Crossing the quality chasm: A new health system for the 21st century*. Washington, DC: National Academy Press.

Jackson, J., Sarac, C., & Flin, R. (2010). Hospital safety climate surveys: Measurement issues. *Current Opinion in Critical Care*, 16(6), 632–638.

Kalisch, B. J., & Aebersold, M. (2006). Overcoming barriers to patient safety. *Nursing Economics*, 24(3), 143–148.

Kaufman, G., & McCaughan, D. (2013). The effect of organisational culture on patient safety. *Nursing Standard*, 27(43), 50–56.

Kirk, S., Marshall, M., Claridge, T., Esmail, A., & Parker, D. (2006). Evaluating safety culture. In K. Walshe, & R. Boaden (Eds.), *Patient safety: Research into practice* (pp. 173–182). New York, NY: Open University Press.

Kizer, K. W. (1999). *Large system change and a culture of safety*. Chicago, IL: National Patient Safety Foundation.

Levy, S. M., Senter, C. E., Hawkins, R. B., Zhao, J. Y., Doody, K., Kao, L. S., . . . , & Tsao, K. (2012). Implementing a surgical checklist: More than checking a box. *Surgery*, 152(3), 331–336.

Luxhoj, J. T., & Kauffeld. (2003). Evaluating the effect of technology insertion into the National Airspace System. *Rutgers Scholar*, 5, np.

Manser, T., Foster, S., Flin, R., & Patey, R. (2013). Team communication during patient handover from the operating room: More than facts and figures. *Human Factors*, 55(1), 138–156.

Martin, G., Oziernanski, P., Willars, J., Charles, K., Minion, J., McKee, L., & Dixon-Woods, M. (2014). Walkrounds in practice: Corrupting or enhancing a quality improvement intervention? A qualitative study. *Joint Commission Journal on Quality & Patient Safety*, 40(7), 303–310.

McLaughlin, C. P., & Kaluzny, A. D. (2006). Defining quality improvement. In C. P. McLaughlin, & A. D. Kaluzny (Eds.), *Continuous quality improvement in health care* (3rd edn., pp. 3–64). Sudbury, MA: Jones and Bartlett Publishers.

Mearns, K., Kirwan, B., Reader, T., Jackson, J., Kennedy, G., & Gordon, R. (2013). Development of a methodology for understanding and enhancing safety culture in air traffic control. *Safety Science*, 53, 123–133.

Nadler, G., & Hibino, S. (1994). The systems principle: Seven-eighths of everything can't be seen. *Breakthrough thinking: The seven principles of creative problem solving* (pp. 197–229). Rocklin, CA: Prima Publishing.

Najjar, S., Hamdan, N., Baillien, E., Vluegels, A., Euwema, N., Sermeus, W., & Vanhaecht, K. (2013). The Arabic version of the hospital survey on patient safety culture: A psychometric evaluation in a Palestinian sample. *BMC Health Services Research, 13*, 193.

Naveh, E., Katz-Navon, T., & Stern, Z. (2005). Treatment errors in healthcare: A safety climate approach. *Management Science, 51*(6), 948–960.

Nieva, V. F., & Sorra, J. (2003). Safety culture assessment: A tool for improving patient safety in healthcare organizations. *Quality and Safety in Health Care, 12*(Suppl), ii17–ii23.

Nolan, T. W. (2000). System changes to improve patient safety. *British Medical Journal, 320*, 771–773.

Parker, D., Lawrie, M., Carthey, J., & Coultous, M. (2008). The Manchester patient safety framework: Sharing the learning. *Clinical Risk, 14*(4), 140–142.

Pfeiffer, Y., & Manser, T. (2010). Development of the German version of the hospital survey on patient safety culture: Dimensionality and psychometric properties. *Safety Science, 48*(10), 1452–1462.

Phipps, D., & Ashcroft, D. M. (2012). An investigation of occupational subgroups with respect to patient safety culture. *Safety Science, 50*(5), 1290–1298.

Raduma, M., Flin, R., Yule, S., & Close, S. (2012). The importance of preparation for doctors' handovers in an acute medical assessment unit: A hierarchical task analysis. *BMJ Quality & Safety, 21*(3), 211–217.

Reason, J. (1997). *Managing the risks of organizational accidents*. Burlington, VT: Ashgate.

Reason, J. (1998). Achieving a safety culture: Theory and practice. *Work Stress, 12*(3), 293–306.

Reason, J. (2000). Human error: Models and management. *British Medical Journal, 320*, 768–770.

Richter, A., & Koch, C. (2004). Integration, differentiation and ambiguity in safety cultures. *Safety Science, 42*(8), 703–722.

Rosen, A., Singer, S. J., Shibei, Z., Shokeen, P., Meterko, M., & Gaba, D. M. (2010). Hospital safety climate and safety outcomes: Is there a relationship in the VA? *Medical Care Research & Review, 67*(5), 590–608.

Sammer, C. E., Lykens, K., Singh, K. P., Mains, D. A., & Lacken, N. A. (2010). What is patient safety culture: A review of the literature. *Journal of Nursing Scholarship, 42*(2), 156–165.

Sarac, C., Flin, R., Mearns, K., & Jackson, J. (2010). Measuring hospital safety culture: Testing the HSOPSC scale. *Proceedings of the Human Factors and Ergonomics Society Annual Meeting, 54*(12), 850–854.

Schein, E. H. (1985). *Organizational culture and leadership* (1st edn.). San Francisco, CA: Jossey-Bass.

Schein, E. H. (1990). Organizational culture. *American Psychologist, 45*, 109–119.

Schein, E. H. (2004). *Organizational culture and leadership* (3rd edn.). San Francisco, CA: Jossey-Bass.

Schmele, J. A. (1993). Research and total quality. In A. F. Al-Assaf, & J. A. Schmele (Eds.), *The textbook of total quality in healthcare* (pp. 239–257). Delray, FL: St. Lucie Press.

Sexton, J. B., Helmrich, R. L., & Neilands, T. B. (2006). The safety attitudes questionnaire: Psychometric properties, benchmarking data, and emerging research. *BMC Health Services Research, 6*(44). doi:10.1186/1472-6963-6-44

Singer, S. J., Gaba, D. M., Falwell, A., Lin, S., Hayes, J. & Baker, L. (2009). Patient safety climate in 92 US hospitals: Differences by work area and discipline. *Medical Care, 47*(1), 23–31.

Singer, S. J., Gaba, D. M., & Geppert, J. J. (2003). The culture of safety: Results from an organization-wide survey in 15 California hospitals. *Quality and Safety in Health Care, 12*(2), 112–118.

Singer, S. J., Meterko, M., Baker, L., Gaba, D. M., Falwell, A., & Rosen, A. (2007). Workforce perceptions of hospital safety culture: Development and validation of the patient safety climate in healthcare organizations survey. *Health Services Research, 42*(5), 1999–2021.

Smith, D. R., Muto, T., Sairenchi, T., Ishikawa, Y., Sayama, S., & Yoshida, A. (2010). Hospital safety climate, psychosocial risk factors and needlestick injuries in Japan. *Industrial Health, 48*(1), 85–95.

Smits, M., Dinglehoff, I. C., Wagner, C., Wal, G., & Groenewegen, P. P. (2008). The psychometric properties of the "hospital survey on patient safety culture" in Dutch hospitals. *BMC Health Services Research, 8*, 230.

Sorra, J. S., and Battles, J. (2014). Lessons from the AHRQ survey on patient safety culture in Europe. In P. E. Waterson (Ed.), *Patient safety culture: Theory, methods, and application* (pp. 263–284). Aldershot, UK: Ashgate.

Sorra, J., & Dyer, N. (2010). Multilevel psychometric properties of the AHRQ hospital survey on patient safety culture. *BMC Health Services Research, 10,* 199.

Taylor, T., Dominini, F., Agnew, J., Gerin, D., Morlock, L., & Miller, M. (2012). Do nurse and patient injuries share common antecedents? An analysis of associations with safety climate and working conditions. *BMJ Quality & Safety, 21,* 101–111.

Turner, B. A. (1978). *Man-made disasters.* London, UK: Wykeham.

van Noord, I., de Bruijne, M., & Twisk, J. (2010). The relationship between patient safety culture and the implementation of organizational patient safety defences at emergency departments. *International Journal for Quality in Health Care, 22*(3), 162–169.

Verbeek-van Noord, I., de Bruijne, M., Zwijnenberg, N., Jansma, E., van Dyck, C., & Wagner, C. (2014). Does classroom-based crew resource management training improve patient safety culture: A systematic review. *Sage Open Medicine, 2.* http://smo.sagepub.com/content/2/2050312114529561. abstract (accessed June 20, 2015).

Vincent, C. A., Neale, G., & Woloshynowych, M. (2001). Adverse events in British hospitals: Preliminary retrospective record review. *British Medical Journal, 322*(7285), 517.

Vincent, C. A., Taylor-Adams, S., & Stanhope, N. (1998). Framework for analyzing risk and safety in clinical medicine. *British Medical Journal, 316*(1), 1154–1157.

Vlayen, A., Hellings, J., Claes, N., Peleman, H. & Schrooten, W. (2012). A nationwide hospital survey on patient safety culture in Belgian hospitals: Setting priorities at the launch of a 5-year patient safety plan. *BMJ Quality & Safety, 21*(9), 760–767.

Voluntary Hospitals of America (2000). Strategies for leadership: An organizational approach to patient safety. https://www.premierinc.com/safety/topics/patient_safety/downloads/31_AHA_VHA_patient_safety_assessment_tool.pdf (accessed June 7, 2015).

Wagner, C., Smits, M., Sorra, J. S., & Huang, C. C. (2013). Assessing patient safety culture in hospitals across countries. *International Journal for Quality in Health Care, 25*(3), 213–221.

Waring, J. J. (2005). Beyond blame: Cultural barriers to medical incident reporting. *Social Science & Medicine, 60*(9), 1927–1935.

Waterman, A. D., Gallagher, T. H., Garbutt, J., Waterman, B. M., Fraswer, V., & Burroughs, T. E. (2006). Hospitalized patients' attitudes about and participation in error prevention. *Journal of General Internal Medicine, 21*(4), 367–370.

Waterson, P. E. (Ed.). (2014). *Patient safety culture: Theory, methods and application.* Aldershot, UK: Ashgate.

Waterson, P. E., Griffiths, P., Stride, C., Murphy, J., & Hignett, S. (2010). Psychometric properties of the hospital survey on patient safety: Findings from the UK. *Quality and Safety in Health Care, 19*(5), e2.

Weick, K., & Sutcliffe, K. (2001). *Managing the unexpected: Assuring high performance in an age of complexity.* San Francisco, CA: Jossey-Bass.

West, P., Sculli, G., Fore, A., Okam, N., Dunlap, C., Neily, J., & Mills, P. (2012). Improving patient safety and optimizing nursing teamwork using crew resource management techniques. *Journal of Nursing Administration, 42*(1), 15–20.

Wilson, R. M., Runciman, W. B., Gibberd, R. W., Harrison, B. T., Newby, L., & Hamilton, J. D. (1995). The quality in Australian health care study. *Medical Journal of Australia, 163*(9), 458–476.

Yule, S., Flin, R., Paterson-Brown, S., & Maran, N. (2006). Non-technical skills for surgeons in the operating room: A review of literature. *Surgery, 139*(2), 140–149.

Zohar, D. (1980). Safety climate in industrial organizations: Theoretical and applied implications. *Journal of Applied Psychology, 65*(1), 96–102.

Zohar, D., Livne, Y., Tenne-Gazit, O., Admi, H., & Donchin, Y. (2007). Healthcare climate: A framework for measuring and improving patient safety. *Critical Care Medicine, 35*(5), 1312–1317.

Zohar, D., & Luria, G. A. (2005). A multilevel model of safety climate: Cross-level relationships between organization and group-level climates. *Journal of Applied Psychology, 90*(4), 616–628.

21

Managing Uncertainty in High-Risk Environments

Gudela Grote

Introduction

High-risk environments like medicine, aviation, or firefighting are characterized by particularly high amounts of uncertainty, which individuals, teams, and organizations are required to cope with, while at the same time being pressured by regulators and the public to demonstrate full control over all related work processes. This affords the need to concurrently foster stability and flexibility in organizational functioning. Processes involved in achieving this balance will be discussed by reviewing a wide range of literatures including organizational theory, organizational behavior, work psychology, social psychology, and human factors. After a short introduction into general literature on the management of uncertainty in organizations, the review will turn to research concerned with high-risk environments and will be organized by level of analysis, starting at the individual level and continuing on to the team and organizational levels.

At the individual level, different concepts capturing people's attitudes toward and ways of coping with uncertainty will be presented. Decision-making under uncertainty and related individual differences in attitudes and behavior will be discussed. The concept of the psychological contract will be introduced as one approach to handling uncertainties regarding safety-related expectations at the workplace. At the team level, research on leadership and coordination will be reviewed. Relevant concepts comprise shared and inclusive leadership, adaptive coordination, psychological safety, and propensity to speak up. At the organizational level, decisions on the appropriate mix between stability- and flexibility-enhancing mechanisms have to be taken. This also involves consideration of interactions between organizational-, team-, and individual-level processes, which will be outlined with respect to rules and standardization, substitutes for leadership and safety culture. From the review of these multifaceted literatures a detailed picture of the intricacies involved in managing uncertainty at the individual, team, and organizational level emerges, while also opening up important avenues for future research.

The Wiley Blackwell Handbook of the Psychology of Occupational Safety and Workplace Health, First Edition. Edited by Sharon Clarke, Tahira M. Probst, Frank Guldenmund, and Jonathan Passmore. © 2016 John Wiley & Sons Ltd. Published 2020 by John Wiley & Sons Ltd.

A Historic Account of Uncertainty as a Core Variable in Organization Research

Ever since the shift from viewing organizations as closed systems to acknowledging their nature as open systems that co-exist with and depend on their environment, especially environmental uncertainties, have been a core concern in organization research: "Uncertainty appears as the fundamental problem for complex organizations, and coping with uncertainty as the essence of the administrative process" (Thompson, 1967, p. 159). There is a multitude of definitions of uncertainty (cf. Grote, 2009), but Galbraith's definition is probably the one most widely used in organization research: Uncertainty is the absence of information and more specifically, "the difference between the amount of information required to perform a task and the amount of information already possessed by the organization" (Galbraith, 1973, p. 5).

From the perspective of a decision-making framework, uncertainty can arise due to incomplete information, inadequate understanding of available information, and undifferentiated alternatives, that is, alternatives that are equally attractive or unattractive (Lipshitz & Strauss, 1997). Uncertainty may concern the probability of an event (state uncertainty), a lack of information about the outcomes of an event and the underlying cause–effect relationships (effect uncertainty), or a lack of information about response options and their likely consequences (response uncertainty) (Milliken, 1987). In Milliken's original work, the three contents of uncertainty were described in terms of environmental uncertainty; so for instance, effect uncertainty is understood only as uncertainty about impacts of environmental events on the organization. But the distinction can also be used more broadly to define the different contents of what the decision-maker is uncertain about, that is, any state, any effect, or any response in the organization or in the environment (Grote, 2009). While incomplete information is a factor that can be determined objectively, both undifferentiated alternatives and inadequate understanding are sources of uncertainty that imply an interaction between characteristics of the decision to be taken, the environment in which the decision is embedded, and the decision-maker him- or herself (Sitkin & Pablo, 1992). Because of these differences, sometimes only incomplete information is defined as uncertainty, whereas the other two elements are subsumed under a separate category ambiguity, referring to the multiplicity of meanings that can be imposed on a situation (Daft & Lengel, 1984; Leifer & Mills, 1996; Weick, 1979).

In the literature on managing uncertainties in organizations, two longstanding debates concern (a) the significance of objective versus subjective accounts of uncertainty and (b) whether organizations and the decision-makers within them merely react and adapt to environmental uncertainties or actively shape their environments as well (cf. Grote, 2009). Regarding the first debate, the focus on decision-makers in organizations and their having to face uncertainties has fueled arguments against objective accounts of uncertainty, in favor of perceptions of uncertainty by the actors themselves as adequate measures (Jauch & Kraft, 1986). Contributing factors for inadequate understanding, such as ambiguous information, need to be identified with reference to the actors affected. Many landmark studies on contingencies between uncertainty and organization design therefore only used perceptual measures of uncertainty (e.g., Lawrence & Lorsch, 1967).

The second debate delves into basic beliefs by researchers and practitioners alike about the relationship between organizations and their environment (Jauch & Kraft, 1986). One of Pfeffer and Salancik's (1978) main intentions in developing resource dependence theory was to show both organizations' links with their environments and how they can actively shape these links. In doing so, organizations do not react to or act upon given realities, but they enact their environments through processes of selective attention and interpretation. Or as Weick (1979, p. 130) puts it: "Enactment is the only process where the organism directly engages an external environment. All processes subsequent to enactment work on edited raw materials. . ." Enacting situations is part of sense-making (Weick, 1995) that is, literally making sense out of things happening through placing them in a particular framework and deriving their meaning from that. Environments are socially constructed on the basis of actors' subjective theories and preconceptions that are used to make sense of any ambiguous information. Any meaning that is derived from this sense-making process subsequently shapes actors' behavior. It is through the cyclical sense-making and enactment processes that actors can either improve their own conditions or, in contrast, can become the authors of their own problems (Weick, 1979). Self-fulfilling prophecies are an extreme case of sense-making, because starting from specific assumptions about the world, people act in ways that will make these assumptions come true. "People create and find what they expect to find" (Weick, 1995, p. 35). Sense-making is particularly powerful under conditions of high uncertainty when incomplete or ambiguous information requires assumption-based reasoning and interpretation in order to develop a basis for action (Lipshitz & Strauss, 1997).

In organizations, gaining and maintaining control is an important overarching aim of managing uncertainty (Pfeffer & Salancik, 1978). Control is usually described as exercising influence or power in order to reach certain goals, often also with the implication of influence or power over other people. In order for influence to be exerted effectively, there has to be sufficient predictability and understanding or transparency of the situation (Brehmer, 1992; Sutton & Kahn, 1987), that is: little uncertainty. Turning this argument around, uncertainty reduces effective control because it reduces transparency and predictability. Additionally, there may even be uncertainty as to which means of influence there are and what effects they have on what outcomes, which is implied in the notion of response uncertainty introduced earlier. While lack of transparency and predictability can be fully described in terms of uncertainty, lack of influence is predominantly determined by other factors, such as the distribution of power within and across organizations and the competence level of the actors.

How control is achieved differs in terms of both objective and subjective perspectives on uncertainty. Barley and Kunda (1992) argued that just how uncertainties are understood and which form of uncertainty management is chosen depends on the prominence of normative versus rational ideologies; that is, ideologies that build on normative control such as culture, versus ideologies that build on rational control, such as Taylor's scientific management. "The fact that we expect all organizations to seek the same state – self-control – does not mean that we expect all of them to attain it in the same way, with identical design, structures, or behavior. It is essential that we find universals, but equally essential to find patterns in variations" (Thompson, 1967, p. 161). Such different approaches will be discussed in the next section.

Different Approaches to Managing Uncertainty

In organization theory and strategic management, frameworks for contingent use of different strategies for managing uncertainty have been developed (cf. Grote, 2009). "Uncertainty about the firm's future is the core of strategy; it is the essential reason to engage in strategic planning (...) A first step toward making planning truly strategic will occur if top management calls for, and participates in, a no-nonsense consideration of uncertainty" (Allaire & Firsirotu, 1989, p. 16).

One prominent distinction is that between minimizing uncertainties versus coping with uncertainties (Grote, 2009). Which approach to choose is assumed to be related to the amount of uncertainty with which the organization is faced: minimizing uncertainty only works well with generally low levels of uncertainty (e.g., Burns & Stalker, 1961; Thompson 1967; Van de Ven, Delbecq, & Koenig, 1976; for a comprehensive review see Wall, Cordery, & Clegg, 2002, and Grote, 2009). Scientific treatment of organization design at the turn of the twentieth century (Taylor, 1911; Weber, 1947) was built on the assumption that organizations are closed systems, thereby protected from external uncertainties. Internal uncertainties were to be minimized by minute planning and continuous monitoring of the execution of these plans, providing minimal degrees of freedom to the people in charge of carrying out the plans and taking any deviation from the plans as signs for the necessity of even more planning and monitoring. A fundamentally different approach that has been promoted by organization theorists and work scientists for several decades now is to enable all members of an organization to cope with uncertainties locally (e.g., Cherns, 1987; Perrow, 1967; Weick, Sutcliffe & Obstfeld, 1999). From this perspective, planning is understood primarily as a resource for situated action (Suchman, 1987) and local actors need to be given sufficient degrees of freedom in order to control variances and disturbances at their source and to learn from failure. There are also a number of newer studies which have been carried out within a contingency framework, for example, concerning manufacturing flexibility (Anand & Ward, 2004; Ketokivi, 2006), project management (Faraj & Sambamurthy, 2006; Levitt et al., 1999; Shenhar, 2001), and organizational governance and control (Folta, 1998; Hendry & Kiel, 2004; Santoro & McGill, 2005). Usually, more uncertainty has been found to be associated with more internal flexibility and less hierarchical forms of leadership and control, as would be predicted by the basic contingency model (Van de Ven et al., 1976).

However, recently the main concern in management thinking has been to overcome dichotomies and to search for a middle ground between the extremes of either avoiding or embracing uncertainty as the sole strategy. Thus, the question becomes which uncertainties to avoid and which to embrace. Over the last century, with increasingly fast and global competition, an ever more clear understanding has developed that organizations are continuously faced with uncertainties from within and from without, which can only partially be reduced. How to live with uncertainties or even take advantage of them without losing the stability created by reducing uncertainty, has become an important issue not only in research on organizations but also in practical management guidelines (e.g., Brown & Eisenhardt, 1997; O'Reilly & Tushman, 2004). The fundamental objective is to balance stability and flexibility in accordance with internal and external demands, which requires addressing and managing strategic contradictions such as short-term performance and long-term adaptability or differentiation and integration (Smith & Tushman, 2005). Recent research into extremely innovative companies has provided interesting examples of how this balance can be achieved (e.g., Benner & Tushman, 2003; Brown & Eisenhardt, 1997). Concepts such as loose coupling (Weick, 1976), enabling bureaucracy (Adler & Borys, 1996), ambidexterity (Tushman & O'Reilly, 1996), or semistructures (Brown & Eisenhardt, 1997) all refer to organizations' capability to be stable and flexible simultaneously, for example, by coordinating activities through norms, values, and shared expertise rather than through standardization, by building parallel organizational units for stability and flexibility, or by defining routine procedures for probing new ideas. These concepts point to ways for fulfilling requirements of concurrent stability and flexibility that neither minimizing nor coping with uncertainty can accomplish alone.

Uncertainty in High-Risk Environments

Uncertainty is at the heart of risk. Only very recently, though has uncertainty regained a significant place in debates on risk. In an early economic definition by Knight (1921), risk was distinguished from uncertainty by postulating that risk is measurable, while uncertainty is not. Subsequently, risk has dominated the debate, usually based on definitions where uncertainty is quantified into probabilities, which presumably renders a separate discussion of uncertainty obsolete. By virtue of renewed concerns with improving our grasp of very rare events, as illustrated by the popularity of Taleb's (2007) book "The Black Swan," uncertainty has re-entered academic and practical discourse in risk management (e.g., Aven & Renn, 2009; Paté-Cornell, 2012; Power, 2004, 2007). Even for high-risk industries, it is now acknowledged that organizations need both the stability created by minimizing uncertainty and the flexibility achieved by coping with uncertainty. The concepts of high-reliability organization (e.g., Weick et al., 1999) and of resilience engineering (e.g., Hollnagel, Woods, & Leveson, 2006) are prominent examples of this change in thinking.

Grote (2015) has argued that for effective management of risk it is important to go a step further still by not only acknowledging existing uncertainties, but accepting also that in certain circumstances deliberate increases in uncertainty are conducive to safety. To illustrate her argument, she points to examples such as speaking up in critical situations, where a course of action is questioned and new alternatives introduced to recalibrate decision-making, or the use of flexible rules that put certain constraints on actors, while also leaving room for deliberate exploration of options for action. Management of uncertainty in high-risk environments thus requires one to establish a balance between stability and flexibility through systematically considering reducing, maintaining *and* increasing uncertainty as options. These three options are founded on fundamentally different conceptions of risk control, though. *Reducing uncertainty* to a level of acceptable risk is the main thrust in classic risk mitigation. The overall objective is to create stable systems that allow for a maximum of central control. Measures such as standardization and automation help to streamline work processes. *Maintaining uncertainty* follows from acknowledging the limits to reducing uncertainty in complex systems, which forms the basis for the concepts of high reliability organizations and resilience engineering just mentioned. Flexibility as a source for resilience, that is the capability of systems to recover from perturbations, is sought. For this purpose, control capacity needs to be decentralized, for example, by means of empowering local actors. *Increasing uncertainty*, finally, aims also at flexibility, but not only in response to perturbations, but also in support of innovation. An important conceptual basis is complexity theory (cf. for example, Anderson, 1999) and self-organization as one of the theory's fundamental principles. Self-organizing local agents cannot be directly controlled, but only indirectly influenced in their adaptive behavior by shaping contexts, for instance through setting incentives and constraints for experimentation.

Carroll (1998), referring to Schein (1996), has pointed out that the different conceptions tend to be prevalent in different professional (sub)cultures in organizations. While engineers and executives believe in uncertainty reduction through design and planning, operative personnel are very aware of the need for resilience in the face of only partially controllable uncertainties. Social scientists finally will also argue for openness to learning and innovation, thereby even adding uncertainty. As a consequence, building a shared understanding of the legitimacy of all three options of reducing, maintaining and increasing uncertainty across professional boundaries is paramount to developing a more comprehensive approach to managing uncertainty in high-risk environments.

In the following, literature at the individual, team, and organizational level will be reviewed in order to provide pertinent examples of research on managing uncertainty in high-risk environments and to suggest avenues for future research.

An important caveat relates to the nature of risks considered in the review. It has been argued that process risks (or process safety) should be distinguished from personal risks (or personal safety, often also called occupational safety) (Grote, 2012; Hopkins, 2009). Personal safety concerns any potential harm to workers inflicted in the context of executing their work. This harm may stem from the primary work task, for example, the danger for a nurse to get ill her- or himself while taking care of patients, or it may be part of the larger work environment, such as having to work at great heights or in a very noisy location. Common occupational injuries, such as sprains, fractures, cuts, and bruises may even result from activities not directly related to work at all like walking down stairs. Protection against these hazards is mostly a secondary task, sometimes even interfering with the primary task, as, for instance, in the case of hearing protection preventing detection of task-relevant signals such as unusual machine noises or preventing proper communication with coworkers (Reddy, Welch, Ameratunga, & Thorne, 2014). In process safety, the risks and uncertainties to be managed are directly linked to the primary work task of the organization, such as curing patients, producing energy or transporting goods and people. Breaches of process safety do not necessarily cause harm to the workers involved, as in the case of the death of a patient due to false medication (see Bishop, Fleming & Flin, Chapter 20, this volume). Personal and process safety may or may not be closely related depending on the primary work task. Pilots put their own just as much as passengers' lives at risk when operating an aircraft. In building construction, structural safety as the core requirement of the work process and personal safety are quite unrelated, except when structures fail during construction. Furthermore, causal mechanisms involved in promoting personal versus process safety most likely differ due to differences in the visibility and complexity of risks, required competence for risk handling, available incentives for safe behavior, and conflicts between safety and production requirements (Anderson, 2005; Hale & Heijer, 2006). However, to date there is little conceptual and empirical knowledge on how measures aimed at process safety or personal safety achieve their effects and how they interact. This constitutes a significant need for future research.

In the following discussion I will concentrate on process safety for which the management of uncertainty is considered more relevant due to the high levels of uncertainty inherent in process-related risks. However, yet again it would be worthwhile to empirically study the assumption that process safety generally makes higher demands on managing uncertainty.

Managing uncertainty at the individual level

Regarding the question of how uncertainties are managed by individuals, decision-making under uncertainty is probably the most frequently discussed issue. Besides a general understanding of how uncertainty is dealt with in decision-making, consideration of individual differences is important, especially with respect to differences in risk propensity. Finally, the psychological contract will be introduced as a way for individuals to handle uncertainties regarding safety-related expectations at the workplace.

Decision-making under uncertainty   The most pervasive prescriptive conception of decision-making is the maximization of subjective expected utility, which postulates that the alternative with the highest expected payoff gets chosen. In order to use this model, knowledge of probabilities and utilities is needed and certain prerequisites have to be fulfilled like absence of apriori preference for (un)certainty or framing effects, that is preferences being influenced by how choices are presented, for example, in terms of gains or losses. Research has provided convincing evidence that these requirements are often not met, which substantially reduces the viability of the model (Mellers, Schwartz & Cooke, 1998; Shafir & LeBoeuf, 2002). For instance, certainty is often preferred in decisions on gains, but uncertainty is preferred when losses are to be decided upon (Kahneman & Tversky, 1979).

Another frequently used formal conception of decision-making is the maximization of multi-attribute utility based on the knowledge of all relevant alternatives and all dimensions and their relative weights for distinguishing among the alternatives. Simon (1955) pointed out half a century ago that people's cognitive capacities are limited, which he termed bounded rationality, leading them to accept "satisficing" choices, for instance based on an alternative's acceptable level on one crucial dimension. In recent years, especially Gigerenzer has advocated the view that the use of simple decision heuristics is often fully adequate even if abundant cognitive resources are available. He postulates that expert intuition is about knowing which information is important and ignoring the rest, that is only using those cues which have the highest discriminatory power (Gigerenzer, 2007; Gigerenzer & Goldstein, 1996).

The debate whether deviations from the formal prescriptive decision models make human decision-making irrational or whether the formal models are built on a rather restricted and possibly even irrelevant understanding of rationality is still on-going (Weber & Johnson, 2009). Recent research has stressed adaptive functioning as the ultimate criterion for good decision-making instead of some normative one best way (Kahneman & Klein, 2009; Kerr & Tindale, 2004). This view has been advocated in particular by researchers following the so-called naturalistic decision-making approach, which focuses on studying real-life decision-making by professional groups instead of conducting laboratory experiments (Klein, 2008). Most recently, the apparent contradictions between heuristics-based intuitive decision-making and formal rational decision-making have been built into dual-process models (Evans, 2008; Kahnemann, 2011). These models assume the parallel and situation-dependent operation of both types of decision-making, sometimes called System 1 and System 2. While System 1 refers to intuition and is characterized by implicit, automatic, low effort, holistic, fast, and emotional processes, System 2 entails reasoning with explicit, controlled, high effort, analytic, slow, and cognitive processes.

However, as Grote (2015) outlines, many fundamental questions remain: Is one of the models to be preferred as the better way of making decisions? Is switching between the two modes of functioning necessary in certain conditions? What would be conditions for such switches and how could decision-makers be helped in making them? With respect to the first question whether one model should generally be considered superior to the other, the debate about studies involving a short scenario describing a woman called "Linda" is instrumental. In an experimental setup participants are asked to first read a short text about Linda, describing her as having leftist political attitudes, and then to indicate whether they consider it more probable for her to be a bank teller or a bank teller and a feminist. The answer usually is the latter which implies – in mathematical terms completely irrational – the decision that two events combined are more likely than one of them alone. Kahneman (2011) argues that this finding reflects the workings of System 1, while still maintaining that this is by any account faulty decision-making because it defies mathematical logic. Gigerenzer (2007) on the other hand, postulates that under the given circumstances it is perfectly rational to decide for the formally less likely option because based on the additional information provided in the description of Linda the less likely option is the more plausible one.

An example closer to the current topic of managing uncertainty in high-risk environments concerns differences between experts' and lay people's risk perception. The general finding is that laypeople in essence follow System 1 decision-making while risk experts follow System 2. After many decades where the System 2 expert view was taken as the more rational and therefore more substantial perspective, it seems that gradually consensus is building to accept both views as legitimate, resulting in the need to integrate them through broad public dialogue (Renn, 2008).

Individuals in high-risk environments are frequently confronted with having to make decisions with high degrees of uncertainty implied and much of the research on naturalistic decision-making has in fact been undertaken in such environments. However, a systematic exploration of System 1 and System 2 thinking and of what might constitute appropriate switches between the two is still missing. This would be a worthy endeavour in order to advance our understanding of the underpinnings of managing uncertainty in decision-making, where reducing uncertainty through reasoning is not always the best approach, but has to be complemented with expertise-based intuition that acknowledges uncertainty as inevitable or possibly even positive for the decision process.

Individual differences related to uncertainty management There are a number of approaches to studying differences in the way individuals handle uncertainty in decision-making and in other tasks. Sorrentino, Short, and Raynor (1984) differentiate between persons that are uncertainty-orientated and motivated by situations that involve exploratory behaviors and persons that are certainty-orientated and prefer familiar situations. Building on this research Lind and Van den Bos proposed a theory of uncertainty management (Lind & Van den Bos, 2002) which links individuals' need for uncertainty reduction to fairness judgments. In particular, they argued and provided empirical evidence for the importance of fairness in situations that cannot be directly controlled by the individual. Subjective uncertainty is reduced when people perceive decision-makers as fair and therefore trust in good outcomes for themselves without having immediate influence on those outcomes. One recent study by Pierro, Giacomantonio, Kruglanski, and van Kippenberg (2014) which was conducted within this framework, provided evidence of the relevance of leaders' procedural fairness especially for those individuals who have a high need for cognitive closure, which is a construct related to individuals' desire to reduce uncertainty suggested by Kruglanski and Webster (1996). Interestingly, there seems to be little research in high-risk environments that has taken on these individual-level variables related to different preferences for reducing, maintaining, or increasing uncertainty. One exception is the work by Brashers who has investigated uncertainty management with respect to health-related risk communication (Brashers, 2001; Brashers & Hogan, 2013). He argues for the importance of not only focusing on uncertainty reduction, but on helping people live with uncertainties and benefit from optimism and hope that can be associated with uncertainty, for instance when coping with chronic illness.

While earlier research was built on the assumption that there are stable differences between people regarding their motivation to seek or avoid risk (e.g., MacCrimmon & Wehrung, 1990; Zuckerman & Kuhlman, 2000), recent studies have provided converging evidence on an interactionist view that considers individual differences in behavior as a function of person and situational factors. In a recent review of individual differences in risk taking, Figner and Weber (2011) for instance, summarize the evidence for gender differences in risk propensity that also indicates domain-specific effects such that women take more risks in the social domain while men take more risks in financial, recreational and ethical decisions. Additionally, they argue that these differences are more related to differences in risk perception based on different familiarity with these domains than on differences in basic risk attitudes. Similarly, Nicholson, Soane, Fenton-O'Creevy, and Willman (2005) show that on the one hand risk propensity is linked to personality factors – more open and extravert persons take more risks – but that yet again there are situational influences also which they use to suggest several types of risk propensity. While health and safety risks feature in the various measures used to study individual differences in risk propensity they mostly concern the private domain, such as driving fast or smoking.

Psychological contract on safety A very different approach to uncertainty management at the individual level concerns uncertainties in the employment relationship, which have been much discussed in recent decades due to economic developments related to globalization. Rousseau (1989) proposed the concept of psychological contract – mutual perceptions and beliefs about informal obligations between employees and their employer – as a way to manage employment uncertainties, for example, by shifting attention away from job security to ensuring employability. There is some research that indicates that increasing uncertainty embedded in employment relationships can also impact safety-related behavior (e.g., Hopkins, 2000; Rousseau & Libuser, 1997). This raises the question whether safety itself can be part of psychological contracts. This idea has recently been taken up by Walker (Walker & Hutton, 2006; Walker, 2013) to capture mis(matches) between safety-related expectations and offers. She developed a questionnaire to measure the "psychological contract of safety," which includes a set of items related to employee obligations (e.g., follow safety rules), and employer obligations (e.g., listen to employee safety concerns). Responses to this questionnaire were shown to be linked to safety climate and self-reported safety behavior. However, one can argue that this questionnaire actually does not capture the social exchange relationship which is core to psychological contracts, but rather is another way to ask about adequate provision of safety management measures by an employer and the use of these provisions by employees, which at best concerns the simple exchange of, for instance, being provided with personal protection equipment and actually wearing it.

An extension of this original attempt to measure safety-related psychological contracts could prove interesting, though. Especially with respect to personal safety, the rather counter-intuitive behavior of employees that expose themselves to hazards despite the organization's expressed interest in and provisions for preventing harm for their employees, may have its origin in unresolved conflicts in the employment relationship.

Managing uncertainty at the team level

The team literature is vast and well-documented by increasingly specialized reviews (e.g., Crawford & LePine, 2013; Humphrey & Aime, 2014; Mathieu, Tannenbaum, Donsbach, & Alliger, 2014). The following discussion focuses on literature that helps to better understand leadership and coordination in teams aimed at balancing stability and flexibility of work processes in response to internal and external uncertainties. Concepts reviewed comprise shared leadership, adaptive coordination concerning, for instance, switches between implicit and explicit coordination, and two important prerequisites for effective team work: psychological safety and the propensity to speak up.

Team leadership In meta-analyses and reviews of research on team leadership (e.g., Burke, Stagl, Klein et al., 2006; Day, Gronn, & Salas, 2004; Friedrich, Vessey, Schuelke, Ruark, & Mumford, 2009), leadership is defined very broadly as exerting influence on others in order to determine and achieve objectives (Yukl, 2006). Furthermore, leadership is understood in functional terms, that is, a leader is called upon to adaptively fulfill those functions in a team that are needed for task accomplishment and are not taken up by other team members (Zaccaro, Rittman, & Marks, 2001). Thereby, the process of leadership is emphasized rather than the formal leadership role. This view is extended by the concept of shared leadership, which argues that leadership functions can be fulfilled not only by the formal leader but by any team member based on situational requirements and individual competencies (Carson, Tesluk, & Marrone, 2007; Friedrich et al., 2009; Pearce & Conger, 2003). Shared leadership is also part of what Weick and Sutcliffe (2001) have termed deference to expertise, which they identified as an important component of organizing for high reliability.

Along with this general emphasis on adaptability of leadership behavior, in much of the recent literature the necessity for leaders to support flexible team processes is stressed. Kozlowski, Watola, Jensen, Kim, and Botero (2009), for instance, look at changing demands on leadership as teams move through the various stages of team development. Similarly, Morgeson, DeRue, and Karam (2010) distinguish leadership functions that are relevant during action phases versus transition phases in teams. Looking at leadership in different kinds of high-risk teams especially, both Klein, Ziegert, Knight, and Xiao (2006) and Bigley and Roberts (2001) provide excellent accounts of how leaders navigate their teams through rapidly changing circumstances, delegating leadership tasks and taking them back as their overall responsibility demands. Theirs are also examples of the much rarer studies that explicitly mention both flexibility- and stability-related functions of leadership: stability is seen to be established by leadership at the organizational level through standards, routines, or role definitions which reduce uncertainty, while team leaders' main contribution is to enhance flexibility within these stable structures and help teams cope with or even increase uncertainty as the situation requires.

Two issues that should be addressed in future research concern more attention to the requirements of particular tasks with which teams are charged (Burke, Stagl, Klein et al., 2006) and the distribution of responsibility between formal leaders and team members (Denis, Langley, & Sergi, 2012). One can assume that depending on the demands on flexibility and stability inherent in certain tasks, different mixes of shared leadership and leadership by the formal leader are required. Also, the higher the risks that have to be managed by the team, the more important questions of responsibility become, possibly favoring leadership modes where responsibility is clearly assigned to the formal leader, thereby reducing uncertainty for the team.

Furthermore, there is an increasing awareness that often it is not single teams that operate in high-risk environments, but rather multi-team systems, where leadership within and between teams needs to be distinguished (Zaccaro & DeChurch, 2011). Bienefeld and Grote (2012), for instance, found in aircrews that during a simulated emergency landing pursers' leadership role as boundary spanner between cockpit crew and cabin crew became crucial for mission success, coupled with increased shared leadership in the cabin. Similarly, Davison, Hollenbeck, Barnes, Sleesman, and Ilgen (2012) reported on research where formally assigned boundary-spanning activities were more successful than decentralized boundary-spanning in a simulated military task. Lanaj, Hollenbeck, Ilgen, Barnes, and Harmon (2013) argued more generally that decentralized decision-making may be less successful in multi-team systems compared with single systems. Again, much more research is needed to explore different leadership mechanisms for the more complex settings of multi-team systems and the particular demands on stability and flexibility they create.

Team coordination When turning to the coordination literature, one finds balancing between stability and flexibility being stressed particularly in relation to the requirement for adaptive coordination, for instance by switching between different coordination mechanisms in response to changing situational and task demands (Burke, Stagl, & Salas, 2006; Rico, Sánchez, Manzanares, Gil, & Gibson, 2008). Two coordination mechanisms that have received much attention in this respect are explicit versus implicit coordination (e.g., Entin & Serfaty, 1999; Espinosa, Lerch, & Kraut, 2004; Rico et al., 2008). Explicit coordination is the deliberate and resource-intensive establishment of common ground and subsequent decision-making based on the information acquired and evaluated in the team, which entails coping with or even increasing uncertainty for the team. Implicit co-ordination, on the other hand, relies on reduced uncertainty through shared assumptions and knowledge about the team, the task and the context, enabling team members to coordinate their action in an effortless manner with little demands on information acquisition and assessment (e.g., Wittenbaum, Stasser, & Merry, 1996). As implicit coordination is less resource-intensive it is considered most suited for very demanding tasks. However, if these tasks entail unexpected elements, explicit coordination may become necessary, indicating a delicate balance between stability and flexibility (Faraj & Xiao, 2006; Waller, Gupta, & Giambatista, 2004; Xiao et al., 1996). Heedful interrelating (Weick & Roberts, 1993) has been found to be effective in bridging these conflicting demands (Grote, Kolbe, Zala-Mezö, Bienefeld-Seall, & Künzle, 2010).

From a coordination perspective, the previously discussed dynamic delegation of leadership (Bigley & Roberts, 2001; Klein et al., 2006) can be regarded as switching between unilateral leadership and mutual adjustment among all team members, which in organization theory are understood to be different types of personal coordination (Van de Ven et al., 1976). Still building on organization theory, one can also consider switching between personal coordination (leadership, mutual adjustment) and impersonal coordination (standardization, technology), where as outlined earlier impersonal coordination mechanisms are less suited for handling uncertainty than personal coordination (Van de Ven et al., 1976). The relevance of the interplay between personal and impersonal co-ordination has long been recognized in the substitutes for leadership theory (Kerr & Jermier, 1978), stating that under certain conditions leadership can be replaced, for instance, by standardization. A complementary perspective is expressed in the definition of leadership as the influential increment over and above mechanical compliance (Katz & Kahn, 1978). However, the creation of substitutes should itself be considered as an act of leadership, though possibly at a higher level in the organization (Dionne, Yammarino, Howell, & Villa, 2005), which will be taken up again in the next section. Substitutes may be stability-enhancing, such as standardization and routinization, but they may also be flexibility-enhancing, such as individual and team empowerment. Systematic research on these presumed effects of substitutes and the interaction between different substitutes is largely lacking. Furthermore, substitution may affect different leadership functions differently (Dionne, Yammarino, Atwater, & James, 2002). For instance, higher levels of team member competence may require less effort by the formal leader for assuring information use in problem solving, but he or she is still needed to support information search and structuring. This very behavior pattern was found in well-performing anaesthesia teams consisting of more experienced nurses and less experienced, but formally responsible residents (i.e., physicians training at a hospital to become a specialist in a particular field of medicine) (Künzle, Zala-Mezö, Kolbe, Wacker, & Grote, 2010; Künzle, Zala-Mezö, Wacker et al., 2010).

Another example of the interplay between personal and impersonal coordination concerns implicit coordination. Organizational rules as a form of impersonal coordination ease the demands on personal coordination by reducing uncertainty. They help build a shared understanding of the task which enables implicit coordination (March, Schulz, & Zhou, 2000). This conceptual reasoning has formed the basis for several studies of adaptive coordination: for both medical teams and cockpit crews, it was found that there was indeed more implicit coordination in work phases with higher standardization (Grote et al., 2010; Zala-Mezö, Wacker, Künzle, Brüesch, & Grote, 2009).

Prerequisites for effective team leadership and coordination in high-risk teams From the perspective of managing uncertainty in teams, two concepts are particularly relevant as prerequisites for effective team processes: speaking up and psychological safety. Speaking up has been defined as "discretionary communication of ideas, suggestions, concerns, or opinions about work-related issues with the intent to improve organizational or unit functioning" (Morrison, 2011, p. 375). By questioning ongoing work or bringing in new options for decision-making, speaking up increases uncertainty. The uncertainty resulting from speaking up will be beneficial in as much as individuals and teams have sufficient cognitive resources for shifting into a mode of divergent thinking during their ongoing activity, but are also capable of converting back to convergent thinking in order to adapt their course of action in a timely manner (Grote, 2015).

In the past decade, a growing body of research has investigated individual, situational, or organizational conditions that can foster or undermine people's willingness to speak up, whereby status and leadership have been identified as the most prominent predictors of speaking up (Morrison, 2011). There are a number of studies that have addressed speaking up specifically in high-risk environments, indicating that speaking up is related to better team performance (e.g., Edmondson, 2003; Kolbe et al., 2012; Nembhard & Edmondson, 2006). Furthermore, Kolbe et al. (2012) showed that speaking up is an important mechanism to help teams switch from a more implicit mode of coordination to explicit coordination by initiating clarification of plans or changes in the procedures followed. Also, reasons for not speaking up have been studied. For instance, Bienefeld and Grote (2012) found that the most common reason for cockpit crew members' silence was their desire to maintain good team relationships. An important reason for silence indicated by cabin crew members, on the other hand, was fear of punishment. Finally, feelings of futility, that is, the belief that speaking up will not make a difference, was mentioned frequently by the lower status aircrew members, first officers, and flight attendants, respectively. These reasons conform to the two broader categories mentioned by Morrison (2014), efficacy and psychological safety.

The sense of feeling (un)safe as a crucial factor for the willingness to speak up is core to the concept of psychological safety, which denotes the cognitive and emotional state that it is safe to voice concerns or admit mistakes (Edmondson, 1999). Psychological safety has been found to be an important mediating factor between status, leadership, and speaking up in high-risk teams and in teams more generally (Bienefeld & Grote, 2014; Detert & Burris, 2007; Edmondson, 1999, 2003; Nembhard & Edmondson, 2006). Leaders are the target of upward voice and through their behavior they can strongly influence team members' willingness to speak up (Ashford, Sutcliffe, & Christianson, 2009; Detert & Burris, 2007; Edmondson, 1999, 2003; Morrison & Rothman, 2009). Leaders can create feelings of psychological safety if they signal that they can be trusted and that they will not punish team members for admitting unintentional mistakes or for voicing their concerns. Nembhard and Edmondson (2006) named this type of leader behavior "leader inclusiveness," a construct related to participative leadership (e.g., Yukl, 2006) and team leader coaching (Edmondson, 2003), but different in that it more specifically describes leader behavior that breaks down status barriers to enable open communication.

The interaction between speaking up and psychological safety is interesting as an example for the interplay between stability- and flexibility-enhancing mechanisms. The duality of reducing and increasing uncertainty is in fact embedded in psychological safety itself:

lower uncertainty regarding individuals' personal standing and support in their teams leads to possibly higher uncertainty in work processes, as people question established routines more frequently (Bienefeld & Grote, 2012; Morrison, 2011). To date, research has not systematically addressed this dual nature of psychological safety (Edmondson & Lei, 2014), which points to an interesting avenue for future research.

Managing uncertainty at the organizational level

At the organizational level, contingencies for stability and flexibility requirements, as discussed in organizational theory and strategy management, are relevant for the management of uncertainty. Importantly, stability and flexibility should not be treated as two ends of one dimension, but rather as two analytically distinct dimensions, derived from the need to simultaneously cater for stability and flexibility in some situations.

The mechanisms operating on the individual and team level described above can be systematically used in organizations to achieve the appropriate balance between stability and flexibility. One can assume that stability- and flexibility-enhancing effects differ for (a) different leadership and coordination mechanisms; (b) different variants of one mechanism; or (c) even different elements of the same mechanism (Grote, Kolbe, & Waller, 2012). An example for (a) is the combination of few structural mechanisms and formal leadership, where the uncertainty resulting from few rules is reduced and control is established by the team leader's decisions. An example for (b) is different kinds of rules; rules may specify required actions in great detail, thereby nurturing behavior control, but rules may also leave the actor with substantial uncertainty – and at the same time flexibility – by only providing information on the priorities of goals to be pursued or on the process to follow in order to define the right course of action (Grote, Weichbrodt, Günter, Zala-Mezö, & Künzle, 2009; Hale & Swuste, 1998). An example for (c) is psychological safety, as discussed earlier. More research on the distinct stability- and flexibility-enhancing qualities of specific mechanisms would be beneficial from a theoretical as well as practical point of view to help organizational decision-makers in designing the most appropriate working conditions for individuals and teams in high-risk environments and beyond.

Establishing the best mix of stability- and flexibility-enhancing mechanisms also entails careful consideration of interactions between organizational-, team-, and individual-level characteristics. As stated earlier, *rules and standardization* are generally considered to reduce uncertainty at lower levels of the organization (March, Schulz, & Zhou, 2000). Rules may be introduced at the organizational level, but also at team level (Bunderson & Boumgarden, 2010; Okhuysen & Bechky, 2009), either by decisions in the team or through processes of behavioral routinization at the individual and team level (Gersick & Hackman, 1990). If there are few rules in place either at the organizational or team level, more coordination via mutual adjustment among team members and/or via personal leadership is required to cope with remaining uncertainties. Additionally, independent of where in the organization rules are defined, different rule types can be chosen, which reduce uncertainty to a lesser (goal and process rules) or larger (action rules) extent (Grote et al., 2009; Hale & Swuste, 1998). How different rule types defined at different levels in the organization interact, still awaits investigation. Possibly, setting priorities by means of goal rules at the organizational level combines well with more specific rules at the team level. However, crucial risks may have to be controlled by strict organizational-level rules also, such as the rule in all airlines that a go-around (i.e., aborted landing) can be initiated at all times by both pilots, independent of rank (captain, first officer) and assigned role (pilot flying, pilot non-flying).

The concept of *substitutes for leadership* (Kerr & Jermier, 1978) also entails interaction between different levels of analysis. For example, decisions at the organizational level to rely on standardized work procedures or to empower employees for independent decision-making both establish substitutes for leadership at team level, with very different effects however. In the first case uncertainty is reduced and stability enhanced for teams, while in the second case, teams are enabled to cope with uncertainties without much interference from supervisors, thus becoming "self-managed". Interestingly, Bunderson and Boumgarden (2010) found that self-managed teams performed better if they themselves had developed operational standards, indicating a need for stability, which may be more adequately responded to at team level rather than higher up in the organization. More research would be useful to better understand these processes.

The impact of *safety culture*, finally, can also be understood in terms of interactions between organizational-, team-, and individual-level mechanisms. Following general definitions of organizational culture (e.g. Schein, 1985), safety culture can be defined as "the sum of all safety-related assumptions and norms that are shared by the majority of an organisation's members, and which find their expression in the way safety is actually dealt with in all areas of the organisation" (Müller, Brauner, Grote, & Künzler, 1998, p. 25; see also Guldenmund, Chapter 19, this volume). A basic feature of culture is that it supports coordination and integration via centralization of norms and values, not via fixed rules and standards. Thus, organizational and team culture can provide stability in otherwise flexible and adaptive work processes with high levels of decision latitude given to individual actors (Weick, 1987). When, on the other hand, coordination is achieved through high levels of standardization and strict planning at the organizational and team level, team norms fostering rule following and obedience are helpful to enforce standards and plans, but are not essential to ensure sufficient integration for effective organizational functioning (Grote, 2007, 2012). Similarly, homogeneous teams, (e.g., made up of people with the same professional background), by their very nature share many norms and assumptions. Here, attention has to be paid to the fact that cultures can become too strong, penalizing any deviance or speaking-up. In heterogeneous teams, building shared cultural norms may be difficult to start with, while at the same time being important to ensure coordination and integration. Moreover, culture can be assumed to play quite a different role in promoting process safety and personal safety (Grote, 2012). When personal risks are fairly distinct from process risks, protection against personal risks creates a task separate from the primary work task. In that case the "Safety First" principle needs to be stressed and firmly grounded in organizational and team norms and values in order to promote personal safety. For process safety, alignment between task requirements and safety requirements is generally easier because they are more tightly interlinked with the primary work task itself, like in rail or air transport. Therefore, cultural norms that emphasize and support good task fulfilment will in themselves be beneficial for safety. However, these are assumptions that call for an empirical test before firm conclusions can be drawn.

Future Research

This broad review of the literature has provided many avenues for future research, which are summarized here. Most importantly, the chosen focus on the management of uncertainty allows one to bring together quite disparate research streams, ranging from the impact of an individual's need for closure to organizations' attempts to face uncertainty by establishing ambidextrous structures, for example, by creating separate organizational units for stability and flexibility. This integrative force is hoped to spur research that will significantly improve our understanding of how individuals, teams, and organizations can be supported in their attempts to handle significant risks with high impact on all of us. Among the many more specific research suggestions that have been discussed throughout the chapter, three fields for future research stand out.

First, in the field of decision-making, progress is needed on the interaction between what has been labelled "System 1 and System 2 thinking". The different ways of handling uncertainty implied in these types of thinking could prove an interesting lens to use in such research. Depending on requirements for managing uncertainty in terms of finding an appropriate balance between stability and flexibility, System 1 or System 2 thinking or any mix between the two may be most effective. Learning more about appropriate uses of System 1 and System 2 thinking and about the impact of individual differences in (un) certainty orientation could eventually lead to specifically tailored training programs for different groups of individuals and different high-risk settings.

Second, studying different modes of leadership and coordination across team and organizational levels in terms of their stability- and flexibility-enhancing impact on work processes is a highly relevant endeavour. Again, the management of uncertainty lens could help to integrate research on shared leadership and adaptive coordination in high-risk teams, investigating, for instance, the constraints on formal and shared leadership as well as on implicit and explicit coordination. Furthermore, the effects of different kinds of substitutes for leadership should be analyzed, taking into consideration that some may be more stability-enhancing, such as standardization and routinizations, and others more flexibility-enhancing, such as individual and team empowerment.

Finally, an overarching question in safety research should be addressed, which concerns conceptual and empirical knowledge on how measures aimed at process safety versus personal safety achieve their effects and how they interact. This constitutes a significant need for future research because frequently these two kinds of safety are not sufficiently differentiated and mechanisms operating on either not sufficiently distinguished. Examining the kinds of uncertainty acting toward or against securing process and personal safety could be a good point of departure. For such research, it might also be useful to include not only uncertainties in the work process, but also uncertainties operating at the level of the employment relationship, as expressed for instance in breaches of the psychological contract.

Conclusion

Working in high-risk environments requires particularly careful handling of uncertainties, as human lives are at stake. This, as a general trend, leads decision-makers at strategic and operational levels in organizations to reduce uncertainty wherever possible. Taking research in organizational theory as a starting point – which shows the necessity to balance stability and flexibility in organizations through careful consideration of reducing, maintaining, and increasing uncertainty – this review has attempted to build a convincing case for a more balanced approach to managing uncertainties in high-risk environments. Conceptual and empirical work at the individual, team, and organizational level of analysis has been discussed through an uncertainty management lens. While there is much research to rely on, the review has also indicated many avenues for future investigations to help gain an even better understanding of how different stability- and flexibility-enhancing mechanisms can be employed to promote safety. Not least this research is hoped to change the predominant mind-set in practice that through its focus on uncertainty reduction precludes the flexibility needed to cope with ever more complex socio-technical systems.

References

Adler, P. S., & Borys, B. (1996). Two types of bureaucracy: Enabling and coercive. *Administrative Science Quarterly, 41,* 61–89.

Allaire, Y., & Firsirotu, M. E. (1989). Coping with strategic uncertainty. *Sloan Management Review, 30,* 7–16.

Anand, G., & Ward, P. T. (2004). Fit, flexibility and performance in manufacturing: Coping with dynamic environments. *Production and Operation Management, 13,* 369–385.

Anderson, P. (1999). Complexity theory and organization science. *Organization Science, 10,* 216–232.

Anderson, M. (2005). Behavioural safety and major accident hazards: Magic bullet or shot in the dark? *Process Safety and Environmental Protection, 83,* 109–116.

Ashford, S. J., Sutcliffe, K. M. & Christianson, M. K. (2009). Speaking up and speaking out: The leadership dynamics of voice in organizations. In J. Greenberg & M. Edwards (Eds.), *Voice and silence in organizations* (pp. 175–202). Bingley, UK: Emerald.

Aven, T., & Renn, O. (2009). On risk defined as an event where the outcome is uncertain. *Journal of Risk Research, 12,* 1–11.

Barley, S. R., & Kunda, G. (1992). Design and devotion: Surges of rational and normative ideologies of control in managerial discourse. *Administrative Science Quarterly, 37,* 363–399.

Benner, M. J., & Tushman, M. L. (2003). Exploitation, exploration, and process management: The productivity dilemma revisited. *Academy of Management Review, 28,* 238–256.

Bienefeld, N., & Grote, G. (2012). Silence that may kill: When aircrew members don't speak up and why. *Aviation Psychology and Applied Human Factors, 2,* 1–10.

Bienefeld, N., & Grote, G. (2014). Shared leadership in multi-team systems: How cockpit and cabin crews lead each other to safety. *Human Factors, 56,* 270–286.

Bigley, G., & Roberts, K. H. (2001). The incident command system: High-reliability organizing for complex and volatile environments. *Academy of Management Journal, 44,* 1281–1299.

Brashers, D. E. (2001). Communication and uncertainty management. *Journal of Communication, 51,* 477–497.

Brashers, D. E., & Hogan, T. P. (2013). The appraisal and management of uncertainty: Implications for information-retrieval systems. *Information Processing and Management, 49,* 1241–1249.

Brehmer, B. (1992). Dynamic decision making: Human control of complex systems. *Acta Psychologica, 81,* 211–241.

Brown, S. L., & Eisenhardt, K. M. (1997). The art of continuous change: Linking complexity theory and time-based evolution in relentlessly shifting organizations. *Administrative Science Quarterly, 42,* 1–34.

Bunderson, J. S., & Boumgarden, P. (2010). Structure and learning in self-managed teams: Why "bureaucratic" teams can be better learners. *Organization Science, 21,* 609–624.

Burke, C. S., Stagl, K. C., Klein, C., Goodwin, G. F., Salas, E., & Halpin, S. M. (2006). What type of leadership behaviors are functional in teams? A meta-analysis. *Leadership Quarterly, 17,* 288–307.

Burke, C. S., Stagl, K. C., & Salas, E. (2006). Understanding team adaptation: A conceptual analysis and model. *Journal of Applied Psychology, 91,* 1189–1207.

Burns, T., & Stalker, G. M. (1961). *The management of innovation.* London, UK: Tavistock.

Carroll, J. S. (1998). Organizational learning activities in high-hazard industries: The logics underlying self-analysis. *Journal of Management Studies, 35,* 699–717.

Carson, J. B., Tesluk, P. E., & Marrone, J. A. (2007). Shared leadership in teams: An investigation of antecedent conditions and performance. *Academy of Management Journal, 50,* 1217–1234.

Cherns, A. (1987). Principles of sociotechnical design revisited. *Human Relations, 40,* 153–162.

Crawford, E. R., & LePine, J. A. 2013. A configural theory of team processes: Accounting for the structure of taskwork and teamwork. *Academy of Management Review, 38,* 32–48.

Daft, R. L., & Lengel, R. H. (1984). Information richness: A new approach to managerial behavior and organizational design. *Research in Organizational Behavior, 6,* 191–233.

Davison, R. B., Hollenbeck, J. R., Barnes, C. M., Sleesman, D. J., & Ilgen, D. R. (2012). Coordinated action in multiteam systems. *Journal of Applied Psychology, 97,* 808–824.

Day, D. V., Gronn, P., & Salas, E. (2004). Leadership capacity in teams. *Leadership Quarterly, 15,* 857–880.

Denis, J.-L., Langley, A., & Sergi, V. (2012). Leadership in the plural. *Academy of Management Annals, 6,* 211–283.

Detert, J. R., & Burris, E. R. (2007). Leadership behavior and employee voice: Is the door really open? *Academy of Management Journal, 50,* 869–884.

Dionne, S. D., Yammarino, F. J., Atwater, L. E,. & James, L. R. (2002). Neutralizing substitutes for leadership: Leadership effects and common source bias. *Journal of Applied Psychology, 69,* 307–321.

Dionne, S. D., Yammarino, F. J., Howell, J. P., & Villa, J. (2005). Substitutes for leadership, or not. *Leadership Quarterly, 16,* 169–193.

Edmondson, A. (1999). Psychological safety and learning behavior in work teams. *Administrative Science Quarterly, 44,* 350–383.

Edmondson, A. C. (2003). Speaking up in the operating room: How team leaders promote learning in interdisciplinary action teams. *Journal of Management Studies, 40,* 1419–1452.

Edmondson, A. C., & Lei, Z. (2014). Psychological safety: The history, renaissance, and future of an interpersonal construct. *Annual Review of Organizational Psychology and Organizational Behavior, 1,* 23–43.

Entin, E. E., & Serfaty, D. (1999). Adaptive team coordination. *Human Factors, 41,* 312–325.

Espinosa, A., Lerch, F. J., & Kraut, R. E. (2004). Explicit vs. implicit coordination mechanisms and task dependencies: One size does not fit all. In E. Salas & S. M. Fiore (Eds.), *Team cognition: Understanding the factors that drive process and performance* (pp. 107–129). Washington, DC: American Psychological Association.

Evans, J. S. B. T. (2008). Dual-processing accounts of reasoning, judgment, and social cognition. *Annual Review of Psychology, 59,* 255–278.

Faraj, S., & Sambamurthy, V. (2006). Leadership of information systems development projects. *IEEE Transactions Engineering Management, 53,* 238–249.

Faraj, S., & Xiao, X. (2006). Coordination in fast-response organization. *Management Science, 52,* 1155–1169.

Figner, B., & Weber, E. U. (2011). Who takes risks when and why? Determinants of risk taking. *Current Directions in Psychological Science, 20,* 211–216.

Folta, T. B. (1998). Governance and uncertainty: The trade-off between administrative control and commitment. *Strategic Management Journal, 19,* 1007–1028.

Friedrich, T. L., Vessey, W. B., Schuelke, M. J., Ruark, G. A., & Mumford, M. D. (2009). A framework for understanding collective leadership: The selective utilization of leader and team expertise within networks. *Leadership Quarterly, 20,* 933–958.

Galbraith, J. (1973). *Designing complex organizations.* Reading, MA: Addison-Wesley.

Gersick, C., & Hackman, J. R. (1990). Habitual routines in task-performing groups. *Organizational Behavior and Human Decision Processes, 47,* 65–97.

Gigerenzer, G. (2007). *Gut feelings: The intelligence of the unconscious.* London, UK: Penguin.

Gigerenzer. G., & Goldstein, D. G. (1996). Reasoning the fast and frugal way: Models of bounded rationality. *Psychological Review, 103,* 650–669.

Grote, G. (2007). Understanding and assessing safety culture through the lens of organizational management of uncertainty. *Safety Science, 45,* 637–652.

Grote, G. (2009). *Management of uncertainty: Theory and application in the design of systems and organizations.* London, UK: Springer.

Grote, G. (2012). Safety management in different high-risk domains – all the same? *Safety Science, 50,* 1983–1992.

Grote, G. (2015). Promoting safety by increasing uncertainty: Implications for risk management. *Safety Science, 71,* 71–79.

Grote, G., Kolbe, M., & Waller, M. J. (2012). *On the confluence of leadership and coordination in balancing stability and flexibility in teams.* Paper presented at the 72nd Annual Meeting of the Academy of Management, Boston, August 2012.

Grote, G., Kolbe, M., Zala-Mezö, E., Bienefeld-Seall, N., & Künzle, B. (2010). Adaptive coordination and heedfulness make better cockpit crews. *Ergonomics, 52,* 211–228.

Grote, G., Weichbrodt, J. C., Günter, H., Zala-Mezö, E., & Künzle, B. (2009). Coordination in high-risk organizations: the need for flexible routines. *Cognition, Technology & Work, 11,* 17–27.

Hale, A., & Heijer, T. (2006). Is resilience really necessary? The case of railways. In E. Hollnagel, D. D. Woods, & N. Leveson (Eds.), *Resilience engineering: Concepts and precepts* (pp. 125–148). Aldershot, UK: Ashgate.

Hale, A. R., & Swuste, P. (1998). Safety rules: Procedural freedom or action constraint? *Safety Science, 29,* 163–177.

Hendry, K., & Kiel, G. C. (2004). The role of the board in firm strategy: Integrating agency and organisational control perspectives. *Corporate Governance: An International Review, 12,* 500–520.

Hollnagel, E., Woods, D. D., & Leveson, N. (Eds.) (2006). *Resilience engineering: Concepts and precepts.* Aldershot, UK: Ashgate.

Hopkins, A. (2000). *Lessons from Longford: The Esso gas plant explosion.* Sydney, Australia: CCH.

Hopkins, A. (2009). Thinking about process safety indicators. *Safety Science, 47,* 460–465.

Humphrey, S. E., & Aime, F. (2014). Team microdynamics: Toward an organizing approach to teamwork. *Academy of Management Annals, 8,* 443–503.

Jauch, L. R., & Kraft, K. L. (1986). Strategic management of uncertainty. *Academy of Management Review, 11,* 777–790.

Kahneman, D. (2011). *Thinking, fast and slow.* New York, NY: Farrar, Straus, and Giroux.

Kahneman, D., & Klein, G. (2009). Conditions for intuitive expertise: A failure to disagree. *American Psychologist, 64,* 515–526.

Kahneman, D., & Tversky, A. (1979). Prospect theory: An analysis of decision under risk. *Econometrica, 47,* 263–291.

Katz, D., & Kahn, R. L. (1978). *The social psychology of organizations.* New York, NY: John Wiley & Sons, Inc.

Kerr, S., & Jermier, J. M. (1978). Substitutes for leadership: Their meaning and measurement. *Organizational Behavior and Human Performance, 22,* 375–403.

Kerr, N. L., & Tindale, R. S. (2004). Group performance and decision making. *Annual Review of Psychology, 55,* 623–655.

Ketokivi, M. (2006). Elaborating the contingency theory of organizations: The case of manufacturing flexibility strategies. *Production and Operation Management, 15,* 215–228.

Klein, G. (2008). Naturalistic decision making. *Human Factors, 50,* 456–460.

Klein, K. J., Ziegert, J. C., Knight, A. P., & Xiao, Y. (2006). Dynamic delegation: Shared, hierarchical, and deindividualized leadership in extreme action teams. *Administrative Science Quarterly, 51,* 590–621.

Knight, F. H. (1921). *Risk, uncertainty and profit.* Boston, MA; New York, NY: Kelley.

Kolbe, M., Burtscher, M. J., Wacker, J., Grande, B., Nohynkova, R., Manser, T., Spahn, D. R., & Grote, G. (2012). Speaking up is related to better team performance in simulated anesthesia inductions: An observational study. *Anesthesia and Analgesia, 115,* 1099–1108.

Kozlowski, S. W. J., Watola, D. J., Jensen, J. M., Kim, B. H., & Botero, I. C. (2009). Developing adaptive teams: A theory of dynamic team leadership. In E. Salas, G. F. Goodwin, & C. S. Burke (Eds.), *Team effectiveness in complex organizations: Cross-disciplinary perspectives and approaches* (SIOP Frontier Series) (pp. 113–155). New York, NY: Taylor & Francis.

Kruglanski, A. W., & Webster, D. M. (1996). Motivated closing of the mind: Seizing and freezing. *Psychological Review, 103,* 263–283.

Künzle, B., Zala-Mezö, E., Kolbe, M., Wacker, J., & Grote, G. (2010). Substitutes for leadership in anaesthesia teams and their impact on leadership effectiveness. *European Journal of Work and Organizational Psychology, 19,* 505–531.

Künzle, B., Zala-Mezö, E., Wacker, J., Kolbe, M., Spahn, D. R., & Grote, G. (2010). Leadership in anaesthesia teams: The most effective leadership is shared. *Quality and Safety in Health Care, 19,* 1–6.

Lanaj, K., Hollenbeck, J. R., Ilgen, D. R., Barnes, C. M., & Harmon, S. J. (2013). The double-edged sword of decentralized planning in multiteam systems. *Academy of Management Journal, 56,* 735–757.

Lawrence, P. R., & Lorsch, J. W. (1967). Differentiation and integration in complex organizations. *Administrative Science Quarterly, 12*, 1–47.

Leifer, R., & Mills, P. K. (1996). An information processing approach for deciding upon control strategies and reducing control loss in emerging organizations. *Journal of Management, 22*, 113–137.

Levitt, R. E., Thomsen, J., Christiansen, T. R., Kunz, J. C., Jin, Y., & Nass, C. (1999). Simulating project work processes and organizations: Toward a micro-contingency theory of organizational design. *Management Science, 45*, 1479–1495.

Lind, E. A., & Van den Bos, K. (2002). When fairness works: Towards a general theory of uncertainty management. *Research in Organizational Behavior, 24*, 181–224.

Lipshitz, R., & Strauss, O. (1997). Coping with uncertainty: A naturalistic decision-making analysis. *Organizational Behavior and Human Decision Processes, 69*, 49–163.

MacCrimmon, K. R., & Wehrung, D. A. (1990). Characteristics of risk-taking executives. *Management Science, 36*, 422–435.

March, J., Schulz, M., & Zhou, X. (2000). *The dynamics of rules: Change in written organizational codes.* Stanford, CA: Stanford University Press.

Mathieu, J. E., Tannenbaum, S. I., Donsbach, J. S., & Alliger, G. M. (2014). A review and integration of team composition models: Moving toward a dynamic and temporal framework. *Journal of Management, 40*, 130–160.

Mellers, B. A., Schwartz, A., & Cooke, A. D. J. (1998). Judgment and decision-making. *Annual Review of Psychology, 49*, 447–477.

Milliken, F. J. (1987). Three types of perceived uncertainty about the environment: State, effect, and response uncertainty. *Academy of Management Review, 12*, 133–143.

Morgeson, F. P., DeRue, D. S., & Karam, E. P. (2010). Leadership in teams: A functional approach to understanding leadership structures and processes. *Journal of Management, 36*, 5–39.

Morrison, E. W. (2011). Employee voice behavior: Integration and directions for future research. *Academy of Management Annals, 5*, 373–412.

Morrison, E. W. (2014). Employee voice and silence. *Annual Review of Organizational Psychology and Organizational Behavior, 1*, 173–197.

Morrison, E. W., & Rothman, N. B. (2009). Silence and the dynamics of power. In J. Greenberg & M. Edwards (Eds.), *Voice and silence in organizations* (pp. 175–202). Bingley, UK: Emerald.

Müller, S., Brauner, C., Grote, G., & Künzler, C. (1998). *Safety culture: A reflection of risk awareness.* Zurich, Switzerland: Swiss Re.

Nembhard, I. M., & Edmondson, A. C. (2006). Making it safe: The effects of leader inclusiveness and professional status on psychological safety and improvement efforts in health care teams. *Journal of Organizational Behavior, 27*, 941–966.

Nicholson, N., Soane, E., Fenton-O'Creevy, M., & Willman, P. (2005). Personality and domain-specific risk taking. *Journal of Risk Research, 8*, 157–176.

Okhuysen, G., & Bechky, B. A. (2009). Coordination in organizations: An integrative perspective. *Academy of Management Annals, 3*, 463–502.

O'Reilly, C. A., & Tushman, M. L. (2004). The ambidextrous organization. *Harvard Business Review, 82*, 74–81.

Paté-Cornell, E. (2012). On "Black Swans" and "Perfect Storms": Risk analysis and management when statistics are not enough. *Risk Analysis, 32*, 1823–1833.

Pearce, C. L., & Conger, J. A. (2003). *Shared leadership: Reframing the how's and why's of leadership.* Thousand Oaks, CA: Sage.

Perrow, C. (1967). Framework for comparative analysis of organizations. *American Sociological Review, 32*, 194–208.

Pfeffer, J., & Salancik, G. R. (1978). *The external control of organization: A resource dependence perspective.* New York, NY: Harper and Row.

Pierro, A., Giacomantonio, M., Kruglanski, A. W., & van Knippenberg, D. (2014). Follower need for cognitive closure as moderator of the effectiveness of leader procedural fairness. *European Journal of Work and Organizational Psychology, 23*, 582–595.

Power, M. (2004). *The risk management of everything: Rethinking the politics of uncertainty.* London, UK: Demos.

Power, M. (2007). *Organized uncertainty: Designing a world of risk management.* Oxford, UK: Oxford University Press.

Reddy, R., Welch, D., Ameratunga, S., & Thorne, P. (2014). Development of the hearing protection assessment (HPA-2) questionnaire. *Occupational Medicine, 64,* 198–205.

Renn, O. (2008). *Risk governance: Coping with uncertainty in a complex world.* London, UK: Earthscan.

Rico, R., Sánchez-Manzanares, M., Gil, F., & Gibson, C. (2008). Team implicit coordination processes: A team knowledge-based approach. *Academy of Management Review, 33,* 163–184.

Rousseau, D. M. (1989). Psychological and implied contracts in organizations. *Employee Responsibilities and Rights Journal, 2,* 121–139.

Rousseau, D. M., & Libuser, C. (1997). Contingent workers in high-risk environments. *California Management Review, 39,* 103–123.

Santoro, M. D., & McGill, J. P. (2005). The effect of uncertainty and asset co-specialization on governance in biotechnology alliances. *Strategic Management Journal, 26,* 1261–1269.

Schein, E. H. (1985). *Organizational culture and leadership.* San Francisco, CA: Jossey-Bass.

Schein, E. H. (1996). Three cultures of management: The key to organizational learning. *Sloan Management Review, 38,* 9–20.

Shafir, E., & LeBoeuf, R. A. (2002). Rationality. *Annual Review of Psychology, 53,* 491–517.

Shenhar, A. J. (2001). One size does not fit all projects: Exploring classical contingency domains. *Management Science, 47,* 394–414.

Simon, H. A. (1955). A behavioral model of rational choice. *Quarterly Journal of Economics, 6,* 99–118.

Sitkin, S. B., & Pablo, A. L. (1992). Reconceptualizing the determinants of risk behavior. *Academy of Management Review, 17,* 9–38.

Smith, W. K., & Tushman, M. L. (2005). Managing strategic contradictions: A top management model for managing innovation streams. *Organization Science, 16,* 522–536.

Sorrentino, R. M., Short, J. C., & Raynor, J. O. (1984). Uncertainty orientation: Implications for affective and cognitive views of achievement behavior. *Journal of Personality and Social Psychology, 46,* 189–201.

Suchman, L. A. (1987). *Plans and situated actions: The problem of human–machine communications.* Cambridge, UK: Cambridge University Press.

Sutton, R. I., & Kahn, R. L. (1987). Prediction, understanding, and control as antidotes to organizational stress. In J. W. Lorsch (Ed.), *Handbook of organizational behavior* (pp. 272–283). Englewood Cliffs, NJ: Prentice-Hall.

Taleb, N. N. (2007). *The Black Swan: The impact of the highly improbable.* New York, NY: Random House.

Taylor, F. W. (1911). *The principles of scientific management.* New York, NY: Harper and Row.

Thompson, J. D. (1967). *Organizations in action.* New York, NY: McGraw-Hill.

Tushman, M. L., & O'Reilly, C. A. (1996). Ambidextrous organizations: Managing evolutionary and revolutionary change. *California Management Review, 38,* 8–29.

Van de Ven, A. H., Delbecq, A. L., & Koenig, R. J. (1976). Determinants of coordination modes within organizations. *American Sociological Review, 41,* 322–338.

Walker, A. (2013). Outcomes associated with breach and fulfilment of the psychological contract of safety. *Journal of Safety Research, 47,* 31–37.

Walker, A., & Hutton, D. M. (2006). The application of the psychological contract to workplace safety. *Journal of Safety Research, 37,* 433–441.

Wall, T. D., Cordery, J. L., & Clegg, C. W. (2002). Empowerment, performance, and operational uncertainty: A theoretical integration. *Applied Psychology: An International Review, 51,* 146–169.

Waller, M. J., Gupta, N., & Giambatista, R. C. (2004). Effects of adaptive behaviors and shared mental models on control crew performance. *Management Science, 50,* 1534–1544.

Weber, M. (1947). *The theory of social and economic organization.* Trans. by A. M. Henderson and T. Parsons. New York, NY: Oxford University Press.

Weber, E. U., & Johnson, E. J. (2009). Mindful judgment and decision-making. *Annual Review of Psychology, 60*, 53–85.

Weick, K. E. (1976). Educational organizations as loosely coupled systems. *Administrative Science Quarterly, 21*, 1–19.

Weick, K. E. (1979). *The social psychology of organizing* (2nd edn.). Reading, MA: Addison-Wesley.

Weick, K. E. (1987). Organizational culture as a source of high-reliability. *California Management Review, 29*, 112–127.

Weick, K. E. (1995). *Sensemaking in organizations.* Thousand Oaks, CA: Sage.

Weick, K. E., & Roberts, K. H. (1993). Collective mind in organizations: Heedful interrelating on flight decks. *Administrative Science Quarterly, 38*, 357–381.

Weick, K. E., & Sutcliffe, K. M. (2001). *Managing the unexpected: Assuring high performance in an age of complexity.* San Francisco, CA: Jossey-Bass.

Weick, K. E., Sutcliffe, K. M., & Obstfeld, D. (1999). Organizing for high reliability: Processes of collective mindfulness. *Research in Organizational Behavior, 21*, 81–123.

Wittenbaum, G. M., Stasser, G., & Merry, C. J. (1996). Tacit coordination in anticipation of small group task completion. *Journal of Experimental Social Psychology, 32*, 129–152.

Xiao, Y., Hunter, W. A., Mackenzie, C. F., Jefferies, N. J., Horst, R. L., & the LOTAS Group (1996). Task complexity in emergency medical care and its implications for team coordination. *Human Factors, 38*, 636–645.

Yukl, G. (2006). *Leadership in organizations* (6th edn.). Upper Saddle River, NJ: Pearson Prentice-Hall.

Zaccaro, S. J., & DeChurch, L. A. (2011). Leadership forms and functions in multi-team systems. In S. J. Zaccaro, M. A. Marks, & L. A. DeChurch (Eds.), *Multi-team systems: An organization form for dynamic and complex environments* (pp. 253–288). New York, NY: Routledge.

Zaccaro, S. J., Rittman, A. L., & Marks, M. A. (2001). Team leadership. *Leadership Quaterly, 12*, 451–483.

Zala-Mezö, E., Wacker, J., Künzle, B., Brüesch, M., & Grote, G. (2009). The influence of stand-ardisation and task load on team coordination patterns during anaesthesia inductions. *Quality and Safety in Health Care, 18*, 127–130.

Zuckerman, M., & Kuhlman, D. M. (2000). Personality and risk-taking: Common biosocial factors. *Journal of Personality, 68*, 999–1029.

22

Risk Management

A. Ian Glendon

Introduction

While having particular links with the chapters in this volume devoted to managing uncertainty (Grote, Chapter 21), and safety culture (Guldenmund, Chapter 19; Bishop, Fleming, & Flin, Chapter 20), this chapter also complements the chapter on "managing risk" in the third edition of *Human Safety and Risk Management* (Glendon & Clarke, 2015). As in the latter, to represent contemporary research and theoretical developments in risk management, much of the material for the present chapter is sourced from a review of papers in contemporaneous issues of the *Journal of Risk Research* (*JRR*), and *Risk Management: A Journal of Risk, Crisis and Disaster*. These journals were selected to reflect a global perspective on risk and riskmanagement issues, as well as representing a wide range of risk issues authored by researchers from 47 countries. *JRR* in particular has been a key repository of current research, conceptual thinking, and documented contemporary risk management practice and development. Arguably, *JRR* is the prime forum in which the most general level of contemporaneous scientific debate has been conducted on risk related concepts that have risk management (RM) implications.

Consistent with Beck's (1992) assertion that risk is an inevitable concomitant of wealth production, the modern risk management (MRM) paradigm encapsulates a much broader perspective than the traditional and somewhat formulaic "policies and matrix" approach to RM, in essence becoming an all-of-business model. Qualitative graphical representations of an all-of-business RM approach include the company dynamic response map (Arena et al., 2013). Organizations adopting an MRM approach heed environmental conditions and the organizational context – a perspective harking back to the notion developed in the 1960s, that the most successful organizations were those whose internal operations most effectively matched their environmental conditions (Lawrence & Lorsch, 1969). Within a core values context, MRM incorporates an awareness of the organization's history, evaluates the internal and external environments, undertakes stakeholder assessment, and specifies the organization's purpose, intentions, and goals. More traditional RM processes include assessment, treatment, evaluation, and monitoring of

The Wiley Blackwell Handbook of the Psychology of Occupational Safety and Workplace Health, First Edition. Edited by Sharon Clarke, Tahira M. Probst, Frank Guldenmund, and Jonathan Passmore. © 2016 John Wiley & Sons Ltd. Published 2020 by John Wiley & Sons Ltd.

risks and incorporating these processes within the regulatory framework (Jondle, Maines, Burke, & Young, 2013). The RM process has been expanded to incorporate eight stages: (World Economic Forum, 2014)

1 identify risks;
2 prioritize top risks;
3 undertake risk assessment (RA);
4 identify RM options;
5 design RM strategy;
6 design crisis management strategy;
7 implement strategy;
8 monitor progress and update strategy.

A variety of organizational, programmatic, and socio-legal phenomena reflect the risk society rubric initially popularized by Beck (1992). Ultimately, almost any and every human behavior and activity can be described and defined in terms of risk-based dialogues. It is increasingly evident that, because they impact on all aspects of our lives through institutions, organizations, communities, and jurisdictions, risk issues are also matters intimately concerned with life and living, affecting not just human societies, but also the natural environment, its flora and fauna. The World Economic Forum (WEF) has noted a trend in organizations away from individual risk planning in technical terms toward a more holistic approach to a range of less well specified risks (WEF, 2014), akin to Grote's distinction between personal and process orientations to risk (see Chapter 21, this volume). Of conceptual interest is the WEF's equating of "risks" as exclusively downside, perhaps also reflecting an aspect of the risk society. Contemporary risks to organizations and communities are frequently interdependent and interconnected, requiring flexible, holistic, collaborative, and resilient solutions. Chief risk officers at director level are often the strategic RM standard-bearers in defending organizational vulnerabilities. Designating cabinet-level national risk officers has also been proposed (Michel-Kerjan, 2012).

Risk management is increasingly influenced by theoretical perspectives from a variety of disciplines, including psychology, thereby providing further links with most other chapters in this volume. For example, framing effects derived from prospect theory provide contexts for decision-making (DM), and have consistently revealed that a loss-making frame typically produces risk-taking behavior, while gain-frames tend to generate risk-averse behavior. As well as creating biases in decisions about risk, framing contexts also affect DM under uncertainty (see Grote, Chapter 21, this volume). Heuristics (mental "short cuts") and cognitive or attributional biases have also featured in many studies of DM under conditions of risk and uncertainty (see Grote, Chapter 21, this volume). Cognitive and affective approaches to risk and uncertainty are perhaps best represented in dual process theories, popularized by Kahneman (2011), in which System 1 thinking is affect-driven, while System 2 thinking is rational-cognitively driven.

Traditional Occupational Health and Safety Risks

A Swiss study of workplace safety comparing nine risk-assessment (RA) techniques in an academic/research environment reviewed: preliminary hazards analysis, failure modes and effects analysis, hazard and operability studies, fault tree analysis, event tree analysis, checklists, human reliability analysis, and decision matrix (Groso, Ouedraogo, & Mayer, 2012). The authors opined that as well as ranking risks, identifying critical areas, and prioritizing safety actions, RAs should combine severity, accident probability, hazard detectability, and worsening factors (Groso et al., 2012). ISO 31000, systems thinking, heuristic biases, and mental models were the framework for an organizational safety review by Kubicek, Bhanugopan, and Fish (2013). After reviewing the role of risk perception (RP), human factors, safety management systems, safety RM, culturally diverse organizations, safety behavior, DM, human error, emotional intelligence, and teams, the authors stressed the importance of organizational culture in managing risk within organizations (Kubicek et al., 2013).

An Italian survey of occupational accidents, safety behaviors, and psychosocial risk factors among highway emergency response workers revealed that RP and safety climate predicted adherence to safety procedures, reporting accident risk, and personal protective equipment use (Prati & Pietrantoni, 2012). Occupational psychosocial risks (e.g., stress and other psychological conditions either generated or exacerbated by workplace factors) also featured in Iavicoli et al.'s (2014) review of European Union (EU) policy framework, referring to hard and soft law. Assessing management standards for work-related stress, the authors argued that flexible European-level psychosocial work risk policies were needed for good practice, surveillance, and benchmarking (Iavicoli et al., 2014). More extensive coverage of workplace psychosocial risks and psychosocial safety climate can be found in Zadow and Dollard (Chapter 18, this volume).

Accident sequences, causation models, probabilistic distributions, complexity, attributions and biases, featured in Hudson's (2014) theoretical analysis, which reviewed multiple attributional biases, blame, the fundamental attributional error, asymmetric hindsight bias, preventive management, chaotic behavior, organizational, cultural factors, and "non-causal" contributory factors (e.g., fatigue). While most accident causation sequences are deterministic, four percent are non-linear and non-deterministic, for which management implications are problematic. While in hindsight these may appear linear, non-complex and deterministic, attributional biases tend to favor simplistic causation models. As the legal profession only ever sees post hoc cases, it adopts a superficially attractive but incorrect model (Hudson, 2014). Prospect theory and framing formed the conceptual basis for Kluge, Badura, and Rietz's (2013) experimental simulation of production-related risks involving safety violations, individual differences (IDs), risky DM, risk-taking, production, and consequences. As well as being impacted by IDs, risky DM, and skill, violations were affected by framing effects of production outcomes when work performance was sub-aspirational (Kluge et al., 2013). Individual and collective responsibility for work-related risks featured in a Dutch survey to test four hypotheses on risk society, blame culture, resentment, and narcissism (Mascini, Achterberg, & Houtman, 2013). Work-related risk was individualized due to utilitarian individualism and individual responsibilization of work-related risks (Mascini et al., 2013).

The literature reviewed in this brief section has highlighted that even traditional workplace risks are subject to an increasing variety of approaches, models, and methodologies. Contemporaneous research paradigms reinforce the expansion of current perspectives on organizational health and safety issues, which will be discussed in the following sections in this chapter. These relate to research papers reviewed in relation to policy impacts, risk communication, conceptualizing and measuring risk, behavioral aspects of risk, supply chain risk management, and transport risk.

Policy Impacts

Various aspects of policy on risk issues were addressed by several papers. A social dialectic on policy-making legitimacy covering uncertainty, policy-making, risk governance (RG), public awareness, claims-making, and individualization of risk, led Brown and Olofsson

(2014) to maintain that social problems were increasingly likely to be framed as risks. Individualization of responsibility for risk was also a theme of Hamilton's (2014) review of "workfare" policy, process, government activation, entrepreneurial self, discourse of blame, and self-sufficiency. Invoking the normative power of neoliberal welfare state transformation, the author found that over a 30-year period, contractual reciprocity ideas had mobilized to gradually legitimize the principle that individuals should manage life-course risks (Hamilton, 2014). Reporting on an International Conference on Risk and Responsibility that, inter alia, addressed cross-cultural comparisons, and pan-European DM, Hesselbein (2015) described government's role and responsibility for physical risks, RG, risk communication (RC), crisis, uncertainty, risk regulation (RR) balance, compromise, stakeholder power imbalances, public skepticism, and tolerability. Observing that governments often introduced new RR after incidents (regulatory index), a dispute resolution process was needed in which RG could take account of scientific RA, public RP, framing, stakeholders, and values (Hesselbein, 2015).

Reviewing conceptual and evaluative studies in the first five years of EU impact assessments (IAs), Torriti and Löfstedt (2012) compared the theory and practice of IAs. Considering risk-based regulation, competition, cooperation, policy learning, policy options, risk economics, and stakeholder opinions in developing policy proposals, the authors reported that to reduce the discrepancy between rationale and practice, greater emphasis was required on crucial aspects of IAs, including value of statistical life, carbon price, and integrating scenario analysis with macroeconomic modeling (Torriti & Löfstedt, 2012). In a review of regulatory control policy, Löfstedt (2015) employed case studies of Bisphenol A in plastic food containers within the food and environmental sectors to explore the impact of the precautionary principle (PP), chemicals, pharmaceuticals, and endocrine disruptors, within the EU adversarial model of regulation and use of emotions by campaigning journalists. Because academics and stakeholders might amplify research findings in the theatre of media coverage rather than presenting them within a broader context, scientific uncertainty may be translated into "facts." With all EU member states having their own positions, politicization of regulatory DM was inevitable. The issue of whether greater transparency was related to higher public trust was deemed to be problematic, as the author argued for science-based regulation in which risk–risk trade-offs were not ignored (Löfstedt, 2015). However, in considering organizational culture and framing issues to address risk prevention, DM, mitigation, paradigm blindness, worldview, uncertainty, expertise, failure, and policy process, Fischbacher-Smith (2012) observed that multiple effects made it hard to resolve political tensions with scientific knowledge and that there was a need to accept limitations of understanding.

The Dutch Risk and Responsibility Program and International Risk Governance Council (IRGC) risk framework were used by Macrae (2014) to review concern assessment, over-regulation, and responses to disasters. The author argued for framing concern response as part of a political value statement to provide political leadership and allay public fears (Macrae, 2014). Three case examples from the New Zealand Environmental Risk Management Authority informed Corin, McNeill, and Atapattu's (2012) consideration of community involvement and stakeholder engagement in risk-assessment DM. To reconcile public views with science-based risk assessments, the authors urged allowing subjective democratic decisions to bridge the gap between practitioners and public (Corin et al., 2012). Sociological fateful moments (Giddens) and RA formed the framework for a Norwegian study of public services case studies (Braut, Rake, Aaestad, & Njå, 2012). Considering risk image, DM, planning, comprehension, risk and vulnerability analysis, uncertainty, expertise, and risk dynamic, the authors recommended training practitioners to establish a risk image for DM during fateful moments (e.g., accidents, crises), with focus on uncertainty, developed on their experience (Braut et al., 2012). Policy networks mediating risk society and a culture of fear, as well as actor network theory, formed the conceptual framework for a Dutch case study of school safety (Binkhorst & Kingma, 2012). Using grounded theory for a stakeholder analysis (school, local government, police), to address the problematization of school safety, local leadership was required to develop firm safety measures, and to balance risks and reputation. The authors noted the desirability of taking account of soft cultural factors as well as hard material elements (Binkhorst & Kingma, 2012).

Linking with themes from the chapters in this volume on safety culture (see Guldenmund, Chapter 19, and Bishop et al., Chapter 20), reliability and culture were thematic in papers from Norway, Australia, Canada, the USA, and the UK-Netherlands. The theory and mindset of high reliability organizations (HROs), as well as sense-making, mindfulness, failure potential, risk perspectives, and resilience were considered by Khorsandi and Aven (2014), who advocated a risk perspective that replaced probability with uncertainty in defining risk. This would support HRO implementation better than traditional perspectives (e.g., probabilistic risk assessment), it being more critical to identify correct thinking processes rather than to focus on the outcomes of those processes (Khorsandi & Aven, 2014). An ethnographic approach involving storytelling and using safety imagination, as a route to organizational learning for hazardous industry HROs was adopted by Hayes and Maslen (2015). Narrative themes included expert judgments, tacit knowledge, sense-making, and major incidents. It was concluded that organizations should incorporate story-based learning for more effective DM, embed stories in work practices, and learn by using incident reporting as story sharing (Hayes & Maslen, 2015).

Two examples from the current author's direct experience in two different countries illustrate how incidents and the prior potential for harm in seemingly innocuous environments might be incorporated within an organization's story-based learning. The first example involves a new elevator (lift) door design, which resulted in an arrangement that could be confusing for visitors to the organization who wished to use the elevators. The elevator entrance design was part of a refurbished covered entrance area for two adjacent buildings, incorporating a security and information desk. Two elevators were encased in a glass tube that ran the height of the buildings right down to the ground-floor entrance area, where access doors for maintenance had been incorporated into the design. These doors were kept locked at all times unless maintenance access was required. On a day when maintenance work was being undertaken and the glass doors had been opened for access, a visitor unfamiliar with the elevator door layout opened the glass door and sustained serious injury as a result of falling into the elevator shaft. The subsequent investigation revealed that the security staff, whose desk was a few meters from the elevators' glass maintenance door, reported frequently observing visitors in the very busy concourse area trying the locked maintenance access doors before realizing that the elevator doors were on the other side of the shaft and proceeding to use the elevator successfully. After the accident, the small notice advising users of the location of the elevator doors was replaced by colored tape, a very large notice, and a large arrow to inform users of the location of the elevator doors. This case could have been used in group discussions within the organization to consider, inter alia, what the incident revealed about the safety culture of the organization, what safety values were inculcated in its employees, either directly or by default, and what reporting mechanisms and practices might (or might not) have existed. The case study might also be used as an opportunity for members of other organizations to determine whether a similar type of incident could happen in their organization, and what steps might be taken to obviate such threats to safety.

The second illustrative case involved the author contacting his organization's safety committee to urge that they strategically post some notices in a multistory car park in which there was the possibility of injury as a result of low levels of illumination, particularly during busy periods at the beginning and end of each working day. The suggested form of words sought to employ well-established principles of describing the desired behavior, and explaining the reason for the requested behavior as simply as possible: "SEE AND BE SEEN: USE DIPPED HEADLIGHTS AT ALL TIMES IN THIS CAR PARK." The eventual response was that the safety committee did not see the need for such a sign as it was assumed that people exercised due caution when using the car park and there had been no incidents to date. Resisting the temptation to compose a reply to the effect that I had not appreciated that they were waiting for an incident to occur before taking action, on the grounds that this might prejudice any future attempts to persuade the safety committee of some threat to safety, I opted for silence. Many years later, a pedestrian was duly injured in an incident in the car park, soon after which a sign was posted at the entrance, although it was indicative rather than directive. Casual observation suggested that less than 50 percent of drivers used dipped headlights when negotiating the tight corners in the car park, and even at nighttime drivers could occasionally be seen not switching on their lights until they had exited the car park. Neither of these incidents was broadcast within the respective organizations, and I only heard about them through "grapevine" communication. Thus, it appeared that neither organization was either able or willing to use these stories to enhance safety culture among their employees, at least in any widespread way, thereby missing a potentially valuable opportunity to inculcate higher safety values within their respective workforces.

ISO standards and RM models were the framework for Lalonde and Boiral (2012) to review crises, threats, and strategy as practice in HROs. Noting the practice base for RM, the authors advocated questioning assumptions about implementing ISO standards, taking account of both internal and external organizational environments, and remaining vigilant in monitoring standards (Lalonde & Boiral, 2012). Self-assessment and improvement methodology within the context of ISO 31000 was the basis for Jondle et al.'s (2013) organizational culture case analysis of the Veritas Institute. Reviewing the incorporation of RA within organizational ethics, espoused and enacted values, corporate risk universe, and MRM, the authors described five characteristics of an ethical business culture as: values-driven (core), adopting a long-term perspective, leadership effectiveness, stakeholder balance, and process integrity. Values included respect for scientific method, respect for the past, vigilance, fairness/respect for all stakeholders, personal and corporate responsibility for actions and consequences, collaborative effort, openness, transparency, and honesty (Jondle et al., 2013). Operationalizing chronic unease within safety critical industries to develop a model incorporating pessimism, propensity to worry, vigilance, requisite imagination, and flexible thinking, Fruhen, Flin, and McLeod (2014) reported that a specific type of strain was needed to manage risks in HROs.

The papers reviewed in this section and the personal examples provided, indicate that the complexities of risk decision-making extend from the local level at which policies and practices are implemented, right up the organizational hierarchy to government and international agencies with risk-related responsibilities. Particularly problematic is likely to be translating scientific and experiential information into policy, regulation, management, and governance of risk through the prism of political values at all levels.

Risk Communication

While a substantial proportion of all papers within the sample frame made reference to risk communication (RC) issues, 15 had RC or the social amplification of risk framework (SARF) as a prime focus. Initiating a special *JRR* issue on RC, based on a 1989 National

Research Council report, Kasperson (2014) argued for greater RC differentiation, for example, in relation to hazards resulting from agentic activity (e.g., smoking), or environmentally induced hazards (e.g., radioactive waste disposal). Four key RC issues addressed were: (1) how to learn from major successes and failures; (2) how to assess and communicate uncertainty to decision-makers and the public; (3) how risk governance could handle declining social trust; and (4) adopting new RC principles. RC principles advocated by Kasperson (2014) were: (1) more sustained, better funded, more ambitious RC goals and outputs; (2) broaden and deepen RC to internalize conflicting interests, values and lifestyles; (3) focus on relevant uncertainties; and (4) revamp RC goals, structure, and format in the face of high distrust.

Eight authors formulated responses on the basis of Kasperson's ideas. Using DM case examples, Árvai (2014) argued that the disconnect between how RC is defined and practiced should be a dialogue, not a one-way process, nor be used to "correct" RPs, for example, seeking to align lay views with those of experts. RC should clarify the risk context, specify key risk attributes, and assist creative thinking about risk problems and RM options, including risk–risk trade-offs (Árvai, 2014). In similar vein, inveigling against normative RC (trying to persuade people to do something), or the contrast between information provision versus seeking to change views, Siegrist (2014) sought to elucidate RC goals as including increasing acceptance of technology, making better and more informed decisions, and instilling social trust of governments. Observing the wide range of views of what constituted RC, the author noted how RC was simpler in some areas (e.g., preparing poultry safely) than others (e.g., nuclear power). Evidence-based RC was required for better understanding and when communicating uncertainties (Siegrist, 2014).

Noting the role of science as a change agent, Fischhoff (2014) observed the problematic nature of translating research findings into client usable data. Creating trust involved getting to know the client and their business. The RC process also required representing *all* social, behavioral, and decision sciences' contributions to risk issues, as well as creating realistic expectations (Fischhoff, 2014). From an RP context, Bostrom (2014) noted that RC enhancements included: development and application of pragmatic and evidence-driven approaches, new engagement strategies, and efforts to communicate uncertainty. Using case examples (e.g., direct ownership of community wind farms) to address a range of issues, including inclusive RG, trust in the DM process, and two-way communication, Renn (2014) observed that personal experience was increasingly being replaced by institutional (e.g., scientific) advice. Arguing that the ultimate RC goal was to assist public and stakeholders to understand the rationale of risk-based decisions and arrive at a balanced judgment reflecting evidence relevant to their interests, the author identified four factors crucial for trusting relationship between laypersons and RMs: (1) acknowledge the necessity of RM strategy; (2) benefit accruing to self and others; (3) assured self-efficacy; and (4) emotional identification (Renn, 2014). Reviewing the role of social trust, uncertainty, and RG, within a fair participatory process, McComas (2014) characterized RC as a dynamic process responding to an ever-changing environment. A process was required for making ethical RC decisions beyond the court system, which would prioritize and provide a context for judging uncertainties (McComas, 2014).

The example of climate change (CC) risks being distorted by corporate sponsored "denials" to discredit CC science, provided the context for Wardman's (2014) polemic on culture, effectiveness, scientific progress, self-interest, and stakeholders, in which people were disempowered by misinformation (e.g., on CC risks). Arguing that RC was socio-culturally contingent, involving a multiplicity of ideals, practices, and artifacts, it was suggested that reducing sociocultural complexity might help to provide a focus on a few explanatory factors that could lead to generic solutions (Wardman, 2014). Other case examples informed Pidgeon's (2014) review of uncertainty, complexity, SARF, and the unwinding of social identities – thereby individualizing responsibility for risks (e.g., employment, personal finance, status, personal security, healthcare, social standing). The author pointed to a lack of strategic capacity to address many risk challenges, including global financial system dysfunctions, extreme inequalities, and environmental threats, using traditional RA and decision analysis. Problems extended to uncertainty assessment, methods for situating values in stakeholder and public engagement, and fostering citizen deliberation for a wider public good (Pidgeon, 2014).

Using scenarios, images, uncertainty, and probability to probe deliberate versus incidental use of RC affect (fear, outrage) in RP and DM, Visschers et al. (2012) revealed that affect may be induced incidentally and therefore be hard to control. Moral considerations implied a need for prior assessment of RC's affect-inducing potential (Visschers et al., 2012). An experimental design employing videoed messages about RC crises informed Frisby, D. D. Sellnow, Lane, Veil, and T. L. Sellnow's (2013) review of efficacy, instruction, RC, message design and effectiveness, self-protection, and crisis management. Reminding readers of the traditional four learning styles (perceivers, thinkers, divergers, feelers), and stressing the critical nature of self-efficacy, the authors argued for developing messages that appealed to all learning styles. Crisis managers should work closely with media when public health or safety was threatened (Frisby et al., 2013). The Q-sort methodology was used by Johnson and Waishwell (2014) to identify the universe of relevant statements on cancer clusters, public health, RP, beliefs, and disparate perspectives. A principal components analysis revealed five distinct perspectives: cancer causation, best information, cancer frequency, study success, and empathy/competence. Similar to Frisby et al. (2013), the authors recommended audience segmentation to maximize the RC effect (Johnson & Waishwell, 2014).

Using scenarios to explore RA, RP, target person, and unrealistic optimism for high- and low-probability risks, Lermer, Streicher, Sachs, and Frey (2013) observed distributional and singular approaches to risk perspectives, and probabilistic reasoning. Higher RA estimates were found for abstract targets and lower estimates for specific targets (Lermer et al., 2013). To explore media-government interactional risk dynamics, Howarth (2013) used moral panic, SARF, advocacy coalition framework, discourse coalition framework, and social representation/cultivation analysis. The author advocated a more robust framework for analyzing media-political risk to conceptualize: risk type, the nature of media–government relationships, wider context, interactional dynamics, and any deeper emblematic nature of disturbance (Howarth, 2013). SARF and the social attribution of risk amplification provided the conceptual framework for Duckett and Busby (2013) to explore asymmetries in RP, risk controversies, and risk politics. Characterizing amplification and attenuation narratives as attributive claims created within a context of competing interests, the authors identified SARF as how social actors' inter-subjectivity understood the position of the other (Duckett & Busby, 2013).

The papers reviewed in this section have highlighted the complexity of risk communication (RC), including the great variety of risk issues that require to be communicated, the uncertainties and ambiguities surrounding most risk issues, the range of potential stakeholders likely to be involved, timing of communication, and the multiple contextual features (e.g., political, legal) that must be taken into account. Extending the debate on science and knowledge introduced in the previous section, in addition to addressing traditional features of all communication forms – what? when? how? to whom? etc. – RC must take account of such factors as public trust in agencies, stakeholder engagement in risk processes, and emotional involvement in risk issues.

Conceptualizing and Measuring Risk

A few papers addressed various generic aspects of the risk concept. An epistemological framework provided Solberg and Njå (2012) with an opportunity to study the nature of risk, including time, state of affairs, events, consequences, uncertainty, and human value for outcomes. A consideration of risk ontology (what exists?) in terms of future (possibilities) and present (actual) states, led the authors to conclude that risk does not exist except as possible future states. As all risk definitions are problematic, all risk claims must be subjective (Solberg & Njå, 2012). Appraisal theory was the foundation for investigating RP, heuristics and biases, and integrating cognitive and affective approaches to risk by Keller et al. (2012), who concluded that it was possible to apply various risk appraisal models. The efficacy of risk matrices and risk rating systems as RA tools for making qualitative risk assessments was examined by Levine (2012) within the context of a cyber attack on an information systems network. It was noted that logarithmically scaled matrices could better differentiate between hazards with a large dynamic risk range, and when risk categorization was straightforward (Levine, 2012). A decision-theoretic approach, combining historical approaches with risk (toxicological, action-based), provided the framework for Scholz, Blumer, and Brand (2012) to explore risk typologies (dynamic vs. static), within the context of vulnerability, robustness, resilience, and adaptive capacity. The authors determined that risk equated to the evaluation of uncertain loss potential, and that vulnerability was comparable with resilience. Adaptive RM required the elimination of future events if their value was below the vulnerability threshold (Scholz et al., 2012). A concurrent validity study, using clinical files and psychometric (personality) assessment to measure risk within the Historical, Clinical, and Risk Management (HCR-20) violence RA scheme, was described by Jung, Ledi, and Daniels (2013). Reviewing RA, forensics, offenders, criminal history, and level of service measure, the authors reported that while many HCR-20 items had concurrent validity, the RM scales performed least well (Jung et al., 2013).

The nature of RA/RM expertise was addressed in two papers. In considering the role of social scientists' expertise in risk issues, Wendling (2012) noted that demands of policy-makers included: (1) analyzing perceptions to build robust models; (2) guaranteeing validity; (3) communicating, mediating, and educating; (4) being a team member; and (5) providing early warnings. The author regarded social scientists' five roles to be: (1) deconstructing rhetoric and framing; (2) analyzing risk in political systems; (3) opening debate; (4) representing vulnerable stakeholders; and (5) post hoc monitoring of RA and RM outcomes (Wendling, 2012). These criteria might usefully be combined with those suggested by Fischhoff (2014) described above. A macro-sociological (Pareto, Machiavelli) and risk-decision theory framework to address realism, risk, and uncertainty, was the foundation for Marshall and Ojiako's (2013) review of the RM profession. The authors opined that to control overconfidence, the RM profession should stress the corrigibility of risk subjectivities by referring to sociological understanding that reflected widespread risk ignorance (Marshall & Ojiako, 2013).

These few papers have indicated something of the complexity of measuring risk, clearly revealing that simplistic two-dimensional measures can no longer be considered adequate. The nature of expertise required of risk practitioners and researchers suggests a divide between what is currently researched and the toolbox of skills and techniques required for real-world RM.

Behavioral Aspects of Risk

While a wide variety of risk-related behaviors, either explicitly or implicitly, characterized many of the papers reviewed in this chapter, various types of risk behaviors were a prime focus for a few contributions. An evolutionary framework for a series of experiments on mating primes to explore male versus female risk-taking in mating, gambling, reckless driving, mood, and risky behavior in general was adopted by Greitemeyer, Kastenmüller, and Fischer (2013). It was revealed that while males were driven to take physical, financial, health, ethical, and recreational risks by mating imperatives and for reputation enhancement, females were more likely to take risks in the social domain (Greitemeyer et al., 2013), a point also made by Grote (see Chapter 21, this volume). With prospect theory as the conceptual basis, a betting game was used in a Chinese study of cognitive biases, prior experience, and gender differences in risk-taking behaviors (Lam & Ozorio, 2013). The authors found that while males were more likely to bet more after a win, females were more likely to bet more after a loss (Lam & Ozorio, 2013). To better understand risk-taking attitudes in Chinese youth, Cheung, Wu, and Tao (2014) examined sensation seeking, culture, and various risk domains – ethics, finance, health and safety (H&S), recreational, and social. Hyper core self-evaluations of overconfidence and hubristic pride significantly predicted risk-taking attitudes in ethics, finance, and H&S domains. The authors recommended developing courses to reduce overconfidence (Cheung et al., 2014).

Connell's theory of hegemonic masculinity and the cultural theory of risk were the conceptual bases for a South African study of masculinities, cultural worldviews, and societal RPs on environment, crime, and social instability (Reardon & Govender, 2013). Traditional masculine types endorsed a hierarchical/individualist worldview and were less concerned about various risks than were those representing the progressive masculine type. Worldview mediated the masculinity effect on societal RP. RM interventions were recommended to take cultured, subjective, and gendered worldviews into account (Reardon & Govender, 2013). Also using cultural theory, a Swedish survey examined the so-called "White Male Effect," and sociocultural differences (Olofsson & Öhman, 2015). Considering vulnerability, values, demographics, IDs, and social heterogeneity, it was revealed that gender was a less important determinant of RP in Sweden, but that the strength of association varied with risk type or behavior, with contributory age, gender, and sexual orientation effects (Olofsson & Öhman, 2015). The cultural paradigm formed the basis for a South Korean survey of cultural influences on RP, using both emic and etic risk structures (Yang, 2015). Koreans expressed most concern about economic risks, crime, environmental risks, and uncontrollable risks, the author noting that the psychometric paradigm could not account for contextual effects (e.g., culture) on RP (Yang, 2015).

In a Dutch experimental study modeling natural and anthropogenic risks within a risk awareness framework, Cremers, Stubbé, van der Beek, Roelofs, and Kerstholt (2014) reviewed risk awareness, RP, information search, self-efficacy, affect, RC, and risk dilemmas. Identifying game playing as a means to increase risk awareness, the authors noted the need to empower citizens to take more responsibility for their own safety by enhancing their risk awareness and self-efficacy (Cremers et al., 2014). A social constructionist interpretive sociological perspective on danger and risk for industrial sites used documentation to create an historical account (Flanquart, 2012). The French leisure case, which involved regulations restricting access during renovations to a harbor, sandy beach, and cove, revealed different RPs of authorities and the community (Flanquart, 2012).

A case study based on decision analysis and game theory was the subject matter for a Canadian study on risk DM (Farmer, 2014). Considering expected utility, DM criteria, dilemmas (social ethics), and monetary values of consequences, it was concluded that choosing the best outcome could be achieved by quantifying qualitative criteria (Farmer, 2014). A French experimental study based on a prisoner's dilemma formula ("chickie run") explored cautious and risky behaviors within the context of extreme sports leisure pursuits (Collard & Oboeuf, 2013). Somewhat counterintuitively, while combat sports players took more risks, extreme sports specialists played more cautiously, perhaps because they took greater account of environmental factors and estimated the odds prior to engagement (Collard & Oboeuf, 2013). Content analysis using computer linguistic analysis of 53 shark-diving websites explored message sensation value (MSV), threat, RC, emotion, and motivation to engage in risky behaviors (Lapinski, Neuberger, Gore, Muter, & Van Der Heide, 2013). Reviewing threat information (susceptibility, severity), self-efficacy, and response efficacy, it was found that few sites provided explicit threat information (only implicit), efficacy-related messages dominated, RC was overwhelmingly positive rather than negative, and that there was little traditional MSV representation (Lapinski et al., 2013).

To study reputation risk in a US survey of young adults' college risk behaviors, Newby and DeCamp (2015) used a combined conceptual framework comprising culture of fear (Furedi), risk society (Beck), and stigma (Goffman). Exploring responses on topics that included deviance, crime, state of fear, cheating on tests, and driving under the influence (usually of alcohol), it was revealed that fear of harm and of harming others plus risk-taking stigma inhibited risk-taking behavior (Newby & DeCamp, 2015). Reputation risk was also the subject of a UK study of micro-enterprise risk among musicians, including competition risk, RP, and stakeholders (Portman-Smith & Harwood, 2015). Reputation managing strategies included working with agents, behavioral adaptation, collaboration, venue choice, technology use, and always being reliable (Portman-Smith & Harwood, 2015).

Leadership theory and leadership styles were the focus of an Israeli survey of managers' crisis management preparedness, with locus of control, and sensation seeking as trait measures (Sheaffer & Brender-Ilan, 2014). Impulsive sensation seekers with external locus of control and transactional style leaders were crisis prone. Transformational leadership and feminine traits were associated with effective crisis management preparedness (see also Smith, Jordan, & Wallace, Chapter 2, and Wong, Kelloway, & Makhan, Chapter 5, this volume). Developing transformational leadership in low-level managers was recommended to manage crises more effectively (Sheaffer & Brender-Ilan, 2014). A Swedish survey of military officers and soldiers considered international missions, risk-taking, individual risk propensity, age and gender differences (Börjesson, Österberg, & Enander, 2015). The authors advocated military leaders balancing safety-orientated and risk-promoting behaviors (Börjesson et al., 2015). The ethnographic paradigm was the framework for a UK interview study of aid workers (Roth, 2015), which explored voluntary risk-taking, edgework, danger acceptance, individualized risk-taking, and self-governance. Risk-taking was reported as an opportunity to escape from boring and unfulfilling jobs to achieve something with immediate and important results. Security measures that focused on protection rather than acceptance might undermine the attraction of aid work by increasing the distance between intermediary organizations and aid beneficiaries (Roth, 2015).

The papers in this section have revealed a variety of contexts within which risk behaviors may be studied, and the complexity of motivations that characterize such behaviors. Enhanced understanding of such behaviors can be derived from evolutionary explanations for observed behaviors, using models that adequately reflect the context for the risk behavior studied.

Supply Chain Risk Management

In terms of organizational functions in relation to RM, the supply chain featured strongly in those papers reviewed. Referring to the supply chain operations reference model (SCORM), key performance indicators, risk breakdown structure (RBS), risk breakdown matrix (RBM), and risk escalation process in the manufacturing sector, an Italian study applying a base case to a hypothetical structure revealed an unpredictable supply-chain environment for risk identification, RA, and process mapping (Cagliano, De Marco, Grimaldi, & Rafele, 2012). The authors recommended integrating supply chain (SCORM) and RM tools (RBS, RBM) to inform the risk escalation process and increase risk communication (Cagliano et al., 2012). A Tunisian food industry supply-chain risk management (SCRM) case study considered risk prioritization, RA, and the impact of risk variables (autonomous, influent, depending, reliant), as well as supply network, indirect influence, and integrated approach (Hachicha & Elmsalmi, 2014). The authors' interpretive structural hierarchical model flow chart showed interrelationships between risk sources (types) as: environment (6), supplier (4), manufacturer (7), wholesaler (4), distributor (3), retailer (3), and customer (3). The final map showed eight key risk variables (Hachicha & Elmsalmi, 2014). A Brazilian automotive industry risk profile SCRM case study revealed 11 risk drivers and risk sources as: network, organizational, industrial, and environmental (Ceryno, Scavarda, & Klingebiel, 2014). To reduce uncertainty, six risk-mitigation strategies were advocated: financial RM, avoidance, control, cooperation, imitation, and flexibility (Ceryno et al., 2014).

A review of SCRM approaches identified operational, financial, and integrated forms (Bandaly, Shanker, Kahyaoglu, & Satir, 2013). Risk sources were identified as: process uncertainty, information systems failures, labor uncertainty, supplier un/reliability, distribution, network, demand uncertainty, currency exchange rate fluctuations, marketplace randomness, natural disasters, socio/political, major accidents, wilful attacks, and regulations. Ways in which DM is managed under conditions of uncertainty are described by Grote (see Chapter 21, this volume). The four risk domains were: internal operations, external stakeholders, environment, and market. Financial SCRM types were avoidance, prevention, and mitigation. The authors recommended that responsibilities be assigned to functional areas (Bandaly et al., 2013). An earlier review by these authors identified a risk taxonomy framework (avoidance, prevention, mitigation), risk domains (internal operations, external stakeholders, market environment), RA, risk events, risk identification, and vulnerabilities (Bandaly, Satir, Kahyaoglu, & Shanker, 2012). The SCRM planning process proposed was to navigate a sequence toward RM strategy (Bandaly et al., 2012).

Using fuzzy analytic hierarchy process, risk typology, and fuzzy set theory to rank supply-chain risk categories using expert knowledge, Radivojević and Gajović (2014) considered risk modeling, RA analysis, processing, decision support, operational/technological risks (system risks, complexity, hierarchical structure), as well as risk categories and levels (low, medium, high). Risk types were: internal/external, known-in-advance/inherently unknowable, time-dependent, process-dependent, and response-dependent (secondary). Risk categories were: operational/technological, economy/competition, natural hazard, social, and legal/political (Radivojević & Gajović, 2014). A pharmaceuticals SCRM case study involving experimental simulation, failure mode effects and criticality analysis, and scenario analysis, reported on risk minimization, desirability function, and hospital access (Elleuch, Hachicha, & Chabchoub, 2014). Reviewing SCRM risk identification, RA, RM decisions and implementation, and risk monitoring, the authors recommended combining RM techniques to identify and manage supply chain multiple risks (Elleuch et al., 2014).

While not SCRM cases, two papers respectively addressed product development (Malaysia), and project RM (Italy). A life-cycle RM approach facilitated Abdul-Rahman, Mohd-Rahim, and Chen's (2012) study of software development failure, risk mitigation, information technology, time and cost overruns, and risk anticipation. It was concluded that risk mitigation strategies were more effective if employed in RM (e.g., user involvement/commitment) than in technical components of a project (Abdul-Rahman et al., 2012). By categorizing and selecting risk techniques and knowledge management, Cagliano, Grimaldi, and Rafele (2015) applied their taxonomy to 31 risk techniques. The authors stressed the need to select the appropriate project RM technique on the basis of RM process phase, project life-cycle phase, and corporate maturity toward risk (Cagliano et al., 2015).

As a fundamental feature of modern economies, supply chains provide multiple options for encountering hazards. They thereby proffer opportunities to identify and manage risks and threats to health and safety in a wide variety of dynamic environments.

Transport Risk

Given that an estimated 1.3 million lives are lost globally through road traffic accidents alone – a figure that is predicted to rise (WHO, 2013), it might seem surprising that transport risk did not rate as one of the WEF's major risk categories. With 29 papers addressing some aspect of transport safety, this topic is the last substantive risk category to be reviewed here.

Two Norwegian studies addressed generic transport issues. A mailed survey exploring risk mitigation attitudes (worry, risk sensitivity, risk perception) generated a model explaining demand for risk mitigation and transport priorities (Lund, Nordfjærn, & Rundmo, 2012). A case-study workshop discussion identified non-quantifiable DM variables, uncertainties, gaps, stakeholders, dilemmas, cost–benefit analysis (CBA), and security RA for public transport (Hagen, Valdal, Pettersen, & Gjerstad, 2015). The authors developed a risk-based evaluation accommodating non-monetary benefits and costs that prioritized evaluation criteria: expenses, feasibility, passenger perceptions, legal and ethical challenges, and side effects. The paper evaluated risk-reduction effects from: video surveillance, an intrusion detection alarm system, armed guards, an electric perimeter fence, and 24/7 activity on site (Hagen et al., 2015). RM strategies were based on: analysis (traditional), precaution (PP), and discourse (participatory, consensual).

A majority of the transport theme papers considered road traffic risks. Road accidents/crashes were the focus for four papers. From Chile, Jimenez and Bronfman's (2012) review of road accidents and environmental pollution enabled statistical modeling of mortality rates for an analysis of "premature deaths" from vehicle accidents and emissions. Considering cross-sector comparisons, the authors advocated a combination of RC, RR, and individual awareness strategies (Jimenez & Bronfman, 2012). In a review of road tunnel safety in Greece, accident severity increase, quantitative risk assessment (QRA) models incorporating hazard identification (HAZID), event tree, fault tree, consequence estimations, societal risks, and complexity, were developed by Kazaras and Kirytopoulos (2014). It was concluded that as some items were inadequately addressed by QRA models, interactions between equipment systems were increasingly likely as accident scenarios (e.g., firefighting or fire-detection and ventilation, communications), these should be enhanced with common-cause failure analysis (Kazaras & Kirytopoulos, 2014). Road tunnel safety also featured in Abrahamsen, Røed, and Jongejan (2013) study of risk acceptance, in which incidence rate and fatality frequency were outcome variables. After reviewing three

RA levels to evaluate risk acceptability, the authors recommended combining selected quantitative and qualitative RA methods (Abrahamsen et al., 2013). Using a network approach, an Italian study of crash data modeled density diagrams per road crash risk type (Dell'Acqua, Francesca Russo, & Biancardo, 2013). From an analysis of crash types, risk maps, and crash risk bands, the authors identified factors associated with crashes as infrastructure and environmental conditions, mean lane width, horizontal curvature, and mean speed. To reduce deaths and injuries, it was necessary to address multiple factors and to check outcomes against the predictive model (Dell'Acqua et al., 2013).

Cross-cultural comparisons were the focus of a further three papers. Comparable surveys in Turkey and Norway on willingness to take different risks in traffic led Şimşekoğlu, Nordfjærn, and Rundmo (2012) to advocate taking account of country differences in risk perceptions, attitudes, and behaviors when designing road traffic RM strategies. A contemporaneous survey of Turkish and Norwegian road users examined road traffic culture, RP, risk willingness, speeding, rule violations, beliefs, and attributions (Nordfjærn, Şimşekoğlu, & Rundmo, 2012). These authors found that while risk-taking willingness predicted risky behavior in both cultures, fatalism was the most important predictor of risky driving in Turkey, where visual (written information) road traffic orientation was the strongest predictor of reduced risky behavior (Nordfjærn, Şimşekoğlu, & Rundmo, 2012). Errors and violations as aspects of expatriates' driver behavior in Norway and Iran were surveyed by Nordfjærn, Hezaveh, and Mamdoohi (2015). The authors opined that road infrastructure and regulation enforcement in developed countries did not facilitate emotional violations (e.g., horn use, chasing another driver) as much as in less developed countries (Nordfjærn, Hezaveh, & Mamdoohi, 2015).

Group comparisons of safe/unsafe driving behaviors and attitudes within Norway were surveyed by Nordfjærn, Jørgenson, and Rundmo (2012). It was concluded that high-risk professional drivers required RM to address safety priorities and reduce insensitivity to traffic risks (Nordfjærn, Jørgenson, & Rundmo, 2012). A Spanish survey exploring speed and risk, external factors, distraction, and alcohol use, concluded that different groups of pre-drivers required different strategies to reduce risk, dependent on gender and injury experience (Arnau-Sabatés, Garcia, Martínez Muñoz, & Montané Capdevila, 2013).

From Australia, three studies using self-report data examined various aspects of driver behavior. The dual process model of risky behavior provided the conceptual basis for McNally and Titchener (2012) to study young driver safety, RP, and cognitive and affective evaluations. Identifying inconsistent RPs for transport-related behaviors, the authors concluded that driver interventions may need to be individually targeted (McNally & Titchener, 2012). Attentional control theory was the framework for Wong, Mahar, & Tichener (2014) to study trait anxiety (TA) experimentally. It was concluded that while central executive processing efficiency was the key determinant of driving lapses, TA was also important, and that processing efficiency mediated the effect of TA on driving lapses (Wong et al., 2014). Drink driving was the focus of the study by MacKenzie, Watling, and Leal (2014) of risk-taking, attitudes, personality ("Big Five"), perceived legitimacy, and enforcement. It was revealed that attitudes partially mediated the relationship between risk-taking and drink-driving likelihood, and that more work was needed to change driver attitudes (MacKenzie et al., 2014).

A survey of risky driving, social cognitive factors, RP, personality, sensation seeking, and normlessness among a sample of Turkish drivers revealed that risk-taking personality traits had a strong relationship with unsafe driver behavior (Nordfjærn, Şimşekoğlu, Can, & Somer, 2015). The authors recommended tailoring campaigns to address specific personality traits, where RP exerted less of an influence (Nordfjærn, Şimşekoğlu, et al. 2015). Risky/reckless driving, media effects, video games, and music provided the focus of a number of Austrian experiments considering arousal when driving (Greitemeyer, 2013). The general learning model provided the framework for the author to report that effects of media exposure on risk behavior depended on whether the content was prosocial or neutral (Greitemeyer, 2013). The sociological theory of emotion formed the basis for a Swedish focus groups study exploring risk sense-making, experience, and control among young drivers (Wall, 2014). It was found that empathic and reflexive role-taking emotions revealed the value of social interaction for risk sense-making. Indirect social interactions with other road users, including acknowledging their values and judgments, were important for young road users' learning and development (Wall, 2014). As well as underscoring the complexity and multiplicity of variables in driving, the papers on driver behavior indicated the importance of tailoring RM interventions to address individual (e.g., personality traits), group (e.g., learning stage), and cultural factors (e.g., stage of development, cultural predispositions) for maximum effectiveness.

Aviation safety was the topic for a further six papers. Two US studies used a Bayesian approach to interrogate aviation crash databases. Adopting an RA framework, Wagner and Barker (2014) explored five types of airport runway excursions, which while less frequent than runway incursions, are more likely to have fatal outcomes. Noting that as it uses nominal values for likelihood and consequence, the traditional risk matrix lacked granularity, with risk categories often poorly defined. The authors argued that enhancements were needed. With the most critical features being human error and adverse weather, to mitigate human error risks it was recommended to use redundancy in landing and take-off systems by automation (Wagner & Barker, 2014). An object oriented probabilistic model to analyze loss-of-control (LOC) accident type was used by Ancel et al. (2015) to review accident causation, risk factor prioritization, mitigation portfolio study, and multi-causal shaping factors. Preliminary results showed that the model with human factors emphasis was adequate for representing LOC accidents and creating a predictive analysis platform for assessing various NASA technologies' effects on decreasing future LOC accidents (Ancel et al., 2015).

Airport and runway safety was the focus of another US study using decision analysis, risk hierarchy, quantitative risks-CBA, a seven-step RA, stakeholder interests (e.g., National Transport Safety Bureau), program evaluation, and a multi-layered approach as analysis tools (Rogerson, Lambert, & Johns, 2013). The authors argued for a layered perspective to assess and plan safety program effectiveness, including benefits and costs uncertainties (Rogerson et al., 2013). From simulation and airport radar system data analysis, a study from China considered RA probability and severity estimates for bird strike (Ning, Wang, & Chen, 2013). The authors urged improvement of the effectiveness of current methods by combining bird strike RA with avian sensors at airports (Ning et al., 2013).

Using a hazard index developed from an algorithm, based on aircraft characteristics, route, environmental conditions, and traffic type, Čokorilo, De Luca, and Dell'Acqua (2014) developed a cluster analysis of accidents. The authors constructed a predictive model for aviation accidents based on multivariate analysis (Čokorilo et al., 2014). Helicopter crash statistics for maritime air transport were the focus for a Serbian crash data analysis (Čokorilo, Mirosavljević, Vasov, & Stojiljković, 2013). Using fault tree analysis and RA, the study considered interactions between pilot, aircraft, environment, and operation. Implementing a safety management system to address the four safety factors was recommended, as well as balancing technology, regulation, and training (Čokorilo et al., 2013).

Two papers addressed aspects of military transport safety. A Dutch study considered Air Force helicopter safety, RA, perceived control critical to RP, risk severity/frequency, and risk/benefits assessment (Bakx & Richardson, 2013). Using multi-dimensional risk theory at shop floor and HQ organizational levels, the authors created a fictional risky mission scenario to conduct a between-groups analysis. It was noted that RM tools might not be enough to secure safety as they could obscure perceptual differences, so should not be used to justify decisions. It was recommended not to use over-simplified (e.g., bi-dimensional) risk models (Bakx & Richardson, 2013). A US study of aircraft carrier safety used qualitative reasoning in a review of safety risk models (Luxhøj, 2014). The author's object-oriented Bayesian network identified nine subsets, 70 causal factors, and 15 mitigations. Reviewing risk evaluation, probabilistic models, mishap likelihood, and human factors, the unmanned aircraft system (UAS) represents a revolutionary change in aviation. The integrative safety risk model analysis prioritizes the most important causal factors and assesses mitigating effects systematically for multiple UAS applications. A top-down system-of-systems higher-order model can also be created (Luxhøj, 2014).

Three papers focused on aspects of maritime transport safety. A simulation scenario analysis using a probabilistic accident risk model incorporating RA, risk mitigation, and wait times, was the framework for a study of maritime traffic in the Istanbul Strait (Özbaş, Or, & Altıok, 2013). To reduce risk and wait times for a win–win outcome, it was noted that pilots and scheduling were critical, and the authors advocated taking account of broader economic and political demands (Özbaş et al., 2013). Maritime collisions were the focus of a Norwegian study examining employee participation, safe culture, specialized and generalized barriers, mindfulness, normalization of deviance, and the logistics chain (Kongsvik, Haavik, & Gjøsund, 2014). A framework based around socio-technical systems, HROs, and safety barrier analysis (SBA) informed a case study approach that included HAZID, interviews, documentary analysis, and search conferences. It was concluded that SBA could involve employees to strengthen barriers as well as improving motivation and awareness. For more comprehensive input to analyses, methods should be triangulated, while employee involvement assisted in creating an informed culture (Kongsvik et al., 2014). From the Netherlands, a study of water transport of hazardous materials used qualitative RA modeling, risk rating, and risk graphs to explore a series of case studies (van der Vlies, 2014). Included were sluices, dams, major disasters, external safety policy, and QRA. The author reported a big disadvantage of quantitative risk modeling to be that very few risk-mitigating measures could be weighed quantitatively, which meant that many measures were not implemented despite being beneficial. The need to incorporate "soft" risk-mitigating measures was advocated, as well as recommending the use of this method for other forms of transportation (van der Vlies, 2014).

A single study, from Sweden, addressed the topic of rail safety. After conducting stakeholder interviews and undertaking documentary analysis, a case study modeling DM processes was developed to examine safety features of 28 rail tunnels (Cedergren, 2013). In a critique of the IRGC approach, the author discussed resilience, rail infrastructure, stakeholder disagreements, RA, and political influences. RG deficits included: missing early risk signals, failing to resolve conflicts, not reassessing change, and not appreciating element interactions. Resilience engineering was the system's ability to continue operating or recover a stable state after a major mishap or event. It was noted that DM was determined by power relations between stakeholders, and that double binds (choices between equally bad outcomes) restricted system resilience. In complex socio-technical systems, micro-level decisions could affect macro-level events. The author advocated building in resilience at the design stage and combining RG and resilience engineering to reduce risk DM (Cedergren, 2013).

The papers reviewed in this section have revealed the multi-dimensional nature of transport-related risks, including the multiple stakeholders involved in all transport modes and the increasing complexity of transport systems, leading to inevitable occasional systemic breakdowns. Generally lacking in studies investigating transport-related risks are opportunities for those managing risk within a particular transport mode to identify potentially useful practices and policies in other transport modes that can be used as learning opportunities. A number of risk-related problems (e.g., fatigue, shift work, regulation) are common across transport modes (Glendon, 2011).

Future Research

Global risks are becoming more center stage in risk-related debates (Huang, 2012). Society is becoming increasingly risk averse (Beck, 1992), perhaps because of the greater visibility of risks and communications about them, as well as phenomena such as risk amplification and systems implications of events or issues identified as risks. There is continuing divergence between populations and authorities in respect of risk perception and risk management priorities (Mudu & Beck, 2012). Three current trends in risk research identified by these authors were: (1) increased adoption of multidisciplinary approaches; (2) the problematic distinction between risk proximity and distance; and (3) the socially constructed and multi-scalar definitions of key terms (e.g., risk, danger, vulnerability) across various dimensions. The nature of risk is changing, for example, becoming more focused on risks associated with developing technologies and entangled with emotional responses to risk, such as worry and fear (Räsänen, Näsi, & Sarpila, 2012). Increasingly, risks are "boundaryless" insofar as while a certain type of risk might be deemed to "inhabit" a particular location or environment, the complexity of contemporary systems inevitably means that organizations or domains cannot remain isolated, but are best represented as a series of overlapping subsystems, like a Venn diagram. For example, because many people drive as a major component of their work, road traffic risks overlap with occupational risks, as do multiple risks encountered by employees in their daily lives, including potentially stressful and anxiety-creating encounters with significant others, including family members. To survive and thrive, organizations need to take account of increasing complexity in their business and operational environments, inter alia, including political, social, environmental, financial, ethical, and communication factors. Thus, for an organization RM needs to be envisaged as a complex tapestry in which these various threads are woven. Reflecting this complexity, the risk and RM literature has become increasingly diverse in terms of context, methodology, and subject matter. Now, nearly all disciplines and professions embrace risk concepts and have their own perspective on what constitutes "risk management". For this reason RM insights are likely to be gleaned from a broad spectrum of research and practice.

Discussion of risk, particularly within the academic research literature, has become increasingly conceptual. On the one hand this reflects the dimensional complexity of this multi-faceted and problematic concept. On the other hand, it is frequently difficult to derive usable generic RM strategies from published studies. As noted by the WEF (2014), "traditional concepts of risk have become inappropriate as a basis of modern global governance" (p. 27). There needs, inter alia, to be a greater synergy between risk researchers and practitioners (e.g., business leaders, politicians). The researcher/practitioner divide has been observed in other disciplines (e.g., organizational psychology), and efforts seeking to bridge this divide often founder on the fundamentally different motivations of the two main parties, which in turn are driven by their respective employment and personal agendas as well as by their separate agency relationships to the concrete representation of the risks about which they write or have to deal with. Among the best examples of such a divide in the risk domain is the debate on widespread devastating effects of anthropogenic climate change, in which many political agents continue to close their eyes to the overwhelming scientific evidence, illustrating the lack of ability and willingness of political leaders to address risks that will play out beyond their immediate term (WEF, 2014).

At a macro-level, the task of building capacity to address the global complexities of RM, including risk–risk trade-offs, can seem overwhelming when expressed in words (e.g., Jovanović & Pilić, 2013; WEF, 2014). That RM is not a panacea for progress or even a route to the diminution of risks, was highlighted by Huber and Rothstein (2013), who observed that: "consultants, public inquiries and organizational scholars that optimistically see risk management as the solution to the deeply organizational roots of accidents and disasters are likely to be disappointed if further thought is not given to the organizational roots of risk management itself" (p. 671).

Conclusions

A repeating theme in the literature is the criticality of participant and multiple stakeholder involvement and engagement in risk decision-making, and in risk management, and risk governance issues more broadly. Trust or the lack of trust, in government agencies, scientists, and other experts, have been common threads (Glendon & Clarke, 2015). It is becoming increasingly axiomatic that affected publics should have a genuine voice in the risks that they are exposed to. A basis for such engagement might be the principles of procedural justice, for example, as extemporized by Rawls (2001). Closely aligned with the above is that risk communication needs to become increasingly two-way (or multi-way), so that rather than being seen as "experts" delivering information to lay publics, risk communication can reciprocate public worries and fears to risk governance agencies. Where information needs to be delivered to publics, then it should be tailored to groups to take adequate account, inter alia, of differences in culture, values, and group differences in message receptiveness.

The complexity of risk issues has been reflected in the plethora of sophisticated risk assessment methodologies, models, and statistical procedures that continue to emerge. Particularly post-2000, we have entered the era of high-risk expertise. Organizations increasingly seek to incorporate all potential sources of risk within their risk management portfolios to enhance business survival and success, so that key performance indicators are commonly aligned with safety (and perhaps also environmental) performance indicators.

References

Abdul-Rahman, H., Mohd-Rahim, F. A., & Chen, W. (2012). Reducing failures in software development projects: Effectiveness of risk mitigation strategies. *Journal of Risk Research*, 15(4), 417–433. doi:10.1080/13669877.2011.634520

Abrahamsen, E. B., Røed, W., & Jongejan, R. (2013). A practical approach for the evaluation of acceptable risk in road tunnels. *Journal of Risk Research*, 16(5), 625–633. doi:10.1080/1366 9877.2012.761268

Ancel, E., Shih, A. T., Jones, S. M., Reveley, M. S., Luxhøj, J. T., & Evans, J. K. (2015). Predictive safety analytics: Inferring aviation accident shaping factors and causation. *Journal of Risk Research*, 18(4), 428–451. doi:10.1080/13669877.2014.896402

Arena, M., Azzone, G., Cagno, E., Ferretti, G., Prunotto, E., Silvestri, A., & Trucco, P. (2013). Integrated risk management through dynamic capabilities within project-based organizations: The company dynamic response map. *Risk Management: A Journal of Risk, Crisis and Disaster*, 15(1), 50–77. doi:10.1057/rm.2012.12

Arnau-Sabatés, L., Garcia, M. J., Martínez Muñoz, M., & Montané Capdevila, J. (2013). The relationship between awareness of road safety measure and accident involvement in pre-drivers: The basis of a road safety programme. *Journal of Risk Research, 16*(5), 635–650, doi:10.1080/13669877.2012.761272

Árvai, J. (2014). The end of risk communication as we know it. *Journal of Risk Research, 17*(10), 1245–1249. doi:10.1080/13669877.2014.919519

Bakx, G. C. H., & Richardson, R. A. L. (2013). Risk assessments at the Royal Netherlands Air Force: An explorative study. *Journal of Risk Research, 16*(5), 595–611. doi:10.1080/13669877.2012.726249

Bandaly, D., Satir, A., Kahyaoglu, Y., & Shanker, L. (2012). Supply chain risk management – I: Conceptualization, framework and planning process. *Risk Management: A Journal of Risk, Crisis and Disaster, 14*(4), 249–271. doi:10.1057/rm.2012.7

Bandaly, D., Shanker, L., Kahyaoglu, Y., & Satir, A. (2013). Supply chain risk management – II: A review of operational, financial and integrated approaches. *Risk Management: A Journal of Risk, Crisis and Disaster, 15*(1), 1–31. doi:10.1057/rm.2012.8

Beck, U. (1992). *Risk society: Towards a new modernity.* London, UK: Sage.

Binkhorst, J., & Kingma, S. F. (2012). Safety vs. reputation: Risk controversies in emerging policy networks regarding school safety in the Netherlands. *Journal of Risk Research, 15*(8), 913–935. doi:10.1080/13669877.2012.686049

Börjesson, M., Österberg, J., & Enander, A. (2015). Risk propensity within the military: A study of Swedish officers and soldiers. *Journal of Risk Research, 18*(1), 55–68. doi:10.1080/13669877.2013.879489

Bostrom, A. (2014). Progress in risk communication since the 1989 NRC report: Response to "Four questions for risk communication" by Roger Kasperson. *Journal of Risk Research, 17*(10), 1259–1264. doi:10.1080/13669877.2014.923032

Braut, G. S., Rake, E. L., Aaestad, R., & Njå, O. (2012). Risk images as basis for decisions related to provision of public services. *Risk Management: A Journal of Risk, Crisis and Disaster, 14*(1), 60–76. doi:10.1057/rm.2011.18

Brown, P. R., & Olofsson, A. (2014). Risk, uncertainty and policy: Towards a social-dialectical understanding. *Journal of Risk Research, 17*(4), 425–434. doi:10.1080/13669877.2014.889204

Cagliano, A. C., De Marco, A., Grimaldi, S., & Rafele, C. (2012). An integrated approach to supply chain risk analysis. *Journal of Risk Research, 15*(7), 817–840. doi:10.1080/13669877.2012.666757

Cagliano, A. C., Grimaldi, S., & Rafele, C. (2015). Choosing project risk management techniques: A theoretical framework. *Journal of Risk Research, 18*(2), 232–248. doi:10.1080/13669877.2014.896398

Cedergren, A. (2013). Designing resilient infrastructure systems: A case study of decision-making challenges in railway tunnel projects. *Journal of Risk Research, 16*(5), 563–582. doi:10.1080/13669877.2012.726241

Ceryno, P. S., Scavarda, L. F., & Klingebiel, K. (2014). Supply chain risk: Empirical research in the automotive industry. *Journal of Risk Research.* Advance online publication. doi:10.1080/13669877.2014.913662

Cheung, H. Y., Wu, J., & Tao, J. (2014). Predicting domain-specific risk-taking attitudes of mainland China university students: A hyper core self-evaluation approach. *Journal of Risk Research.* Advance online publication. doi:10.1080/13669877.2014.948903

Čokorilo, O., De Luca, M., & Dell'Acqua, G. (2014). Aircraft safety analysis using clustering algorithms. *Journal of Risk Research, 17*(10), 1325–1340. doi:10.1080/13669877.2013.879493

Čokorilo, O., Mirosavljević, P., Vasov, L., & Stojiljković, B. (2013). Managing safety risks in helicopter maritime operations. *Journal of Risk Research, 16*(5), 613–624. doi:10.1080/13669877.2012.737828

Collard, L., & Oboeuf, A. (2013). Do dangerous sports specialists play more dangerously? An experimental study on sample selection. *Journal of Risk Research, 16*(1), 39–50. doi:10.1080/13669877.2012.725671

Corin, S. E., McNeill, A., & Atapattu, A. (2012). Democracy and risk-based decision-making: The next step in public involvement. *Journal of Risk Research*, 15(8), 1021–1026. doi:10.1080/1 3669877.2012.686055

Cremers, A., Stubbé, H., van der Beek, D., Roelofs, M., & Kerstholt, J. (2014). Does playing the serious game B-SaFe! make citizens more aware of man-made and natural risks in their environment? *Journal of Risk Research*. Advance online publication. doi:10.1080/13669877.2014.9 19513

Dell'Acqua, G., Francesca Russo, F., & Biancardo, S. A., (2013). Risk-type density diagrams by crash type on two-lane rural roads. *Journal of Risk Research*, 16(10), 1297–1314. doi:10.1080 /13669877.2013.788547

Duckett, D., & Busby, J. (2013). Risk amplification as social attribution. *Risk Management: A Journal of Risk, Crisis and Disaster*, 15(2), 132–153. doi:10.1057/rm.2013.2

Elleuch, H., Hachicha, W., & Chabchoub, H. (2014). A combined approach for supply chain risk management: Description and application to a real hospital pharmaceutical case study. *Journal of Risk Research*, 17(5), 641–663. doi:10.1080/13669877.2013.815653

Farmer, Y. (2014). Using vNM expected utility theory to facilitate the decision-making in social ethics. *Journal of Risk Research*. Advance online publication. doi:10.1080/13669877.2014. 923024

Fischbacher-Smith, D. (2012). Getting pandas to breed: Paradigm blindness and the policy space for risk prevention, mitigation and management. *Risk Management: A Journal of Risk, Crisis and Disaster*, 14(3), 177–201. doi:10.1057/rm.2012.6

Fischhoff, B. (2014). Four answers to four questions (about risk communication). *Journal of Risk Research*, 17(10), 1265–1267. doi:10.1080/13669877.2014.940598

Flanquart, H. (2012). An unwelcome user? Or how to negotiate the use of a risky space. *Journal of Risk Research*, 15(10), 1261–1279. doi:10.1080/13669877.2012.609316

Frisby, B. N., Sellnow, D. D., Lane, D. R., Veil, S. R., & Sellnow, T. L. (2013). Instruction in crisis situations: Targeting learning preferences and self-efficacy. *Risk Management: A Journal of Risk, Crisis and Disaster*, 15(4), 250–271. doi:10.1057/rm.2013.7

Fruhen, L. S., Flin, R. H., & McLeod, R. (2014). Chronic unease for safety in managers: A conceptualisation. *Journal of Risk Research*, 17(8), 969–979. doi:10.1080/13669877 .2013.822924

Glendon, A. I. (2011). Safety and risk in transportation. In R. J. Burke, S. G. Clarke, & C. L. Cooper (Eds.). *Occupational health and safety: Psychological and behavioral aspects of risk* (pp. 239–275). Farnham, UK: Gower.

Glendon, A. I., & Clarke, S. G. (2015). *Human safety and risk management: A psychological perspective* (3rd edn.). Boca Raton, FL: CRC Press/Taylor & Francis.

Greitemeyer, T. (2013). Exposure to media with prosocial content reduces the propensity for reckless and risky driving. *Journal of Risk Research*, 16(5), 583–594. doi:10.1080/13669877.201 2.726248

Greitemeyer, T., Kastenmüller, A., & Fischer, P. (2013). Romantic motives and risk-taking: An evolutionary approach. *Journal of Risk Research*, 16(1), 19–38. doi:10.1080/13669877.201 2.713388

Groso, A., Ouedraogo, A., & Mayer, T. (2012). Risk analysis in research environment. *Journal of Risk Research*, 15(2), 187–208. doi:10.1080/13669877.2011.634513

Hachicha, W., & Elmsalmi, M. (2014). An integrated approach based-structural modeling for risk prioritization in supply network management. *Journal of Risk Research*, 17(10), 1301–1324. doi:10.1080/13669877.2013.841734

Hagen, J. M., Valdal, A. K., Pettersen, K., & Gjerstad, B. (2015). Evaluation of comprehensive security systems for public transport – A methodological approach. *Journal of Risk Research*. do i:10.1080/13669877.2014.961512

Hamilton, M. (2014). The "new social contract" and the individualisation of risk in policy. *Journal of Risk Research*, 17(4), 453–467. doi:10.1080/13669877.2012.726250

Hayes, J., & Maslen, S. (2015). Knowing stories that matter: Learning for effective safety decision-making. *Journal of Risk Research*. doi:10.1080/13669877.2014.910690

Hesselbein, C. (2015). Finding the middle of the road: Report on the International Conference on Risk and Responsibility. *Journal of Risk Research*. doi:10.1080/13669877.2014.911200

Howarth, A. (2013). The weakest link in existing studies: Media–government risk interactions. *Journal of Risk Research, 16*(1), 1–18. doi:10.1080/13669877.2012.713387

Huang, T. (2012). Toward the NGO-involved schooling: A study on teachers' risk perception and teachings. *Journal of Risk Research, 15*(9), 1159–1169. doi:10.1080/13669877.2012.713384

Huber, M., & Rothstein, H. (2013). The risk organisation: Or how organisations reconcile themselves to failure. *Journal of Risk Research, 16*(6), 651–675. doi:10.1080/13669877.2012.761276

Hudson, P. (2014). Accident causation models, management and the law. *Journal of Risk Research, 17*(6), 749–764. doi:10.1080/13669877.2014.889202

Iavicoli, S., Leka, S., Jain, A., Persechino, B., Rondinone, B. M., Ronchetti, M., & Valenti, A. (2014). Hard and soft law approaches to addressing psychosocial risks in Europe: Lessons learned in the development of the Italian approach. *Journal of Risk Research, 17*(7), 855–869. doi:10.1080/13669877.2013.822911

Jimenez, R. B., & Bronfman, N. C. (2012). Comprehensive indicators of traffic-related premature mortality. *Journal of Risk Research, 15*(9), 1117–1139. doi:10.1080/13669877.2012.705314

Johnson, B. B., & Waishwell, L. (2014). Q method can identify diverse perspectives on "helpful" information on cancer clusters and inform risk communication generally. *Journal of Risk Research, 17*(9), 1125–1145. doi:10.1080/13669877.2013.879491

Jondle, D., Maines, T. D., Burke, M. R., & Young, P. (2013). Modern risk management through the lens of the ethical organizational culture. *Risk Management: A Journal of Risk, Crisis and Disaster, 15*(1), 32–49. doi:10.1057/rm.2012.11

Jovanović, A. S., & Pilić, V. (2013). Dealing with risk–risk interdependencies and trade-offs in relation to development and use of new technologies. *Journal of Risk Research, 16*(3–4), 393–406. doi:10.1080/13669877.2012.729528

Jung, S., Ledi, D., & Daniels, M. K. (2013). Evaluating the concurrent validity of the HCR-20 scales. *Journal of Risk Research, 16*(6), 697–711. doi:10.1080/13669877.2012.726247

Kahneman, D. (2011). *Thinking, fast and slow*. London, UK: Penguin.

Kasperson, R. (2014). Four questions for risk communication. *Journal of Risk Research, 17*(10), 1233–1239. doi:10.1080/13669877.2014.900207

Kazaras, K., & Kirytopoulos, K. (2014). Challenges for current quantitative risk assessment (QRA) models to describe explicitly the road tunnel safety level. *Journal of Risk Research, 17*(8), 953–968. doi:10.1080/13669877.2013.822916

Keller, C., Bostrom, A., Kuttschreuter, M., Savadori, L., Spence, A., & White, M. (2012). Bringing appraisal theory to environmental risk perception: A review of conceptual approaches of the past 40 years and suggestions for future research. *Journal of Risk Research, 15*(3), 237–256. doi:10.1080/13669877.2011.634523

Khorsandi, J., & Aven, T. (2014). A risk perspective supporting organizational efforts for achieving high reliability. *Journal of Risk Research, 17*(7), 871–884. doi:10.1080/13669877.2013.822912

Kluge, A., Badura, B., & Rietz, C. (2013). Communicating production outcomes as gains or losses, operator skill and their effects on safety-related violations in a simulated production context. *Journal of Risk Research, 16*(10), 1241–1258. doi:10.1080/13669877.2013.788059

Kongsvik, T., Haavik, T., & Gjøsund, G. (2014). Participatory safety barrier analysis: A case from the offshore maritime industry. *Journal of Risk Research, 17*(2), 161–175. doi:10.1080/13669877.2012.761275

Kubicek, A., Bhanugopan, R., & Fish, A. (2013). Perceiving safety and risk in culturally diverse organizations: Toward a conceptual model. *Risk Management: A Journal of Risk, Crisis and Disaster, 15*(3), 199–223. doi:10.1057/rm.2013.5

Lalonde, C., & Boiral, O. (2012). Managing risks through ISO 31000: A critical analysis. *Risk Management: A Journal of Risk, Crisis and Disaster, 14*(4), 272–300. doi:10.1057/rm.2012.9

Lam, D., & Ozorio, B. (2013). The effect of prior outcomes on gender risk-taking differences. *Journal of Risk Research, 16*(7), 791–802. doi:10.1080/13669877.2012.737824

Lapinski, M. K., Neuberger, L., Gore, M. L., Muter, B. A., & Van Der Heide, B. (2013). Shark bytes: Message sensation value and emotional appeals in shark diving websites. *Journal of Risk Research, 16*(6), 733–751. doi:10.1080/13669877.2012.737822

Lawrence, P. R., & Lorsch, J. W. (1969). *Developing organizations: Diagnosis and action.* Reading, MA: Addison-Wesley.

Lermer, E., Streicher, B., Sachs, R., & Frey, D. (2013). How risky? The impact of target person and answer format on risk assessment. *Journal of Risk Research, 16*(7), 903–919. doi:10.1080/13669877.2012.761267

Levine, E. S. (2012). Improving risk matrices: The advantages of logarithmically scaled axes. *Journal of Risk Research, 15*(2), 209–222. doi:10.1080/13669877.2011.634514

Löfstedt, R. (2015). A possible way forward for evidence-based and risk-informed policy-making in Europe: A personal view. *Journal of Risk Research, 17*(9), 1089–1108. doi:10.1080/13669877.2014.919518

Lund, I. O., Nordfjærn, T., & Rundmo, T. (2012). Associations between risk judgments and demand for transport risk mitigation. *Journal of Risk Research, 15*(9), 1171–1182. doi:10.1080/13669877.2012.705317

Luxhøj, J. T. (2014). A conceptual Object-Oriented Bayesian Network (OOBN) for modeling aircraft carrier-based UAS safety risk. *Journal of Risk Research.* Advance online publication. doi:10.1080/13669877.2014.913664

MacKenzie, J. E., Watling, C. N., & Leal, N. L. (2014). What aspects of demographic, personality, attitudes and perceptions of law enforcement influence self-reported likelihood of drink driving? *Journal of Risk Research.* Advance online publication. doi:10.1080/13669877.2014.923026

Macrae, D. (2014). Managing a political crisis after a disaster: How concern assessment can address the political aspects involved in framing a solution. *Journal of Risk Research.* Advance online publication. doi:10.1080/13669877.2014.910693

Marshall, A., & Ojiako, U. (2013). Managing risk through the veil of ignorance. *Journal of Risk Research, 16*(10), 1225–1239. doi:10.1080/13669877.2013.788056

Mascini, P., Achterberg, P., & Houtman, D. (2013). Neoliberalism and work-related risks: Individual or collective responsibilization? *Journal of Risk Research, 16*(10), 1209–1224. doi:10.1080/13669877.2012.761274

McComas, K. A. (2014). Perspective on "Four Questions for Risk Communication." *Journal of Risk Research, 17*(10), 1273–1276. doi:10.1080/13669877.2014.940600

McNally, B., & Titchener, K. (2012). The role of affective processes on young drivers' risk perceptions: A dual process model approach. *Journal of Risk Research, 15*(1), 39–51. doi:10.1080/13669877.2011.601321

Michel-Kerjan, E. (2012). How resilient is your country? Extreme events are on the rise. Governments must implement national risk-management strategies. *Nature, 491*(7425), 497.

Mudu, P., & Beck, E. (2012). Navigating scientific routes to risk assessment: A tortuous path. *Journal of Risk Research, 15*(10), 1217–1222. doi:10.1080/13669877.2012.730227

Newby, B., & DeCamp, W. (2015). Bad reputation: Stigma as an inhibitor of risk behaviors. *Journal of Risk Research, 18*(5), 843–860. doi:10.1080/13669877.2014.910681

Ning, H-s., Wang, J-k., & Chen, W-s. (2013). Lévy flight-based real-time bird strike risk assessment for airports. *Journal of Risk Research, 16*(5), 513–521. doi:10.1080/13669877.2012.705313

Nordfjærn, T., Hezaveh, A. M., & Mamdoohi, A. R. (2015). An analysis of reported driver behaviour in samples of domestic and expatriate Iranians. *Journal of Risk Research, 18*(5), 566–580. doi:10.1080/13669877.2014.910684

Nordfjærn, T., Jørgensen, S. H., & Rundmo, T. (2012). Safety attitudes, behaviour, anxiety and perceived control among professional and non-professional drivers. *Journal of Risk Research, 15*(8), 875–896. doi:10.1080/13669877.2012.670132

Nordfjærn, T., Şimşekoğlu, Ö., Can, S., & Somer, O. (2015). Social cognition and personality traits related to risky driving in a Turkish sample. *Journal of Risk Research, 18*(4), 452–466. doi:10.1080/13669877.2014.907330

Nordfjærn, T., Şimşekoğlu, Ö., & Rundmo, T. (2012). A comparison of road traffic culture, risk assessment and speeding predictors between Norway and Turkey. *Risk Management: A Journal of Risk, Crisis and Disaster, 14*(3), 202–221. doi:10.1057/rm.2012.5

Olofsson, A., & Öhman, S. (2015). Vulnerability, values and heterogeneity: One step further to understand risk perception and behaviour. *Journal of Risk Research, 18*(1), 2–20. doi:10.1080/13669877.2013.879485

Özbaş, B., Or, İ., & Altıok, T. (2013). Comprehensive scenario analysis for mitigation of risks of the maritime traffic in the Strait of Istanbul. *Journal of Risk Research, 16*(5), 541–561. doi:10.1080/13669877.2012.726239

Pidgeon, N. (2014). Complexity, uncertainty and future risks. *Journal of Risk Research, 17*(10), 1269–1271. doi:10.1080/13669877.2014.940599

Portman-Smith, C., & Harwood, I. A. (2015). "Only as good as your last gig?" An exploratory case study of reputational risk management amongst self-employed musicians. *Journal of Risk Research, 18*(4), 483–504. doi:10.1080/13669877.2014.910679

Prati, G., & Pietrantoni, L. (2012). Predictors of safety behaviour among emergency responders on the highways. *Journal of Risk Research, 15*(4), 405–415. doi:10.1080/13669877.2011.634519

Radivojević, G., & Gajović, V. (2014). Supply chain risk modeling by AHP and fuzzy AHP methods. *Journal of Risk Research, 17*(3), 337–352. doi:10.1080/13669877.2013.808689

Räsänen, P., Näsi, M., & Sarpila, O. (2012). Old and new sources of risk: A study of societal risk perception in Finland. *Journal of Risk Research, 15*(7), 755–769. doi:10.1080/13669877.2012.657218

Rawls, J. (2001). *Justice as fairness: A restatement*. Cambridge, MA: Belknap.

Reardon, C. A., & Govender, K. (2013). Masculinities, cultural worldviews and risk perceptions among South African adolescent learners. *Journal of Risk Research, 16*(6), 753–770. doi:10.1080/13669877.2012.737823

Renn, O. (2014). Four questions for risk communication: A response to Roger Kasperson, *Journal of Risk Research, 17*(10), 1277–1281. doi:10.1080/13669877.2014.940601

Rogerson, E. C., Lambert, J. H., & Johns, A. F. (2013). Runway safety program evaluation with uncertainties of benefits and costs. *Journal of Risk Research, 16*(5), 523–539. doi:10.1080/13669877.2012.725674

Roth, S. (2015). Aid work as edgework – voluntary risk-taking and security in humanitarian assistance, development and human rights work. *Journal of Risk Research, 18*(2), 139–155. doi:10.1080/13669877.2013.875934

Scholz, R. W., Blumer, Y. B., & Brand, F. S. (2012). Risk, vulnerability, robustness, and resilience from a decision-theoretic perspective. *Journal of Risk Research, 15*(3), 313–330. doi:10.1080/13669877.2011.634522

Sheaffer, Z., & Brender-Ilan, Y. (2014). Are sensation seekers in control? A study in crisis preparedness. *Risk Management: A Journal of Risk, Crisis and Disaster, 16*(1), 1–24. doi:10.1057/rm.2014.1

Siegrist, M. (2014). More questions than answers: A response to "Four questions for risk communication" by Roger Kasperson (2014). *Journal of Risk Research, 17*(10), 1241–1243. doi:10.1080/13669877.2014.913668

Şimşekoğlu, Ö., Nordfjærn, T., & Rundmo, T. (2012). Traffic risk perception, road safety attitudes, and behaviour among road users: A comparison of Turkey and Norway. *Journal of Risk Research, 15*(7), 787–800. doi:10.1080/13669877.2012.657221

Solberg, Ø., & Njå, O. (2012). Reflections on the ontological status of risk. *Journal of Risk Research, 15*(9), 1201–1215. doi:10.1080/13669877.2012.713385

Torriti, J., & Löfstedt, R. (2012). The first five years of the EU Impact Assessment system: A risk economics perspective on gaps between rationale and practice. *Journal of Risk Research, 15*(2), 169–186. doi:10.1080/13669877.2011.634512

van der Vlies, V. (2014). A qualitative approach to risk management of hazardous materials in the Netherlands: Lessons learned from 7 sluice cases. *Journal of Risk Research*. Advance online publication. doi:10.1080/13669877.2014.940595

Visschers, V. H. M., Wiederman, P. M., Gutscher, H., Kurzenhäuser, S., Seidl, R., Jardine, C. G., & Timmermans, D. R. M. (2012). Affect-inducing risk communications: Current knowledge and future directions. *Journal of Risk Research, 15*(3), 257–271. doi:10.1080/13669877.2011.634521

Wagner, D. C. S., & Barker, K. (2014). Statistical methods for modeling the risk of runway excursions. *Journal of Risk Research, 17*(7), 885–901. doi:10.1080/13669877.2013.822913

Wall, E. (2014). Sense-making of risk and role-taking emotions: How young Swedes construe road traffic risk. *Journal of Risk Research, 17*(10), 1285–1299. doi:10.1080/13669877.2013.879487

Wardman, J. K. (2014). Sociocultural vectors of effective risk communication. *Journal of Risk Research, 17*(10), 1251–1257. doi:10.1080/13669877.2014.942498

Wendling, C. (2012). What role for social scientists in risk expertise? *Journal of Risk Research, 15*(5), 477–493. doi:10.1080/13669877.2011.636837

Wong, I. Y., Mahar, D., & Titchener, K. (2014). Driven by distraction: Investigating the effects of anxiety on driving performance using the Attentional Control Theory. *Journal of Risk Research*. Advance online publication. doi:10.1080/13669877.2014.919516

World Economic Forum (WEF) (2014). *Global risks 2104: Insight report* (9th edn.). Geneva, Switzerland: World Economic Forum.

World Health Organization (WHO) (2013). *The top 10 causes of death*. Fact sheet no. 310 (Updated May 2014). Geneva, Switzerland: WHO. http://www.who.int/mediacentre/factsheets/fs310/en/ (accessed June 11, 2015).

Yang, J. (2015). The influence of culture on Koreans' risk perception. *Journal of Risk Research, 18*(1), 69–92. doi:10.1080/13669877.2013.879490

Index

The Wiley Blackwell Handbook of the Psychology of Occupational Safety and Workplace Health, First Edition.
Edited by Sharon Clarke, Tahira M. Probst, Frank Guldenmund, and Jonathan Passmore. © 2016 John
Wiley & Sons Ltd. Published 2020 by John Wiley & Sons Ltd.

Printed and bound by CPI Group (UK) Ltd, Croydon, CR0 4YY

27/10/2024

14580362-0004